MRI of the
Neonatal Brain

Commissioning Editor: Deborah Russell
Project Development Manager: Kim Benson
Project Manager: Katharine Eyston
Designer: Andy Chapman

MRI of the Neonatal Brain

Edited by

Mary A Rutherford, MD MRCPCH

Honorary Senior Lecturer and Consultant in Paediatrics
Robert Steiner Magnetic Resonance Unit and Department of Paediatrics and Neonatal Medicine,
Imperial College School of Medicine, Hammersmith Hospital, London, UK

W. B. SAUNDERS

London · Edinburgh · New York · Philadelphia · St Louis · Sydney · Toronto 2002

WB SAUNDERS
An imprint of Elsevier Science Limited

First published 2002
   Reprinted 2002

ISBN 0 7020 2534 8

British Library Cataloguing in Publication Data
A catalogue record for this book is available from the British Library

Library of Congress Cataloging in Publication Data
A catalog record for this book is available from the Library of Congress.

Note
Medical knowledge is constantly changing. As new information becomes available, changes in treatment, procedures, equipment and the use of drugs become necessary. The editors and the publishers have taken care to ensure that the information given in this text is accurate and up to date. However, readers are strongly advised to confirm that the information, especially with regard to drug usage, complies with the latest legislation and standards of practice.

Existing UK nomenclature is changing to the system of Recommended International Nonproprietary Names (rINNs). Until the UK names are no longer in use, these more familiar names are used in this book in preference to rINNs, details of which may be obtained from the *British National Formulary.*

Printed in China by RDC Group Limited
W/02

The
publisher's
policy is to use
**paper manufactured
from sustainable forests**

Contents

Contributors

Hortensia Alvarez MD
Radiology Assistant, Service de Neuroradiologie
Diagnostique et Thérapeutic, Bicêtre Hôpital, Université
Paris-Sud, Le Kremlin Bicêtre, France

Malcolm Battin MB CHB MRCP(UK) FRCPCH FRACP
Senior Lecturer in Neonatology, Neonatal Unit, National
Women's Hospital and University of Auckland, New
Zealand

Laurence E Becker MD FRCPC
Professor, Departments of Laboratory Medicine, Pathology
and Pediatrics, Hospital for Sick Children, Toronto,
Ontario, Canada

Susan Blaser MD FRCPC
Assistant Professor, University of Toronto; Pediatric
Neuroradiologist, Diagnostic Imaging, Hospital for Sick
Children, Toronto, Ontario, Canada

Serena Counsell BSC MSC
Superintendent Research Radiographer, Robert Steiner
Magnetic Resonance Unit, Hammersmith Hospital,
London, UK

Frances M Cowan LRCP&SI MBBS MRCP(UK) DCH MRCGP PHD
MRCPCH
Senior Lecturer in Neonatal Neurology,
Department of Paediatrics and Neonatal Medicine,
Imperial College School of Medicine, Hammersmith
Hospital, London, UK

I Jane Cox MA
Non-Clinical Lecturer, Imperial College School of
Medicine, Hammersmith Hospital, London, UK

Lilly Dubowitz
Honorary Senior Lecturer, Department of Paediatrics and
Neonatal Medicine, Hammersmith Hospital, London, UK

E Lee Ford-Jones MD FRCPC
Associate Professor of Pediatrics, University of Toronto;
Division of Infectious Diseases, Hospital for Sick Children,
Toronto, Ontario, Canada

Floris Groenendaal MD PHD
Consultant in Neonatology, Department of Neonatology,
Wilhelmina Children's Hospital, University Medical Center,
Utrecht, The Netherlands

Venita Jay MBBS FRCPC
Associate Professor, University of Toronto; Neuropathologist,
Hospital for Sick Children, Toronto, Ontario, Canada

Pierre Lasjaunias MD PHD
Professor of Anatomy; Chairman of Neuroradiology, Service
de Neuroradiologie Diagnostique et Thérapeutic, Bicêtre
Hôpital, Université Paris-Sud, Le Kremlin Bicêtre, France

Elia F Maalouf MBCHB MRCP MRCPCH MD
Consultant in Neonatal Paediatrics, Neonatal Unit,
Homerton Hospital, London, UK

Claude Manelfe
Chef de Service, Service de Neuroradiologie Pediatrique,
Purpan Hospital, Toulouse, France

Ernst Martin MD
Professor of Paediatric Neuroradiology and MR Research,
Department of Diagnostic Imaging, University Children's
Hospital Zurich, Switzerland

Maeve McPhillips
Consultant Paediatric Radiologist, Department of Radiology,
Royal Hospital for Sick Children, Edinburgh, Scotland, UK

Linda C Meiners MD PHD
Neuroradiologist, Department of Radiology, University
Hospital Groningen, Utrecht, The Netherlands

Eugenio Mercuri MD PHD
Lecturer in Paediatric Neurology, Department of Paediatrics
and Neonatal Medicine, Hammersmith Hospital, London, UK

Francesco Muntoni MD
Professor in Paediatric Neurology, Department of
Paediatrics, Hammersmith Hospital, London, UK

Zoltan Patay MD PHD
Consultant Neuroradiologist, Department of Radiology,
King Faisal Specialist Hospital and Research Centre, Riyadh,
Kingdom of Saudi Arabia

Jacqueline M Pennock M PHIL
Senior Scientific Officer (Retired), Enniskillen, County
Fermanagh, Northern Ireland

Nicola Robertson MB CHB
Consultant Neonatologist, Imperial College School of
Medicine, Robert Steiner Magnetic Resonance Unit,
Hammersmith Hospital, London, UK

Georges Rodesch MD
Radiology Assistant, Service de Neuroradiologie
Diagnostique et Thérapeutic, Bicêtre Hôpital, Université
Paris-Sud, Le Kremlin Bicêtre, France

Andrea Rossi MD
Staff Neuroradiologist, Department of Pediatric
Neuroradiology, G Gaslini Children's Research Hospital,
Genoa, Italy

Mary A Rutherford MD MRCPCH
Honorary Senior Lecturer and Consultant in Paediatrics,
Robert Steiner Magnetic Resonance Unit and Department
of Paediatrics and Neonatal Medicine, Imperial College
School of Medicine, Hammersmith Hospital, London, UK

Annick Sévely MD
Radiologist, Department of Neuroradiology, Purpan
Hospital, Toulouse, France

Waney Squier BSC MBCHB MRCP FRCPATH
Consultant Neuropathologist and Honorary Clinical
Lecturer, Department of Neuropathology, Radcliffe
Infirmary, Oxford, UK

Paolo Tortori-Donati MD
Professor of Neuropathology; Head of Pediatric
Neuroradiology, G Gaslini Children's Research Hospital,
Genoa, Italy

Linda S de Vries MD PHD
Professor in Neonatal Neurology, Department of
Neonatology, Wilhelmina Children's Hospital, University
Medical Center, Utrecht, The Netherlands

Foreword

At no other time in human life are the clinical manifestations of neurological disease as subtle as they are in the newborn infant. Many neural structures that later govern the highest cognitive activities of the human brain are functionally silent in the infant. This structural–functional disconnect is even more pronounced in the premature newborn, in whom serious cerebral pathology is unfortunately common. Thus, the need for high-resolution imaging of the neonatal brain is great indeed, and in response to that need a virtual explosion of research and application of such imaging has occurred in the past 25 years. Therein lies the timeliness of this comprehensive, up-to-date book on imaging the neonatal brain. Dr Mary Rutherford and her colleagues have succeeded in a most decisive way in creating such a book.

The book is divided in a logical manner into four major sections. Part I deals with practical issues, Part II with anatomy and development of the immature brain, Part III with pathology, and Part IV with disorders in the newborn infant. A total of 18 well-organized chapters, most of which are within Part IV, are followed by a detailed and informative glossary of physics terms.

The chapters are written by experts in the field and are presented in a uniform organizational style. The chapter summaries are succinct and very useful. The images, the core of the book, are superb and abundant. However, importantly, the chapters place the images in the context of clinical aspects, which are discussed clearly but succinctly throughout.

Although all the chapters are valuable, many deserve special note. For example, the discussions of normal development of both the preterm and term brain include insights gained not only from conventional MRI but also from diffusion-based, volumetric and functional MRI, and from MR spectroscopy. The chapter on the asphyxiated term infant is a classic and reflects the large personal contributions of Dr Rutherford. Similarly, the chapter on cerebral infarction by Mercuri, Dubowitz and Rutherford draws appropriately heavily on the authors' superb contributions. The chapters on ischemic lesions of the preterm infant by de Vries et al., hemorrhagic lesions by Rutherford, and vascular malformations by Lasjaunias et al. are also particularly notable. Chapters on imaging brain structure in the fetus and visual function in the newborn show us some of the future promise of this field.

Dr Rutherford is to be congratulated for her personal contributions, for assembling a superb group of authors, and for orchestrating all the contributions into an outstanding book on neonatal brain imaging. It should prove useful to anyone involved in the evaluation and care of the newborn.

Joseph J Volpe, MD
Children's Hospital/Harvard Medical School
Boston, MA
May 21, 2001

Preface

It is a pleasure to introduce this volume, which collects together experience from specialists and clinicians working in many of the leading children's hospitals of the world.

The field of neonatal and infant magnetic resonance is now expanding rapidly. The technical problems in providing magnetic-compatible equipment for life support and monitoring have now been overcome, and we are now seeing images and spectra from infants of 24 weeks of gestation and upwards. But more than that, there have also been rapid advances in fetal imaging and it is now possible to see a full continuum of normal development.

Much is owed to the early pioneers in this field, such as Jaap Valk and Marjo van der Knaap (Amsterdam), Charles Raybaud (Marseille), Robert Zimmerman (Philadelphia), James Barkovich (San Francisco), Rosalind Dietrich (UCL), Ernst Martin (Zurich), Ossie Reynolds (London) and Britton Chance (Philadelphia), who took a long-term view and recognised the possibilities of magnetic resonance even before the technical capabilities were developed.

There is a shift in diagnosis from adults to children and almost as big a shift from children to neonates. The normal brain undergoes a quite remarkable series of changes, which can be observed in detail with magnetic resonance, and these present a background for the wide spectrum of pathology in the newborn. Twenty years on, since the advent of clinical MR, there are few areas presenting such new and interesting opportunities as neonatal MR and it is a pleasure to commend Mary Rutherford's book, which provides a platform and a basic foundation for all those practising and performing research in this field.

A David Edwards
Professor of Paediatrics and Neonatal Medicine,
Hammersmith Hospital, London

Acknowledgments

This book would not have been possible without the help and hard work of a great many people: Graeme Bydder, Jackie Pennock, Frances Cowan, Dulcie Rodrigues, Serena Counsell, Joanna Allsop, Jane Schweiso, Helen Lewis, Alison Fletcher, Lilly Dubowitz, Eugenio Mercuri, Nadeem Saeed, Joseph Hajnal, David Edwards, Alasdair Hall, Elia Maalouf, Malcolm Battin, Moreneke Ajayi Obe, Nigel Kennea, Christine Foglia, Sabrina Laroche, Phil Duggan, Peter Reynolds, Phil Amess, Michael Harrison, Eleri Adams, Layla Al Nakib, Niran Al Naqeeb, Jane Cox, Nikky Robertson, Angela Oatridge, Nazma Virji, Adnan Manzur, Francesco Muntoni, Dennis Azzopardi, Neena Modi, Neil Murray, Merran Thomson, Maria Flavia Frisone, Daniella Ricci, Amy Herlihy, David Herlihy, David Larkman, David Gilderdale, Alan Collins, Janet Sargentoni, Don Hanrahan, Jacob Kuint, and Olaf Dietrich.

We are very grateful to Marconi Medical Systems and the Medical Research Council for their continuing support.

Most importantly we would like to thank all the parents and their babies from whom we have learned so much.

Dedication

To Rob, Joseph, Alice, Rose and William with all my love.

Part *I*

Practical issues

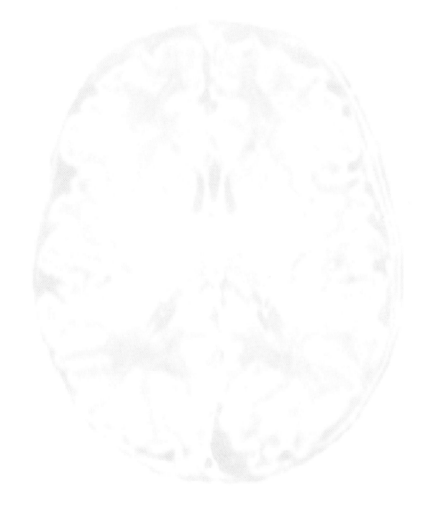

Patient preparation, safety and hazards in imaging infants and children

Jacqueline M Pennock

Contents

Introduction

'The two greatest obstacles we face in imaging infants and children are the proper preparation of the subject and the selection of the right combination of imaging parameters to achieve the desired result'[3].

Magnetic resonance (MR) systems are designed to accommodate the adult population; however, with a little effort and careful planning they can be successfully used to scan infants and children. This chapter offers advice about patient preparation and imaging protocols for those faced with the prospect of scanning infants up to 2 years of age in scanners used mainly for adults.

Examples of the documentation we use for each pediatric examination are included as a guide for the reader with only occasional access to a scanner. We find this information extremely useful for follow-up studies, quality assurance in our sedation program, and dealing with potential medico-legal problems.

Imaging team

Examining a sick infant is a team effort and involves close co-operation between clinical and imaging staff as well as the mother and infant. A highly motivated and unified clinical team helps make a potentially distressing event easier for the mother and child (Fig. 1.1). Our current core team consists of two pediatricians, a radiologist, pediatric nursing staff in the children's out-patients and a radiographer with training in pediatric imaging.

Our team members are involved in all aspects of patient care including setting up new imaging protocols and reporting images.

Assessment of patients for imaging

Before an MR appointment is made the infant is seen by a pediatrician who takes a medical history including details of previous operations and possible implants. If, for example, a

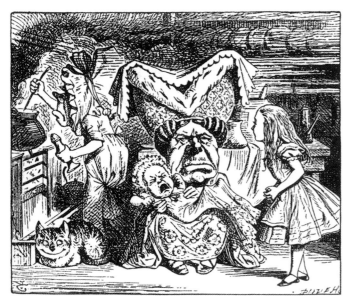

Fig. 1.1 'the Duchess was sitting on a three-legged stool in the middle, nursing a baby; the cook was leaning over the fire, stirring a large cauldron which seemed to be full of soup'. Care and understanding are required for preparing an anxious mother and child for imaging.

ventriculo-peritoneal shunt or a patent ductus arteriosus clip is present then its magnetic compatibility is checked before an appointment is given. The book by Shellock and Kanal lists many items, which have been tested for attraction/deflection forces during exposure to static magnetic fields. These authors are also accessible through the world wide web and provide a quick reply to questions and problems concerned with safety[14].

At this initial assessment the pediatrician explains the MR procedure, the sedation protocol and gives instructions on feeding and or fasting before the scan. We recommend that the infant has no food for 4 h and no drink for 2 h before sedation. The parents are asked to prevent their infant from falling asleep for at least 2 h before the scan. If possible we schedule appointments to coincide with the natural sleeping pattern of the infant.

Organizing the day

Scheduling naturally sleeping and sedated infants can be difficult and requires a degree of flexibility. It is much easier to have exclusively pediatric scanning sessions. Studying babies even when sedated takes more time than adults and they cannot be rushed (Fig. 1.2).

Patients coming from home are given appointment times and admitted to a children's day care ward whereas in-patients are booked at times convenient to the ward. We offer the parents the opportunity to be with their child

throughout the preparation for the scan and encourage them to accompany the baby to the imaging unit so that they can see their child is asleep and comfortable in the scanner. They can stay beside their infant in the scanner if they wish; however, they are often happy to have some time to themselves while we look after their child. Parents going into the scanner room need to be carefully metal checked.

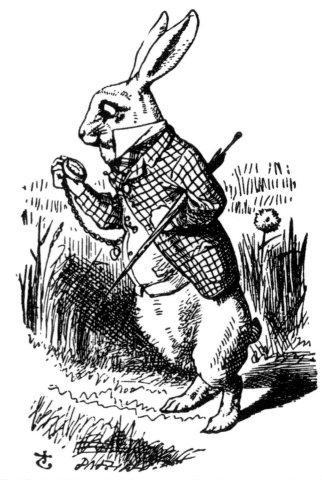

Fig. 1.2 'the Rabbit actually *took a watch out of its waistcoat-pocket*, and looked at it and then hurried on'. It is not possible or desirable to rush mothers and babies through a scanning day.

Preparation of the MR unit and scanning room

Although the sleeping child is unaffected by the sight of an MR scanner, for a new and anxious parent it can be a distressing experience (Fig. 1.3). We attempt to make the scanning room a less intimidating place before a pediatric session by changing the standard hospital linen to brightly colored baby blankets, with flannelette sheets and duvets for cosiness and warmth. We have our own washing machine in the unit so the bedding is washed on site and does not disappear into the depths of the hospital laundry. Removable plastic nursery

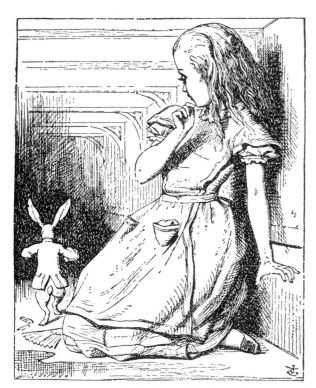

Fig. 1.3 'The rabbit started violently, dropped the white kid gloves and the fan and skurried away into the darkness as hard as he could go'. At first sight an MR scanner can be a frightening piece of machinery.

rhyme characters can be placed around the magnet for the baby scanning day. A comfortable plastic chair placed next to the magnet is useful for parents to nurse the baby to sleep before the scan.

We put some toys and books in the waiting room for brothers and sisters to play with while their sibling is being examined. We also have coffee and tea facilities available in the waiting room. These details are designed to provide a relaxed environment for parents and their infants.

Clinical safety in the MR unit

To manage any emergencies arising from scanning sick and sedated infants adequate resuscitation equipment must be available in the MR unit and all the members of the imaging team must be trained in its use.

The minimal requirements for resuscitation are a positive-pressure oxygen delivery system with the appropriate flow meters, wall suction with an assortment of catheters suitable for small children, and physiological monitoring. Back-up portable oxygen cylinders and suction boxes should be available outside the scanning unit. An emergency resuscitation box containing 'in date' drugs and appropriately sized and magnetically safe laryngoscopes,

oral airways and positive pressure bags should be in the scanning room or close at hand[1].

Physiological monitoring devices

These may be either situated in the scanning room or outside in the control room. Monitors in the scanning room may need to be shielded to prevent radiofrequency (RF) interference. If free standing, they should be attached to the wall with a plastic chain, well behind the 5-Gauss line.

Although our equipment is checked for safety on a regular basis we take the extra precaution of checking that all the equipment used for scanning babies is in the unit and working before we start each day's scanning (Table 1.1).

Prior to sedation

SAFETY IN THE PRESENCE OF A MAGNETIC FIELD

It is essential that all patients and accompanying persons are thoroughly screened before entering the magnetic field. Various types of screening are necessary and we use a series of metal check forms for visitors and different types of patients. A well-taken clinical history should reveal any metal or electronically activated implants in the child. However, before any sedation is given, a formal metal check form for the baby (Table 1.2) should be completed by an informed and MR-aware member of staff.

At the same time earrings and hair ornaments as well as clothes with metal buttons and religious artifacts should be removed. Baby-grows and clothes with metal poppers are not suitable attire for an MR scan. A hospital flannelette nightie with tie or velcro fastenings is ideal, leaving the feet free for attaching pulse oximeter probes and the chest accessible for ECG leads.

It is also essential that the person accompanying the baby throughout the procedure completes and signs a metal check form (Table 1.3). In our unit all new members of staff complete and sign a screening form as part of their clinical induction for relevant medical history on arrival in the unit. Staff who visit the unit only on pediatric days may need to be under constant vigil and are always reminded to empty their pockets and remove watches before they enter the scanner room (Fig. 1.4).

CLINICAL CARE

On the day of the MR appointment the mother and child are seen in the day care ward by the pediatrician and the

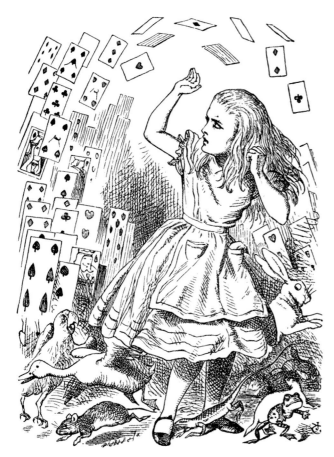

Fig. 1.4 'At this the whole pack rose up into the air and came flying down upon her; she gave a little scream, half of fright and half of anger and tried to beat them off…'. The missile effect on pocket contents and other ferromagnetic materials in the presence of a magnetic field is both dangerous and terrifying and can be fatal.

pediatric nurse. The infant is weighed and his or her body temperature, pulse rate and respiratory rate are recorded by the pediatric nurse on the drug chart (Table 1.4). The pediatrician performs a physical examination on the child and checks for signs of upper respiratory tract infection or any other current illness which may preclude sedation.

The infant's normal sleep pattern and general levels of activity are also noted and any sleep-related problem such as snoring, stridor or apnea is documented (Table 1.5). Supplemental oxygen may be needed when the child is sedated if there is a history of chronic lung disease, prematurity or snoring.

Sedation

Chloral hydrate is the most popular and frequently used sedative in radiology today[8]. It is readily available, easily administered and has a relatively wide margin of safety[4,8]. We have scanned over 1000 infants whose problems cover all five physical status categories of the American Academy of

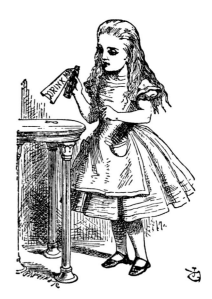

Fig. 1.5 'so Alice ventured to taste it, and finding it very nice she soon finished it off'. However chloral hydrate does not taste very nice.

Pediatrics[1] with chloral hydrate[2,8]. Occasionally, children over 1 year of age become hyperactive with oral chloral hydrate and if this happens we use nasal midazolam 0.2–0.5 mg/kg[9,11,12] or pethidine compound 0.06 ml/kg intramuscularly and oral trimeprazine (alimemazine) (Vallergan) 4 mg/kg. Other drugs have been used with or without chloral but whatever the decision, it is recommended that each unit sets up its own formulary and keeps the number of drugs used to a minimum[3].

Oral chloral hydrate is best given on an empty stomach as it is rapidly absorbed and most children are asleep within 15–30 min of administration. We recommend that chloral is given slowly from a syringe into the side of the mouth with the infant semi-upright in the mother's arms. However, it tastes awful and some infants will spit it out. With patience and care it is usually possible to ensure that most of the dose is swallowed (Fig. 1.5).

Infants with muscle disorders or generalized hypotonia are given a smaller dose of sedation, calculated on an individual basis.

We have found vomiting to be a problem only in the period immediately after the administration of the chloral, and not when the child is asleep if the infant has been properly prepared.

Chloral hydrate suppositories are useful for the child who is upset by the oral preparation. However, rectal applications may cause a bowel movement and then additional drugs may be required.

The doses and preparations we have found to be most successful are given in Table 1.6.

Infants less than 6 weeks of age are scanned whenever possible during natural sleep after a feed. If, however, these young babies do not sleep then a smaller dose of either oral or rectal chloral hydrate can be given (Table 1.6).

The dose and route of sedation are determined by the pediatrician (Table 1.4). The sedation should only be given when the radiographer performing the imaging has confirmed that the scanner is free and working, and that he or she is ready to scan the infant.

Transfer to the MR unit

When the sedation has been given and the infant is settled we attach a pulse oximeter probe and put the baby into a small baby cot with wheels. The mother and the baby are then taken to a quiet area in the MR unit until the baby falls asleep.

Immediately before entering the scanning room we do a final metal check and ask the accompanying person to empty their pockets and remove watches, etc. It is also worthwhile checking the baby again before putting him or her into the scanner as religious artifacts may have been put back on the baby or hidden in their clothes.

Monitoring

Monitoring of sedated and naturally sleeping infants during an MR scan is mandatory. MR-compatible monitoring systems are available for this purpose and can be purchased separately or directly from the MR manufacturer. The monitoring equipment accessories should be of the correct size for the infant and approved and tested by the MR manufacturer.

We use both pulse oximetry and ECG. ECG electrodes should be carefully placed on the chest and have no contact with each other. The ECG leads should be plaited and pass along the long axis of the body and out of the coil and have as little contact with the skin as possible.

The pulse oximeter should be attached to the infant's foot so that the probe and lead are outside the receive coil. Coiled monitoring wires may cause skin burns in rapidly changing magnetic fields[10].

Immobilization

Sedation alone may not keep an infant still enough to obtain diagnostic images. Swaddling further reduces body movement and helps to keep the infant warm. We routinely scan babies on their side, this position reduces the artifact from breathing and snoring and also prevents inhalation of secretions. If, however, the baby objects then it is better to let

them settle into their preferred position and accept that getting the images straight can be achieved with the pilot scans.

We cover a vacuum-pack bag (Vac-fix)[15] containing tiny polystyrene granules with a muslin baby nappy and curl the bag around the baby's head. When the air is evacuated from the bag the head is cradled in a firm but gentle mold. This device also protects the ears from the noise of the gradients (Fig. 1.6) and heat loss through the scalp is minimized. In very small babies it may be necessary to provide extra warmth and well-insulated gel or wheat-filled heated bags are suitable for this purpose.

Before the baby is slid into the scanner the monitoring is checked. Infants who snore or suffer from broncho-pulmonary dysplasia or have pronounced hypotonia may require oxygen to maintain their saturation levels. In these cases we attach a small ventilation mask to the oxygen supply and place the mask close to the infant's face before sliding them into the magnet and the oxygen flow can then be adjusted without bringing the baby in and out of the magnet.

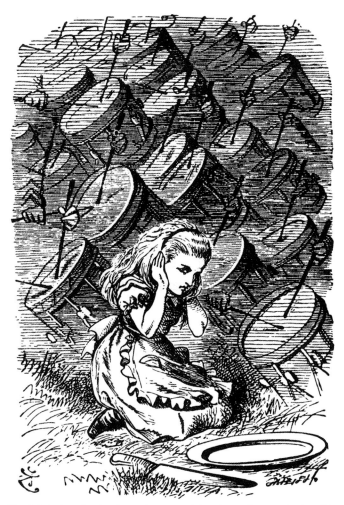

Fig. 1.6 'and put her hands over her ears, vainly trying to shut out the dreadful uproar'. Gradient noise can disturb a sleeping infant.

During the scan

Oxygen saturation and heart rate are recorded at 5-min intervals throughout the scan by the pediatrician (Table 1.7). He or she knows the clinical state of each infant and is responsible for the procedures of evacuation, resuscitation and the management of any reaction to the sedative and/or contrast agents.

Although each member of the group has his or her own skill we have an agreed protocol for the responsibilities of all team members to cover emergencies including a quench of the magnet. An example of the protocol we use in the event of a respiratory or cardiac arrest is given in Table 1.8.

Any unexpected event, although extremely rare, should be well documented and a careful explanation given to the parents. Precautions need to be taken so that infants over 6 months of age do not wake up and come out of the bore of the scanner and fall off the scanner table on to the floor.

Recovery from sedation

Most sedated infants will waken up naturally as they are brought out of the magnet; however, if this is not the case the baby should either stay in the MR unit or return to the ward with supervised monitoring continued until he or she is rousable.

The recommended discharge criteria after sedation are that the child must return to the baseline established prior to receiving sedation and this will depend on the developmental level of the child[1].

Discharge can be considered safe if the baby is rousable and orientated with stable vital signs and able to take a drink.

We give the parents written instructions about care of their child after the examination with information on the sedation, other relevant details and a telephone number in case of an emergency (Table 1.9).

Technical considerations

COILS

The signal to noise ratio on an MR image is greatly improved by using the smallest coil ('closest fit') for the part being examined (Fig. 1.7). Preterm and term neonates can be imaged in the adult knee coil (typical internal diameter 19 cm).

If small children are expected to become a significant proportion of your work load then purchasing a head coil with an internal diameter of 24 cm is recommended for infants aged from 2 months to 2 years of age. We have

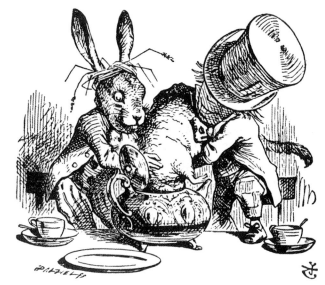

Fig. 1.7 'the last time she saw them, they were trying to put the Dormouse into the teapot'. Always use the smallest coil for the part being examined.

found our home-made split coil made from clear perspex excellent for this age group (Fig. 1.8). The improvement in the signal to noise ratio, the shorter scanning times and ease of positioning the infant within this coil makes it an excellent investment.

SEQUENCE CHOICE AND IMAGING PROTOCOLS

It is not possible to rush infants through an MR examination and there is always the risk that the baby will waken at any time. Before the infant is put into the scanner we make sure we have the relevant clinical information, and if possible a provisional diagnosis so that the appropriate sequences can be entered onto the computer prior to the examination.

At birth the water content of the infant's brain is 92–95% and during the first 2 years of life falls to the proportions of the adult brain, that is 80–85%[7]. This is associated with a markedly increased T1 and T2 and the standard sequences for the adult brain are not appropriate for imaging infants. It is important to adjust the available adult sequences to accommodate the changes in T1 and T2 as physiological myelination and growth take place. A list of sequence parameters for imaging the central nervous system in infants up to the age of 2 years is given in Table 1.10 for systems operating at 1.0 Tesla.

The brain changes rapidly from birth to 2 years of age[16,17] and being aware of these changes and their appearance on your own machine will help in the differentiation between normal development and the presence of pathology. Compiling a file of 'normal' images throughout the brain with a variety of sequences at different ages is a useful and informative exercise.

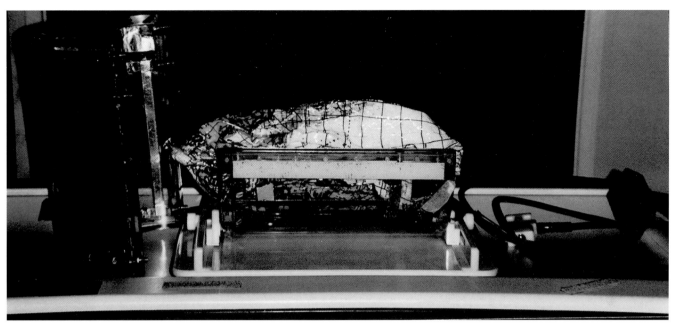

Fig. 1.8 The 'in house' transparent split coil with an internal diameter of 24 cm. Inside the coil is an inflatable plastic globe filled with small polystyrene balls which is our home-made fixation device.

IMAGING PROTOCOLS

In preterm and term infants we start all examinations with a short TR, short TE spin echo sequence in the transverse plane. It takes less than 5 min and provides information on ventricular size and shape, brain swelling, hemorrhage and cystic change.

The second sequence is usually a long TR, long TE spin echo or a fast spin echo in the same plane and with the same slice thickness and field of view. These two sequences may give enough information for a diagnosis. If the baby remains asleep we obtain other useful sequences. An example of the parameters of conventional sequences is given in Table 1.11.

OTHER SEQUENCES IN SPECIFIC CONDITIONS

The image contrast in diffusion-weighted sequences depends on the molecular motion of water. These sequences show regions of focal infarction and diffuse anoxic–ischemic brain injury during the early phase which are not obvious on T1 and T2 weighted spin echo or inversion recovery images[6].

If a new-born infant has a history of suspected infarction or hypoxic–ischemic encephalopathy and is being scanned within 48 h of the event we follow the short TR TE spin echo sequence with diffusion-weighted sequences.

Angiographic sequences are not so useful in the new-born infant as cerebral blood flow is slow and the blood vessels are small. However, they may be very useful in the older infant for defining the blood flow.

The FLAIR (fluid attenuated inversion recovery) sequence is particularly sensitive for the detection of subdural hematomas in the new born[13]. In the older infant this sequence provides excellent information on regions of gliosis and pathology at the CSF interface[18].

SPECIAL CONSIDERATIONS

Sick ventilated infants can be imaged safely in a distant MR unit provided the same level of care is available as that in the neonatal intensive care unit. Extra preparation and safety precautions are necessary including a specific metal check form (Table 1.12). Monitoring of body temperature may be required and this is not a problem as long as the temperature probe has been tested for use in a magnetic field. Arterial and venous lines need to be lengthened so that pumps and monitoring devices can be parked safely behind the 5-Gauss line. Ventilator tubing and oxygen lines should be prepared and *in situ* before the baby arrives in the unit.

In our hospital the baby is brought from the intensive care unit in a standard Vickers transport incubator. The incubator is parked and locked in a corner of the room well beyond the 5-Gauss line and attached to the wall by a plastic chain. The infant is ventilated from the Vicker neovent unit via long extension tubes from the incubator to the baby. Appropriate adjustment of the inspiratory and expiratory pressure is required to take account of the large dead space. Alternatively infants can be imaged using an MR-compatible ventilator (Siemens).

CONTRAST AGENTS

The use of gadolinium-based contrast agents may be indicated in defined clinical conditions in infants, for example in infections and suspected tumors.

If there is a possibility that a contrast agent will be required then an intravenous line should be inserted prior to sedation and after the application of a topical anesthetic cream such as EMLA.

Table 1.1 List of equipment to be checked at the beginning of each pediatric session

Check that	Checked
Piped medical gases have appropriately sized flow meters attached	
Extra portable gas cylinders are close by and full	
Portable suction is available, working and catheters are available	
The insulation on the transmit and receive coils is not damaged	
All monitoring equipment is working and sufficient probes and leads available	
The insulation on ECG and pulse oximetry leads is not broken	
Contents of pediatric resuscitation box are there	
Drugs are not out of date	
Scanner working	
Other......	

Table 1.2 Final metal safety check for imaging infants (use in combination with Table 1.12 if relevant). Some categories from Shellock and Kanal[14].

Name: Date:		
Categories	Yes	No
Cardiac pacemaker – any type		
Heart surgery (e.g. patent ductus) or other		
Ventriculo-peritoneal shunt		
Other surgery		
Any type of surgical clip or staples		
Aneurysm clip		
Any type of biostimulator or neurostimulator pump		
Any type of internal electrode including pacing wires, cochlear implant, other		
Swan–Ganz catheter		
Any type of electronic, mechanical or magnetic implant		
Hearing aid or any type of ear implant		
Any type of foreign body, shrapnel or bullet		
Implanted drug infusion device		
Orbital/eye prosthesis		
Any type of implant held in place by a magnet		
Artificial limb or joint		
Any implanted orthopedic item		
Allergies		
Remove earrings and all jewelry		
Remove ornaments		
Change into hospital gown		

If the answer to any of the above questions is 'YES' please give details.

Please note: that a device not known to be safe must be assumed to be unsafe. In the cases operated by microprocessors (e.g. implantable pumps) device malfunction caused by field effects on the circuitry must be considered. Other devices such as ventricular shunts, orthodontic braces may be safe, but may degrade image quality significantly.

Name:............................. Date:......................

Signed:.. (Parent or guardian)

.... MR personnel

Table 1.3 Imaging safety check list for parent/guardian/accompanying person. Some categories from Shellock and Kanal[14]. This form is offered as a guideline and can be changed to meet individual requirements.

Name: Date:		
Categories	Yes	No
Cardiac pacemaker any type		
Aneurysm clip		
Any type of biostimulator or neurostimulator pump		
Any type of internal electrode including pacing wires, cochlear implant, other		
Implanted insulin pump		
Any type of electronic, mechanical or magnetic implant		
Hearing aid		
Implanted drug infusion device		
Any type of foreign body, shrapnel or bullet		
Any type of ear implant		
Artificial eye		
Occupation as a metal worker, grinder, welder		
Any type of implant held in place by a magnet		
Vascular access port		
Intraventricular shunt		
Artificial limb or joint		
Any implanted orthopedic item		
Pregnancy		
Before entering the scanning room		
please remove your watch		
please take out metal hair ornaments		
please empty your pockets (some coins are ferromagnetic)		

If the answer to any of the above questions is 'YES' please give details.

Please note: that a device not known to be safe must be assumed to be unsafe. In the cases operated by microprocessors (e.g. implantable pumps) device malfunction caused by field effects on the circuitry must be considered.

Name:... Date:........................

Signed:... (Parent or guardian)

.... MR personnel

Table 1.4 Drug chart and vital signs before MR procedure

Name: Date:

Vital signs

Temperature	Respiratory rate	Pulse rate	Body weight
Drug prescribed	Dose/kg	Actual dose	Route oral/rectal

Time of administration:

Problems with administration:

None	Coughing	Vomiting	Bowel movement	Other

Pediatrician/nurse: Date:

Table 1.5 Pediatric record form for magnetic resonance studies

Name Date of birth Consultant	Examination date Time
Part to be examined	
Reason for MR study	
Is contrast required yes/no	EMLA applied or iv *in situ*
Previous MR studies yes/no	When
Relevant past medical history	Previous operations yes/no Implants yes/no Details Checked for magnetic compatibility yes/no
Previous sedation yes/no Problems yes/no Details	
On-going problems	

Oxygen requirement	Feeding/swallowing difficulties	Snoring	Other
Present condition enter times below please			

Last food	Last drink	Last sleep	Last bowel movement

Signs of respiratory tract infection yes/no	Other illness yes/no
Current medication	
Metal check internal yes/no	Metal check external yes/no (hair, ears, jewelry, clothes changed)
Intravenous lines long enough yes/no	
Magnet safe yes/no	
Signed	

Table 1.6 Age-related doses for oral chloral hydrate

Age	Dose
Up to 6 weeks post term (46 weeks PMA)	nil or chloral hydrate 30–50 mg/kg
47 weeks PMA – 6 months	chloral hydrate 50–80 mg/kg
7 months – 2 years	chloral hydrate 80–100 mg/kg (maximum dose 2 g)

PMA, postmenstrual age

Readily available preparations of chloral hydrate:

Oral	200 mg/5 ml flavored with blackcurrant
	1000 mg/5 ml – unflavored
Suppositories	12.5, 25 and 50 mg available on most neonatal units
	100, 250 and 500 mg available on special request

Table 1.7 Oxygen saturation measurements during MR imaging

Name:		Date of birth:		Date:	
Start time					
Baseline O$_2$ saturation					
Baseline pulse rate					

Time from start of scan (min)	O$_2$ saturation	Pulse rate	Time from start of scan (min)	O$_2$ saturation	Pulse rate
5			35		
10			40		
15			45		
20			50		
25			55		
30			60		

Monitoring normal/abnormal (specify)   Oxygen required yes/no
                                                        Amount

Contrast given   type   dose
Adverse reaction
Time of wakening: Normal O$_2$ saturation in air   Drinking
yes/no
Injection site checked yes/no   Sent to ward/home
Discharge letter given to parents   yes/no

Signed by pediatrician: . . . .

Time: . . . .

Table 1.8 Protocol for evacuation of MR scanner

In the event of a respiratory or cardiac arrest:
- Remove the infant from the magnet and the MR room
- Assigned person closes door to MR room (to prevent access by unauthorized personnel (such as cardiac arrest team)
- Place on a stretcher outside the MR room
- Assigned person puts out cardiac arrest call
- Pediatrician starts cardio-pulmonary resuscitation
- Assigned person attaches mobile pulse oximeter
- Assigned person makes ready suction with correct-sized catheter, drugs, oxygen with mask and ambu bag, intubation equipment, intravenous access equipment, etc.

In our hospital the assigned person is the radiographer.
A written report of any incident must be produced. Careful explanation to the parents is also required.

Table 1.9 Patient information sheet

Hospital address and name of department
Telephone numbers
Dear parents/carers
Your infant   has been sedated today with a drug called . . . .
He/she also had an injection of a contrast agent to enhance the images.
There were/were not any problems.
Your child may remain sleepy for up to 8 h but you should be able to waken her/him easily and he/she may be irritable for up to 24 h after this sedation.
Eating and drinking instructions: we suggest that you feed your baby with juice, formula or breast milk. If there is no signs of vomiting then continue with your usual routine.
If you are anxious about any aspects of the baby's activity please do not hesitate to ring the hospital at the above telephone number.
The results of the MR scan take a few days to prepare and then they will be forwarded to your doctor.

Signed: Pediatrician

Table 1.10 Sequence parameters for systems operating at 1.0 Tesla. These should be adjusted for different field strengths.

Inversion recovery (IR) sequences:

Age	Type	TR	TE	TI
29–34 weeks	IR medium TI	7000	30	1500
35–39 weeks		6500	30	1200
40 weeks – 3 months		3800	30	950
> 3 months – 24 months		3500	30	800
< 3 months	FLAIR long TI	6000	240	2100
> 3 months	FLAIR long TI	6000	160	2200

Spin echo sequences at 1.0 Tesla:	TR	TE
All ages T1 weighted spin echo	860	20
Up to 2 years of age T2 weighted spin echo	3000	120
Fast spin echo (FSE) 16 echo train length	3500	208

Table 1.11 Imaging protocols: these will vary from center to center and depend on the clinical problem, the state of the infant, the type and strength of the magnetic field. However, the ones given below have been tried and tested in our department

	T1 weighted spin echo	T2 weighted spin echo	Fast spin echo	Inversion recovery
Slice orientation	Transverse	Transverse	Transverse	Transverse
Phase encoding axis	left–right	left–right	left–right	left–right
Number of slices	24	24	24	18
Echo time (TE)	20	120	208	30
Inversion time (TI)				1500–800
Repeat time (TR)	860	3200	3500	6000–3500
Field of view	22–23	22–23	22–23	22–23
Phase resolution	192	128	256	128
Phase sampling ratio	256	256	256	256
*Number of signal averages	2	1 or 2	4–16	1 or 2
Slice thickness	4 mm	5 mm	4 mm	5 mm
Receive coil	Smallest available			

* The number of signal averages will depend on time constraints and the size of the receiver coil.

Table 1.12 Neonatal metal check form to be completed before entry to the scanning room

Name: Ward:

For in-patients (i.e. infants coming from the ward and or the neonatal intensive care unit and supplements metal check form given in Table 1.2)

Please check the following items on or in the baby and remove if necessary

	Action
Searle arterial lines (these contain an electronic O$_2$ monitor)	Babies with these *in situ* **must not** be put into the scanner
Scalp needles	Cause susceptibility artifacts which degrade images
Electronic name tabs	Remove
Name tabs with metal closures	Remove
Clothes with metal poppers	Take off
Ward monitoring leads **must be taken off** and	Take off and replace with MR-compatible leads
Religious artifacts	Take off

This is to confirm that the baby named above has been checked and the appropriate action has been taken

Signed . . . .   Date . . . .

Checked by:

This form is to be completed before entering the scanning room

Summary

■ '*Imaging infants is a formidable task to do well*'; '*the least read chapter in most imaging text books is the one on preparation and management*'[3].

■ This important group of patients deserve the extra effort and time involved in a technology which continues to evolve and offers diagnostic information not available with any other imaging techniques,

and most importantly, without known biological hazard.

■ I have included line drawings of John Tenniel in Lewis Carroll's *Alice in Wonderland* and *Through the Looking-Glass, and What Alice Found There*[5] in the hope that these 'images' will catch your eye and entice you to read this chapter!

Acknowledgments

We are grateful to Macmillan Children's Books for permission to use the line drawings of John Tenniel from *Alice in Wonderland* and *Through the Looking Glass, and What Alice Found There*.

This chapter was written with the advantage of 18 years experience of MRI after 2 years retirement in County Fermanagh, Northern Ireland. It was a task tinged with sadness as well as pleasure and the remembering of the many marvellous and caring people I worked with at Hammersmith Hospital in the Robert Steiner MR unit and the department of Paediatrics. Thank you Frank Doyle, Robert Steiner, Graeme Bydder, David Bryant, David Gilderdale, Lilly Dubowitz, Frances Cowan and Mary Rutherford for all the good times.

References

1. American Academy of Pediatrics, Committee on Drugs (1992) Guidelines for monitoring and management of pediatric patient during and after sedation for diagnostic and therapeutic procedures. *Pediatrics* **89**, 1110–1115.
2. American Academy of Pediatrics, Committee on Drugs and Committee on Environmental Health (1993) Use of chloral hydrate for sedation in children. *Pediatrics* **92**, 471–473.
3. Ball WS Jr (1997) Patient management for neuroimaging. In: Ball WS Jr (Ed.) *Pediatric Neuroradiology*. Philadelphia, Lippincott–Raven, pp. 3–16.
4. Bisset III George S and Ball Jr William S (1991) Preparation, sedation and monitoring of the pediatric patient in the magnetic resonance suite. *Seminars in Ultrasound, CT and MRI* **12**, 376–378.
5. Carroll Lewis, with illustrations by John Tenniel (1872) In: *Alice in Wonderland*, Macmillan, London, pp. 1, 10, 18, 110, 188, and *Through the Looking Glass, and What Alice Found There*, Macmillan, London, pp. 56.
6. Cowan FM, Pennock JM, Hanrahan JD *et al.* (1994) Early detection of cerebral infarction and hypoxic ischaemic encephalopathy in neonates using diffusion weighted magnetic resonance imaging. *Neuropediatrics* **25**, 172–175.
7. Dobbing J and Sands J (1973) Quantitative growth and development of human brain. *Arch Dis Child* **48**, 757–767.
8. Greenberg SB, Faerber EN, Aspinall CL *et al.* (1993) High-dose chloral hydrate sedation for children undergoing MR imaging: safety and efficacy in relation to age. *Am J Radiol* **161**, 639–641.
9. Harcke HT, Grissom LE and Meister MA (1995) Sedation in pediatric imaging using intranasal midazolam. *Pediatr Radiol* **25**, 341–343.
10. Kanal E, Shellock FG and Talagala L (1990) Safety considerations in MR imaging. *Radiology* **176**, 593–606.
11. Louon A and Reddy VG (1994) Nasal midazolam and ketamine for paediatric imaging during computerised tomography. *Acta Anaesthesiol Scand* **38**, 259–261.
12. McCarver-May DG, Kang J, Aouthmany M *et al.* (1996) Comparison of chloral hydrate and midazolam for sedation of neonates for neuroimaging studies. *J Pediatr* **128**, 753–756.
13. Noguchi K, Ogawa T, Seto H *et al.* (1997) Subacute and chronic subarachnoid hemorrhage: diagnosis with fluid-attenuated inversion-recovery MR imaging. *Radiology* **203(1)**, 257–262.
14. Shellock FG and Kanal E (1996) Appendix 1 list of items tested. In: *Magnetic Resonance, Bioeffects, Safety, and Patient management*, 2nd edn. Philadelphia, Lippincott–Raven, pp. 179–215. Internet helpline: http://kanal.arad.upmc.edu/mrsafety.html
15. Vac-fix available from S&S Xray Products Inc., 1101 Linwood St, Brooklyn NY 11208.
16. van der Knaap MS, van Wezel-Meijler G, Barth P *et al.* (1996) Normal gyration and sulcation in preterm and term neonates: appearance on MR images. *Radiology* **200**, 389–396.
17. van der Knaap MS and Valk J (1995) *Magnetic Resonance of Myelin, Myelination and Myelin disorders*, 2nd edn. Heidelberg, Springer.
18. Young IR, Bydder GM and Hajnal JV (1997) Contrast properties of the inversion recovery sequence. In: WG Bradley and GM Bydder (Eds) *Advanced MR Imaging Techniques*, 1st edn. London, Martin Dunitz, pp. 143–162.

Imaging the preterm infant: practical issues

2

Elia F Maalouf and Serena J Counsell

Contents

Introduction

Magnetic resonance imaging (MRI) is an established method for determining the presence and extent of lesions in adults and older infants. However, very few studies have been performed on preterm infants and these have only been undertaken on infants of 29 weeks of gestational age (GA) or more[3,10,13,14]. This is primarily because of difficulties in transporting, temperature maintenance, continuing intensive care and monitoring preterm infants. In order to overcome these problems, a purpose-designed 1.0T system (Oxford Magnet Technology Ltd, Eynsham, Oxford, UK and Marconi (Picker) International Inc., Cleveland, Ohio, USA) has been installed in our neonatal intensive care unit (NICU)[5]. Using this system it is possible to provide the same standard of care for the infants in the scanner as they receive elsewhere in the NICU. As a result it has been possible to study very premature neonates as young as 24 weeks GA[1,2,9].

The neonatal scanner

The integration of an MR scanner into an NICU provides a unique opportunity to image preterm infants and infants in the acute phase of an insult, without compromising their intensive care. The neonatal MR scanner was designed to provide access to the infants at all times whilst they were being scanned. In order to achieve this, the length of the magnet bore was made very short (38 cm) (Fig. 2.1). Active shielding is employed within the magnet but paradoxically this results in a 2 T fringe field at a radius of 50 cm from the center of the bore of the 1 T magnet. The 5-Gauss line is at a distance of 3 m from the center of the bore. The maximum gradient strength is 40 mT/m in all three axes with a maximum gradient slew rate of 40 mT/m/ms. A specially designed transmit/receive quadrature birdcage coil (32 cm × 23 cm) is used for all examinations and allows infants to be studied up to a maximum weight of about 5 kg. The short Z axis of the magnet results in a discoid volume of useful homogenous field (≤10 ppm) (14 cm in the X direction, 14 cm in the Y direction and 4 cm in the Z direction).

Transport of the baby

A specially designed non-magnetic transport trolley has been made of similar dimensions to the incubators used on the ward. The main design objective of the transport trolley was to minimize handling of the baby whilst being able to continue life monitoring, and ventilation where required, during the move from incubator to the imaging system.

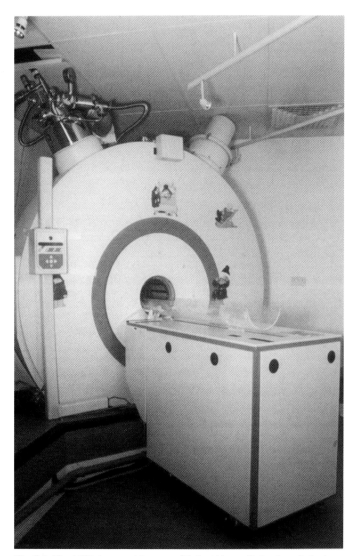

Fig. 2.1 The 1.0 Tesla neonatal scanner (Oxford Magnet Technology, Oxford and Marconi (Picker) International Inc., Cleveland Ohio).

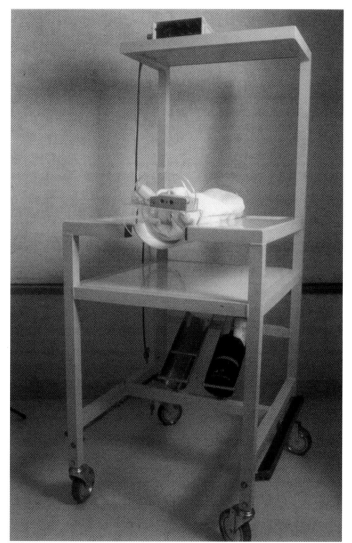

Fig. 2.2 Transport trolley.

The baby is placed on a specially made perspex cradle, which fits into the transport trolley (Fig. 2.2). Using this system, infants are only handled when being moved from their cot or incubator to the trolley and back to their cot from the trolley after scanning. This cradle has a fastening device at one end for securing ventilator tubing and infusion lines. Infusion lines are extended and all infusion pumps and monitoring equipment are placed on shelves on the transport trolley.

As monitoring equipment used on the NICU is not MR compatible, all monitoring is switched to MR-compatible monitoring and the oxygen line is attached to the piped supply at the door of the scanning room. Infusion pumps are attached to a wall-mounted rail within the scanning room but beyond the 5-Gauss line. The perspex cradle is transferred from the trolley to a sliding, dished, perspex bed on the scanner table.

Ventilation

Ventilated infants may be imaged using an MR-compatible ventilator (babyPAC neonatal, pneuPac Limited, UK) (Fig. 2.3), which can be sited adjacent to the scanner. If an MR-compatible ventilator is not available, ventilation may be performed using a ventilator sited in a radio frequency (RF) cupboard, with ports for the ventilator tubing, or by securing the ventilator outside the 5-Gauss line. If these methods are used, ventilator tubing will have to be extended and the positive inspiratory pressure, the end expiratory pressure valve and the gas flow must be adjusted to allow for the 'dead space' of the tubing.

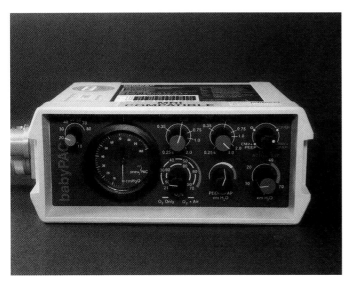

Fig. 2.3 babyPAC MR compatible ventilator.

Immobilization

Effective immobilization of the neonate is vital in order to obtain high-quality MR images. Immobilization is achieved with an Olympic bag, which contains small polystyrene balls and is evacuated with suction to fit snugly around the baby's head. The Olympic bag also helps to muffle sound. Babies who are not ventilated are imaged on their side whenever possible but as a large number of babies are not sedated for imaging, it is most important to find a position that is comfortable for the baby and which can be maintained for the duration of the scan. Ventilated babies need to be imaged supine to accommodate the endo- or nasotracheal tube and ventilator tubing.

Temperature maintenance

In order to maintain the infant's temperature, he or she is swaddled in blankets and the temperature of the scanning room is set at 27°C, the same as the temperature on the neonatal unit. Additional heating for extremely preterm neonates can be provided with bubble wrap, woollen hats and 'gel bags', which retain their heat once warmed in a microwave oven.

Sedation

Sedation with oral chloral hydrate (20–30 mg/kg) is occasionally necessary but the majority of preterm infants and neonates can be successfully imaged following a feed or whilst sedated for ventilation[4].

Monitoring

Physiological data must be recorded throughout an MRI examination when imaging preterm infants. We use a Hewlett Packard Merlin life support system. All monitoring equipment for use in the scanner room must either be MR compatible or be RF shielded. In our case the monitor is sited in an RF-shielded cupboard within the scanning room. Oxygen saturation, heart rate, temperature and, where required, mean arterial blood pressure are monitored throughout the examination.

Oxygen saturation can be measured by pulse oximetry (Nellcor oxiband or oxisensor D-20 transducer with a Nellcor pulse oximeter, Nellcor Incorporated, Pleasanton, CA, USA) and heart rate may be measured using chest ECG leads. ECG leads and electrodes must be MR compatible and we use Blue sensor (Medicotest, Olstykke, Denmark) ECG electrodes and ECG leads with current limiting resistors (NDM Division, American Hospital Supply Corporation, Ohio, USA). RF fields can cause currents in conduction loops, which may cause burns[7] and, therefore, care must be taken to ensure that ECG leads do not form conductive loops and skin contact is kept to a minimum. The electrodes should be placed close together, but not touching, to minimize ECG interference by the magnetic field and ECG leads should be plaited in order to minimize loops across which potential differences may occur[11]. Temperature may be measured by placing an MR-compatible temperature probe in the axilla. In the neonatal scanner, all monitoring devices are connected via a gantry, which prevents loose cables stretching across the floor and causing a potential hazard.

As a safety precaution, an experienced pediatrician remains in the scanning room with the infant during scanning and can view the monitor through the glass window of the RF-shielded cupboard. A further monitor is sited in the scanner control room.

Pulse sequences and scanning parameters

The neonatal brain has a higher water content (92–95%) than the adult brain (82–85%) and so T1 and T2 values are greater[6]. This means that echo times (TE), repetition times (TR) and inversion times (TI) have to be increased. Transverse T1 weighted conventional spin echo (CSE), T2 weighted fast spin echo (FSE) and inversion recovery fast spin echo (IRFSE) images are obtained in each study and in some cases coronal and sagittal T2 weighted FSE images are obtained. T1 weighted CSE images have low gray/white matter contrast but are useful in assessing hemorrhage, brain swelling in hypoxic ischemic encephalopathy and for assessing tissue enhancement after administration of contrast. The T2 weighted FSE sequence is useful to demonstrate pathology and fast imaging techniques are helpful to reduce motion artifact in neonatal imaging. We have found the T2 weighted FSE to be the optimal sequence for demonstrating myelination in the premature brain. The IRFSE sequence provides excellent gray/ white matter contrast and is useful in assessing myelination.

Diffusion weighted and angiographic sequences are performed where indicated and T1 weighted sequences are obtained after intravenous gadolinium (0.1 mmol/kg gadopentate dimeglumine) in selected cases.

Sequence parameters used on the neonatal scanner are listed in Table 2.1.

Safety issues

The number of people in the scanning room should be kept to a minimum but in the case of ventilated babies two pediatricians and a radiographer are essential. We exclude parents from the scanning room but they are welcome to watch from the control room. A metal check form is completed by the pediatrician or nurse caring for the baby and checked by the radiographer before transporting the baby to the magnet. This form includes specific neonatal items such as Serle arterial lines with terminal electrodes, electronic name tags and metal poppers on clothes (see Chapter 1). The door of the neonatal scanning room is kept locked by a magnetic latch system with one push-release button being in the control room and one inside the scanning room.

Emergency resuscitation equipment should be kept either in the scanning room or in the immediate vicinity. Any equipment kept within the scanning room must be MR compatible and so, in many centers, resuscitation equipment is kept just outside of the scanner room. If this is the case, the infant must be brought out of the scanning room for emergency treatment to avoid incompatible equipment being brought into the MR environment. In the neonatal scanner at the Hammersmith Hospital, we keep an MR-compatible laryngoscope, stethoscope, endotrachial (ET) tubes and

introducers and ET suction equipment within the scanner room. If the infant requires anything further they are returned to the NICU for treatment.

Acoustic noise is produced through the vibration of the gradient coils as electric current through the coils is switched on and off. Acoustic noise exposure has been reported to cause increased stimulation in neonates[8]. The neonatal scanner at the Hammersmith Hospital has several noise reduction measures incorporated into the design, including lagging and gradient cable immobilization. To reduce acoustic noise levels still further, an Olympic bag filled with polystyrene balls is evacuated of air and is used as immobilization. As the immobilization bag fits snugly around the infant's head, it is an effective method of reducing the infant's exposure to acoustic noise. Acoustic noise levels in the neonatal scanner during different pulse sequences were measured and found to be below the recommended safe limits and are described in Table 2.2[1].

One study has reported physiological changes in infants undergoing MRI, including raised heart rate, BP or desaturation, probably due to stimulation whilst undergoing MRI[12]. However, in a recent study infants did not show an excessive disturbance in heart rate whilst undergoing MRI[1]. A slight increase in heart rate and temperature was observed towards the end of the scan but these increases were not clinically significant. This study concluded that there have been no detrimental physiological effects on infants undergoing MRI in the neonatal scanner[1].

Table 2.2 Acoustic noise measurements

Pulse sequence	MAXL (dBA)	Leq (dBA)
T1 weighted CSE	70	67
T2 weighted FSE	72	70
IRFSE	71	67
Open incubator	62	–
Transport incubator with alarm and compressor	66	–

MAXL, maximum root mean squared level; Leq, average sound pressure level during the measurement period; dBA, a weighted decibel.

Table 2.1 Pulse sequences parameters

Pulse sequence	TR (ms)	TI (ms)	TE (ms)	Slice thick (mm)	Slice gap (mm)	No. of slices	NSA	Phase matrix	Scan time (mins)	Echo train length
T1 weighted CSE	600	–	20	4	–	9	2	192	3:30	–
T2 weighted FSE	3500	–	208	4	–	9	4	256	3:50	16
IRFSE	3697	950	36	4	1	6	4	256	3:45	16

CSE, conventional spin echo; FSE, fast spin echo; IRFSE, inversion recovery fast spin echo; NSA, number of signal averages.

Summary

- MRI of preterm infants receiving intensive care can be safely performed using a dedicated neonatal scanner situated on a neonatal intensive care unit.

- Excellent image quality can be produced once adaptations to coils for the small head and sequences for the immature brain have been made.

- Meticulous attention to detail has to be made in transferring a sick ventilated infant into the scanner. Two neonatally qualified staff are needed in addition to the radiographer.

- All intensive care monitoring equipment must be MR compatible.

- Temperature maintenance may be achieved by controlling the room temperature and the immediate environment of the infant.

- Some imaging sequences may be unacceptably noisy and noise reduction measures must be made.

- Fast imaging sequences are ideal to decrease the examination time and to avoid the unnecessary use of sedation although some image detail may be sacrificed.

References

1. Battin M, Maalouf EF, Counsell SJ *et al.* (1998a) Physiological stability of preterm infants during magnetic resonance imaging. *Early Human Development* **52**, 101–110.
2. Battin MR, Maalouf EF, Counsell SJ *et al.* (1998b) Magnetic resonance imaging of the brain in very preterm infants: visualization of the germinal matrix, early myelination, and cortical folding. *Pediatrics* **101**, 957–962.
3. Childs A, Ramenghi LA, Evans DJ *et al.* (1998) MR features of developing periventricular white matter in preterm infants: evidence of glial cell migration. *Am J Neuroradiol* **19**, 971–976.
4. Cowan FM (1997) Sedation for magnetic resonance scanning for infants and young children. In: Whitman JG and McCloy R (Eds) *Principles and Practice of Sedation.* London, Blackwell Healthcare, pp. 206–213.
5. Hall AS, Young IR, Davies FJ *et al.* (1997) A dedicated magnetic resonance system in a neonatal intensive therapy unit. In: Bradley WG and Bydder GM (Eds) *Advanced MR Imaging Techniques.* London, Martin Dunitz, pp. 281–290.
6. Johnson MA, Pennock JM, Bydder GM *et al.* (1983) Clinical NMR imaging of the brain in children: normal and neurologic disease. *Am J Roentgenol* **141**(5), 1005–1018.
7. Kanal E and Shellock FG (1990) Burns associated with clinical MR examinations. *Radiology* **175**, 585.

8. Long JG, Lucey JF and Philip AG (1980) Noise and hypoxaemia in the intensive care nursery. *Pediatrics* **65**, 143–145.
9. Maalouf EF, Duggan PJ, Rutherford MA *et al.* (1999) Magnetic resonance imaging of the brain in a cohort of extremely preterm infants. *J Pediatr* **135**, 351–357.
10. McArdle CB, Richardson CJ, Nicholas DA *et al.* (1987) Developmental features of the neonatal brain: MR imaging. Part 1 gray–white matter differentiation and myelination. *Pediatr Radiol* **162**(1), 223–229.
11. Peden CJ, Menon DK, Hall AS *et al.* (1992) Magnetic resonance for the anaesthetist. Part 2: anaesthesia and monitoring in MR units. *Anaesthesia* **47**, 508–517.
12. Philbin MK, Taber KH and Hayman LA (1996) Preliminary report: changes in vital signs of term newborns during MR. *Am J Neuroradiol* **17**, 1033–1036.
13. Sie LT, van der Knapp MS, van Wezel-Meijler G *et al.* (1997) MRI assessment of myelination of motor and sensory pathways in the brain of preterm and term-born infants. *Neuropediatrics* **28**(2), 97–105.
14. Van der Knapp MS, Barkhof F, Ader HJ *et al.* (1996) Normal gyration and sulcation in preterm and term neonates: appearances on MR images. *Radiology* **200**, 389–396.

Part II

Anatomy and development of the immature brain

Magnetic resonance imaging of the brain in preterm infants: 24 weeks' gestation to term

3

Malcolm Battin and Mary A Rutherford

Contents

Introduction

Brain maturation involves a complex sequence of morphological, functional and organizational changes. Although these changes are complex they occur in a sequence that is both organized and predictable. Pathological studies have been important in documenting the process of brain maturation but imaging offers the added advantage of being able to study the live fetus or infant. Furthermore, repeated or serial imaging may be performed, thus permitting longitudinal assessment of maturity both *in utero* and *ex utero*.

Ultrasound is readily available in the neonatal nursery and has been used extensively to assess the preterm infant brain; however, recently interest in using MRI in this age group has increased. Magnetic resonance imaging (MRI) is a non-invasive multiplanar technique that provides detailed images. Qualitative and quantitative assessment of brain development including myelination can be performed and pathological processes including migration disorders and neonatal intracranial hemorrhage are well demonstrated. Sequential imaging provides the means to study not only normal development but also the response of the brain to injury.

Although MRI is a useful technique in the preterm infant, differences exist from adult imaging and these must be addressed in order to obtain optimal images. The immature brain has higher water content than the adult brain and this is associated with a marked increase in T1 and T2 values. Appropriate changes in the pulse sequences are required in order to produce optimum images. In our experience it has been possible to produce good-quality images using the same sequence parameters between 23 weeks and term, although measurements of T2 values have been shown to gradually decrease over this period[9] (Fig. 3.1). T1 and T2 shortening occurs more dramatically from term age over the first year of life in association with myelination[19].

The aim of this chapter is to describe the MRI appearances of the brain in preterm infants imaged between 24 weeks' gestational age (GA) and term (37–42 weeks). MR study of the developing brain is important, not only to illustrate the normal changes that occur but also because it may shed light on the origin of brain lesions causing long-term neurodevelopmental sequelae in the preterm infant. Evaluation of the developing brain using MRI is likely to be of value in the interpretation of isolated images taken later in infancy. MRI has also been shown to produce valuable postmortem data and it is feasible to image the neonatal brain both in and outside of the body after death.

In order to establish the normal variation in a preterm population we have attempted to image every infant born at less than 30 weeks' gestation at the Hammersmith Hospital. The majority of images presented in this chapter were obtained from this cohort of over 150 preterm infants. Images were

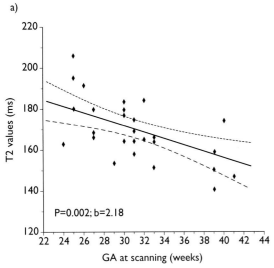

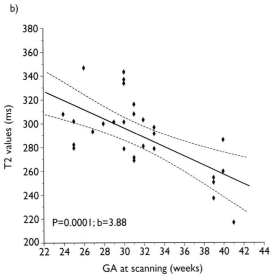

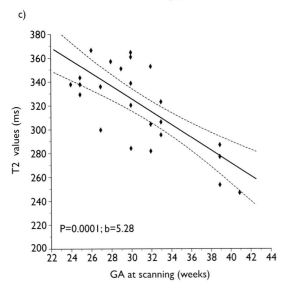

Fig. 3.1 T2 values at 1 Tesla in **(a)** the lentiform nuclei **(b)** the anterior white matter and **(c)** the posterior white matter at the level of the centrum semiovale. (Courtesy of Serena Counsell, Hammersmith Hospital.)

obtained using a 1T (Oxford Magnet Technology/Marconi Medical Systems) neonatal MRI system[14] situated in the neonatal unit (see Chapter 2). The GA for the infants was calculated from the date of the last menstrual period and confirmed with data from early antenatal ultrasound scans. Parental consent for imaging the infants was obtained in each case and ethical approval for this study was given by the Hammersmith Hospitals Research Ethics Committee.

Cortical folding

The most obvious changes in the preterm brain between 24 weeks and term are the increase in overall size and the increase in cortical folding. Cortical development occurs from approximately 8 weeks, initially with replication of neurons and glial cells in the periventricular germinal zones. In the mammalian brain the germinal zone consists of a ventricular zone, which forms first, and a more superficial subventricular zone. The former produces mainly neuronal cells and the latter is responsible for mainly glial cell proliferation[4] (see Fig. 3.14). Although these layers may be distinguishable histologically, they are indistinguishable on MRI. The ventricular zone is largely exhausted by the end of neuronal migration and residual ventricular zone cells become ependymal cells. The subventricular zone remains and persists into adult life as the subependymal layer. The term germinal matrix is usually used to describe the residual subependymal tissue in the caudothalamic notch, which is easily visible with cranial ultrasound. Using MR images it is possible to see that there is a densely cellular layer, the subependymal layer, lining the entire ventricle although it is most obvious overlying the caudate nucleus. It is not possible to differentiate the ependymal layer on MR images as this is only one cell thick.

The layers of the developing cortex are formed initially by neuronal migration along radial glia. Radial glia not only guide neurons but appear to facilitate the columnar organization of the cortex. The first wave of immature neurons to migrate form the preplate of the developing cortex, which is then split into an inner and outer layer by neurons arriving to form the cortical plate. The inner layer of the preplate is known as the subplate and plays an important role in cortical organization. The outer layer is the subpial marginal zone.

The permanent cortical layers form from the inside out, so that layer six which lies medially is laid down first. The mature cortex consists of six distinct layers in most areas of the brain. Neuronal migration to the cerebral cortex is completed by 20–24 weeks' gestation in the human brain. Glial cell migration probably continues for at least 1 year post birth. Between

29 weeks' gestation and term cortical gray matter volume increases from approximately 60 ml to approximately 160 ml[17]. This subsequent increase in cortical gray matter volume is secondary to glial cell migration, neuronal differentiation and organizational changes. Following migration, radial glia proliferate and differentiate into astrocytes and possibly oligodendrocytes within the white matter.

During early gestation the brain is smooth or 'lissencephalic' in appearance but as growth proceeds the typical convoluted pattern develops allowing a considerable increase in the surface area of the brain. Normal convolution probably relies on a full complement of neurons within the developing cortical plate. Primary sulci begin as a shallow groove with widely separated side walls and straight ends. The groove then becomes deeper and the side walls become progressively steeper approximating and eventually meeting each other. These secondary sulci may show V-shaped or bifid ends. With continued maturation, the gyri and sulci become complex and side branches develop as seen in the adult brain. Each of the gyri and matching sulci are named according to their site within the brain.

The anatomical development of the major sulci and gyri in the brain has been well documented by Chi *et al.*[5] who studied 507 brains obtained from fetuses and infants from 10 to 44 weeks' gestational age. The gyral development evolves in an ordered fashion up until term.

In pathological series, the first fissure to develop is the interhemispheric fissure, which appears at 8 weeks' gestation. It starts anteriorly and proceeds posteriorly separating the two cerebral hemispheres by 10 weeks' gestation. At 14 weeks the Sylvian fissure begins as a shallow depression formed by the progressive indentation of the cortex in the region of the insula. By 19 weeks the Sylvian fissure is deeper and the insula can be identified. At 20 weeks the central sulcus is first seen. The parieto-occipital fissure, which divides the parietal from the occipital lobe, is first seen at 16 weeks and is documented on antenatal ultrasound in all infants by 24 weeks' gestation. The calcarine sulcus appears at about 16 weeks and joins the parieto-occipital fissure anteriorly. Together they form a Y shape that is easily visible on parasagittal ultrasound scan. The calcarine sulcus is seen on ultrasound in the majority of infants by 24–25 weeks and in all infants by 26–27 weeks. The cingulate sulcus is present in the anterior frontal lobe by 18 weeks' gestation on ultrasound but may lag behind as in 25% of infants it is not visible until 24–25 weeks. The callosal sulcus separates the cingulate gyrus from the corpus callosum and appears at 14 weeks' gestation but is not a constant finding on ultrasound until 24 weeks' gestation. The process of cortical folding is also recognizable on postnatal ultrasound[15,27,30] and may be used as a guide to GA. Murphy *et al.*[24] used ultrasound to

study the development of sulci on the lateral and medial surfaces of the brain in preterm infants between 24 weeks and 34 weeks.

Using MRI Martin *et al.*[22] described a four-stage grading system for the structural maturation of the brain surface. In stage 1 there is lissencephaly; in stage 2 the primary gyri are well identified and separated by shallow sulci; in stage 3 the infolding of the brain surface is more pronounced; and in stage 4 the adult pattern with well-developed tertiary gyri and sulci is seen. This system, however, is not detailed enough to be used for assessment of sulcation in a population of premature or extremely premature infants. Systematic study of sulcal and gyral development using MRI has been reported in infants from 30 weeks onwards by Van der Knapp *et al.*[29] and subsequently in infants as immature as 25 weeks' gestation[3]. The gyral development score is a scoring system used to describe cortical folding. A score of 1–5 is given for different areas of the brain depending on the depth, width, the relationship to adjacent sulci, and the complexity of sulcation and gyration. Using this scoring system an increase in cortical folding can be seen in each area which correlates well with increasing age (Fig. 3.2).

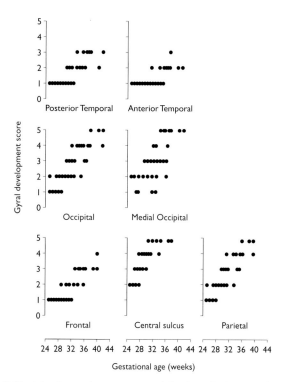

Fig. 3.2 Gyral development score versus gestational age for the posterior part of the temporal lobe, the anterior part of the temporal lobe, the occipital lobe minus the medial area, the medial occipital lobe, the frontal lobe minus the central sulcus, the central sulcus and the parietal lobe minus the central sulcus. The graphs demonstrate the different rates of cortical development in the different brain regions. (Reproduced from Battin *et al.*[3] by permission of *Pediatrics*.)

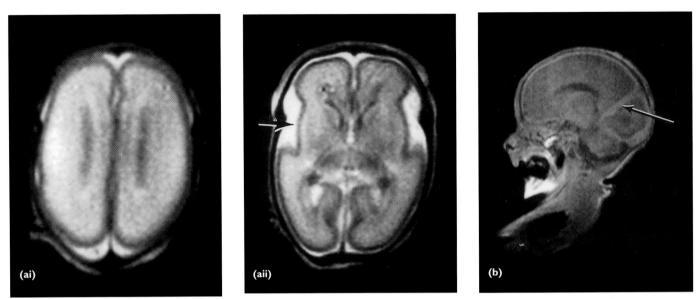

Fig. 3.3 Cortical folding at 25 weeks' gestation. **(a)** T2 weighted fast spin echo sequence (FSE 3000/208) in the transverse plane. **(i)** At the level of the centrum semiovale, the brain surface is smooth. The central sulcus is not seen but at a lower level **(ii)** there is a widely open very rudimentary Sylvian fissure (arrow). **(b)** T1 weighted spin echo (SE 600/20) in the sagittal plane, the parieto-occipital fissure (*arrow*) can be demonstrated.

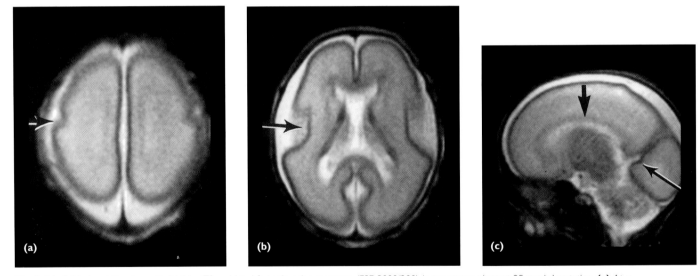

Fig. 3.4 Individual variation in cortical folding. T2 weighted fast spin echo sequence (FSE 3000/208) in transverse plane at 25 weeks' gestation. **(a)** At a supraventricular level, in the transverse plane the brain surface is smooth but the central sulcus is visible, as a rudimentary shallow infolding of the cortex (*arrow*). **(b)** At a mid-ventricular level the Sylvian fissure is widely open (but less than in Fig. 3.3) and the insula cortex exposed (*arrow*). **(c)** The sagittal image shows early development of the calcarine fissure (*long arrow*). The corpus callosum can be seen as low signal intensity (*short black arrow*).

MRI can be performed as early as 23 weeks' gestation and at this stage a rim of cortex is demonstrated as high signal intensity compared to the underlying white matter on T1 and low signal intensity on T2 weighted images. In our cohort of infants there was some variation in cortical maturity in infants born at the same gestation (Figs 3.3 and 3.4). Delays in cortical folding may have important neurodevelopmental consequences or may just reflect normal individual variation.

Visual analysis of cortical folding is sufficient for identifying major abnormalities or discrepancies in maturation (Fig. 3.11). Occasionally, the evolution of abnormal folding can be detected with serial imaging in the very preterm

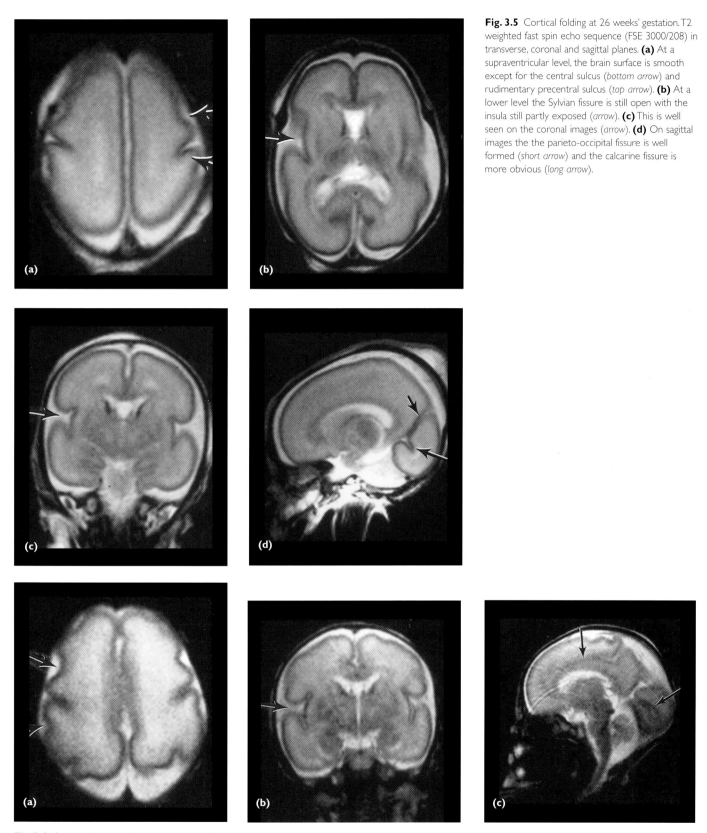

Fig. 3.5 Cortical folding at 26 weeks' gestation. T2 weighted fast spin echo sequence (FSE 3000/208) in transverse, coronal and sagittal planes. **(a)** At a supraventricular level, the brain surface is smooth except for the central sulcus (*bottom arrow*) and rudimentary precentral sulcus (*top arrow*). **(b)** At a lower level the Sylvian fissure is still open with the insula still partly exposed (*arrow*). **(c)** This is well seen on the coronal images (*arrow*). **(d)** On sagittal images the the parieto-occipital fissure is well formed (*short arrow*) and the calcarine fissure is more obvious (*long arrow*).

Fig. 3.6 Cortical folding at 28 weeks' gestation. T2 weighted fast spin echo (FSE 3000/208) sequence in **(a)** transverse, **(b)**, sagittal, and **(c)** coronal planes. **(a)** At a supraventricular level, in the transverse plane the central sulcus has developed further and is now deeper with more closely applied edges and a narrow opening. The precentral sulcus is also more developed but is still shallow and has a wide opening (*long arrow*). There are also signs of postcentral sulcus forming posteriorly to the central sulcus (*arrowhead*). **(b)** On the coronal image the Sylvian fissure is still open but is beginning to close (*arrow*). **(c)** On the sagittal image the calloso-marginal gyrus is just evident and the calcarine sulcus is well developed demonstrating a 'long stem to the Y' (*right arrow*). The cingulate sulcus is well demonstrated but not yet branched (*top arrow*).

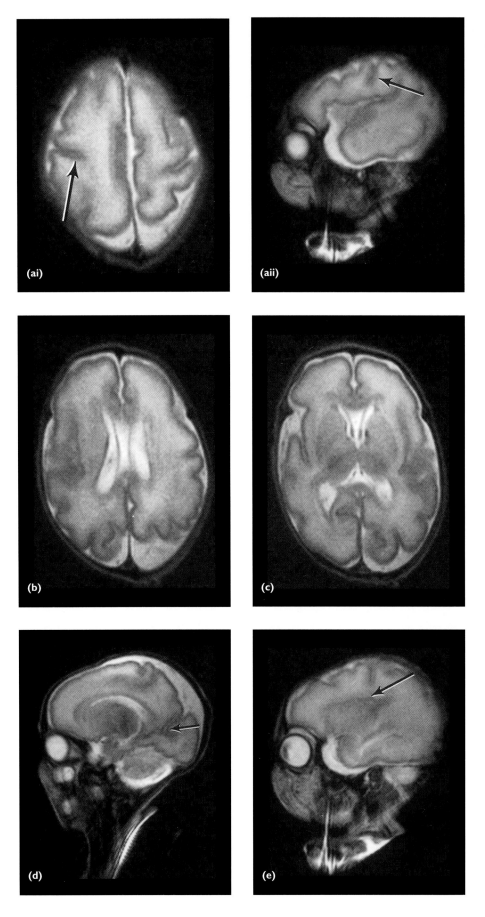

Fig. 3.7 Cortical folding at 30 weeks' gestation. T2 weighted fast spin echo (FSE 3000/208) sequence in transverse and sagittal planes. These images are slightly rotated giving some asymmetry between the appearances demonstrated. **(ai,ii)** Both the pre- and postcentral sulci are obvious and the central sulcus is deep and narrow but unbranched in appearance (*arrow*). **(b)** At a lower level there are numerous shallow sulci forming in the parietal lobes. There is a normal wide posterior extracerebral space. **(c)** Closure of the Sylvian fissure is well advanced. This is also demonstrated on the sagittal image **(aii)**. **(d)** On the sagittal image the parieto-occipital and calcarine sulcus are well developed (*arrow*). The corpus callosum is seen as low signal intensity. **(e)** By 30 weeks the cingulate sulcus has a slightly curvy appearance (*arrow*).

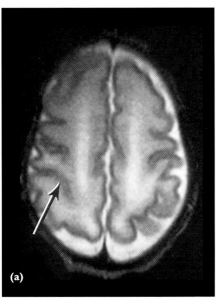

Fig. 3.8 Cortical folding at 32 weeks' gestation. T2 weighted fast spin echo (FSE 3000/208) sequence in transverse, sagittal and coronal planes. **(a)** The central sulcus is becoming more complex (*arrow*). **(bi,ii)** The Sylvian fissure is almost closed (*arrow*). **(c)** The frontal and anterior temporal lobes remain relatively smooth (*arrows*). **(d)** The cingulate sulcus demonstrates secondary branches (*arrow*). The parieto-occipital and calcarine fissures continue to develop and are very well demonstrated (*short arrows*).

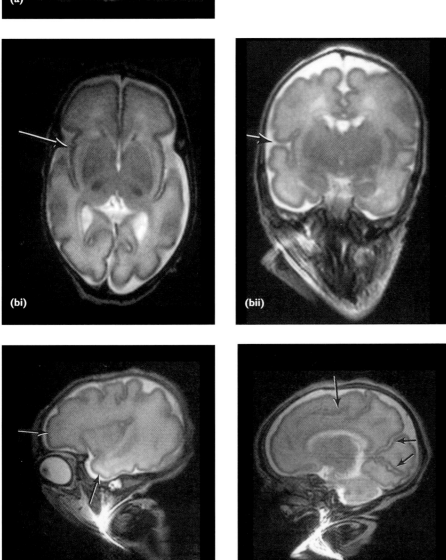

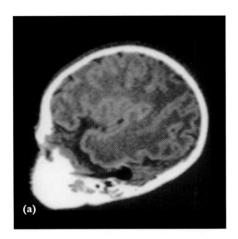

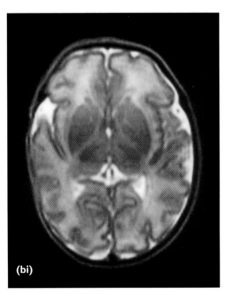

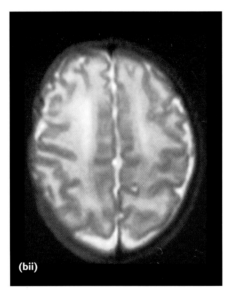

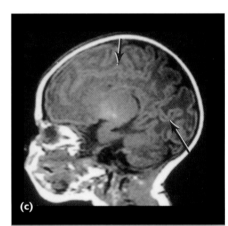

Fig. 3.9 34 weeks' gestation. T2 weighted fast spin echo (FSE 3000/208) sequence in transverse plane **(bi,ii)** and T1 weighted spin echo (SE 600/20) sequence in sagittal plane **(a, c)**. The sulci are complex. The Sylvian fissure is closed **(a, bi)**. The frontal lobes remain less folded **(bi)**. The cingulate sulcus is branched (*short arrow*). The calcarine is complex and branched (*long arrow*) **(c)**.

infant (Fig. 3.12). Visual analysis of images of term-equivalent preterm infants is not sufficient to detect a milder delay or abnormality in cortical folding (Fig. 3.10).

COMPUTERIZED QUANTIFICATION OF CORTICAL FOLDING

In order to study cortical development in more detail we have developed a computerized method for quantifying cortical folding[25]. We use T2 weighted fast spin echo images as these give optimum contrast between the cortex and underlying white matter. The process involves drawing a cortical contour as a template for each slice of the brain. The program then measures the length and curvature of this cortical contour. A curvature code is produced. The program also allows a measure of cortical density to be obtained and the product of this and the curvature code gives a cortical con-

volution index. Using this program we have shown an exponential increase in the whole cortical convolution index (measuring all slices through the brain but excluding the cerebellum) from 24 weeks until term (Fig. 3.13).

It has been suggested that gyral development proceeds in a programmed fashion and that there is little effect of illness on this pattern[23]. However, this has been questioned by Hüppi[16]. At term-equivalent age, preterm infants show less cortical folding than infants born at term (Fig. 3.13)[1,25]. This is not explained by a smaller brain size as the brain volumes between the two groups are not significantly different (Fig. 3.13). These findings imply that the brain of the preterm infant is developing in a different way *ex utero*. The differences in cortical development compared with those infants born at term may be associated with the increase in neurocognitive and neurobehavioral disorders seen in ex-preterm children[7,28].

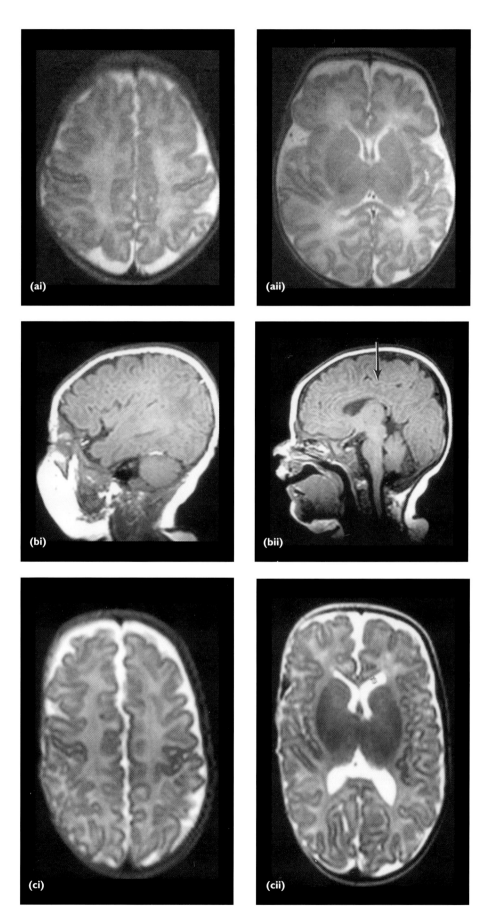

Fig. 3.10 Term gestation. Infant born at term. T2 weighted fast spin echo sequence (FSE 3000/208) in transverse plane. **(ai,ii)** Although the brain shows a pattern approaching that of an adult the numbers of gyri are less and sulci are not as deep as in the adult. The posterior corpus callosum is seen as low signal intensity **(ii)**. **(bi,ii)** T1 weighted spin echo sequence (SE 600/20) in sagittal plane. The cingulate sulcus is easily visible the whole length of the brain on MRI **(ii)** (*arrow*). It has been described as having a cobblestone appearance on ultrasound. The corpus callosum is difficult to differentiate from the surrounding brain. **(ci,ii)** T2 weighted images (FSE 3000/208) sequence. Infant born at 27 weeks and imaged at term-equivalent age. Although the shape of the brain is highly suggestive that this infant was born preterm there is no obvious difference in the cortical folding. The shape also gives the impression on a single image that there is less white matter then the term-born infant.

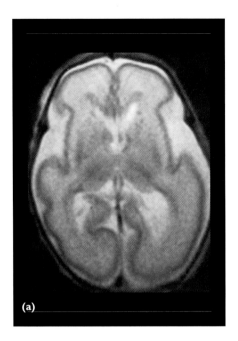

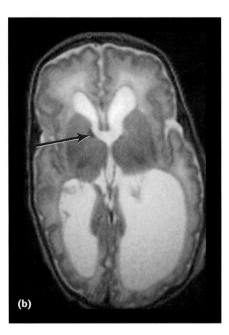

Fig. 3.11 Delayed cortical folding. T2 weighted images (FSE 3000/208). Infant born, one of twins, at 27 weeks' gestation. **(a)** The initial image on day 2 shows appropriate cortical folding. **(b)** Infant imaged at term. The image is markedly abnormal. There is a small area of low signal intensity corresponding to a previous germinal matrix/subependymal hemorrhage (*arrow*). This infant developed severe ventricular dilation secondary to a large intraventricular hemorrhage. The cortical development is inappropriate for term with very shallow sulci. In infants with ventricular dilatation the cortex appears to unfold as a result of increased intraventricular pressure (Fig. 3.13).

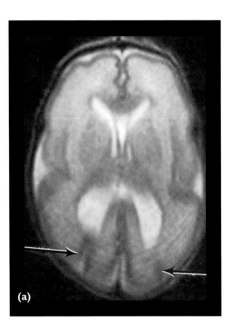

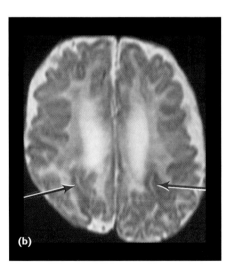

Fig. 3.12 Abnormal cortical folding. T2 weighted images (FSE 3000/208). sequence. Surviving twin born at 27 weeks' gestation. **(a)** Imaged at 4 weeks of age. There are bilateral abnormal cortical folds posteriorly, the right-sided fold extending up to the ventricular wall (*arrows*). This image is slightly artifacted. **(b)** Imaged at 6 months of age (uncorrected). There has been generalized maturation of cortical folding but there are bilateral abnormal sulci in the posterior temporal lobes (*arrows*).

Ventricular system and extracerebral space

Very preterm infants <26 weeks' gestation may have a transient mild dilation of the posterior horns of the lateral ventricles, a developmental colpocephaly (Fig. 3.16). The ventricles are smooth in outline but may show some asymmetry. In most cases the left ventricle is larger than the right. The reason for this asymmetry is unclear but has also been noted on fetal MRI[12] and on ultrasound. On repeat scan at term-equivalent age the asymmetry may persist or no longer be apparent. In the very preterm infant there is a marked widening of the posterior parietal extracerebral space (Figs 3.5–3.8). This may persist until approximately 36 weeks; it is minimally widened in Fig. 3.9 at 34 weeks, but is only occasionally seen at term-equivalent age. The space has been termed benign external hydrocephalus[13] but probably represents a normal development process. This posterior widening gradually disappears and is not usually apparent at term-equivalent age.

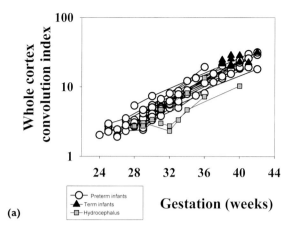

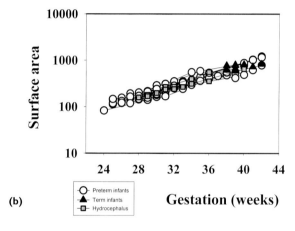

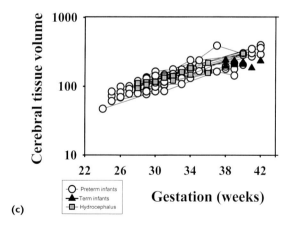

Fig. 3.13 Cortical development from 24 weeks' gestation until term-equivalent age. **(a)** Cortical folding measured as a whole cortex convolution index (WCCI). **(b)** Cortical surface area. **(c)** Brain volume (without ventricles). (Courtesy of Dr Ajayi Obe, Hammersmith Hospital.)

At term-equivalent age there may be an increase in the anterior extracerebral space with widening of the anterior interhemispheric fissure (Fig. 3.26)[20]. This is often attributed to atrophy of the brain but it may not be secondary to a

reduction in brain size (Fig. 3.13) and tends not to persist beyond 1 year of age.

Germinal matrix

The germinal matrix or subependymal layer is situated at the surface of the lateral ventricles. It consists of a loose stroma and is highly vascularized with irregular endothelial lined vessels. From 10 to 20 weeks' gestation it is responsible for neuroblast and glioblast production and thereafter glioblast production alone, from the subventricular zone. The matrix includes the transient ventricular zone and the subventricular zone and increases in volume from 13 weeks' gestation to a maximum at about 26 weeks' gestation. It then regresses although it persists for longer in the caudothalamic notch and in the roof of the temporal horn. On cranial ultrasound the term 'germinal matrix' is usually applied to the tissue seen in the caudothalamic notch. On MRI the germinal matrix may be visualized as a prominent structure at the lateral margin of the lateral ventricles, overlying the caudate (Fig. 3.14) and at the roof of the temporal horns of the lateral ventricles. The subependymal layer also appears to extend as a much thinner layer all around the ventricles. It is characterized by a high signal intensity on T1 weighted images and more obviously as a low signal intensity on T2 weighted images (Fig. 3.14)[20].

The germinal matrix can be identified by virtue of its shape and location adjacent to the lateral ventricles as well as its signal characteristics. This appearance of high signal on T1 weighted and low signal on T2 weighted images in the germinal matrix is also described on fetal imaging[12] and persists until between 30 and 32 weeks' gestation, continuing for longer on the T2 weighted images (Fig. 3.15).

Germinal matrix is easier to identify on MRI than on ultrasound. Using MRI it is possible to identify thicker rests of germinal tissue, over the caudate heads and at the roof of the temporal horn of the lateral ventricles. It is also possible to detect the thinner cellular layer that lines the entire ventricular system. On ultrasound the germinal matrix is only really identified over the caudate heads. This is partly because cranial ultrasound is not routinely used in the transverse plane and therefore matrix in the temporal horns cannot be detected. In addition, the subependymal layer elsewhere around the ventricles may to be too thin for detection by ultrasound.

Germinal matrix hemorrhage has similar characteristics to germinal matrix with a short T1 and T2 but is distinguished from normal matrix by its irregular shape, asymmetry and persistence of susceptibility effect (Fig. 3.16) (see Chapter 9). Preterm infants may show small lesions consistent with

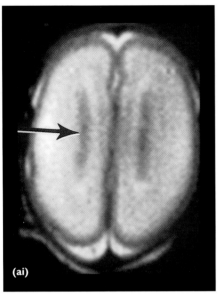 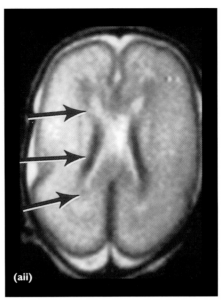 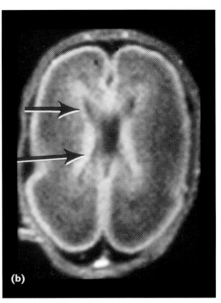

Fig. 3.14 Germinal matrix/subependymal layer at 25 weeks. **(a)** T2 weighted fast spin echo sequence (FSE 3000/208) at **(i)** a supraventricular level, and **(ii)** a high ventricular level. The germinal matrix is seen as low signal intensity and lines most of the lateral ventricular wall overlying the caudate nucleus (*middle arrow*). A thinner band of low signal intensity seen around the remaining areas of ventricle consistent with densely cellular area of subependymal tissue (*top and bottom arrows*) **(a ii)**, which is responsible for glial cell migration. **(b)** T1 weighted sequence (SE 600/20) in the transverse plane, high ventricular level. The germinal matrix is seen as high signal intensity on T1 weighted images (*arrow*). The subependymal layer elsewhere is seen as a thinner band of high signal intensity (*short arrow*).

hemorrhage within the subependymal layer with or without evidence of hemorrhage in more classical sites of matrix over the caudate nuclei (Fig. 3.17). In addition, infants with multiple hemorrhagic lesions may appear to have white matter lesions but in fact the lesions are in the subependymal layer and partial volume effects give the appearance of white matter lesions, particularly superiorly (Fig. 3.17).

White matter

The high water content of the premature infant brain produces relatively long T1 and T2 times and gives rise to a low signal on T1 weighted images in the white matter. As previously mentioned, provisional data suggest that these values gradually decrease between 24 weeks and term. Term-born infants demonstrate a steady decrease in the brain water content throughout the first 2 years of life.

Within the white matter of the centrum semiovale (CSO) and periventricular area, several well-defined layers of alternating signal intensity are observed in the brain of preterm infants. At 24 and 25 weeks' gestation four layers can be identified in the CSO. These represent the cortex, subcortical white matter, an intermediate zone representing migrating cells and a periventricular zone representing developing white matter. This periventricular zone lies adjacent to the subependymal layer or germinal matrix (Fig. 3.18).

At a low ventricular level the bands are incomplete but areas are observed around the anterior horns of the lateral ventricles that form the shape of a 'cap' (Figs. 3.19 and 3.23) and around the posterior horns of the lateral ventricles forming the shape of an 'arrowhead'. These 'caps' and 'arrowheads' are in continuity with the multilayered periventricular appearance described above. Caps have an additional area of low signal intensity on T2 weighted images (high signal intensity on T1 weighted images) (Figs 3.19 and 3.23).

Arrowheads differ from the caps by their posterior site and characteristic shape. They also do not have alternating layers of long and short T2 within them. Infants born at ≤27 weeks' gestation may not demonstrate high signal intensity within bands, caps and arrowheads when first imaged but this develops on follow-up imaging with increasing GA[20]. Histologically, these sites correspond to regions with dense white matter fibers converging from different regions of the brain.

In posterior white matter it is possible to see the developing optic radiation with a cellular layer either side (Fig. 3.19). In summary, layers of high and low signal intensity are found within the unmyelinated white matter of the CSO and periventricular regions. These may be described as 'bands' in the CSO and periventricular white matter, 'caps' around the anterior horns of the lateral ventricles and 'arrowheads' around the posterior horns of the lateral ventricles.

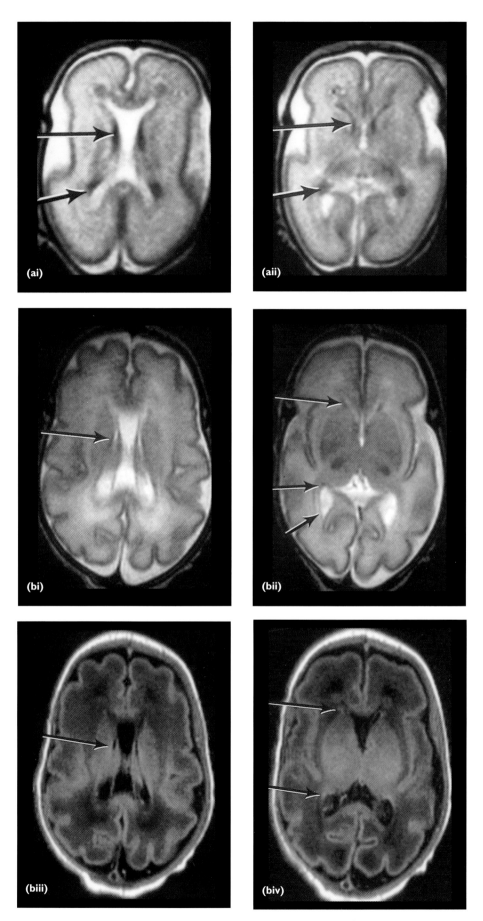

Fig. 3.15 Involution of the germinal matrix. T2 weighted fast spin echo (FSE 3000/208) and T1 weighted spin echo sequence (TE 600/20). **(a)** Mid-ventricular level **(i)** and low ventricular level **(ii)**. At 25 weeks' gestation germinal matrix is visible as low signal intensity in the anterior horns continuing posteriorly over the caudate heads (*long arrow*). It is also seen in the roof of the temporal horns (*short arrow*). **(b)** T2 weighted fast spin echo sequence (FSE 3000/208) **(i,ii)** and T1 weighted spin echo sequence (SE 600/20) **(iii,iv)**. At 31 weeks the germinal matrix has involuted and is barely visible on T1 weighted images (*arrows*) but is more obvious on the T2 weighted images **(bi)** (*arrow*) **(bii)** (*top and middle arrows*). There is a persistent low signal lining the ventricles **(bii)** (*bottom arrow*) consistent with the densely cellular subependymal layer.

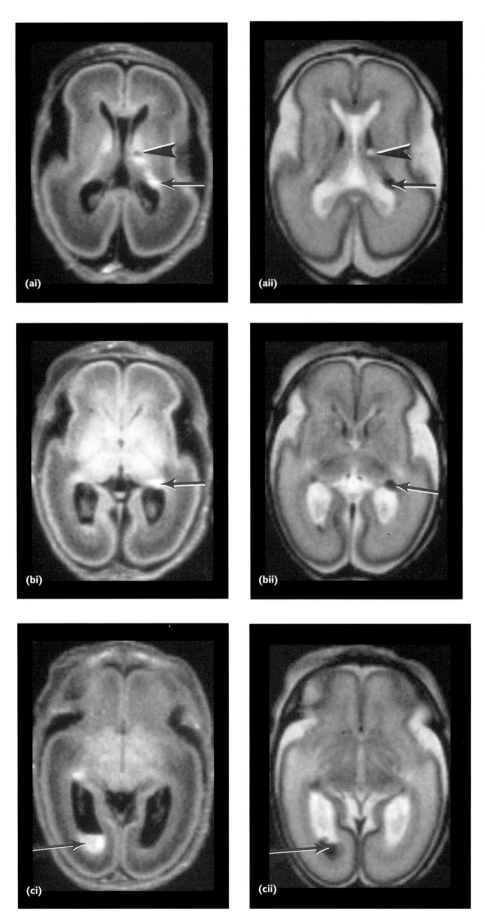

Fig. 3.16 Germinal matrix hemorrhage. Preterm infant born at 25 weeks imaged at 2 days. **(i)** T1 weighted spin echo sequence (SE 600/20), and **(ii)** T2 weighted fast spin echo (FSE 3000/208) sequence. Imaged at a mid-ventricular level **(a)**, low ventricular level **(b)**, and through the occipital horns **(c)**. Subependymal germinal matrix hemorrhage is seen as areas of asymmetrical irregular signal intensity within the germinal matrix, high on T1 weighted images and low on the T2 weighted images (*short arrows*). There is a small cystic lesion on the left (*arrowhead*). There is additional hemorrhage within the ventricles (*long arrows*). The ventricles are slightly dilated at this level although this may just be secondary to the normal colpocephaly at this gestation.

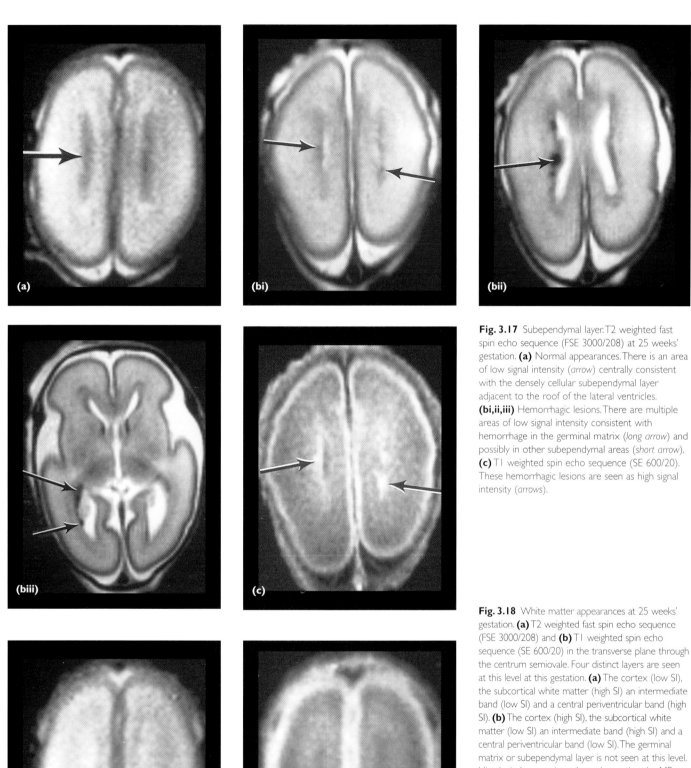

Fig. 3.17 Subependymal layer. T2 weighted fast spin echo sequence (FSE 3000/208) at 25 weeks' gestation. **(a)** Normal appearances. There is an area of low signal intensity (*arrow*) centrally consistent with the densely cellular subependymal layer adjacent to the roof of the lateral ventricles. **(bi,ii,iii)** Hemorrhagic lesions. There are multiple areas of low signal intensity consistent with hemorrhage in the germinal matrix (*long arrow*) and possibly in other subependymal areas (*short arrow*). **(c)** T1 weighted spin echo sequence (SE 600/20). These hemorrhagic lesions are seen as high signal intensity (*arrows*).

Fig. 3.18 White matter appearances at 25 weeks' gestation. **(a)** T2 weighted fast spin echo sequence (FSE 3000/208) and **(b)** T1 weighted spin echo sequence (SE 600/20) in the transverse plane through the centrum semiovale. Four distinct layers are seen at this level at this gestation. **(a)** The cortex (low SI), the subcortical white matter (high SI) an intermediate band (low SI) and a central periventricular band (high SI). **(b)** The cortex (high SI), the subcortical white matter (low SI) an intermediate band (high SI) and a central periventricular band (low SI). The germinal matrix or subependymal layer is not seen at this level. Histological comparisons have shown that the MR appearances of these white matter bands relate to the relative density of cells within them[10]. The intermediate band is densely cellular consisting of cells that are migrating outwards to the cortex. This corresponds to the known migration of glial cells at this gestation. Neuronal migration is thought to be complete by 20 weeks' gestation. These migrating glial cells have also been demonstrated histologically[10]. The periventricular layer is fiber rich and represents developing white matter.

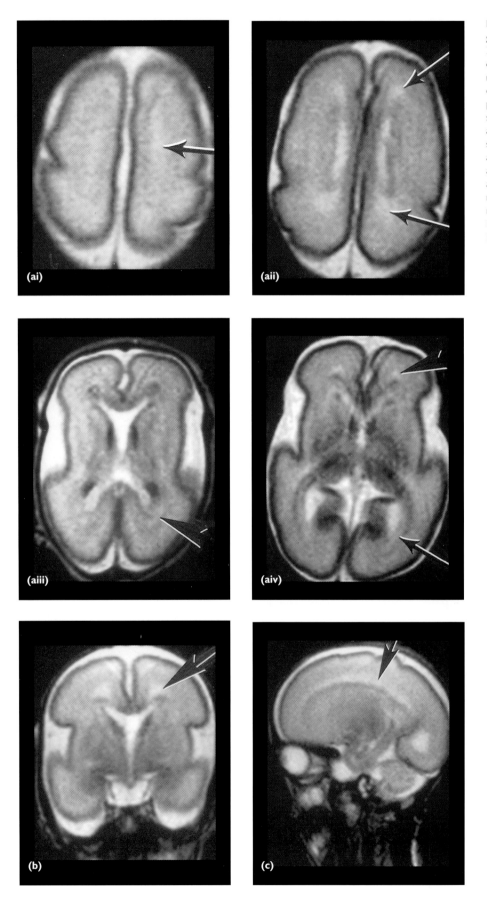

Fig. 3.19 White matter appearance at 27 weeks' gestation. T2 weighted fast spin echo sequence (FSE 3000/208). **(a)** Transverse images at level of **(i)** centrum semiovale, **(ii)** high ventricular level, **(iii)** mid-ventricular level, **(iv)** low ventricular level; **(b)** coronal plane through the basal ganglia; **(c)** parasagittal plane. The developing white matter is seen as a high signal intensity region (*arrows*) adjacent to the low signal intensity germinal or subependymal layer. This takes the form of arrowheads posteriorly (*arrowhead*) **(a iii)** and caps anteriorly (*arrowhead*) **(a iv)**. The more lateral adjacent low signal intensity representing a layer of migrating cells is less obvious. The developing optic radiation can be seen as a thin layer of high signal intensity between the subependymal layer and the lateral layer of migrating cells (*arrow*) **(a iv)**.

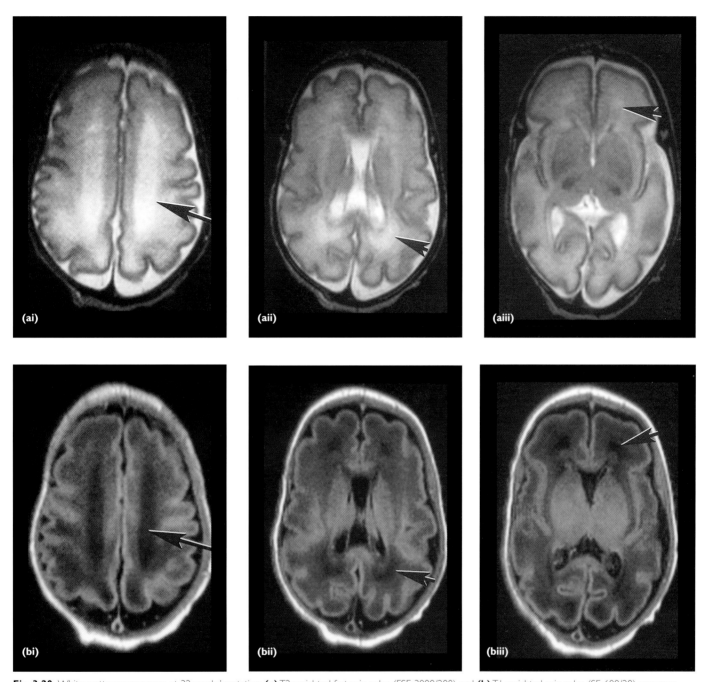

Fig. 3.20 White matter appearances at 32 weeks' gestation. **(a)** T2 weighted fast spin echo (FSE 3000/208) and **(b)** T1 weighted spin echo (SE 600/20) sequence. Transverse plane at high **(i)** mid **(ii)** and low **(iii)** ventricular level. The periventricular layer of developing white matter is wider and more obvious than at 27 weeks' gestation (*arrows*) **(ai, bi)**. It is clearly seen anteriorly forming part of the 'cap' (*arrowhead*) **(aiii, biii)** and posteriorly to from the 'arrowheads' (*arrowhead*) **(aii, bii)**.

The MRI appearances described are thought to be part of the normal developmental features of the white matter since, as we have seen them on first MRI in over 95% of infants born at less than 30 weeks' gestation respectively[3]. The periventricular bands were also demonstrated in another imaging study of preterm infants[6]. In Maalouf *et al*'s study loss of bands, caps or arrowheads was associated with cerebral pathology such as large hemorrhagic infarction and posthemorrhagic hydrocephalus[20]. The bands, caps and arrowhead appearances do become less obvious with increasing GA. Child *et al.*[6] have described multiple bands consistent with 'waves' of migrating cells in the white matter. Whilst we see distinct layers of altering signal intensity within the cerebral hemispheres we have not

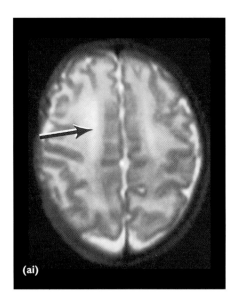
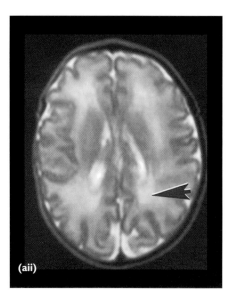
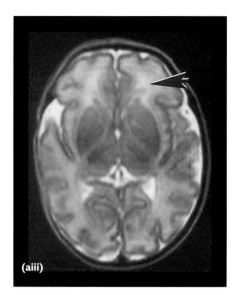

Fig. 3.21 White matter appearances at 34 weeks' gestation. T2 weighted fast spin echo (FSE 3000/208) sequence in the transverse plane through **(i)** the centrum semiovale **(ii)** mid and **(iii)** low ventricular level. The periventricular high signal intensity is less discrete although it can still be distinguished as a layer (*arrow*) **(i)** with posterior arrowheads (*arrowhead*) **(ii)** and anterior caps (*arrowhead*) **(iii)**.

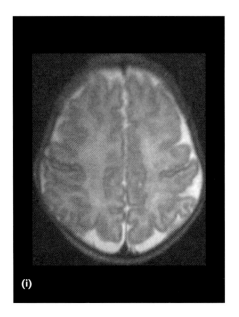
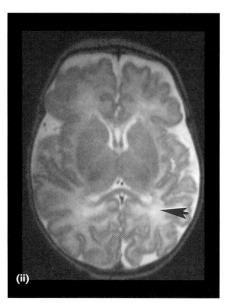

Fig. 3.22 White matter appearances at term-equivalent age. T2 weighted fast spin echo sequence (FSE 3000/208) **(i)** level of the centrum semiovale. There is no periventricular layer of high signal intensity and **(ii)** low ventricular level. There is only minimal high signal intensity in the region of the posterior (*arrowhead*) and anterior periventricular white matter.

identified multiple bands of short T1, short T2 consistent with different bands or waves of cells with MRI or on histology. This may be due to inadequate image definition but it is possible that the effect of multiple bands of cells may sometimes be produced by either motion artifact and or partial volume effects.

We have noted that in some infants approaching term the white matter demonstrates a long T1, long T2 component, the so-called diffuse excessive high signal intensity (DEHSI)

on T2 weighted images[20] (Fig. 3.24). This is probably normal if restricted to the arrowheads and caps but in some infants is more diffuse and extends beyond these areas towards the subcortical white matter. Preliminary studies have shown that DEHSI is associated with the development of abnormal long T2, consistent with glial tissue, in the periventricular white matter at 2 years of age (Fig. 3.25). These later changes could be described as a mild form of periventricular leukomalacia but whilst they may be

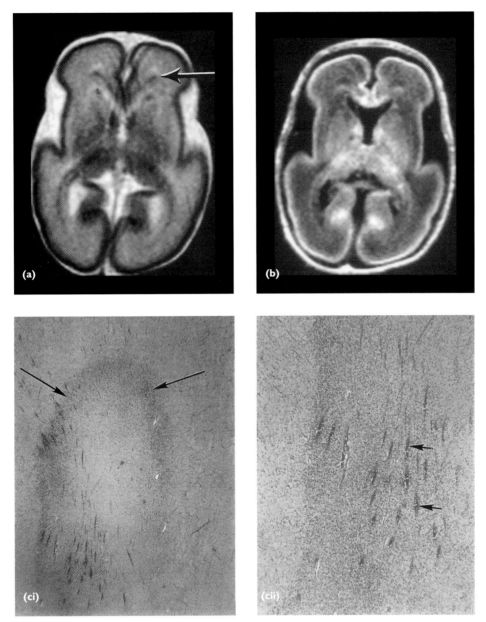

Fig. 3.23 Anterior caps at 27 weeks' gestation. **(a)** T2 weighted fast spin echo (FSE 3000/208). The anterior cap is seen as a medial low and peripheral high signal intensity and **(b)** T1 weighted spin echo (600/20) sequence. The anterior cap has a medial high and a peripheral low signal intensity (*arrow*). **(c)** Histological appearances at **(i)** × 50 magnification. There is a dense band of cells, which appear to be migrating out from the germinal matrix or subependymal layer in the anterior horn (*arrows*). The medial part of the cap corresponds to this relatively cell-rich area. **(ii)** × 250 magnification. The migration is clustered in lines or 'fountains' along small blood vessels (*short arrows*). (Courtesy of Dr W Squier, The Radcliffe Infirmary, Oxford.)

associated with ventricular dilation the ventricular outline is usually normal. The corpus callosum may be thin. These periventricular and corpus callosal changes are a common finding when ex-preterm children and adolescents are imaged[7] but the exact relationship to later neurodevelopmental and neurocognitive deficits remains unclear. It is possible that these relatively focal changes are the visible side of a process that may have effected a much larger amount of developing brain, so-called perinatal teloleukoencephalopathy[21].

In some ex-preterm infants there is ventricular dilation and widening of the extracerebral space at term, findings that suggest cerebral atrophy[20]. However, these findings may not be apparent at later follow-up imaging although children born preterm have smaller heads than term-born controls[7]. Serial measurements of brain and ventricular volume may help clarify this relationship, although in our initial studies there is no difference between the brain volume of ex-preterm infants at term-equivalent age and term-born controls (Fig. 3.13).

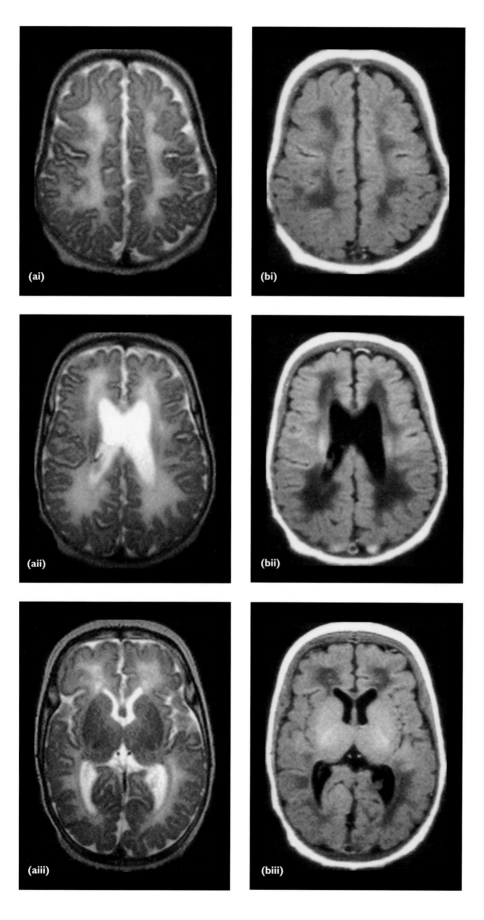

Fig. 3.24 Diffuse excessive high signal intensity. Preterm infant born at 27 weeks' gestation and imaged at term-equivalent age. **(a)** T2 weighted fast spin echo sequence (FSE 3000/208) and **(b)** T1 weighted spin echo sequence (SE 600/20) at the level of the **(i)** centrum semiovale, **(ii)** high ventricular and **(iii)** low ventricular level. The white matter has areas of excessive high signal intensity on the T2 weighted images and excessive low signal intensity on T1 weighted images. This infant subsequently died. No postmortem was performed.

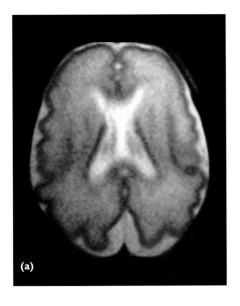
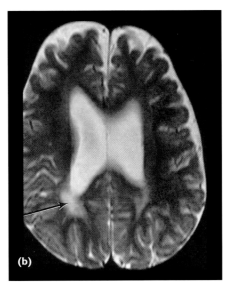

Fig. 3.25 Periventricular white matter abnormalities. **(a)** Neonatal imaging. T2 weighted fast spin echo sequence (FSE 3000/208). At 27 weeks' gestation the posterior periventricular white matter is unremarkable but it is not possible to see the normal arrowhead on the right. **(b)** Follow-up imaging at 2 years of age. Conventional T2 weighted sequence (SE 2700/120). There is some widening of the extracerebral space and moderate dilatation of the ventricles. There is excessive increased signal intensity in the posterior periventricular white matter. It is more marked on the right (*arrow*). This is more dense and more extensive than is seen in normal control infants at this age.

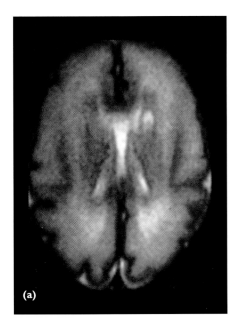
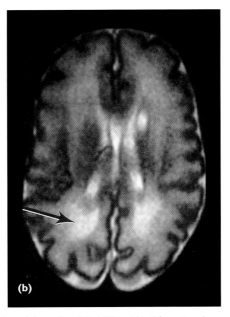
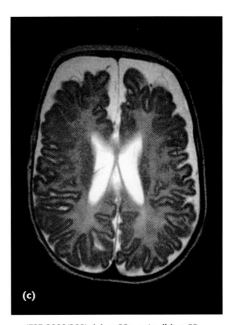

Fig. 3.26 Sequential imaging of the white matter in a 26 weeks' gestation infant. T2 weighted fast spin echo sequence (FSE 3000/208) **(a)** at 29 weeks; **(b)** at 32 weeks; **(c)** and at 6 months uncorrected. There is some high signal intensity within the white matter. This may be slightly excessive in the region of the posterior horns (*arrow*) at 32 weeks but is normal anteriorly **(b)**. At term this infant has markedly widened extracerebral space and anterior interhemispheric fissure. The ventricles were also dilated. The relationship between signal intensity changes in the white matter, ventricular dilatation and widening of the extracerebral space remains unclear.

Myelination

Myelination of white matter enables the more effective transmission of neural impulses. It can be demonstrated histologically to occur in a systematic fashion beginning with the medial longitudinal fasciculus at the end of the first trimester. It is, however, predominantly a post-term process and continues at least until the end of the second year. On MRI, myelination is associated with a shortening of T1 and

T2 and is seen as high signal intensity on T1 weighted sequences and low signal intensity on T2 weighted sequences. In term-born infants, early changes of myelination are best seen on T1 weighted images, particularly on inversion recovery images, in the first 6 months of life and thereafter on T2 weighted images[26]. However, in our experience of imaging preterm infants, evidence of myelination is observed more easily on fast T2 weighted spin echo rather than on T1 weighted scans perhaps due to the better contrast achieved with this sequence. Myelination appears in

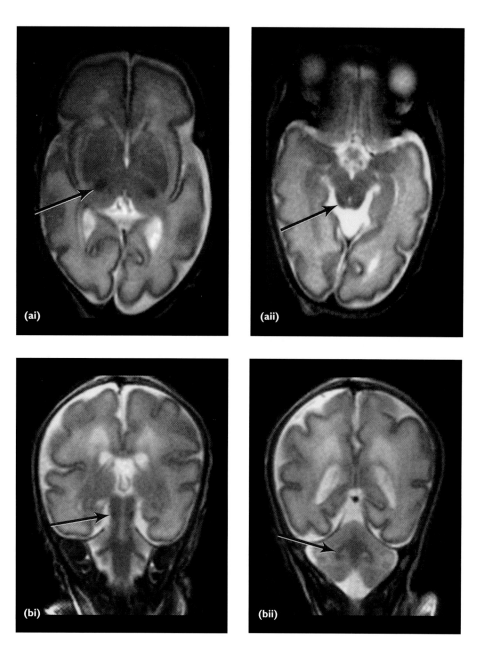

Fig. 3.27 Myelination. Infant imaged at 31 weeks' gestation. T2 weighted fast spin echo sequence (FSE 3000/208). **(a)** Transverse plane **(i)** low-ventricular level. Low signal intensity corresponding to myelination with the region of the ventro-lateral thalamic nuclei is seen (*arrow*). **(ii)** Level of the mesencephalon. Low signal intensity corresponding to myelination within the inferior colliculi and the lateral lemnisci (*arrow*). **(b)** Coronal plane. **(i)** Low signal intensity consistent with myelin in the colliculi (*arrow*). **(ii)** There is low signal intensity within the dentate nuclei of the cerebellum (*arrow*).

the inferior cerebellar peduncles as early as 25 weeks and is followed by the inferior colliculi, posterior brain stem and ventro-lateral nuclei of thalamus. In our cohort we have demonstrated myelin in all these areas in infants using a fast spin echo T2 weighted sequence on first scan (Fig. 3.27).

Between 28 and 35 weeks we have found no evidence for new myelination on MRI[8,17]. Chi *et al.*[5] also report that there is relatively little new myelination between 29 and 40 weeks' gestation and this is also our experience[8]. Using MRI myelination becomes evident in the posterior limb of internal capsule (PLIC) and in the corona radiata by 35 weeks. Histological studies demonstrate the onset of myelination in the PLIC to occur between 32 and 36 weeks' gestation. The preterm infant appears to show myelination within the internal capsule at an earlier post-menstrual age than more mature infants (Fig. 3.28).

The myelin sheath has a high lipid content, which is arranged in alternating layers with protein. The T1 shortening that is observed with the process of myelination probably occurs due to the hydrophilic cholesterol and glycolipid components of the developing myelin sheath[26]. T2 shortening is reported to occur at the time of tightening of myelin around the axon[2] and may correlate best with the development of myelination determined on histological methods.

Myelination is usually only visible in the corpus callosum from 3 months of age. It is difficult to visualize the unmyelin-

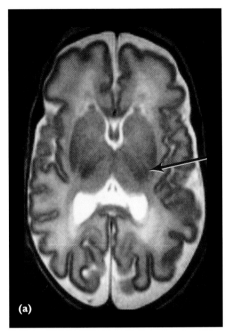 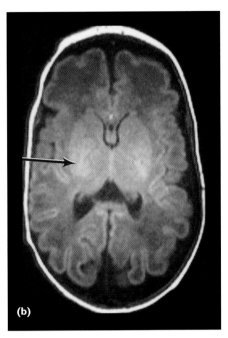 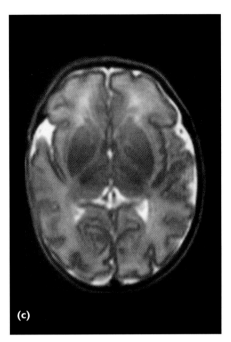

Fig. 3.28 Myelination in the posterior limb of the internal capsule. **(a)** T2 weighted fast spin echo sequence (FSE 3000/208) and **(b)** T1 weighted spin echo (SE 600/20). Preterm infant born at 30 weeks and imaged at 35 weeks. There is obvious myelin within the posterior limb of the internal capsule (*arrow*). This is not usually evident until 37 weeks in infants born at a later gestation. **(c)** T2 weighted fast spin echo sequence (FSE 3000/208). Infant born at 34 weeks and imaged at 35 weeks. There is no evidence of myelin within the posterior limb of the internal capsule.

ated corpus callosum in the transverse plane in term infants prior to myelination (Fig. 3.10). However, the corpus callosum is clearly visualized on heavily T2 weighted imaging as low signal intensity, prior to myelination (Figs 3.4, 3.6 and 3.10). The reasons for this are unclear, but it may be secondary to tightly packed fibers reducing the water content of the structure and thereby decreasing its T2.

Basal ganglia and thalami

The basal ganglia and thalami in very preterm infants are characterized by a short T1 and are uniformly high signal intensity on T1 weighted images. On T2 weighted images the thalami are diffusely low signal intensity but the lentiform nucleus may have a more heterogeneous appearance. The ventro-lateral nuclei of the thalamus is clearly identifiable at 25 weeks' gestation showing as a low signal area on T2 weighted images. This appearance is likely to be due to the increased cellular density of the nuclei and the presence of myelin which can be demonstrated histologically at this age. It is less obviously high signal intensity on T1 weighted images (Fig. 3.29). From 24 weeks until term the basal ganglia and thalami become more isointense on both T1 and T2 weighted images. By 35 weeks' gestation there is only focal high signal intensity on T1 weighted images within the ventro-lateral nuclei and secondary to early myelination in the posterior part of the posterior limb of the internal capsule.

There is additional more diffuse residual high signal intensity in the globus and posterior part of the putamen, inferiorly (see Chapters 4 and 6). On T2 weighted images there is low signal intensity in the ventro-lateral nuclei, which are very clearly seen. There is additional low signal intensity along the lateral border of the lentiform nuclei and in the posterior part of the posterior limb of the internal capsule (Fig. 3.29).

The future

MRI is still a relatively new technique for imaging the very preterm infant. Any new developments in imaging the preterm infant have to be safe and quick as time is of the essence. Fast diffusion weighted imaging may increase our understanding on the formation of white matter tracts in health and disease[18]. Quantification of the brain and its structures will allow us to accurately compare the development of the brain with the development of the child[17]. This may produce more accurate neuroimaging correlates for later neurocognitive disorders. Spectroscopy is providing new insights into metabolic processes in response to injury (Chapter 16). Functional imaging is limited in the newborn but may also throw light on the mechanisms involved in normal and abnormal neurological functioning (Chapter 18). The interpretation of images is greatly aided by accurate histological comparisons although it is becoming increasingly difficult to obtain consent for postmortem with retention of the brain.

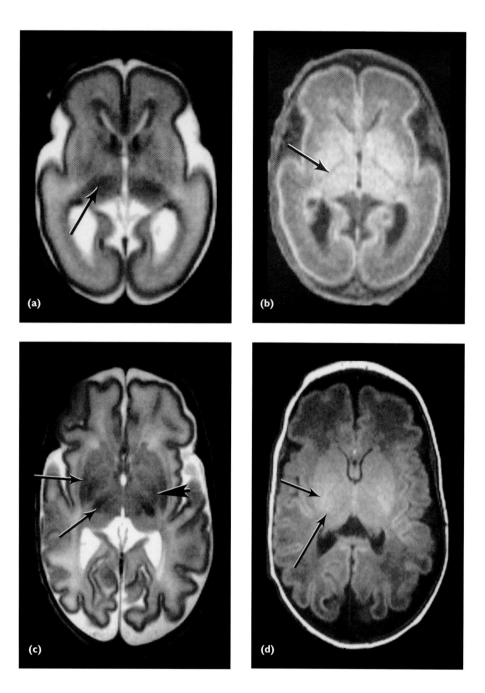

Fig. 3.29 Evolution of the appearances of the basal ganglia and thalami at 25 weeks' gestation. **(a)** T2 weighted fast spin echo sequence (FSE 3000/208). There is diffuse slightly low signal in the thalami with a focal area or lower signal intensity laterally corresponding to the ventro-lateral nuclei (*arrow*). The lentiform nucleus is rather heterogeneous. **(b)** T1 weighted spin echo (SE 600/20). There is diffuse high signal throughout the lentiform nucleus and thalami. It is not possible to see myelin within the ventro-lateral nuclei. The posterior limb is very clearly seen as low signal intensity (*arrow*). 35 weeks' gestation **(c)** T2 weighted fast spin echo sequence (FSE 3000/208). There is very obvious low signal intensity in the ventro-lateral nuclei of the thalami (*bottom arrow*). There is some low signal intensity along the lateral edge of the lentiform nucleus (*top arrow*). On this image there is some low signal intensity along the lateral border of the globus pallidus (*arrowhead*) **(d)** T1 weighted spin echo (SE 600/20). There is less high signal within the lentiform nuclei and thalami. There is a small, slightly indistinct, high signal intensity in the posterior part of the posterior limb of the internal capsule (*short arrow*). The rest of the limb still has a slightly low signal intensity. There is diffuse area of high signal intensity in the region of the ventrolateral nucleus (*long arrow*). This is not seen as clearly as on the T2 weighted imaging. The appearances are asymmetrical on this image. Assessment of any structure should always include the images above and below to avoid asymmetry from rotation being attributed to pathology.

Summary

- Cell-rich regions such as the cortex and subependymal layer or germinal matrix have a short T1 and short T2.

- Sulcation and gyration of the cortex increases in a predictable way.

- Cortical folding can be quantified and appears to be reduced in preterm infants at term-equivalent age.

- MRI can detect bands of migrating glial cells.

- Germinal matrix involution can be documented.

- White matter structures of caps and bands and arrowheads correspond to normal developmental processes within the white matter of the immature brain.

- Diffusion weighted imaging and magnetic resonance spectroscopy should help to further characterize the developing white and gray matter.

References

1. Ajayi-Obe M, Saeed N, Cowan FM *et al.* (2000) Reduced development of cerebral cortex in extremely preterm infants. *Lancet* **356**, 1162–1163.

2. Barkovich AJ, Gressens P and Evrard P (1992) Formation, maturation and disorders of the brain neocortex. *Am J Radiol* **13**, 447–461.

3. Battin MR, Maalouf EF, Counsell SJ *et al.* (1998) Magnetic resonance imaging of the brain in preterm infants: visualization of the germinal matrix, early myelination and cortical folding. *Pediatrics* **101**, 957–962.

4. Blakemore C (1995) Introduction: mysteries in the making of the cerebral cortex. In: *Development of the Cerebral Cortex. Ciba Foundation Symposium* **193**, London, Wiley.

5. Chi Je G, Dooling EC and Gilles FH (1977) Gyral development of the human brain. *Ann Neurol* **1**, 86–93.

6. Childs AM, Ramenghi LA, Evans DJ *et al.* (1998) MR features of developing periventricular white matter in preterm infants: evidence of glial cell migration. *Am J Neuroradiol* **19**, 971–976.

7. Cooke RW and Abernethy LJ (1999) Cranial magnetic resonance imaging and school performance in very low birth weight infants in adolescence. *Arch Dis Child Fetal Neonatal Ed* **81**, F116–121.

8. Counsell SJ, Maalouf EF, Rutherford MA *et al.* (1998) Assessment of myelination in white matter and central grey matter structures in the preterm using a novel neonatal MRI scanner. *ISMRM*, Abstract 91.

9. Counsell SJ, Kennea NL, Herlihy AH *et al.* (2001) T2 relaxation values in the developing preterm brain. *ISMRM*, Abstract 410.

10. Feess-Higgins A and Larroche JC (1987) *Development of the Human Fetal Brain*. Paris, INSERM.

11. Felderhoff-Mueser U, Rutherford M, Squier W *et al.* (1999) Relation between magnetic resonance images and histopathological findings of the brain in extremely sick preterm infants. *Am J Neuroradiol* **20**, 1349–1357.

12. Girard N, Raybaud C and Poncet M (1995) *In vivo* MR study of brain maturation in normal fetuses. *Am J Neuroradiol* **16**, 407–413.

13. Girard N and Raybaud C (2000) Can benign external hydrocephalus be recognised *in utero*? *Child Nervous System* **16**, 70.

14. Hall AS, Young IR, Davies FJ *et al.* (1997) A dedicated magnetic resonance system in a neonatal intensive therapy unit. In: Bradley, WG and Bydder GM (Eds) *Advanced MR Imaging Techniques*. London, Martin Dunitz, pp. 281–289.

15. Huang C-C (1991) Sonographic cerebral sulcal development in premature newborns. *Brain Dev* **13**, 27–31.

16. Hüppi PS, Schuknecht B, Boesch C *et al.* (1996) Structural and neurobehavioral delay in postnatal brain development of preterm infants. *Pediatr Res* **39**, 895–901.

17. Hüppi PS, Warfield S, Kikinis R *et al.* (1998a) Quantitative magnetic resonance imaging of brain development in premature and mature newborns. *Ann Neurol* **43**, 224–235.

18. Hüppi PS, Maier SE, Peled S *et al.* (1998b) Microstructural development of human newborn cerebral white matter assessed *in vivo* by diffusion tensor magnetic resonance imaging. *Pediatr Res* **44**, 584–590.

19. Johnson MA, Pennock JM, Bydder GM *et al.* (1983) Clinical NMR imaging of the brain in children: normal and neurologic disease. *Am J Neuroradiol* **4**, 1013–1026.

20. Maalouf E, Duggan P, Rutherford M *et al.* (1999) Magnetic resonance imaging of the brain in a cohort of extremely preterm infants. *J Pediatr* **135**, 351–357.

21. Leviton A and Gilles F (1996) Ventriculomegaly, delayed myelination, white matter hypoplasia, and 'periventricular' leukomalacia: how are they related? *Pediatr Neurol* **15**, 127–136.

22. Martin E, Kikinis R, Zuerrer M *et al.* (1988) Developmental stages of human brain: an MR study. *J Comput Assist Tomogr* **12**, 917–922.

23. McArdle CB, Richardson CJ, Nicholas DA *et al.* (1987) Developmental features of the neonatal brain: MR imaging. Part1. Gray–white matter differentiation and myelination. *Pediatr Radiology* **162**, 223–229.

24. Murphy NP, Rennie J and Cooke RWI (1989) Cranial ultrasound assessment of gestational age in low birthweight infants. *Arch Dis Child* **64**, 569–572.

25. Saeed N, Ajayi-Obe M, Counsell S *et al.* (1998) Convolution index computation of the cortex using image segmentation and contour following. *ISMRM*, Abstract 2076.

26. Sie LTL, van der Knapp MS, van Wezel-Meijler *et al.* (1997) MRI assessment of myelination of motor and sensory pathways in the brain of preterm and term-born infants. *Neuropediatrics* **28**, 97–105.

27. Slagle TA, Oliphant M and Gross SJ (1989) Cingulate sulcus development in preterm infants. *Pediatr Res* **26**, 598–602.

28. Stewart AL, Rifkin L, Amess PN *et al.* (1999) Brain structure and neurocognitive and behavioural function in adolescents who were born very preterm. *Lancet* **353**, 1653–1657.

29. Van der Knaap MS, Wezel-Meijler G, Barth PG *et al.* (1996) Normal gyration and sulcation in preterm and term neonates: appearance on MR images. *Radiology* **200**, 389–396.

30. Worthen NJ, Gilbertson V and Lau C (1986) Cortical sulcal development seen on sonography: relationship to gestational parameters. *J Ultrasound Med* **5**, 153–156.

Magnetic resonance imaging of the normal infant brain: term to 2 years

4

Frances M Cowan

Contents

Introduction

Magnetic resonance (MR) imaging of the infant brain has given an enormous insight into the maturational processes that take place after birth. The technique has made it possible to see in minute detail changes in cortical folding, involution of the germinal layer, premyelination changes within white matter, myelination, iron deposition, and the growth of different regions of the brain that is not possible with computed tomography or ultrasound.

Establishing normality is especially difficult because the appearance of the normal brain is changing almost weekly. A large number of infants need to be studied with different strength magnets and using different sequences to fully appreciate the range of normal appearances[4–8,11,19,25,28,37–39,41,49,53,54,58,59,61,62,64,71,78–81,86,88,91]. The introduction of new sequences often means that new norms need to be established. Centers must determine normal appearances for different ages on their own system.

Pulse sequences used by our own group for imaging neonates and young infants

We have a 1 Tesla Picker HPQ Vista/Plus system and a 1 Tesla novel short small bore system which is situated in the neonatal intensive care unit. For imaging and multinuclear spectroscopy we have a 1.5 Tesla Picker Eclipse system. All three scanners are used for imaging infants up to term. After term, the neonatal unit magnet cannot be used as the bore is too small[57]. Our MR scans are not angled as steeply as is usual for computed tomography (CT). This makes the appearance of images, particularly the basal ganglia, thalami and internal capsule, different from some published data. These differences must be taken into account when interpreting images. Details of the sequences used on the different systems at different ages are given in Table 4.1. The slice thickness we use is 4–6 mm with no slice gap.

An excellent review of different pulse sequences and their relative merits in the pediatric context is given by Barkovich[8].

Table 4.1 Pulse sequences. Term to 3 months

	IT Picker HPQ		IT NNU magnet		1.5 T Eclipse	
	TR/TE	FOV	TR/TE	FOV	TR/TE	FOV
T1W SE	860/20	24	600/20	20	500/15	30
T2W SE	2700/120	22				
T2W FSE			3500/208	20		
Dual Echo	2500/20–80	25				
Dual FSE					4200/15–210	30
Volume	23/6	26.5 (1.6 slice thickness)				
DWI	Cardiac gated, pulsed gradient					
	SE pulse interval/200 ms					
	b = 600 s/mm²					
	4 data acquisitions					
	2/3 perpendicular planes					
Multislice	Single shot echoplanar					
	b = 1000 s/mm²					
	1 data acquisition					
	3 perpendicular planes					
	TR6200/100					
	matrix 100 x 100					
	TR/TE/TI	FOV	TR/TE/TI	FOV		
IR	3800/30/950	22–24	3697/36/950	20		
FLAIR	8142/150/2100	25				
Sequences used after 3 months						
IR 3 months – 2 years	3400/30/800	22–24				
>2 years	3100/30/700	22–24				

NNU, neonatal unit.

MR imaging of the brain in the term infant: conventional T1 and T2 weighted sequences

THE CORTEX

The brain of the term (37–42 weeks) infant is similar to that of the adult in terms of its cortical folding. By 38 weeks all the sulci are formed though they become deeper over the following few weeks[1] (Figs 4.1–4.5).

The signal intensity (SI) of the cortex is high on T1 weighted (T1W) (Figs 4.1 and 4.4a,b) and low on T2 weighted (T2W) images (Figs 4.2, 4.3, 4.4c and 4.5). In general, the more heavily the images are T1 weighted the higher the relative SI of the cortex (Fig. 4.1) and the more heavily they are T2 weighted, as seen with the fast spin echo (FSE) sequence (Fig. 4.3), the lower the relative SI. Highest signal contrast is seen around the Rolandic or central sulcus, that is the posterior cortex of the precentral gyrus and the anterior cortex of the postcentral gyrus (Figs 4.1–4.3). This feature remains with decreasing conspicuity for up to 2 months on T1W images (Fig. 4.8) and for up to 6 months on T2W images (Fig. 4.12).

As this pattern of SIs is the same as for myelinated white matter (WM) it has been suggested that the cortical signal in the perirolandic region is due to myelination. However, this seems unlikely for a number of reasons[53]. In myelinating WM T1 shortening precedes T2 shortening, whilst in the perirolandic cortex T2 shortening is more prominent and lasts longer. Also there is very little myelin in this tissue at this age. It is seen microscopically from 35 weeks' gestation in the pre- and postcentral gyri but macroscopically only from 40 weeks in the subcortical WM, and not in the cortex. Microscopically, there is slightly more myelin in the precentral than postcentral cortex whilst the MR SIs of the two regions are the same. Finally, myelination increases enormously over the first 6 months after birth at term, during which time the signal differences in this part of the cortex become less obvious.

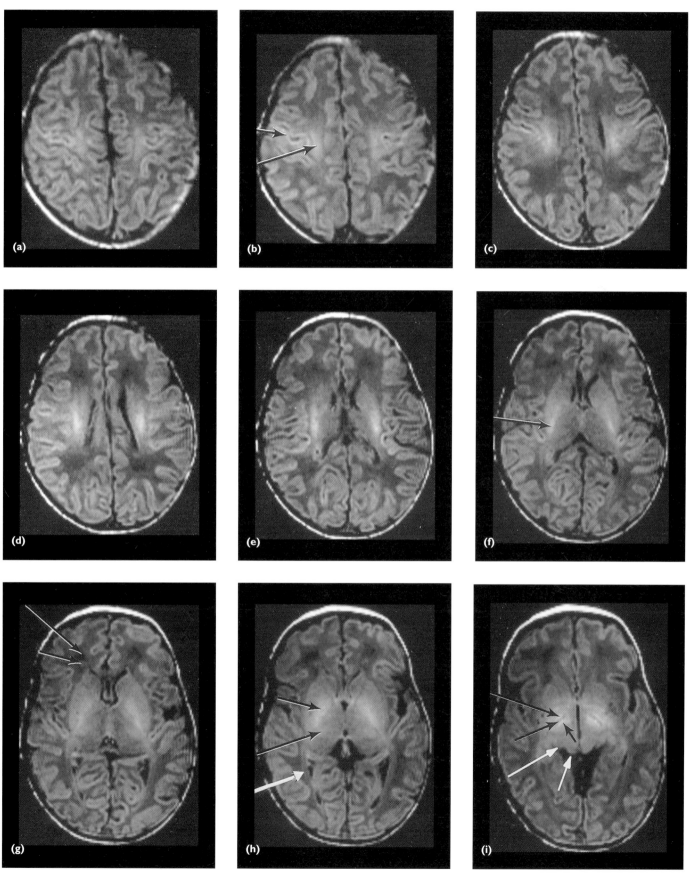

Fig. 4.1 *(See overleaf)*

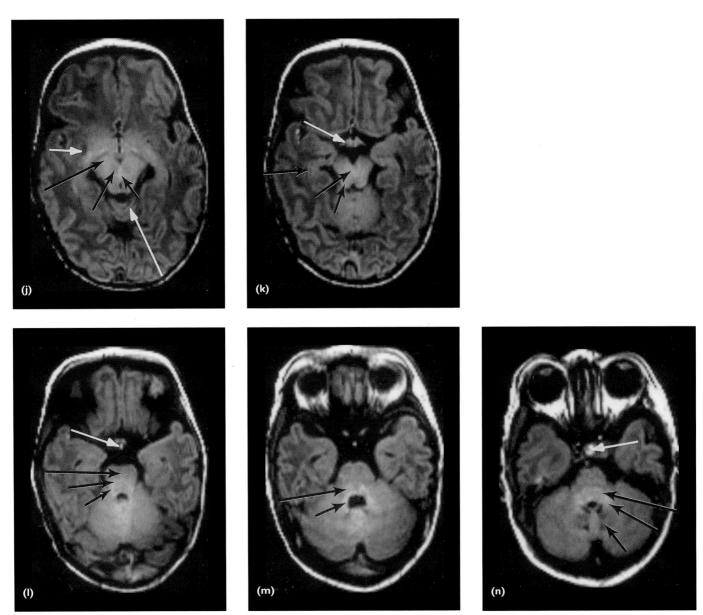

Fig. 4.1 Serial axial IR (IR 3800/30/950) images of an infant at term from high CS level to mid-cerebellar – low temporal lobe level. **(b)** Short T1 in the perirolandic cortex (*short arrow*) and central myelinated WM (*long arrow*). **(f)** Myelinated PLIC. **(g)** Short T1 anterior 'caps' (*short arrow*) and long T1 anterior 'region' (*long arrow*). **(h)** Short T1 in the GP (*short b/w arrow*) and the VLNT (*long b/w arrow*), also seen in (**g**). The high SI in the GP can be marked up to 42 weeks gestational age. The region of the optic radiation (*white arrow*) consist of three bands of low and high SI. **(i)** Characteristic hair pin appearance of the junction of the basal ganglia and mesencephalon with the GP anteriorly (*long b/w arrow*), unmyelinated tracts in the internal capsule (*medium b/w arrow*) and subthalamic nucleus posteriorly (*short b/w arrow*). The superior colliculi are seen (*short white arrow*) and the site of the medial geniculate body is seen laterally (*long white arrow*). **(j)** At mesencephalic level the largely unmyelinated crus is seen (*long b/w arrow*), as are the red nuclei (*medium b/w arrow*) and the medial longitudinal fasciculi (*short b/w arrow*). Vascular spaces are seen (*short white arrow*), as is the vermis of the cerebellum (*long white arrow*). **(k)** The inferior colliculi are clearly seen (*short b/w arrow*), as is the optic tract (*white arrow*). The central high SI within the brain stem is the decussation of the superior cerebellar peduncles (*medium b/w arrow*). The hippocampus is of intermediate SI (*long b/w arrow*). **(l)** The ventral upper pons is largely unmyelinated but of mixed SI from the pyramidal tracts (*long b/w arrow*). The dorsal pons is of high SI. The medial lemniscus (*medium b/w arrow*) and superior cerebellar peduncle (*short b/w arrow*) are marked. The pituitary stalk is well seen (*white arrow*). **(m)** At mid-pons level the medial lemniscus (*long arrow*) is well seen and the superior cerebellar peduncle (*short arrow*) radiates posteriorly. **(n)** In the lower pons the medial lemniscus (*long b/w arrow*), inferior cerebellar peduncle (*medium b/w arrow*) and dentate nucleus (*short b/w arrow*) are marked. The pituitary gland is seen (*white arrow*).

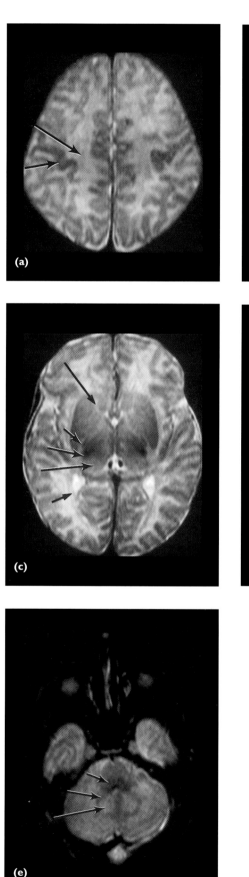

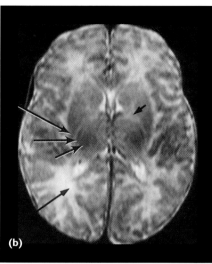

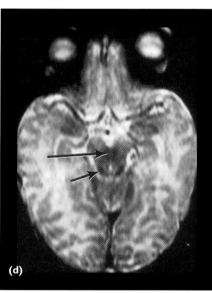

Fig. 4.2 Axial T2W (SE 2700/120) images of an infant at term. **(a)** Low SI in the perirolandic cortex (*short arrow*). The central WM is of slightly lower SI (*long arrow*) than the more frontal and posterior WM consistent with the onset of myelination. **(b)** At mid-basal ganglia level the PLIC has a small region of low SI (*medium b/w arrow*), the GP is of intermediate to high SI (*black arrowhead*) but the posterior putamen (*long b/w arrow*) and the VLNT (*short b/w arrow*) are of low SI. There is an ill-defined 'arrowhead'-shaped region of high SI in the posterior periventricular WM (*black arrow*). **(c)** At low basal ganglia level a portion of the PLIC has a characteristic low SI globular appearance (*short b/w arrow*) high SI around it; small regions of high SI are seen within the ALIC (*long black arrow*). The VLNT is clearly demarcated and of low SI (*medium b/w arrow*). The posterior thalami are of intermediate SI (*long b/w arrow*). The optic radiations appear to consist of three tracts (*short black arrow*). **(d)** In the upper brain stem the superior colliculi (*short arrow*) and the medial longitudinal fasciculi (*long arrow*) are of low SI. **(e)** The medial lemnisci (*short arrow*) and inferior cerebellar peduncles (*medium arrow*) are of low SI and the dentate nuclei (*long arrow*) is of high SI with a low SI rim.

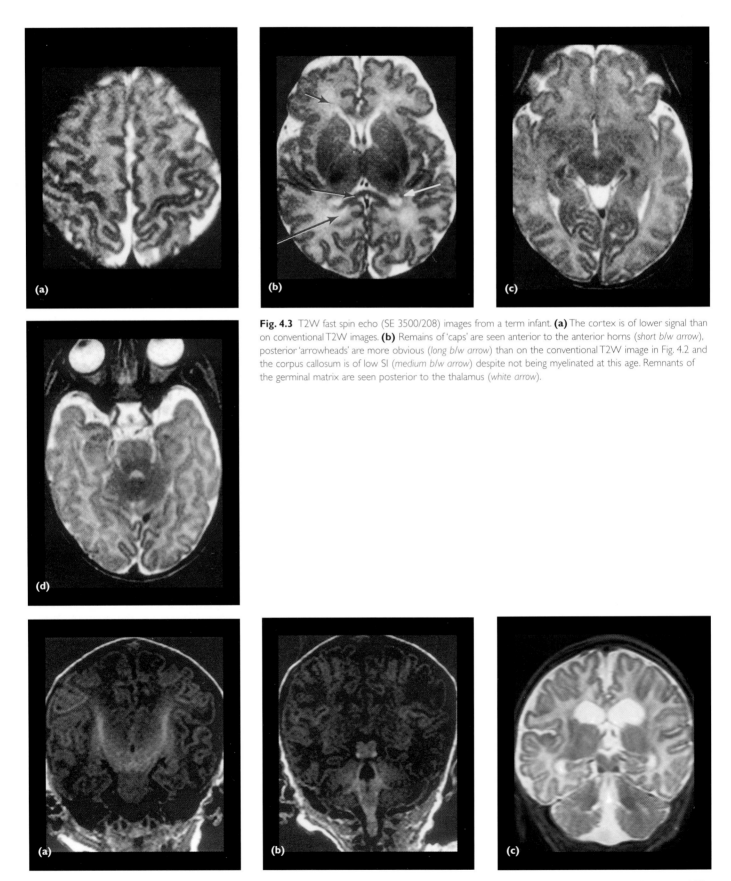

Fig. 4.3 T2W fast spin echo (SE 3500/208) images from a term infant. **(a)** The cortex is of lower signal than on conventional T2W images. **(b)** Remains of 'caps' are seen anterior to the anterior horns (*short b/w arrow*), posterior 'arrowheads' are more obvious (*long b/w arrow*) than on the conventional T2W image in Fig. 4.2 and the corpus callosum is of low SI (*medium b/w arrow*) despite not being myelinated at this age. Remnants of the germinal matrix are seen posterior to the thalamus (*white arrow*).

Fig. 4.4 Coronal views to show the myelinated PLIC (T1W SE images, **a**) as well as the superior and inferior colliculi and tectum (T1W, **b** and T2W SE images, **c**). The inferior colliculi myelinate before the superior colliculi. The inferior cerebral peduncle is also seen to be myelinated on both images.

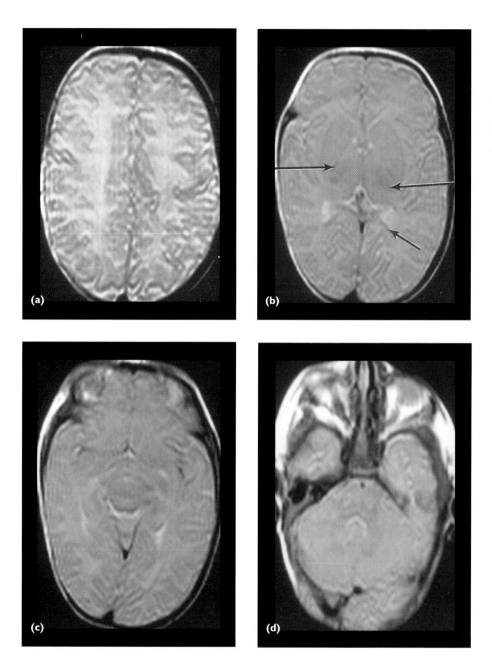

Fig. 4.5 Axial proton density (TR 2500, TE 20 ms) images from an infant at term through **(a)** the centrum semiovale; **(b)** the basal ganglia; **(c)** the mesencephalon; **(d)** the cerebellum. The cortex, myelinated WM (PLIC, *long arrow*), VLNT (*medium arrow*) and the corpus callosum (*short arrow*) are of lower SI than the remaining central gray matter and all are of lower SI than unmyelinated WM. The CSF is of high SI. The contrast in the images is inferior to that of T1 and T2 weighted SE images.

Alternative explanations for the signal appearance of the perirolandic cortex are that it is due to more advanced development of neurons and oligodendroglia as well as greater density of synapses and dendrite formation. All of these may result in decreased free water content and increased lipid content of this particular part of the cortex[9,20–22]. If the water content decreases faster than lipid is laid down then T2 shortening would precede T1 shortening (see below for myelination). Others have suggested that these cortical signal differences are due to the paramagnetic effects of trace elements but this has not been substantiated[40]. Capillary proliferation or changes in protein layering[15] may also account for the difference.

THE GERMINAL MATRIX

The germinal matrix, which gives rise to the cortex, largely involutes by 37 weeks but occasionally remnants of it are seen in the caudothalamic notch and posterior to the thalami at their junction with the optic radiation. Residual germinal matrix at these sites is best seen on FSE T2W sequences (Fig. 4.3). Remnants are also seen in the periventricular WM anterior to the anterior horns[18,57,89]. In older subjects this region shows patchy interruption of the ependyma, subependymal gliosis and finer myelin than in adjacent WM. This zone corresponds to the subcallosal fasciculus and it is thought that defects in the ependymal lining appear in this region during normal development as the germinal matrix disappears[30,54].

WHITE MATTER

In contrast to the relative completeness of the cortical folding, myelination which has been fairly static and confined to the brain stem, globus pallidus (GP) and ventro-lateral nucleus of the thalamus (VLNT) up to term[16,29,34,50,83,92], shows an enormous spurt from about 38 weeks' gestation onwards. This continues over the first year, and to a lesser extent into the second year and even to a small degree, into adolescence.

Myelin is composed of a bilayer of lipids with several large proteins traversing the bilayer. These include myelin basic protein and proteolipid protein. Histologically, myelination starts at about 25 weeks' gestation in the GP, VLNT and some tracts in the posterior limb of the internal capsule (PLIC)[16,32,34,36,50] 10–12 weeks before it is seen in WM tracts on MR images. By 32 weeks myelin is seen microscopically in the ascending thalamocortical tracts and the descending corticospinal tracts and by 35 weeks in the striatum, and pre- and postcentral gyri. By 37 weeks it is apparent in the anterior limb of the internal capsule (ALIC) and optic radiation. At term, myelin is seen macroscopically in the thalamus, ALIC and PLIC, part of the GP, optic and acoustic radiations as well as in the pre- and postcentral subcortical WM. The pattern of myelin seen at term with MR imaging is described in Table 4.2.

The degree to which myelin is seen histologically depends on the stains used[36]. Stains for myelin basic protein show myelin earlier than those that select more for lipid content. It is well recognized that myelin appears earlier and proceeds faster on T1W images than it does on conventional T2W SE images. This difference in timing of the appearance of myelination between the two sequences may be due to the difference in water binding resulting from the process of myelination. The shortening of T1 is temporally related to the increase in cholesterol and glycolipids that is associated with the formation of myelin from oligodendrocytes. The shortening of T2 is associated with the tightening of the spiral myelin around the axon, changes in myelin protein and saturation of polyunsaturated fatty acids in the myelin membrane. These processes are hydrophilic and alter the ratio of bound to free water in the different layers of the myelin[6,8,88].

The internal capsule

On T1W images the PLIC should be myelinated at term (Figs 4.1 and 4.4) and absence of the short T1 appearance has great significance for future neurodevelopment[27,63,74,75,77]. Myelination in the PLIC is best seen on inversion recovery (IR) images where the signal is more extensive in length and breadth and the contrast with the surrounding tissues is greater than with T1W SE images.

In the term infant the PLIC starts to myelinate around 37 weeks. The increase in signal in the PLIC over the next 1–3 weeks is a constant feature that is prognostically very important (see above). It is our experience that the PLIC myelinates a little earlier in infants born very preterm where it often appears by 35 weeks. It is therefore necessary when reporting the stage of myelination of the PLIC to be certain of the infant's gestational age and postnatal age, if born very early.

On conventional T2W SE images at low basal ganglia level only a small region in the most posterior portion of the PLIC appears myelinated (i.e. of short T2). It has a characteristic globular appearance (Fig. 4.2b,c) and is surrounded almost entirely by signal of intermediate intensity that separates it from the putamen and thalamus. On FSE images the region of short T2 is longer (Fig. 4.3b) and may be as extensive as the high SI on the T1W images.

The ALIC is often clearly seen and is of low SI on T1W (Fig. 4.1g,h) and intermediate SI on T2W images with small areas of high SI within the line of the capsule (Figs 4.2b and 4.3b). These areas have the appearance of small cysts and may be due to vascular spaces; their aetiology is not clear.

Table 4.2 Regions of the brain that are myelinated on MR images at 37–42 weeks

Centrum semiovale	Central portion
Visual system	Optic nerves and tracts
	Beginning of the optic radiations
Basal ganglia	Globus pallidus (partly)
Thalami	Ventro-lateral nucleus
Internal capsule	Posterior third
Brain stem and	Medial and lateral leminisci
mesencephalon	Medial longitudinal fasciculi
	Inferior and superior cerebellar peduncles
	Decussation of the superior cerebellar peduncles
	Inferior colliculi
Cerebellum	Peduncles
	Dentate nucleus (partly)

Table 4.3 Unmyelinated white matter on MR images at term

Most WM within the cerebral hemispheres
Anterior 2/3 of the PLIC
ALIC
External capsule
Corpus callosum
Anterior brain stem

Unmyelinated white matter in the hemispheres

The distribution of unmyelinated WM is given in Table 4.3. Within the unmyelinated WM which is generally of intermediate to low SI on T1W and of high SI on T2W images there is some variation (Figs 4.1–4.3). Around the anterior horns are small 'caps' of low SI on T2W images that are probably migrating cells or remnants of them originating in the germinal matrix (see section on the germinal matrix)[18,30,55,57,89]. Adjacent, but more peripherally is an arrow-shaped region of high SI on T2W images and low SI on T1W images. This is relatively cell-poor on histology[33]. These regions are better seen on T1W and T2W FSE images than conventional T2W SE images. Posterior to the occipital horns on axial views (Figs 4.1–4.3) and above the ventricles on coronal views, there are similar regions shaped like 'arrowheads' that stand out from the surrounding WM. These features are much more prominent earlier in gestation and should not be obvious at term[18,57,89]. Indeed 'caps' are only obvious at term if the surrounding WM has an abnormally long T1 and T2. The 'arrowheads' should not be well defined at term even if the periventricular WM is of slightly long T1 and T2[57].

The WM should not be of uniform SI but change slightly at it goes towards the cortex so that the SI becomes closer to that of cortex. However, this is very variable and, especially posteriorly, the high SI on T2W images may be quite marked when using FSE sequences.

The corpus callosum

The corpus callosum is thin, even in thickness (about 2 mm) and fairly flat (Fig. 4.17a)[5,8,49]. It is unmyelinated at term. The bulbous genu and splenium develop towards the end of the first year (Fig. 4.17b,c). It is of intermediate SI on T1W images but may be of low SI on T2W FSE images even though it is not myelinated (Fig. 4.3). The reason for this is unclear but it may be due to the compactness and uniformity of the fibers. However, the internal capsule, which is also made of densely packed fibers, does not have the same very low SI appearance on T2W FSE images.

THE BASAL GANGLIA AND THALAMI

The basal ganglia and thalami are relatively large in the term infant. The head of caudate nucleus, the lentiform nucleus (globus pallidus (GP) and putamen) and thalami are clearly demarcated by the internal capsule (Fig. 4.1e–h). The GP, VLNT and to a lesser extent the posterior putamen are prominent and of high SI on T1W images. The GP and the VLNT contain myelin from as early as 25 weeks[29,32,34,36,92].

The GP on T1W images becomes less obvious in terms of SI from 38 to 42 weeks. The VLNT remains differentiated from the surrounding tissue for several months. The internal capsule, which is myelinated in its posterior third, lies between the putamen and the thalamus. Where the GP descends forwards to the upper mesencephalon it forms the anterior portion of a region in the diencephalon that has a very characteristic hair pin appearance (Fig. 4.1i). The central portion of the hair pin is of low SI on T1W images and consists of the unmyelinated tracts forming the internal capsule. The posterior portion is of high SI and is probably formed by the subthalamic nucleus.

THE HIPPOCAMPUS

The hippocampal region tends to be of high SI on T1W and low SI on T2W images but has a mixture of SIs with complicated cortical folding (Figs 4.1 and 4.2). If the SI is uniform, especially high SI on T1W images, we consider that abnormal. It abuts on the anterior portion of the temporal horn of the lateral ventricle. A small area of myelination may be seen in this region at term on T1W images though the signal is difficult to differentiate from folded cortex.

THE BRAIN STEM

On T1W images the crura containing the pyramidal tracts begin to myelinate in their most lateral portions at term. The red nuclei and substantia nigra are of intermediate to low SI and often cannot be distinguished. The inferior and superior colliculi (the inferior colliculus is more prominent than the superior, Fig. 4.4b,c) and the quadrigeminal plate, medial lemnisci and medial longitudinal fasciculi, and the decussation of the superior cerebellar peduncles are seen. All tend to be of high SI on T1 and low SI on T2W images. The optic chiasm is seen anteriorly (Figs 4.1 and 4.2)[8,32,59,79].

The dorsal pons contains the myelinated medial and lateral lemnisci, the medial longitudinal fasciculi, and the middle cerebellar peduncles. All these structures are of high SI on T1W images and of low SI on T2W images. The ventral portion is generally of intermediate SI though there is some variation in SI in the pons indicating the beginning of MR differentiation of the tracts. Absence of this variation in SI is seen after severe perinatal asphyxia. The pons is prominent and measures about 11 mm in antero-posterior diameter and 14.5 mm in height[53]. The trigeminal nerve may be seen.

CEREBELLUM

The cerebellar hemispheres are of intermediate SI on T1W and T2W images (Figs 4.1–4.3) except for the dentate nuclei, the parasagittal portion of the vermis and the inferior and superior cerebellar peduncles which are of high SI on T1W and low SI on T2W images. In the more mature term

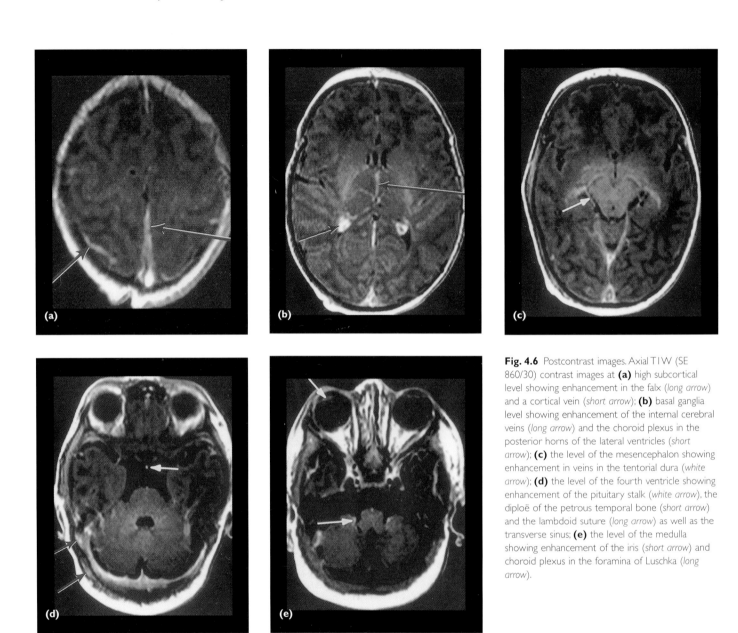

Fig. 4.6 Postcontrast images. Axial T1W (SE 860/30) contrast images at **(a)** high subcortical level showing enhancement in the falx (*long arrow*) and a cortical vein (*short arrow*); **(b)** basal ganglia level showing enhancement of the internal cerebral veins (*long arrow*) and the choroid plexus in the posterior horns of the lateral ventricles (*short arrow*); **(c)** the level of the mesencephalon showing enhancement in veins in the tentorial dura (*white arrow*); **(d)** the level of the fourth ventricle showing enhancement of the pituitary stalk (*white arrow*), the diploë of the petrous temporal bone (*short arrow*) and the lambdoid suture (*long arrow*) as well as the transverse sinus; **(e)** the level of the medulla showing enhancement of the iris (*short arrow*) and choroid plexus in the foramina of Luschka (*long arrow*).

infant the T1 and T2 begin to shorten. The middle cerebellar peduncles are not clearly demarcated from the body of the cerebellum[79,80]. The vermis is about 20 mm in anteroposterior diameter and 22.5 mm in height[53].

Contrast enhancement

Contrast enhancement is normally not seen or is only just apparent in the brain parenchyma, that is the cortex, white matter, basal ganglia and brain stem. However, obvious enhancement is seen in the pineal gland, the pituitary stalk, the dura, the large veins and sinuses and the choroid plexus in the lateral, third and fourth ventricles (Fig. 4.6). Barkovich *et al.*[7] note that enhancement is also seen in the metopic, coronal and lambdoid sutures, the diploë of the

basal skull bones and the iris, regardless of gestational age. Though studies on normal preterm infants are not reported, our own experience with a few infants is that the findings are similar to those reported for the term infant. When giving contrast we use dimeglumine gadopentetate (Magnevist; Schering Ltd, Burgess Hill, East Sussex, UK) in a dose of 0.2–0.4 ml/kg intravenously.

Diffusion weighted imaging of the neonatal brain

DIFFUSION WEIGHTED IMAGES

Diffusion weighted images (DWI) reflect the Brownian motion of water molecules within the brain. This diffusional motion is limited by tissue structure particularly in WM tracts where diffusion of water is freer along the length of axons than across them. Measurements of the diffusion of water therefore depend on the direction of the applied gradients in relation to the direction of the tract. The differences in diffusion in relation to axon (and tract) orientation can be seen on DWIs and is known as anisotropy. Normal WM shows anisotropy within myelinated and unmyelinated tracts. The tracts will appear of high SI if they are perpendicular to the direction of sensitization and of low SI if they are parallel to the direction of sensitization. The whole of the internal capsule shows anisotropy which is clearly seen, as does the external capsule, the corpus callosum, the optic

radiation and other tracts within the cerebral hemispheres long before they are seen to be myelinated on T1 or T2W images. WM in the immediate periventricular region does not show the clear anisotropic features that are seen more centrally and more peripherally. Gray matter does not show anisotropy on visual inspection of images.

The clarity with which the tracts are seen is very dependent on the sequences used[23,66,73,82], the number of data acquisitions and the immobility of the subject. The technique is very sensitive to motion artifact and the images are affected by the T2 weighting of the tissue. Details of the methodology we use are given in Table 4.1 and Refs 23 and 69 (Fig. 4.7). The problem of motion sensitivity, the variation in fiber direction

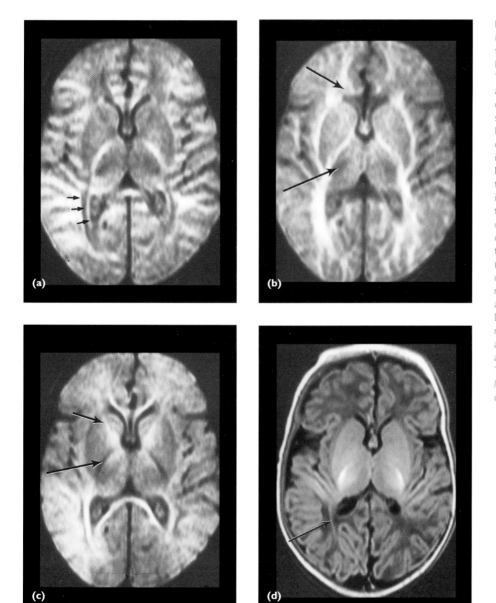

Fig. 4.7 Diffusion weighted images. DW axial images at the level of the basal ganglia sensitized in three directions: **(a)** anterior–posterior; **(b)** left–right; **(c)** head–foot (SE pulse interval/200 ms, TR 1526–1572, b = 600 s/mm², four data acquisitions); and **(d)** an IR image (3800/30/950) for comparison. Tracts at right angles to the direction of sensitization are of high SI and those parallel are of low SI. Note the clear change in SI in the internal capsule, corpus callosum, external capsule and tracts in the unmyelinated WM between **(a)**, **(b)** and **(c)**. No detail of the peripheral tracts is seen in **(c)** with the sensitization in the head–foot direction. The internal capsule is angulated at the genu and therefore the anterior and posterior portions (*short and long arrows*, **c**) are not of the same SI on any one image. The optic radiations seem to contain three tracts which are of high SI, low SI and high SI (*short black arrows*) on **(a)**, all of high SI on **(b)**, and of low SI and high SI on **(c)** and show very early myelination (*arrow*) on **(d)**. The medial portion adjacent to the ventricle remains of high SI on all DW images. The anterior periventricular WM does not show clear anisotropic change (*short arrow*, **b**) and nor does the VLNT although it contains myelin and is of high SI in T1W images **(d)**, of low SI on T2W images (not shown) and on all the DWIs (e.g. *long arrow*, **b**). This lack of anisotropy is probably due to mixed fiber orientation and short T2 effects.

and the proportion of fibers with long T2 components all affect the images and hence affect measurement of the apparent diffusion coefficient (ADC) of water in brain.

Abnormal tissue affected by an acute process often decreases its ADC and loses its anisotropic appearance so it becomes of uniform high SI irrespective of the direction of sensitization[2,23,45,47,69,72,84].

APPARENT DIFFUSION COEFFICIENT MAPS

ADC maps of the normal neonatal brain show the corpus callosum, the optic radiation and the PLIC to be of low SI before they are seen to be myelinated on conventional imaging. Measurements of the ADC in both gray and white matter give higher values than those found in adults. Unlike the adult[70] ADCs are higher in WM than gray matter. There is also a strong correlation with gestational age with the ADCs of gray and hemispheric WM both decreasing and becoming closer to each other towards term[44,66,68]. This is despite the fact that these fibers are not myelinated. The ADC in the PLIC also decreases with increasing gestational age[68] but according to Hüppi et al. the change is minimal though significant[44].

The ADC in the PLIC is lower and nearer to that of the adult than the ADC of the ALIC reflecting the fact that myelination is more advanced in the PLIC. Similarly, at birth the ADC of occipital tracts is lower than the ADC of frontal tracts reflecting the caudo–cephalic progress of WM maturation. Measurements of the ADC within unmyelinated WM also show a rapid decrease over the first 6 post-term months[65,85]. Values also decrease in frontal and occipital WM, the corpus callosum and the lentiform nucleus. The change in ADC is most marked when measured at 90 degrees to tracts. There is little change in ADCs with age when they are measured with gradients parallel to the tract[66,82].

Of note is the fact that the ADC in periventricular WM (but not the PLIC) seems to be higher in healthy preterm infants at term than in newborn full-term infants[44]. This suggests that periventricular WM is less mature in the preterm infant at term than the full-term infant and is in keeping with the observation that the T2 of this WM is long on conventional images[42,52,57]. It is interesting that a difference is not seen in the PLIC which on conventional imaging is not delayed in its myelination in healthy premature infants, and indeed in our experience may be slightly advanced.

These observations show that the diffusion of water is less restricted in all tissues of the brain of the newborn than it is in the adult. It is well known that the fetal and infant brain contains more water than the brain of the older child and adult[29] and that the water content reduces rapidly towards the end of gestation and in early infancy. The rapid changes in ADC during this time reflect this change in water content as well as localized restriction to the diffusional movement of water due to increasing numbers of oligo dendrocytes surrounding axons and later thickening of the myelin sheath and its reduced permeability to water. The changes during the time periods when measurements have been possible, that is the third trimester and in the early postnatal period, are greater frontally than occipitally and are concurrent with the caudo–cephalic progress of myelination. It appears that the WM in the hemispheres of preterm infants at term is less mature than it is in the full-term infants.

DIFFUSIONAL ANISOTROPY

If the entire explanation for anisotropy in WM was myelination of tracts, then one would expect to find that unmyelinated tracts did not show directional changes in ADC. This is not the case. In addition, measurements of quantitative diffusional anisotropy (DA) should inversely parallel the ADCs. Whilst the data from Hüppi et al.[44] support this, the work from Neil et al.[67] does not. Both groups have found that values of DA are greatest in the PLIC, lower in the ALIC (Neil et al.) and lower still in the centrum semiovale. Unlike Hüppi et al., Neil et al. found that measurements of DA in the PLIC, ALIC and corpus callosum did not change during the period from 30 to 40 weeks' gestation. This is in contrast to the ADC values which gradually decreased with age in all tissues though Hüppi found the change in the PLIC to be small. Neil et al. found the DA to increase only within the unmyelinated WM of the centrum semiovale at the end of gestation. Vector maps of fiber orientation show orientation of unmyelinated fibers in the corpus callosum in the term infant. In the periventricular WM bundles of fibers are also seen but they are less tightly organised (Fig. 4.7). Again it is of note that the preterm infant at term has a lower DA in the hemispheric WM and the orientation of fibers seems less organized than in the full-term infant.

The cause of the anisotropy in the newborn brain is uncertain at present but it is becoming clearer. Anisotropic appearances are seen in histologically unmyelinated white matter[90] and may be due to the premyelination state[10] characterized by an increase in axon diameter and axonal membrane changes. This is accompanied by interactions between premyelinated axons and glial cells and by many other ultrastructural and functional changes.

The changes seen on DW images, in measurements of ADC and DA, and on vector maps in the third trimester and early postnatal period, particularly within periventricular WM, offer great potential for visualizing and understanding the processes of WM maturation. However, problems related to knowing the fiber orientation and proportion of long T2 components in the fibers affect all forms of DWI and make image interpretation difficult.

MR changes in the cerebrum, brain stem and cerebellum occurring after term: conventional T1 and T2 weighted sequences

THE CORTEX

There is some increase in the depth and complexity of cortical folding just after term[1,12–14] and the Sylvian (lateral) fissure may close further, but there is little change that is obvious on conventional MR brain imaging. Of note, however, is the fact that the SI of the cortex which is high on T1W images and low on T2W images becomes of intermediate SI by 4–6 months. By this time the WM has myelinated and become of high SI on T1W and later low SI on T2W images. Therefore during the first few months after birth the images go through a phase of relative isointensity compared to earlier and later images. The exact timing of the changes in SI in gray matter and WM depends on the detail of the T1W and T2W sequences that are used. This reduction in SI in the cortex may be due to a reduction in cellularity and an increase in the number of synapses present at this time. It may therefore reflect increasing cortical complexity. Potentially, this could be measured from the changes in T1 and T2 of the tissue. Unfortunately, this is technically difficult as voxels containing only cortex have to be very small and placed in areas where the cortex is very folded to ensure exclusion of the adjacent WM.

As discussed above, the low SI on T2W images (particularly in the perirolandic region) persists for several months more than the high SI seen on T1W images.

WHITE MATTER

The changes in volume and myelination of the WM are dramatic[16,29,34,50,92]. The WM provides the bulk of the brain volume and hence brain growth over the first 2 years. From 29–41 weeks' gestation the rate of increase is 22 ml/week[43]. This increase is accompanied by an increase in head circumference from 34–36 cm at birth of about 0.5 cm/week for the first 3 months and then at decreasing rates to 43–45 cm at 1 year.

Volumetric growth of the brain can be measured from serially acquired images that are registered to each other and subtracted[17,76]. In the adult this process results in an image of almost pure noise[17], but in the infant because of growth and changes in the SI of tissue the subtraction image shows structure[76]. The increase in volume is seen as a rim of tissue around the circumference of the image and demonstrates that there is little change in the size of the basal ganglia and thalami. It also allows the process of myelination to be documented (e.g. along the corpus callosum) and can be used to demonstrate a decrease in T1 and T2 in WM prior to myelination.

Myelination occurs at different rates on T1W and T2W images. Before term myelin is best seen on FSE T2W images. After term for about 8–10 months myelin is better seen on T1W SE and more so on T1W IR images. After that time the major changes on T1W images have occurred and further maturation and detail is again better seen on T2W images.

As a general rule, myelination occurs in a caudal to cephalic direction and in the hemispheres is seen first parietally then occipital, frontally and temporally. The primary tracts myelinate before those in the association areas of the hemispheres. In the brain stem myelination occurs dorsally before ventrally, and in sensory before motor tracts.

Progress of myelination from term to 2 years

On T1W images the internal capsule is myelinated to the genu by 1 month (Fig. 4.8) and in its entirety by 3 months (Fig. 4.9). The splenium of the corpus callosum begins to myelinate at 3 months and the genu by 6 months (Fig. 4.17). The WM of the motor tracts are myelinated out to the subcortical regions by 3 months (Fig. 4.9) and to the primary visual regions of the occipital lobes by 6–7 months (Fig. 4.11). Myelin is seen in the frontal lobes by 5–6 months (Fig. 4.11) and in the temporal lobes by 7–8 months. Subcortical myelin appears in the frontal lobes at 8 months and temporally at 10 months (Fig. 4.13). Little change is seen on T1W images after this time though over the second year there is some extension of myelination in U fibers apparent in the subcortical WM (Fig. 4.15).

On T2W images the changes are slower and more prolonged and hence subtle changes and delays in myelination in the second year are better demonstrated with T2W images. Myelination in the PLIC does not reach the genu before 4–6 months. It starts in the ALIC around 7 months and is not complete before 10 months depending on the particular T2W sequence used. Generally, it will appear sooner on FSE than on conventional SE images. The splenium of the corpus callosum becomes of low SI around 6 months and the genu by 8 months.

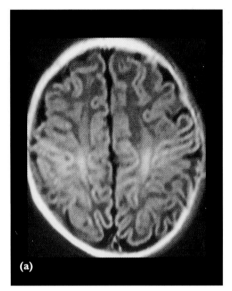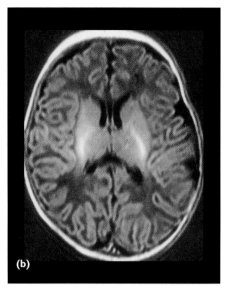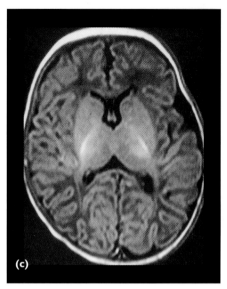

(a)   (b)   (c)

Fig. 4.8 Axial IR (IR 3800/30/950) images at 6 weeks. The PLIC is fully myelinated and the beginning of myelination are seen in the ALIC. Myelin is seen in the central motor tracts. The perirolandic cortex is of high SI.

The WM of the motor tracts starts to become of low SI around 2 months and reaches the subcortical regions by 3–4 months. Low SI is seen in the optic radiations by 2 months and just extends to the calcarine fissure by 4 months. Other regions do not myelinate in terms of the T2 appearances before 9–12 months in the occipital lobes, 11–14 months frontally (Fig. 4.14) and 16–18 months in the temporal lobes. The low SI extends into all the subcortical regions by 2 years (Fig. 4.16).

Details of the timing of the appearance of myelin on T1W and T2W images are given in Table 4.4 and are well described by various authors[4,8,19,28,37–39,58,86–88].

The development of myelination described above is largely descriptive and allows for variations in images produced by different sequences at different field strengths. It is important to know both the general principles that govern the pattern and the rates of myelination of different regions of the brain. For detecting minor variations in myelination it is necessary to know the individual timing of changes in T1 and T2 in the sequences that are available on the particular system being used. We prefer to use FSE sequences up to term, IR sequences from term to 10 months and conventional T2W sequences to 2 years (Table 4.1). Gray and unmyelinated WM should be of almost equal SI at 4 months on T1W images. On T2W images the cortical and most of the central gray matter signal is isointense with myelinated WM around 1 year and the cortical signal becomes higher than myelinated WM between 18 months and 2 years. A very detailed description of the stages of myelination is given by van der Knaap and Valk[88].

The terminal zones

Within myelinating WM there are regions of apparently unmyelinated WM. These are particularly obvious in the periventricular zones posterior and superior to the lateral ventricles (Figs 4.16 and 4.18). They appear as patches of high SI within the low SI WM on T2W images and to a lesser extent regions of low SI within the high SI myelinated WM on T1W images. These regions are normal in infants in the second year and often persist for many years. They were described as 'terminal zones' by Yakovlev and Lecours[92] because these regions do not stain for myelin for many years. They are felt to be normal but do occur in the region of WM most commonly affected in periventricular leukomalacia (PVL) which also produces areas of similar SI and needs to be distinguished from them. Their sites are very much those of the regions noted before term, and at term, within the WM that are of low SI on T1 and high SI on T2W images and correspond to cell-poor areas on histology[32]. These same regions commonly show patchy hyperintensity on T2W images in the elderly in whom on histology the myelin looks pale, there are dilated perivascular spaces, perivascular gliosis and ischemic change[51].

In our experience these regions appear more obvious in very preterm infants without cerebral palsy who are examined at 2 years of age. They are also commonly seen in children imaged for global developmental delay for which no specific cause is found[64]. In these situations the ventricular margin is fairly smooth and of normal shape and there is a band of tissue of low SI on T2W images which separates the regions of long T2 from the ventricular margin.

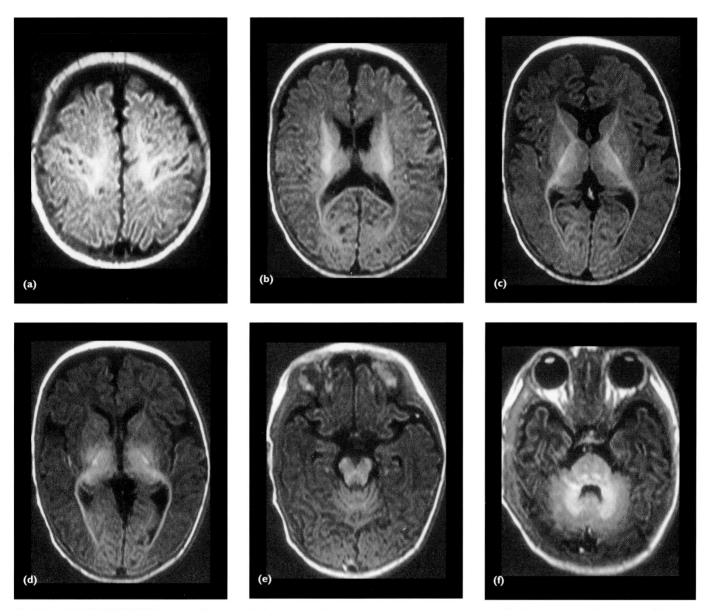

Fig. 4.9 Axial IR (IR 3400/30/800) images at 3 months. Myelination is seen in the subcortical motor tracts, the whole of the internal capsule, the splenium of the corpus callosum, the hippocampus, the optic radiations to the calcarine fissure, the cortico spinal tracts and deep cerebellar WM. The cortex around the central sulcus is no longer of high SI. The inferior portion of the GP and the VLNT are of relatively high SI.

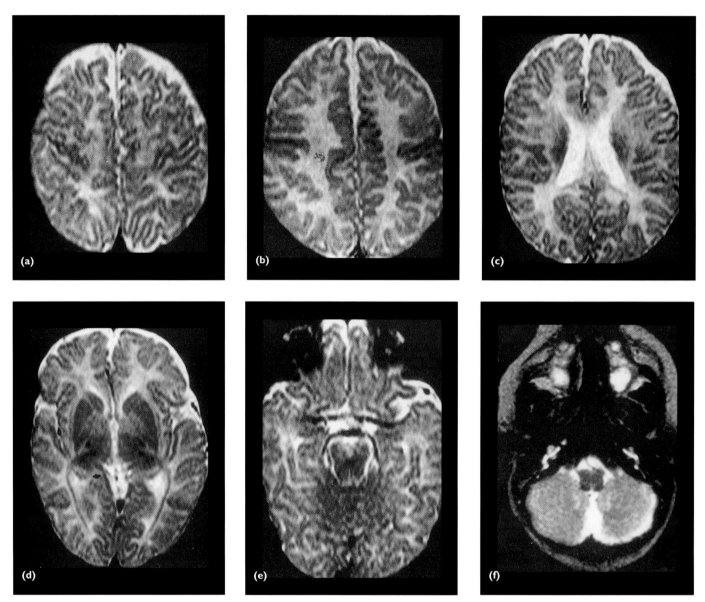

Fig. 4.10 Axial T2W (SE 2700/120) images at 3 months. Myelination is seen in the central periventricular WM, half of the PLIC and in the optic radiations. The cortex of the central sulcus is still of low signal intensity. The GP is of higher SI than the putamen and caudate nucleus.

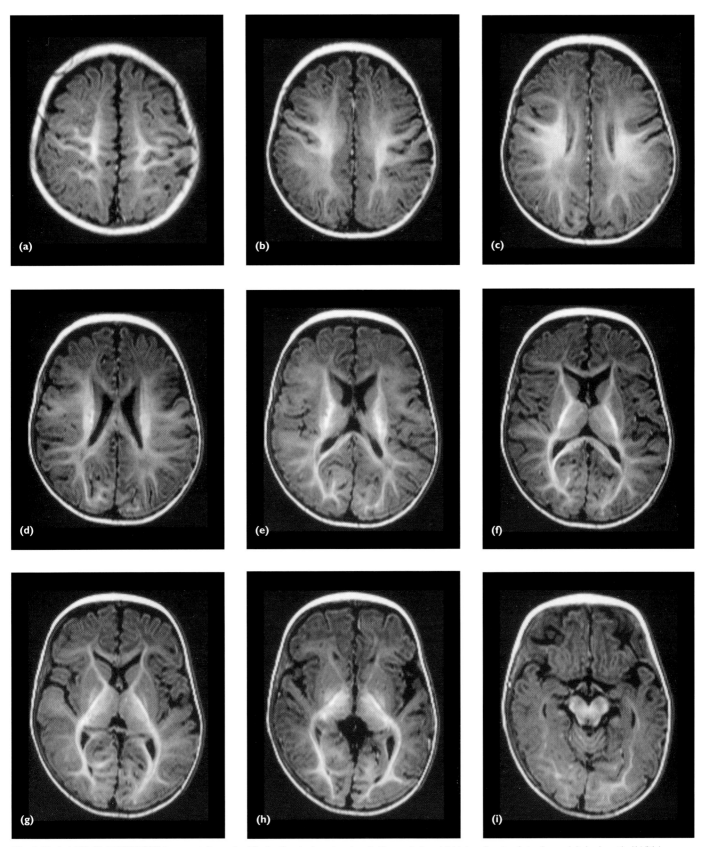

Fig. 4.11 Axial IR (IR 3400/30/800) images at 6 months. Myelination is almost mature in the central parietal lobes, it extends to the occipital subcortical WM, is present in the anterior and posterior portions of the parietal lobes and beginning to appear in the frontal lobes. The internal capsule has an irregular appearance due to fibers transversing it. The GP and VLNT are of higher SI than the rest of the basal ganglia and the posterior thalamus. The corticospinal tracts in the mesencephalon are well myelinated. The peri-aqueductal gray matter is now of low SI.

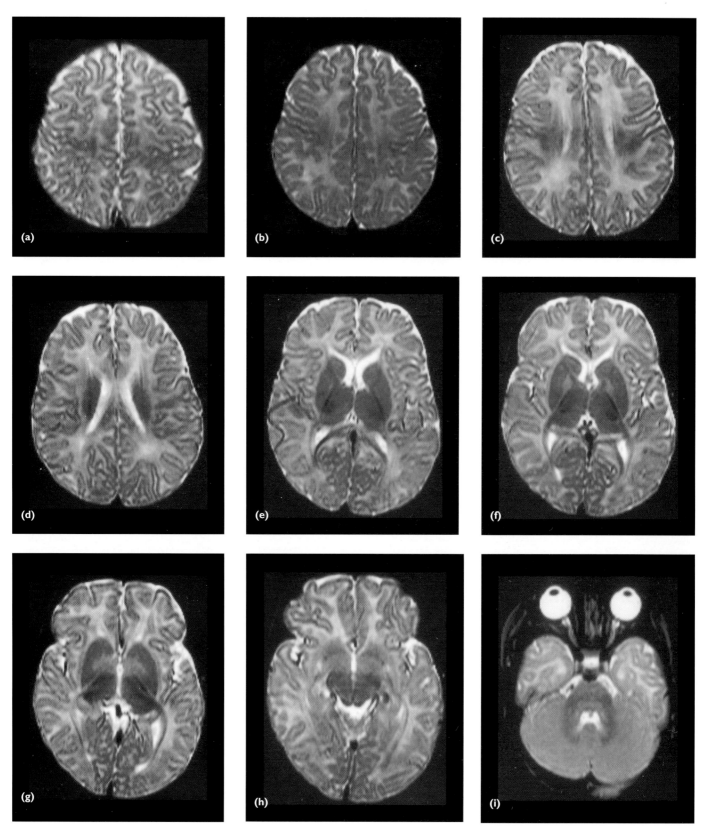

Fig. 4.12 Axial T2W (SE 2700/120) images at 6 months. Myelination is present in the central CS extending out to the subcortical WM of the central sulcus, the whole of the internal capsule, the splenium of the corpus callosum and the hippocampus. The GP and the posterior thalamus are of higher SI than the putamen and caudate nuclei and the VLNT remains of lower SI. The brain stem and cerebellar peduncles are also myelinated but no myelin is seen in the cerebellar folia.

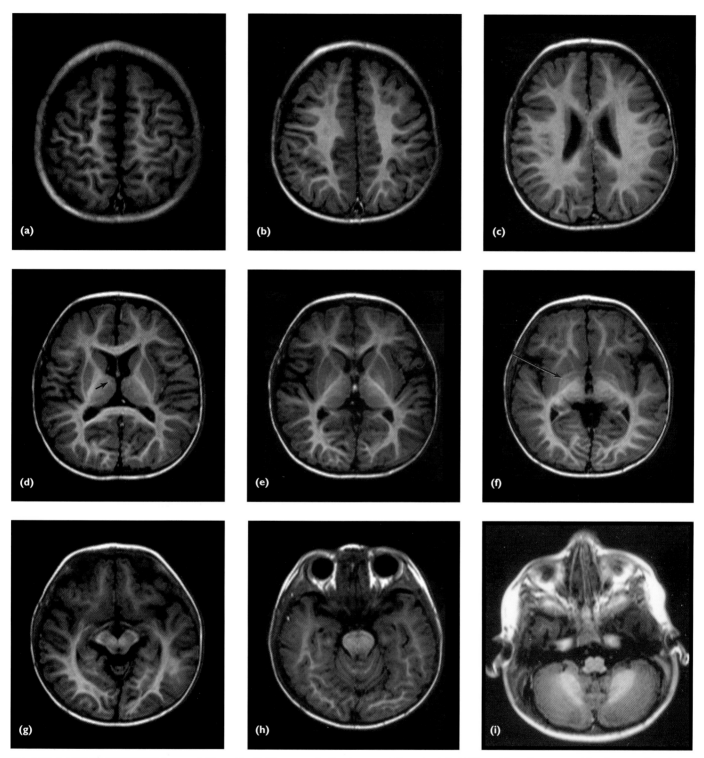

Fig. 4.13 Axial IR (IR 3400/30/800) images at 12 months. At this age myelination is apparent throughout the WM apart from the most peripheral arcuate fibers. In the basal ganglia the border of the GP is clearly demarcated and, as with the VLNT, the GP remains of higher SI than the adjacent tissue. The mamillary bodies are seen in the anterior thalami (**d**, *short arrow*). The anterior commissure is well seen (**f**, *long arrow*). Small cyst-like spaces are seen adjacent to the anterior horns of the lateral ventricles (**d**).

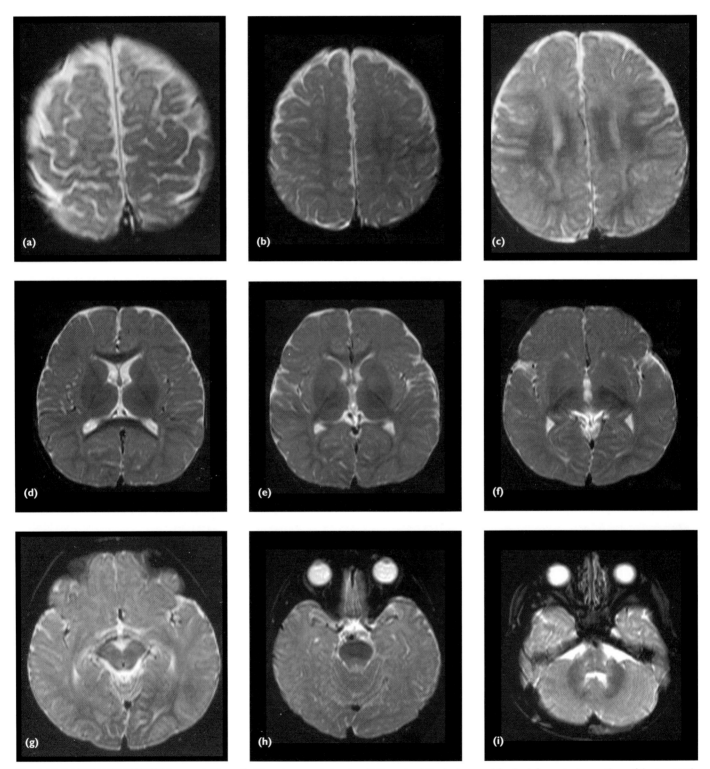

Fig. 4.14 Axial T2W (SE 2700/120) images at 12 months. There is more obvious low SI throughout the brain except for the infero-anterior portions of the temporal lobes. The cortex and myelinated WM are of similar SI at this age. The pons is clearly demarcated again with low SI in the ventral portion and intermediate signal dorsally.

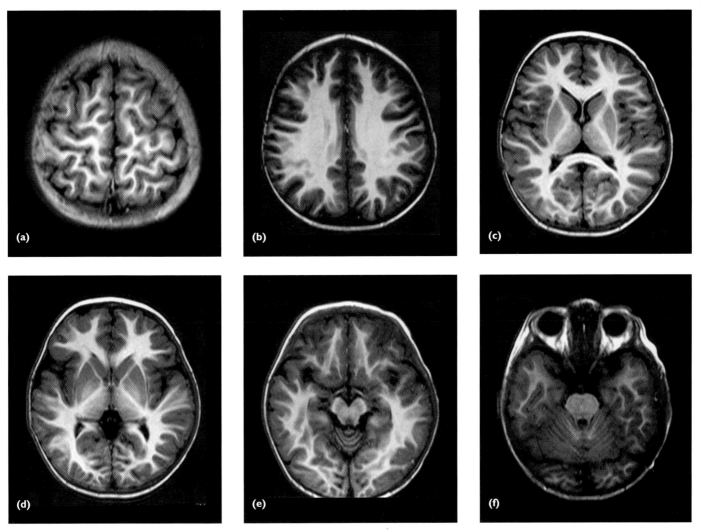

Fig. 4.15 Axial IR (IR 3100/30/700) images at 2 years. The brain has an adult appearance on these images with extensive subcortical myelination though some U fibers are still to myelinate. In the posterior CS there are some patches of slightly lower SI within the myelinated WM.

In PVL associated with a motor deficit, the ventricles have an irregular margin and the high SI on the T2W images abuts on the ventricular margin, unlike the situation seen with normal terminal zones. Usually the high SI in PVL is more marked than is seen with normal terminal zones and with PVL there is usually an abnormal degree of thinning of at least the posterior portion of the body of the corpus callosum. This appearance can also be seen in a few children who had an acute encephalopathy at term with no evidence for preterm damage[24].

Another differential diagnosis for regions of high SI and low SI on T2W and T1W images respectively are vascular spaces. These generally have a distinct linear appearance on the T1W images (see below, Fig. 4.22) and are best seen on the IR images. They can mimic abnormal long T2 in the WM if no T1 image is available.

The corpus callosum

The first postnatal changes that occur are a thickening of the genu and the splenium during the first 2–4 months with the genu being somewhat ahead of the splenium. However, myelination occurs first in the splenium around 4 months and in the genu around 6 months on T1W images. The body also thickens and takes on a more adult appearance around 9 months, often, though not always, with a region of focal thinning at the junction between the body and the splenium. The overall length of the corpus callosum seems to relate

Table 4.4 Distribution of myelin seen on MR images from term to 2 years

T1W images	T2W images
1 month	
PLIC, optic radiation, central CS, optic nerve, cerebellar peduncles, dorsal pons, vermis, dentate nucleus	Posterior 1/3 PLIC, central CS, dorsal pons, peridental WM, vermis
2 months	
Pre- and postcentral sulcus WM, ALIC, anterior pons, hippocampus	PLIC 1/3, CS, optic radiation, middle cerebellar peduncles, dentate nuclei
3 months	
ALIC complete, occipital WM at calcarine fissure, splenium of corpus callosum	1/2 PLIC
4 months	
Beginning of frontal WM	Calcarine WM
5 months	
Genu of corpus callosum	Anterior pons
6 months	
Branching of frontal WM	PLIC complete, ALIC beginning, splenium of corpus callosum
7 months	
Branching of occipital WM	Optic radiation complete
8 months	
Peripheral frontal WM, fine arborization of paracentral and occipital WM	ALIC complete, genu of corpus callosum
10 months	
	ALIC thick, arborization of central motor tracts, branching of occipital tracts
11–12 months	
Temporal WM	Branching of posterior parietal tracts, beginning of frontal tracts
15–18 months	Frontal arborization,
Subcortical WM, U fibers	beginning of temporal WM
24 months	Temporal arborization, subcortical WM, U fibers

the second year of age interesting observations can be made. Characteristic regions of high SI are seen in the posterior portion of the PLIC, the optic radiations, particularly in their distal portions and adjacent to the frontal horns (Fig. 4.18). The PLIC and optic radiations are sites of early myelination and appear to retain long T2 components after myelination. The terminal zones, not surprisingly, are also seen to be of high SI but the cause for the high SI near the frontal horns is uncertain. It may have a common etiology with the cyst-like areas seen well on IR images in infants in the second year (Fig. 4.13) and the histological features noted amongst others by Dooling *et al.*[30] and Leifer *et al.*[55]. Unmyelinated WM is also of high SI (Fig. 4.18a) with this sequence.

THE BASAL GANGLIA AND THALAMI

Between 37 and 42 weeks the high SI on T1W images in the GP and the posterior putamen diminishes considerably but the GP remains of higher SI (Figs 4.8, 4.9, 4.11, 4.13 and 4.15). It becomes clearly demarcated from the rest of the lentiform nucleus. The caudate nucleus remains of intermediate SI. On T2W images the region of the GP is of slightly increased SI throughout the first year. The posterior putamen loses the low SI seen in the neonatal period and becomes of intermediate SI like the caudate nucleus.

The high SI in the VLNT seen on T1W images in the neonatal period persists for longer than the marked high SI in the GP and remains to some extent through the second year (Fig. 4.15). On T2W images the VLNT is of low SI neonatally and remains so, though to a lesser extent through to the second year. The pulvinar of the thalamus is of lower SI on T1W and higher SI on T2W images than the more anterior thalamus.

The iron deposition which reduces the SI of the GP, substantia nigra and red nucleus (and later the dentate nucleus) on T2W images is not seen before 9 years of age.

more to head size and shape than to the presence of disease[5,8,49].

White matter imaging with FLAIR sequences

Myelinated WM is well seen on fluid attenuated inversion recovery (FLAIR) images which have the advantage over T2W SE images of nulling the signal from CSF. We have not found FLAIR sequences to be of particular help in defining normal development in the young infant but in

THE HIPPOCAMPUS

Whilst there may be a very small area of myelinated tissue at term, myelination is always seen by 3 months (Fig. 4.9) and the region is well myelinated on T1W images by 12 months (Fig. 4.13). It is slow to myelinate fully on T2W images even by age 2 years (Fig. 4.16). The overall appearance of this region of the temporal lobe on axial views is of a thick band of folded tissue of mixed SIs lying medial to the temporal horns. The hippocampus is often better seen in the coronal rather than the axial or sagittal planes.

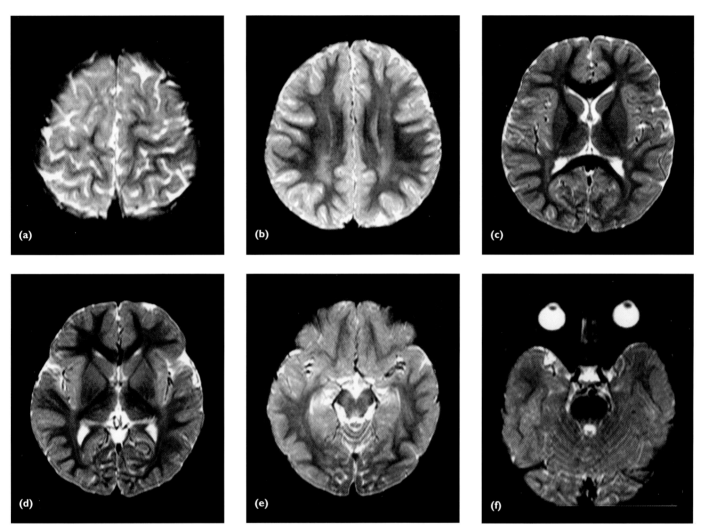

Fig. 4.16 Axial T2W (SE 2700/120) images at 2 years. Myelination has progressed throughout all lobes but has not extended as far in the frontal and temporal lobes as it has on the IR images. Within the myelinated WM are regions of long T2 mainly in the trigones and postero-lateral to the posterior horns of the ventricles. These regions are called terminal zones and may take some years to myelinate fully.

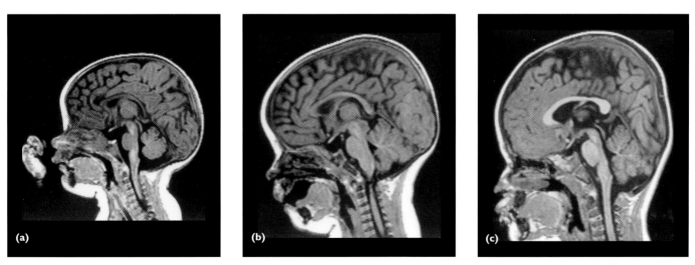

Fig. 4.17 Sagittal T1W (SE 860/20) images of the corpus callosum at: **(a)** term showing a complete, thin, even and unmyelinated corpus callosum; **(b)** 4 months showing thickening of the genu and the posterior body and splenium, but only the latter portions are beginning to myelinate; **(c)** at 10 months showing thickening throughout with some residual thinning of the body at the junction between the posterior portion and the splenium.

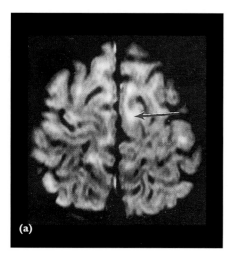 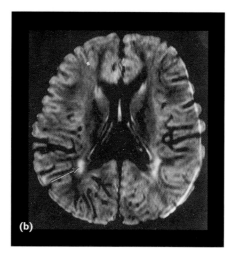 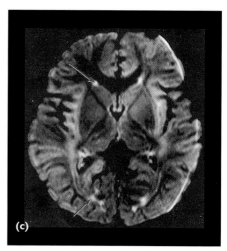

Fig. 4.18 Axial FLAIR (8142/150/2100) images through: **(a)** cortex and subcortical WM; **(b)** high-ventricular level; **(c)** the basal ganglia. Myelinated WM and CSF are of low SI. Unmyelinated WM is best seen in **(a)** and is of high SI (*arrow*). High SI is seen in **(b)** in the posterior periventricular WM of the terminal zones (*arrow*). Regions of high SI are typically seen on FLAIR images adjacent to the anterior horns (*long arrow*) and in the optic radiations (*short arrow*, **c**).

THE BRAIN STEM

From birth to 3 months tracts and nuclei in the brain stem become increasingly obvious particularly on T1W images. The main features of these areas are shown in Fig. 4.19 taken from a 2-month-old infant.

CEREBELLUM

The inferior and superior cerebellar peduncles are already myelinated by term and the middle cerebellar peduncles myelinate in the first 2–3 months. By 3 months high SI is seen in the dentate nucleus, peridental WM and the corpus medullare and the appearances in these regions are similar to those seen in the adult. Myelination on T2W images takes a little longer. More peripheral myelination in the cerebellum extending to the folia begins to appear after 4 months on T1W images and after 8 months on T2W images and the cerebellum has an adult appearance by 18 months (Figs 4.9–4.19)[8,39,80,86,88].

> ### Observations of other areas of the brain seen on MR brain scans from term to 2 years

THE PITUITARY GLAND

The pituitary gland is well seen on T1W mid-line sagittal 4 mm thick slice images[8,25,91]. The anterior portion is of high SI up to 2 months of age. The posterior portion is also of high SI but may not always be seen separate from the anterior portion. Thereafter, the anterior portion is of lower SI than the posterior portion and is easier to differentiate. The gland is described[25] as being upwardly convex for this period.

It gradually becomes flatter in most, but not all, infants though in our experience this is not always the case. It also increases in length slightly from 6 to 7 mm over the first year but the height remains the same at about 3.5–4 mm. It does not grow as fast as the rest of the brain over the first year. The size of the stalk does not change and it should never be as large as the basilar artery. The pituitary infundibulum enhances with contrast.

THE PINEAL GLAND

The pineal gland develops from the caudal portion of the roof of the third ventricle. At birth it has a volume of about 15–40 mm³ and increases to about twice that size by 2 years. It can be seen on very thin 1 mm T1W sagittal or coronal images lying just above the quadrigeminal plate between the thalami and beneath the junction of the posterior body and the splenium of the corpus callosum (Fig. 4.21)[81]. It does not alter in size after the first year[78].

THE VENTRICULAR SYSTEM

The lateral ventricles are small and rounded anteriorly and posteriorly (Figs 4.1–4.3) and are clearly seen extending into the temporal lobes. McArdle *et al.*[62] studied the size of the ventricles in the axial plane in relation to brain diameter. They suggested that the normal ratio of lateral ventricle/brain lies between 0.29 and 0.32 at term at the level of the anterior horns and at mid-ventricular level. The third ventricle is just seen posteriorly but the anterior portion may be more obvious and dips antero-inferiorly towards the pituitary fossa. The aqueduct is narrow but visible

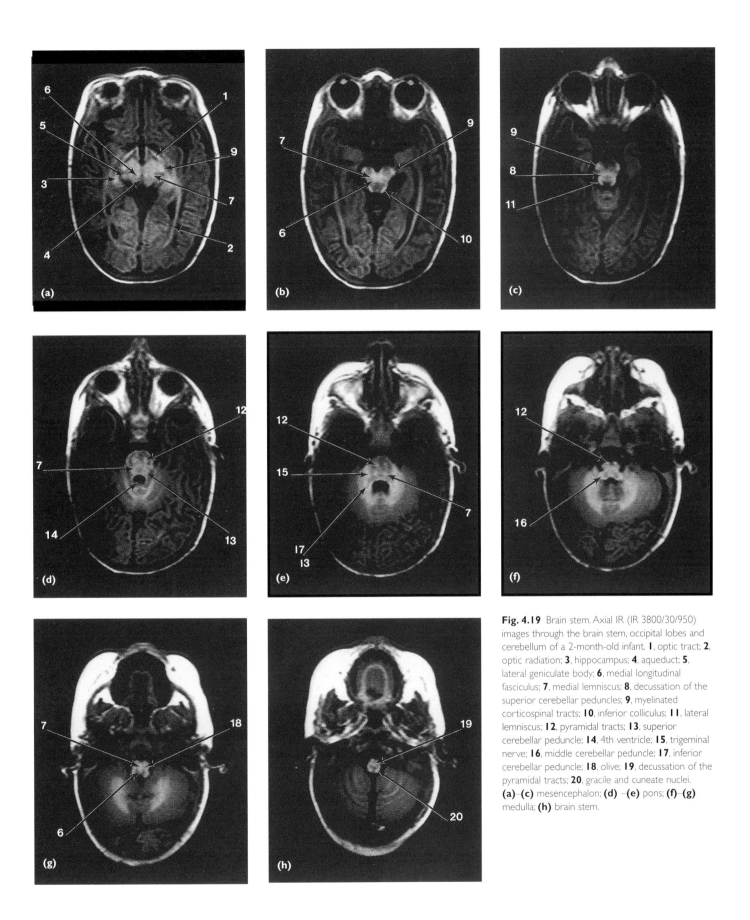

Fig. 4.19 Brain stem. Axial IR (IR 3800/30/950) images through the brain stem, occipital lobes and cerebellum of a 2-month-old infant. **1**, optic tract; **2**, optic radiation; **3**, hippocampus; **4**, aqueduct; **5**, lateral geniculate body; **6**, medial longitudinal fasciculus; **7**, medial lemniscus; **8**, decussation of the superior cerebellar peduncles; **9**, myelinated corticospinal tracts; **10**, inferior colliculus; **11**, lateral lemniscus; **12**, pyramidal tracts; **13**, superior cerebellar peduncle; **14**, 4th ventricle; **15**, trigeminal nerve; **16**, middle cerebellar peduncle; **17**, inferior cerebellar peduncle; **18**, olive; **19**, decussation of the pyramidal tracts; **20**, gracile and cuneate nuclei. **(a)–(c)** mesencephalon; **(d) –(e)** pons; **(f)–(g)** medulla; **(h)** brain stem.

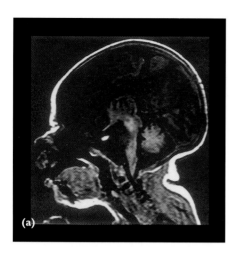
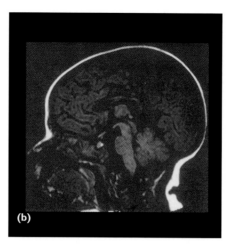

Fig. 4.20 Pituitary gland. Sagittal TIW images (860/20) showing the pituitary gland at **(a)** term and **(b)** 2 months post-term. The gland is initially of uniform high SI usually with an upward convexity. By 2 months the anterior pituitary is of intermediate SI.

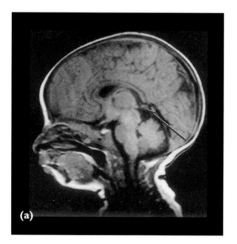
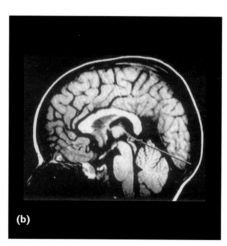

Fig. 4.21 Pineal gland. Sagittal TIW (SE 860/20) images showing the pineal gland marked by an arrow **(a)** at term and **(b)** at 2 years.

(Figs 4.1j and 4.2d). The fourth ventricle is slightly wider than it is deep, and about half the diameter of the pons (Figs 4.1 and 4.19).

THE EXTRACEREBRAL SPACES

These spaces are best assessed on T2W images where the outer cortical margin and the inner table of the skull can be clearly differentiated from CSF[62].

The interhemispheric fissure is narrow and regular (Figs 4.1 and 4.3) but the Sylvian fissures may be prominent. The depth of the insular cortex is 6–10 mm in 35–42 weeks' gestation infants. The width of the subarachnoid space ranges from 0 to 3 mm, being generally 0–3 mm over the convexities and in the interhemispheric fissure and 2–3 mm in the ambient cisterns. The space around the parietal and temporal lobes and the basilar cisterns may appear quite large. It is generally 2–4 mm in the cerebello-pontine angle cistern but the space anterior to the temporal lobe in the middle fossa and anterior to the frontal lobes may be up to

5–6 mm. Some apparently normal term infants may have very wide subarachnoid spaces as large as 12–13 mm posterior to the parietal lobes. In our experience this is an infrequent observation at term but may be a normal finding up to about 36–37 weeks. We see it in almost all ex-premature infants at this age. Enlarged frontal spaces are not uncommon and may be associated with normal development in children scanned because of macrocephaly[26]. A large cisterna magna may be a normal variant but care must be taken to ensure that the cerebellum, in particular the vermis, are of normal size.

VASCULAR SPACES

Vascular spaces are common in the elderly, but they can be seen in the newborn within the tissue of the inferior basal ganglia near the lateral portions of the anterior commissure (Figs 4.1i and 4.22c,e). They usually have a linear shape, and are angled anteriorly and towards the mid-line. There may be several. Care needs to be taken to recognize abnormal vascular spaces, for example in Leigh's disease where the cysts are usually larger and more superior in their distribution.

In the older child regions of long T1 and T2 are seen within the myelinated white matter usually in a periventricular distribution (Fig. 4.22a–d). These have a linear appearance and are also thought to be vascular spaces. They are generally not seen before the WM in the hemispheres is well myelinated. Similar areas, usually smaller and more rounded, can be seen in the basal ganglia (Fig. 4.22b).

Small spaces of cyst-like appearance are common adjacent and antero-lateral to the anterior horns (Fig. 4.22b,d). These have not been described in the literature and their eti-ology is not clear. They may be remnants of subependymal cysts that are not seen until the frontal periventricular WM is well myelinated.

DEVELOPMENTAL SPACES

The cavum septum pellucidum and cavum vergum are still patent in at least 75% of term infants but close rapidly. The cavum septum pellucidum is patent in 6% of children and 1% of adults[11]. Persistance of a large cavum septum pellucidum may be seen as part of the spectrum of mid line developmental anomalies.

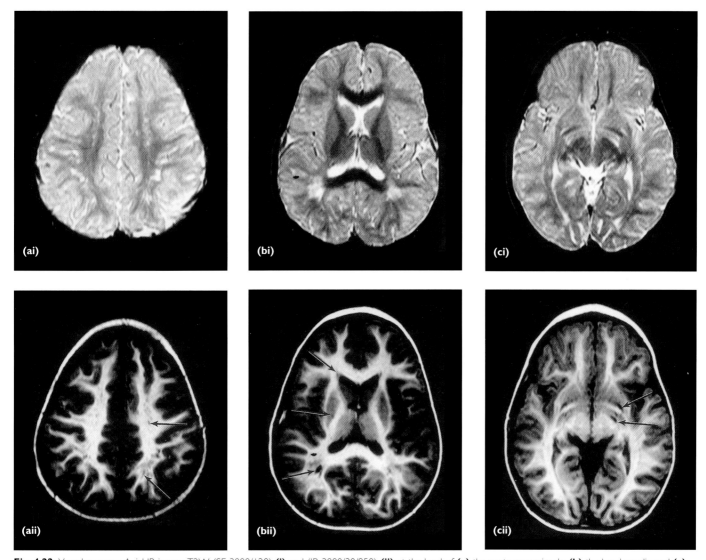

Fig. 4.22 Vascular spaces. Axial IR images T2W (SE 3000/120) **(i)** and (IR 3800/30/950) **(ii)** at the level of **(a)** the centrum semiovale; **(b)** the basal ganglia; and **(c)** the upper mesencephalon. Characteristic small elongated regions of low SI on the IR and high SI on the T2W images are seen (*arrows*) within myelinated WM **(a,b)**, within the lentiform nucleus **(b)** and adjacent to the lateral portions of the anterior commissure **(c)**. In addition there are similar regions adjacent to the anterior horns which are of uncertain etiology.

Functional MR imaging

The subject is covered in more detail in Chapter 16. Studies using functional MR imaging (fMRI) techniques in normal infants are scarce. Most adult studies in this field require the active co-operation of the subject combined with the ability to lie very still, which is clearly not possible in this young age group. Approaches have been limited to studying sensory systems where the stimulus will not disturb the infant. Few entirely normal infants have been studied and none in the awake state.

fMRI attempts to map the distribution of neuronal activity that is involved in a particular active or passive process. It is not a direct measure of neuronal activity but measures changes to local cerebral blood volume, flow or blood oxygenation associated with neuronal activity. The most common imaging method used has the acronym BOLD (blood oxygenation level dependent). Usually spin echo echo-planar sequences with a long TR and long TE or gradient echo sequences are used. The former are less sensitive to motion artifact but problems with motion artifact remain an issue with fMRI[35].

The technique depends largely on detecting changes in local levels of deoxygenated hemoglobin. Cortical venous and capillary blood has a relatively high concentration of deoxygenated hemoglobin. In response to neuronal activation there is a rapid increase in local blood flow which is in excess of that needed to supply oxygen for the increased metabolic demand. This results in a decrease in deoxygenated hemoglobin in the local capillary and venous blood. As deoxyhemoglobin is paramagnetic there is a change in local SI which can be detected by subtraction of pre-stimulus from post-stimulus images. In general, in adult studies, the excess of oxyhemoglobin and decrease in deoxyhemoglobin in the post-stimulus phase results in an increase in SI and therefore a positive BOLD effect.

The studies in newborns and young infants have concentrated on the visual system which can be stimulated in the sleeping and sedated child without disturbance. The visual system is complicated to study. It is thought that the young infant does not use the primary occipital cortex for vision but a subcortical system involving the pulvinar and the superior colliculi[3,31,48]. The infant may only have obligate use of the occipital cortex for vision after 2–4 months.

The results of infant studies have been difficult to interpret as positive, negative and absent responses have been found in the primary visual area in infants with apparently normal visual systems[12–14,60,93]. When the BOLD contrast signal was negative it was often not in the primary visual area but anterior and lateral to it, though in the first month after term a positive BOLD signal was sometimes seen in there. There are probably many explanations for the variation in findings which may partly reflect the processing changes in the visual system in the first months after birth or possibly a relative excess of synapses at this age[93] as compared with later in the first year. Other factors are likely to be non-optimal stimulus paradigms, smaller changes in local blood flow, volume or oxygenation in response to a stimulus than are found in the older child and adult, stimulation of the visual system through closed eyelids, and the effects of sleep or of sedation[46] or motion artifact.

fMRI is an exciting aspect of brain imaging that is only beginning to be applied to the pediatric population. fMRI has shown sites of activity in response to visual stimulation in brains affected by congenital and acquired abnormality of the occipital lobes[14,56]. It is hard to see at present how studies of the normal child in the awake state can be achieved until they are old enough to co-operate. However, the studies of the visual system are encouraging and it should be possible to perform similar work with the auditory and cutaneous systems.

Summary

- MRI gives superb detail of the developing brain. It is essential to have a thorough knowledge of the normal appearances at different ages in order to define the abnormal.

- Structures may look very different depending on the strength of field, the sequence, the plane, and the angle of acquisition. Normal appearances have to be established with the advent of any new MR technique.

- Myelinated structures have a short T1 and short T2. In our experience, prior to term these are best seen using a T2 weighted fast spin echo sequence between term and 1 year using an inversion recovery sequence and after 1 year a T2 weighted spin echo sequence.

- A T1 weighted or inversion recovery sequence in the transverse plane is invaluable in the assessment of the neurologically abnormal neonate at term.

- Diffusion weighted imaging allows definition of white matter tracts prior to MR visible myelination and even prior to histological myelination.

- Volumetric growth of the brain and its intrinsic structures can be objectively quantified using serially acquired images.

- Whilst the normal appearances and sizes of some structures are known, the clinical significance of mild deviations from the normal are seldom well understood.

Abbreviations

ADC	apparent diffusion coefficient
ALIC	anterior limb of the internal capsule
b	diffusion sensitivity parameter
b/w	black and white
BOLD	blood oxygen level dependent
CS	centrum semiovale
CT	computed tomography
DA	diffusional anisotropy
DWI	diffusion weighted imaging
FLAIR	fluid attenuated inversion recovery
fMRI	functional magnetic resonance imaging
FOV	field of view
FSE	fast spin echo
GP	globus pallidus
IR	inversion recovery
MR	magnetic resonance
PLIC	posterior limb of the internal capsule
PVL	periventricular leukomalacia
SE	spin echo
SI	signal intensity
T	Tesla
TE	echo time
TI	inversion time
TR	repetition time
T1W	T1 weighted
T2W	T2 weighted
VLNT	ventro-lateral nucleus of the thalamus
WM	white matter

References

1. Ajayi-Obe M, Saeed N, Cowan FM *et al.* (2000) Reduced development of cerebral cortex in extremely preterm infants. *Lancet* **356**, 1162–1163.
2. Arbelaez A, Castillo M and Mukherji SK (1999) Diffusion-weighted MR imaging of global cerebral anoxia. *Am J Neuroradiol* **20**, 999–1007.
3. Atkinson J (1992) Early visual development: differential functioning of parvocellular and magnocellular pathways. *Eye* **6**, 129–135.
4. Baier P, Forster Ch, Fendel H *et al.* (1998) Magnetic resonance imaging of normal and pathological white matter maturation. *Pediatr Radiol* **18**, 183–189.
5. Barkovich AJ and Kjos BO (1998) Normal postnatal development of the corpus callosum as demonstrated by MR imaging. *Am J Neuroradiol* **9**, 487–491.
6. Barkovich AJ, Kjos BO, Jackson DE *et al.* (1998) Normal maturation of the neonatal and infant brain: MR imaging at 1.5T. *Radiology* **166**, 173–180.
7. Barkovich AJ, Latal-Hajnal B, Partridge JC *et al.* (1997) MR contrast enhancement of the normal neonatal brain. *Am J Neuroradiol* **13**, 1713–1717.
8. Barkovich AJ (2000) Normal development of the neonatal or infant brain, skull and spine. In: *Pediatric Neuro-imaging*, 3rd edn. Philadelphia: Lippincott Williams & Wilkins, pp. 28–45.
9. Becker L, Armstrong DL and Wood CF (1984) Dendritic development in human occipital cortical neurons. *Dev Brain Res* **13**, 117–124.
10. Black JA, Waxman SG, Ransom BR *et al.* (1986) A quantitative study of developing axons and glia following altered gliogenesis in rat optic nerve. *Brain Res* **380**, 122–135.
11. Bodensteiner JB, Schaefer GB and Craft JM (1998) Cavum septi pellucidi and cavum vergae in normal and developmentally delayed populations. *J Child Neurol* **13**, 120–121.
12. Born P, Rostrup E, Leth H *et al.* (1996) Change of visually induced cortical activation pattern during development. *Lancet* **347**, 543.
13. Born P, Leth H, Miranda M *et al.* (1998) Visual activation in infants and young children studied by functional magnetic resonance imaging. *Pediatr Res* **44**, 578–583.
14. Born AP, Miranda MJ, Rostrup E *et al.* (2000) Functional magnetic resonance imaging of the normal and abnormal visual system in early life. *Neuropediatrics* **31**, 24–32.
15. Boyko OB, Burger PC, Shelburne JD *et al.* (1992) Non-heme mechanisms for T1 shortening: pathologic, CT, and MR elucidation. *Am J Neuroradiol* **13**, 143–145.
16. Brody BA, Kinney HC, Kloman AS *et al.* (1987) Sequence of central nervous system myelination in human infancy. I. An autopsy study of myelination. *J Neuropathol Exp Neurol* **46**, 283–301.
17. Bydder GM (1995) Detection of small changes to the brain with serial magnetic resonance imaging. *Br J Radiology* **68**, 1271–1295.
18. Childs A-M, Ramenghi LA, Evans DJ *et al.* (1998) MR features of developmental periventricular white matter in preterm infants: evidence of glial cell migration. *Am J Neuroradiol* **19**, 971–976.
19. Christophe C, Muller MF, Baleriaux D *et al.* (1990) Mapping of normal brain maturation in infants on phase-sensitive inversion-recovery MR images. *Neuroradiology* **32**, 173–178.
20. Conel JL (1941) *The Postnatal Development of the Human Cerebral Cortex, Vol. II. The Cortex of the One-Month Infant.* Cambridge, MA, Harvard University Press.
21. Conel JL (1947) *The Postnatal Development of the Human Cerebral Cortex, Vol. III. The Cortex of the Three-Month Infant.* Cambridge, MA, Harvard University Press.
22. Conel JL (1951) *The Postnatal Development of the Human Cerebral Cortex, Vol. IV. The Cortex of the Six-Month Infant.* Cambridge, MA, Harvard University Press.
23. Cowan FM, Pennock J, Hanrahan JD *et al.* (1994) Early detection of cerebral infarction and hypoxic ischemic encephalopathy in neonates using diffusion-weighted magnetic resonance imaging. *Neuropediatrics* **25**, 172–175.
24. Cowan FM (2000) Outcome after perinatal asphyxia in the term infants. Johnson A (Ed.) *Semin Neonatol* **5**, 1–14.
25. Cox TD and Elster AD (1991) Normal pituitary gland: changes in shape, size and signal intensity during the 1st year of life at MR imaging. *Radiology* **179**, 721–724.
26. de Vries LS, Smet M, Ceulemans B *et al.* (1990) The role of high resolution ultrasound and MRI in the investigation of infants with macrocephaly. *Neuropediatrics* **21**, 72–75.

27. de Vries LS, Groenendaal F, van Haastert IC *et al.* (1999) Asymmetrical myelination of the posterior limb of the internal capsule in infants with periventricular haemorrhagic infarction; an early predictor of hemiplegia. *Neuropediatrics* **30**, 314–319.

28. Dietrich RB, Bradley WG, Zaragoza IV EJ *et al.* (1988) MR evaluation of early myelination pattern in normal and developmentally delayed infants. *Am J Neuroradiol* **9**, 69–76.

29. Dobbing J and Sands J (1973) Quantitative growth and development of human brain. *Arch Dis Child* **48**, 757–767.

30. Dooling EC, Chi JG and Gilles FH (1983) Developmental changes in ventricular epithelia. In: Gilles FH, Leviton A and Dooling EC (Eds) *The Developing Human Brain: Growth and Epidemiologic Neuropathology.* Boston, John Wright, pp. 113–116.

31. Dubowitz LM, Mushin J, de Vries LS *et al.* (1986) Visual function in the newborn infant: is it cortically mediated? *Lancet* **1**, 1139–1141.

32. Feess-Higgins A and Larroche J-C (1987) Development of the human foetal brain – an anatomical atlas. *Inserm CNRS.*

33. Felderhof-Meuser U, Maalouf E, Squier MV *et al.* (1999) Magnetic resonance imaging of the brain in very preterm infants: correlation with histopathological findings. *Am J Neuroradiol* **20**, 1349–1357.

34. Gilles FH, Shankle W and Dooling EC (1983) Myelinated tracts: growth patterns. In: Gilles FH, Leviton A and Dooling EC (Eds) *The Developing Human Brain.* Boston, John Wright, pp. 117–192.

35. Hajnal JV, Myers R, Oatridge A *et al.* (1994) Artefacts due to stimulus correlated motion in functional imaging of the brain. *Magn Reson Med* **31**, 283–291.

36. Hasegawa M, Houdou S, Mito T *et al.* (1992) Development of myelination in the human fetal and infant cerebrum: a myelin basic protein immunohistochemical study. *Brain Dev* **14**, 1–6.

37. Hayakawa K, Konishi Y, Kuriyama M *et al.* (1990) Normal brain maturation on MRI. *Eur J Radiol* **12**, 208–215.

38. Hittmair K, Wimberger D, Rand T *et al.* (1994) MR assessment of brain maturation: comparison of sequences. *Am J Neuroradiol* **151**, 425–433.

39. Hittmair K, Kraker J, Rand T *et al.* (1996) Infratentorial brain maturation: a comparison of MRI at 0.5 and 1.5 T. *Neuroradiology* **38**, 360–366.

40. Hock A, Demmel H, Schicha K *et al.* (1975) Trace element concentration in human brain. *Brain* **98**, 49–64.

41. Holland BA, Haas DK, Norman D *et al.* (1986) MRI of normal brain maturation. *Am J Neuroradiol* **71**, 201–208.

42. Hüppi PS, Schuknecht B, Boesch C *et al.* (1996) Structural and neurobehavioral delay in postnatal brain development of preterm infants. *Pediatr Res* **39**, 895–901.

43. Hüppi PS, Warfield S, Kikinis R *et al.* (1998) Quantitative magnetic resonance imaging of brain development in premature and mature newborns. *Ann Neurol* **43**, 224–235.

44. Hüppi PS, Maier SE, Peded S *et al.* (1998) Microstructural development of human newborn cerebral white matter assessed *in vivo* by diffusion tensor magnetic resonance imaging. *Pediatr Res* **44**, 584–590.

45. Inder T, Hüppi PS, Zientara GP *et al.* (1999) Early detection of periventricular leukomalacia by diffusion-weighted magnetic resonance imaging techniques. *J Pediatr* **134**, 631–634.

46. Joeri P, Huisman T, Loenneker Th *et al.* (1996) Reproducibility of fMRI and effects of pentobarbital sedation on cortical activation during visual stimulation. *Neuroimage Suppl* **3**, S280.

47. Johnson AJ, Lee BCP and Lin V (1999) Echoplanar diffusion-weighted imaging in neonates and infants with suspected hypoxic-ischaemic injury. *Am J Roentgenol* **172**, 1721–1726.

48. Johnson MH (1990) Cortical maturation and the development of visual attention in early infancy. *J Cogn Neurosci* **2**, 81–95.

49. Kier EL and Truwit CL (1996) The normal and abnormal genu of the corpus callosum: an evolutionary, embryologic, anatomic and MR analysis. *Am J Neuroradiol* **17**, 1631–1641.

50. Kinney HC, Brody BA, Kloman AS *et al.* (1987) Sequence of central nervous system myelination in human infancy. II. Patterns of myelination in autopsied infants. *J Neuropathol Exp Neurol* **47**, 217–234.

51. Kitajima M, Korogi Y, Okuda T *et al.* (1999) Hyperintensities of the optic radiation on T2-weighted MR images of elderly subjects. *Am J Neuroradiol* **20**, 1009–1014.

52. Koenig SH, Brown RD III, Spiller M *et al.* (1990) Relaxometry of the brain: why white matter appears bright on MR. *Magn Reson Med* **14**, 482–495.

53. Konishi Y, Hayakawa K, Kuriyama M *et al.* (1993) Developmental features of the brain in preterm and fullterm infants on MR imaging. *Early Hum Dev* **34**, 155–162.

54. Korogi Y, Takahashi M, Sumi M *et al.* (1996) MR signal intensity of the perirolandic cortex in the neonate and infant. *Neuroradiology* **38**, 578–584.

55. Leifer D, Buonanno FS and Richardson Jr EP (1990) Clinicopathological correlations of cranial magnetic resonance imaging of periventricular white matter. *Neurology* **40**, 911–918.

56. Lui WL, Biervert K, Hallmann A *et al.* (2000) Functional MRI in children with congenital structural abnormalities of the occipital cortex. *Neuropediatrics* **31**, 13–15.

57. Maalouf E, Duggan P, Rutherford MA *et al.* (1999) Magnetic resonance imaging of the brain in extremely preterm infants: normal and abnormal findings from birth to term. *J Pediatrics* **135**, 351–357.

58. Martin E, Kikinis R, Zuerrer M *et al.* (1988) Developmental stages of human brain: an MR study. *J Comput Assist Tomogr* **12**, 917–922.

59. Martin E, Krassnitzer S, Kaelin P *et al.* (1991) MR imaging of the brainstem: normal postnatal development. *Neuroradiology* **33**, 391–395.

60. Martin E, Joeri P, Leonneker T *et al.* (1999) Visual processing in infants and children studied using functional MRI. *Pediatric Res* **46**, 135–140.

61. McArdle CB, Richardson CJ, Nicholas DA *et al.* (1987) Developmental features of the neonatal brain: MR imaging. Part 1. Gray–white matter differentiation and myelination. *Radiology* **162**, 223–229.

62. McArdle CB, Richardson CJ, Nicholas DA *et al.* (1987) Developmental features of the neonatal brain: MR imaging. Part 2 Ventricles and extracerebral spaces. *Radiology* **162**, 230–234.

63. Mercuri E, Rutherford M, Cowan F *et al.* (1999) Early prognostic indicators in infants with neonatal cerebral infarction: a clinical, EEG and MRI study. *Pediatrics* **103**, 39–46.

64. Miyazaki M, Hashimoto T, Tayama M *et al.* (1992) Occipital deep white matter hyperintensity as seen by MRI: 1. Clinical significance. *Brain Dev* **14**, 150–155.

65. Morriss MC, Zimmerman RA, Bilaniuk LT *et al.* (1999) Changes in brain water diffusion during childhood. *Neuroradiology* **41**, 929–934.

66. Nomura Y, Sakuma H, Takeda K *et al.* (1994) Diffusional anisotropy of the human brain assessed with diffusion-weighted MR: relation with normal brain development and aging. *Am J Neuroradiol* **15**, 231–238.

67. Neil JJ, Shiran SI, McKinstry RC *et al.* (1998) Normal brain in human newborns: apparent diffusion coefficient and diffusion anisotropy measured by using diffusion tensor MR imaging. *Radiology* **209**, 57–65.

68. Oatridge A, Cowan F, Schwieso J *et al.* (1995) Age related changes in the apparent diffusion coefficient of white and grey matter in the normal infant brain. *SMRM Abst.*, p. 1282.

69. Pennock JM, Cowan FM, Schweiso JE *et al.* (1994) Clinical role of diffusion weighted imaging: neonatal studies. *MAGMA* **2**, 273–278.

70. Pierpaoli C, Jezzard P, Basser PJ *et al.* Diffusion tensor imaging of the human brain. *Radiology* **201**, 637–648.

71. Prenger ER, Beckett WW, Kollias SS *et al.* (1994) Comparison of T2-weighted spin-echo and fast spin-echo techniques in the evaluation of myelination. *J Magn Res Imaging* **4**, 179–184.

72. Robertson RL, Ben-Sira L, Barnes PD *et al.* (1999) MR line-scan diffusion-weighted imaging of term neonates with perinatal brain ischemia. *Am J Neuroradiol* **20**, 1658–1670.

73. Rutherford M, Cowan F, Manzur AY *et al.* (1991) MR imaging of anisotropically restricted diffusion in the brain of neonates and infants. *J Comput Assist Tomogr* **15**, 188–198.

74. Rutherford MA, Pennock JM, Schwieso JE *et al.* (1995) Hypoxic ischaemic encephalopathy: early magnetic resonance imaging findings and their evolution. *Neuropediatrics* **26**, 183–191.

75. Rutherford MA, Pennock J, Schweizo JE *et al.* (1996) Hypoxic–ischaemic encephalopathy: early and late magnetic resonance imaging findings in relation to outcome. *Arch Dis Child* **75**, F145–151.

76. Rutherford MA, Pennock J, Cowan FM *et al.* (1997) Detection of subtle changes in the brains of infants and children via subvoxel registration and subtraction of serial MR images. *Am J Neuroradiol* **18**, 829–835.

77. Rutherford MA, Pennock J, Counsell S *et al.* (1998) Abnormal magnetic resonance signal in the internal capsule predicts poor neurodevelopmental outcome in infants with hypoxic–ischaemic encephalopathy. *Pediatrics* **202**, 323–328.

78. Schmidt F, Penka B, Trauner M *et al.* (1995) Lack of pineal growth during childhood. *J Clin Endocrinol Metab* **80**, 1221–1225.

79. Sie LT, van der Knaap MS, van Wezel-Meijler G *et al.* (1997) MRI assessment of myelination of motor and sensory pathways in the brain of preterm and term-born infants. *Neuropediatrics* **28**, 97–105.

80. Stricker T, Martin E and Boesch C (1990) Development of the human cerebellum observed with high-field-strength MR imaging. *Radiology* **177**, 431–435.

81. Sumida M, Barkovich AJ and Newton TH (1996) Development of the pineal gland: measurement with MR. *Am J Neuroradiol* **17**, 233–236.

82. Takeda K, Nomura Y, Sakuma H *et al.* (1997) MR assessment of normal brain development in neonates and infants: comparative study of T1- and diffusion-weighted images. *J Comput Assist Tomogr* **21**, 1–7.

83. Tanaka S, Mito T and Takashima S (1995) Progress of myelination in the human fetal spinal nerve roots, spinal cord and brainstem with myelin basic protein immunohistochemistry. *Early Hum Dev* **41**, 49–59.

84. Thornton JS, Ordidge RJ, Penrice J *et al.* (1998) Temporal and anatomical variations of brain water apparent diffusion coefficient in perinatal cerebral hypoxic–ischemic injury: relationships to cerebral energy metabolism. *Magn Reson Med* **39**, 920–927.

85. Tofts PB, Leth H, Peitersen B *et al.* (1996) The apparent diffusion coefficient of water in gray and white matter of the infant brain. *J Comput Assist Tomogr* **20**, 1006–1011.

86. van der Knaap MS and Valk J (1990) MR imaging of the various stages of normal myelination during the first year of life. *Neuroradiology* **31**, 459–470.

87. van der Knaap MS and Valk J (1991) Myelination as an expression of the functional maturity of the brain. *Dev Med Child Neurol* **33**, 849–857.

88. van der Knaap MS and Valk J (1995) *Magnetic Resonance of Myelin, Myelination and Myelin Disorders*, 2nd edn. Berlin, Springer, pp. 1–17 and 31–52.

89. van Wezel-Meijler G, van der Knaap MS, Sie LTL *et al.* (1998) Magnetic resonance imaging of the brain in premature infants during the neonatal period. *Neuropediatrics* **29**, 89–96.

90. Wimberger DM, Roberts TP, Barkovich AJ *et al.* (1995) Identification of 'premyelination' by diffusion-weighted MRI. *J Comput Assist Tomogr* **19**, 28–33.

91. Wolpert XM, Osborne M, Anderson M *et al.* (1988) Bright pituitary gland: a normal MR appearance in infancy. *Am J Neuroradiol* **9**, 1–3.

92. Yakovlev PI and Lecours AR (1967) The myelogenetic cycles of regional maturation of the brain. In: Minkowski A (Ed.) *Regional Development of the Brain in Early Life*. Oxford, Blackwell, pp. 3–70.

93. Yamada H, Sadato N, Konoshi Y *et al.* (1997) A rapid brain metabolic change in infants detected by fMRI. *Neuroreport* **8**, 3775–3778.

Part III

Pathology

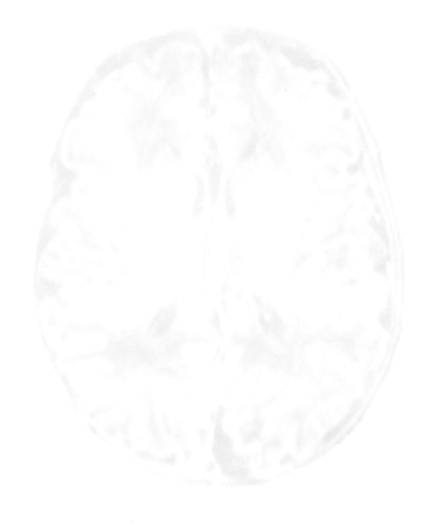

Basic cellular reactions of the immature human brain

5

Waney Squier

Contents

Introduction

An understanding of basic neuropathological processes is fundamental to the interpretation of brain scans. In this chapter basic cellular reactions to injury of the developing human brain are described, with special reference to those processes which may be identified on scans.

Those patterns of injury most characteristic of, and most frequently seen in, the developing brain are described. They have to be interpreted in the light of the changing anatomy of the developing brain. For a comprehensive atlas of the anatomy of the immature brain the reader is referred to Feess-Higgins and Larroche[8].

This chapter deals with reactive processes to a variety of insults. Although hypoxic–ischemic injury (HII) may be a very common cause of damage to the developing brain it is clear that many other insults play a part in prenatal brain damage[3]. These include maternal and fetal infections, iodine deficiency and genetic, including metabolic, diseases.

The postmortem examination

WHY PERFORM A POSTMORTEM EXAMINATION?

- To establish a cause of death
- To diagnose disease
- To assess therapy
- To audit new imaging techniques
- To further understanding of normal and abnormal brain development
- Informed consent for brain retention is required.

Until the last two decades the importance of postmortem examination of the fetus and neonate has been underestimated.

The primary purpose of postmortem examination is to establish a cause of death and to diagnose disease. It can reveal pathology too subtle to be identified by clinical investigations or imaging.

Full examination of all organs, including the placenta, will reveal generalized disease processes which may have detrimental effects on brain development. Examination of the placenta is of particular importance; recent studies show an association of placental pathology, particularly infection, with developmental brain damage[11,12].

Complete postmortem examination requires detailed macroscopic and microscopic examination of the brain. This involves retention of the brain with the informed consent of the parents.

The brain has to be fixed before it can be adequately examined. In small fetuses the brain is very soft and collapses readily on handling and is best preserved by fixation *in situ*. This not only ensures optimal brain fixation but also preserves the relationships of the intracranial structures (Fig. 5.1). In older fetuses (after 30 weeks) and neonates the brain can be removed at postmortem and then fixed for at least 2–3 weeks before macroscopic examination. Blocks are taken and embedded in wax prior to cutting sections and staining for microscopic study.

The most widely used stain in light microscopy is hematoxylin and eosin (H&E). Luxol fast blue and cresyl violet (LBCV), another standard neuropathological method, stains nuclei, RNA and myelin. This stain is less useful in the fetal brain where myelin is sparse.

Immunocytochemical methods employ labelled antibodies to detect specific tissue antigens. These are currently widely used to identify specific cell types and their products.

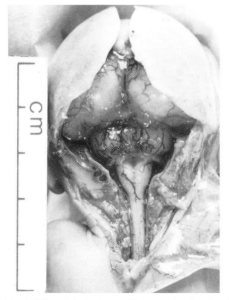

Fig. 5.1 Fetal brain (20 weeks) fixed *in situ*. The posterior fossa has been opened from behind. The anatomy of the hindbrain and its position within the skull is readily seen. Malformations or displacement of hindbrain structures are readily recognized if the brain is examined in this way.

ARTIFACTS

Human tissue is extremely subject to artifactual change. This is because the brain undergoes postmortem autolysis or maceration following death *in utero* or if there is a delay between death and postmortem.

Commonly encountered artifacts include tissue vacuolation, which occurs in macerated brains and is readily confused with edema. Maceration causes cells to break up and nuclei to fragment; these fragments are small and irregular and readily distinguished from karyorrhexis. In many immature brains large areas of ependyma may be shed. This must be distinguished from pathological ependymal loss with associated gliosis.

Cellular reactions of the human brain

- Edema (1 h)
- Cell death: necrosis: apoptosis (1–12 h)
- Gliosis (from 3 days)
- Phagocytosis (from 3 days)
- Capillary proliferation (3–8 days)
- Mineralization (from 1 week)
- Ependymal reaction (2–3 days).

Following injury to the developing brain a series of cellular reactions is set in action, the speed and intensity of these reactions being dependent on the age at the time of injury. Histological examination of the brain in the weeks following injury will allow precise timing, based on the stage of the reactive processes. Some of these cellular reactions leave scars in the brain which persist and are detectable on scans in later life.

EDEMA

The immature brain swells rapidly, within an hour of severe injury. Edema is due to swelling of cell bodies, particularly astrocytes and to accumulation of fluid in the interstitial spaces following leakage through damaged capillary endothelium. Brain swelling causes compression of the lateral ventricles and the cortical sulci. Owing to the ample space around the immature brain and unfused skull sutures herniation is rare in infants.

CELL DEATH

Two main forms of cell death are recognized (Fig. 5.2). The passive form of death is *necrosis*. The cell membrane loses its integrity, calcium floods into the cell and the cytoplasm becomes bright pink in H&E stains. The nuclear membrane

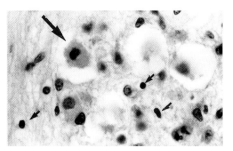

Fig. 5.2 Cell death. A large neuron is dying by necrosis (*arrow*). The cytoplasm stains deeply with eosin, the nucleus has lost all structure and is undergoing lysis. Several adjacent cells show the features of apoptosis with shrunken, rounded and intensely staining nuclei. (*small arrows*) (H&E × 450.)

breaks down with lysis of nuclear chromatin. Necrosis is seen within hours of insult. *Apoptosis* is an active form of cell death mediated by a cascade of intracellular enzyme reactions terminating in breakdown of nuclear DNA. The histological appearances are distinctive. Within hours of injury the nucleus becomes shrunken and rounded and is intensely, uniformly basophilic, appearing deep blue in H&E stains. This appearance is known as *pyknosis*. Subsequently, the nucleus breaks up into a number of rounded fragments or apoptotic bodies. This appearance is termed *karyorrhexis*. Apoptosis is the mechanism of programmed cell death by which cells produced in excess during normal brain development are removed.

GLIOSIS

Astrocytes (the cells responsible for reactive gliosis) have been demonstrated in human brain sections by immunocytochemistry at 15 weeks' gestation[18]. A vigorous glial response can occur as early as 18 weeks' gestation (Fig. 5.3).

Reactive astrocytes are identified within 3 days of an insult; in the early stages they have ample cytoplasm and few processes; dense fibrillary gliosis takes weeks to appear.

PHAGOYCTOSIS

Macrophages are cells which ingest and remove debris from areas of tissue injury and contribute to cyst formation. They develop from microglia, the intrinsic macrophage population of the brain. The earliest reactive changes are seen within hours of injury but mature macrophages with large amounts of cytoplasm containing ingested debris are not seen until several days after injury (Fig. 5.4). They may persist for months or years.

Following hemorrhage, macrophages begin to ingest red cells within 3 or 4 days (Fig. 5.5). Red cells are identified within the cytoplasm where they are degraded and change

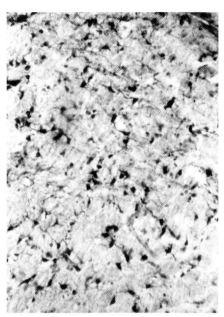

Fig. 5.3 Gliosis. Deep white matter adjacent to an area of trauma in a fetus of 18 weeks. There are many reactive astrocytes, intensely stained for glial fibrillary acidic protein (GFAP). (GFAP × 200.)

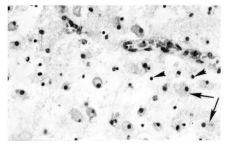

Fig. 5.4 Recent infarction. The tissue is becoming cystic. Many macrophages with large rounded masses of cytoplasm and small nuclei are seen (*arrow*). There are also shrunken, pyknotic glial cells (*arrowhead*). The capillary has plump, reactive endothelial cells. (H&E × 220.)

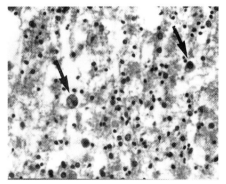

Fig. 5.5 Hemorrhagic infarction. White matter undergoing hemorrhagic infarction. White matter adjacent to a germinal matrix hemorrhage shows cystic breakdown and pyknosis in most of the cells. Macrophages are numerous – two indicated with arrows contain red cells in their cytoplasm. (H&E × 220.)

from red to brown in color. Iron pigment may be demonstrated within macrophages months and years after a bleed (see Chapter 9).

CAPILLARY PROLIFERATION

Capillary endothelium is extremely sensitive to hypoxic–ischemic injury. In the first days after injury the cells become thicker with rounded nuclei; after 5–8 days new capillaries proliferate. Capillary proliferation in the ischemic cerebral cortex is responsible for the MR imaging appearance of 'cortical highlighting' (Fig. 5.6) (see Chapter 6).

MINERALIZATION

Mineral deposition occurs readily in damaged areas of the fetal brain (Fig. 5.7). It is seen within 1 week of injury and

appears in H&E stained sections as deep blue granules in cell bodies and on nerve processes. It persists for many years. Mineral deposition is responsible for the chalky white color of lesions of periventricular leukomalacia when seen by the naked eye and is characteristic of viral infections when it is widely distributed in areas of damage throughout the brain. Mineralization of the deep cerebral nuclei, especially the thalamus, is seen following old ischemic injury.

EPENDYMAL REACTION

The ependyma is a single layer of epithelium which lines all the cerebrospinal fluid (CSF) pathways of the brain. Damage to the ependyma causes focal loss and reactive proliferation of the underlying glial cells. This response causes narrowing of CSF pathways. Abortive regeneration of ependyma forms rosettes buried in the reactive glial tissue (Fig. 5.8).

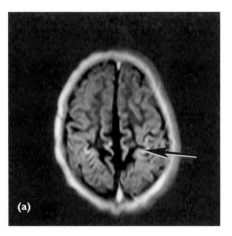

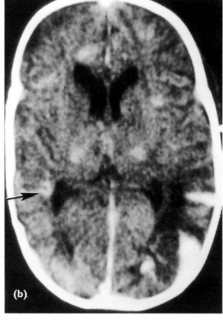

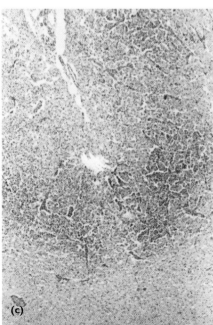

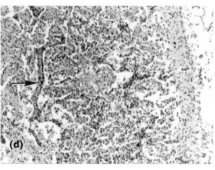

Fig. 5.6 Cortical highlighting. **(a)** T1 weighted (SE 860/20) MR scan of 2-week-old infant with stage II hypoxic–ischemic encephalopathy (HIE) showing areas of abnormal high signal intensity within the cortex (*arrow*). **(b)** CT scan of a 4-month-old child 9 days after trauma and cardiac arrest. The cortex is bright, particularly in the depths of sulci (*arrow*). **(c)** Histology of a corresponding area of the cortex shows tissue necrosis with increased cellularity due to gliosis and prominent capillaries, particularly in the depths of sulci. The increased vascularity causes cortical highlighting in scans. (H&E × 25.) **(d)** At higher power branching, proliferating capillaries are seen in necrotic cortex (*arrow*). (H&E × 45.)

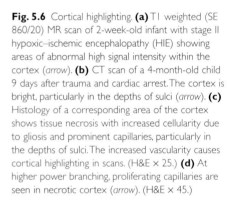

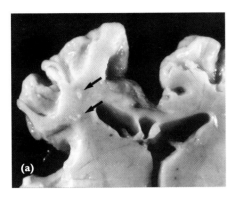

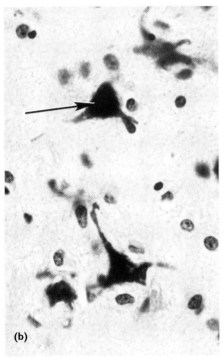

Fig. 5.7 Mineralization. (a) Small cysts in the deep white matter in periventricular leukomalacia (*arrows*). The edge is chalky white due to mineralization. (b) Thalamus in an infant surviving several years after severe asphyxia. There are several calcified nerve cells (*arrow*). (H&E × 450.)

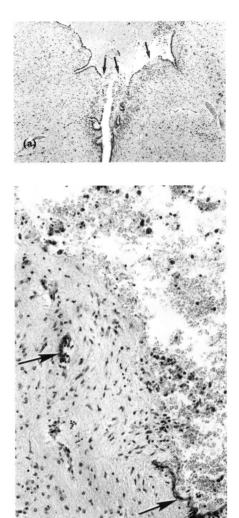

Fig. 5.8 Ependymal reaction. (a) Damaged ependyma in the fourth ventricle. The surface epithelium has been shed in several places (*arrows*). There is fresh blood in the lumen. (H&E × 120.) (b) Higher power picture shows gliotic tissue bulging through ependymal defects. There are fragments of ependyma in this gliotic tissue (*arrows*). (H&E × 200.)

Hemorrhages (see also Chapters 9 and 13)

- Subdural – term infants – trauma
- Subarachnoid – preterm and term – ischemia
- Parenchymal – rare, severe – multiple etiologies
- Periventricular/intraventricular – sick preterm infants – association with parenchymal hemorrhagic infarction.

SUBDURAL HAEMORRHAGE

Hemorrhage into the subdural space typically occurs in term infants and is usually the result of trauma. It results from tearing of superficial veins or sinuses on the surface of the brain. Blood clot in the subdural space gradually liquifies from the center. The edges of the clot are invaded by fibroblasts and capillaries and by 10 days the clot is reduced to a brown vascular membrane. The delicate new capillaries of the membrane may rebleed after even minor trauma.

Macrophages ingest and break down red cells and may remain for months. This explains the low signal intensity from hemosiderin on T2 weighted images which persists for months from a perinatal hemorrhagic lesion (see Chapter 9). The altered blood pigment stains the surface of the brain bright orange or yellow.

SUBARACHNOID HEMORRHAGE

Primary subarachnoid hemorrhage is commonly encountered in premature infants at postmortem but rarely identified with imaging. It is usually mild. It forms a thin, diffuse film over the brain surface. Secondary subarachnoid hemorrhage results from subarachnoid spread of intraventricular blood and forms large collections in the basal subarachnoid spaces. Subarachnoid hemorrhage in the term infant is usually related to severe hypoxia–ischemia or to trauma and may be extensive.

PARENCHYMAL HEMORRHAGE

This is uncommon and may be due to a variety of causes including severe trauma, infections, vasculitis or rupture of a vascular malformation. Parenchymal hemorrhage arising *in utero* may be due to a clotting disorder such as alloimmune thrombocytopenia.

PERIVENTRICULAR GERMINAL MATRIX/ INTRAVENTRICULAR HEMORRHAGE

Periventricular and intraventricular bleeding is characteristic of the sick premature infant and usually occurs within the first 12–72 h of life, but is also observed in a proportion of stillborn infants.

The germinal matrix is the usual source of bleeding. This consists of a dense mass of proliferating cells abundantly supplied with thin-walled capillaries. By 36 weeks' gestation the matrix involutes and periventricular hemorrhage is less common. A small proportion of intraventricular bleeds originate in the choroid plexus, usually in term infants (see Chapter 9). Autoregulation of the cerebral circulation is disturbed in the sick premature infant[17] and the capillary network then becomes susceptible to sudden fluctuations in systemic blood pressure.

GERMINAL MATRIX HEMORRHAGE

Periventricular hemorrhages may be small and confined to the matrix or may rupture through the ependyma into the lateral ventricles (Fig. 5.9).

Matrix hemorrhages are often multiple and bilateral. They tend to occur over the body of the caudate nucleus in very small infants and more anteriorly, at the level of the foramen of Monroe, in infants over 28 weeks.

Localized masses of blood clot undergo evolution over the days and weeks after they occur with central lysis of the clot and invasion of the periphery by macrophages in the first 2–3 days. After prolonged survival the only residual findings

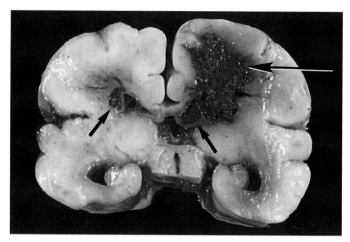

Fig. 5.9 Periventricular–intraventricular hemorrhage. Coronal slice of fixed fetal brain, 24 weeks' gestation. There are bilateral germinal matrix hemorrhages (*arrows*) with intraventricular extension. On the right side a large area of hemorrhagic parenchymal infarction fans out from the germinal matrix hemorrhage (*arrow*).

may be granules of iron pigment, sometimes within macrophages or persistence of a smooth-walled subependymal cyst at the site of the original bleed[7]. Whilst old hemorrhage is easily identified on T2 weighted MR images, subependymal cysts are more difficult to detect.

Alterations in the windowing of the MR images may increase the detection of these cysts, which are usually clearly visible on cranial ultrasound.

INTRAVENTRICULAR HEMORRHAGE

Blood rupturing into the lateral ventricles may be confined to one side or, if more extensive, will spread throughout the ventricular system, through the narrow aqueduct of Sylvius in the mid-brain and into the fourth ventricle. From here blood escapes into the subarachnoid cisterns beneath the brain and cerebellum and surrounds the brain stem. Eventually, blood is washed over the surface of the brain in the CSF and reabsorbed in the arachnoid villi of the sagittal sinus.

Blood in the CSF prompts a brisk reaction in the ependyma and underlying tissues (Fig. 5.8). The ependyma is shed and underlying glial cells proliferate and form masses which protrude into the lumen. Proliferating ependymal cells form rosettes within these gliotic masses which may also contain pigment-bearing macrophages. Narrow parts of the CSF pathways, including the mid-brain aqueduct and the exit foramina of the fourth ventricle, may be obstructed by this reaction and impede the flow of CSF leading to hydrocephalus. When the mid-brain aqueduct is narrowed the lateral and third ventricles dilate. If the exit foramina of the fourth ventricle are obstructed then the lateral, third and fourth ventricles dilate. If blood causes reactive gliosis in the arachnoid villi then resorption of CSF is impaired and there is dilatation of both the intra- and extracerebral CSF spaces causing communicating hydrocephalus.

PARENCHYMAL HEMORRHAGIC INFARCTION

The most serious consequence of germinal matrix/intraventricular hemorrhage is parenchymal hemorrhagic infarction which carries a much more serious prognosis than germinal matrix hemorrhage alone. Parenchymal hemorrhagic infarction occurs in the white matter adjacent to a matrix bleed. The fan-shaped lesion consists of clusters of perivenous hemorrhages extending along veins draining the centrum semiovale (Fig 5.5 and 5.9). The parenchyma is infarcted and, in infants who survive, it is gradually reabsorbed leading to unilateral dilatation of the lateral ventricle (see Figs 9.28f and 9.29a). This distinguishes the lesion from periventricular leukomalacia, which more commonly leads to symmetrical posterior dilatation of the lateral ventricles, which are irregular and 'squared off' in outline (see Chapter 8)[21]. Occasionally, particularly in association with infection, the two conditions appear to co-exist (see Figs 10.8g,h).

White matter damage

■ Multiple etiologies – perfusion failure – hypoxia – infection – inflammation – metabolic disease.
■ Periventricular leukomalacia (PVL) – diffuse with white matter atrophy and gliosis (telencephalic leukoencephalopathy). Focal infarcts of classical PVL. Typically seen between 28 and 36 weeks but can also arise at term.
■ Multicystic leukomalacia – multiple cysts, periventricular or subcortical. Usually associated with abrupt severe interference in blood supply between 30 and 44 weeks. May be mimicked by herpes encephalitis.
■ Posterior limb of the internal capsule.

The white matter is particularly vulnerable to damage between 28 and 36 weeks' gestation. This has usually been ascribed to ischemia due to a tenuous vascular supply but recent studies have shown that the deep white matter has an extensive vascular network[13]. At this stage of development the white matter is undergoing active myelination and the immature oligodendrocytes responsible for myelin synthesis are actively migrating into the area. The vulnerability of those cells to free radical damage may explain white matter damage[1].

Although hypoxia–ischemia may be a common cause of white matter damage it is becoming increasingly apparent

that many other conditions are associated with prenatal cerebral damage[3] Maternal infections have been implicated for some years[10] and recent studies have further supported the role of maternal or placental infection with white matter lesions, possibly mediated by cytokines[5,6,23].

Prenatal white matter damage takes several forms which are related both to the age at insult and the nature of the insult.

PERIVENTRICULAR LEUKOMALACIA

This term encompasses a spectrum of white matter damage, from mild but diffuse injury (sometimes termed telencephalic encephalopathy) to focal areas of cystic infarction. It is a pathological term and its use to describe a variety of imaging appearances is being actively discouraged.

In diffuse leukomalacia the white matter shows only subtle alteration on naked eye examination. The blood vessels are prominent and occasionally flanked by small yellow streaks or patches. Histology shows diffuse infiltration with plump reactive astrocytes and macrophages. Capillaries have thickened endothelium in the early stages and later proliferate[20]. In the chronic stage the white matter is reduced in volume and shows dense fibrillary gliosis. This pattern of injury is probably the result of mild chronic insult (Fig. 5.10).

In more severe leukomalacia focal infarcts appear as white spots several millimeters in diameter, most frequently seen in the deep frontal and parietal white matter (Fig. 5.7a), but also seen in the occipital lobes.

The earliest stage in the microscopical formation of these lesions is an irregular zone of 'coagulation necrosis' in which the tissue loses detailed structure and becomes hyaline and eosinophilic. Nuclei within these zones are pyknotic (Figs 5.11 and 5.12). Later, reactive astrocytes and macrophages

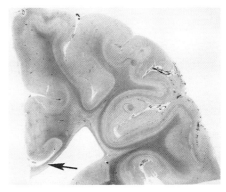

Fig. 5.10 Old periventricular leukomalacia. Section of the hemisphere of a child with cerebral palsy, stained for myelin (LBCV). The deep white matter is reduced in volume and pale due to gliosis. Note the thin corpus callosum (*arrow*) and the dilated square-shaped lateral ventricle.

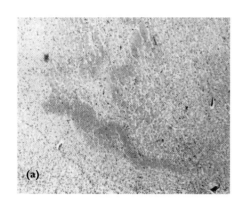

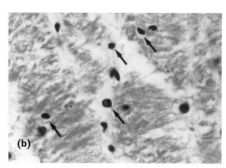

Fig. 5.11 Coagulation necrosis. **(a)** An irregular zone of the white matter stains deeply in an H&E preparation. (× 12.) **(b)** At higher power it can be seen that most of the nuclei in this zone are pyknotic with condensed, deeply staining chromatin (*arrows*). (H&E × 450.)

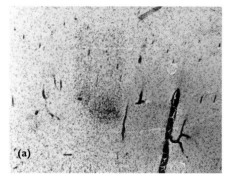

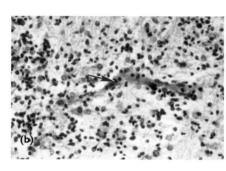

Fig. 5.12 Periventricular leukomalacia (PVL). **(a)** Low power of white matter showing early features of PVL. Capillaries are prominent and congested and there is focal hypercellularity. (H&E × 25.) **(b)** Higher power image shows a reactive capillary with plump endothelial cells (*arrow*) and increased numbers of glial cells and macrophages in the adjacent white matter. (H&E × 230.)

appear in these infarcted zones. Axons around them show rounded 'retraction balls', eosinophilic masses which represent the proximal ends of severed axons. Amyloid precursor protein (APP) is demonstrated in these structures. Mineralization around the periphery of those lesions gives them their chalky appearance (Fig. 5.7a). The central area contains macrophages, which eventually ingest necrotic debris leading to central cavitation.

MULTICYSTIC LEUKOMALACIA

The damaged white matter breaks down into multiple cystic cavities, often predominantly subcortical (Fig. 5.13). The cyst walls consist of glial fibers, and white matter is severely reduced in volume. There is extensive neuronal loss in the overlying cortex, the deep gray nuclei and brain stem are also gliotic. Most cases with a documented history seem to occur following abrupt interference in cerebral blood supply between 30 and 44 weeks' gestation.

POSTERIOR LIMB OF THE INTERNAL CAPSULE

Attention has been drawn to this structure in hypoxic–ischemic damage in neonates by the striking changes identified on MRI scans. In cases where pathology has been correlated with MRI appearances the changes are less striking under the microscope. There is severe edema with little cellular change (Fig. 5.14). Edema in a tightly packed fiber bundle may cause changes of a mechanical nature which are responsible for the MRI appearance[9].

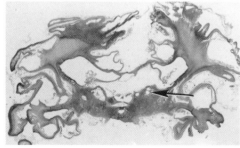

Fig. 5.13 Multicystic leukomalacia. Coronal section of brain. The subcortical white matter has been almost totally replaced by huge cysts. There are smaller cysts in the thalamus, which is shrunken and gliotic (*arrow*).

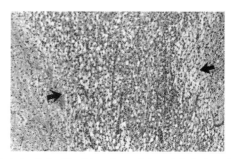

Fig. 5.14 Posterior limb of the internal capsule in an infant whose MRI scan showed marked signal change. The fiber bundle (*between arrows*) shows intense edema, represented by multiple tiny spaces. (H&E × 45.)

Gray matter damage

- Cerebral cortex – mature infants – watershed zones – ulegyria
- Deep gray nuclei – thalamus and lentiform nuclei – status marmoratus
- Brain stem.

CEREBRAL CORTEX

The cerebral cortex is damaged by an insult of sufficient severity at any stage but it is characteristically most vulnerable in the term infant. Damage commonly involves the watershed areas: those are the end fields of supply of the major cerebral arteries. The parasagittal cortex is particularly frequently involved. The hippocampus may also suffer.

As in other brain areas the damaged cortex undergoes a stereotyped sequence of cellular reactions. Capillary proliferation in the cortex is often found with abundant capillaries growing in from the adjacent leptomeninges. This accounts for the characteristic appearance of cortical highlighting seen on scans 1 week after injury (Fig. 5.6).

Within the cortex further regional vulnerability is seen. The depths of sulci are particularly likely to be damaged in the mature infant (see Fig. 6.9 and Figs 6.19–6.21). As the lesions evolve the cortex in the depths becomes atrophic while the spared crests of gyri retain their normal thickness (Fig. 5.15). These give a macroscopical appearance likened to 'mushroom gyri' and termed ulegyria. This lesion is not described in the immature cortex.

DEEP GRAY NUCLEI

The thalamus and lentiform nuclei are particularly vulnerable to HII. This form of damage occurs at term[19] in infants with severe acute insults following, for example, placental abruption. It does occur in very much younger infants[4] and may occur antenatally[14]. The exact site of damage within the basal ganglia and thalami appears to be different in the preterm infant[2].

The histological appearances are of cell death, reactive gliosis and capillary proliferation and mineralization. In long-term survivors there is atrophy of these structures, which are densely gliotic. Calcified neuronal profiles may persist (Fig. 5.7b).

STATUS MARMORATUS

Some infants who survive asphyxial damage may show a further peculiar appearance in the deep nuclei. The shrunken nuclei contain irregular bundles of myelinated fibers. This change does not develop at once but only occurs after 6–9 months when active myelination of the deep cerebral structures occurs.

The appearances of status marmoratus on MR imaging have not been described (Fig. 6.20).

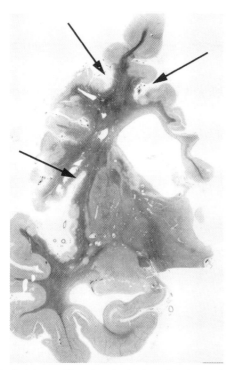

Fig. 5.15 Cortical damage. There is extensive loss of cortex particularly in the depths of sulci: ulegyria (*arrows*). There has also been loss of white matter with some subcortical cysts. Note the large square lateral ventricle.

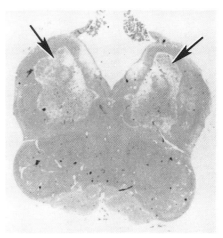

Fig. 5.16 Cardiac arrest encephalopathy. There is symmetrical necrosis of the tegmental nuclei in the medulla (*arrow*), 3 weeks after a severe hypoxic–ischemic episode.

BRAIN STEM

The brain stem nuclei mature very early and are vulnerable to HII. Intrauterine HII to these nuclei is one of the causes of Moebius syndrome.

A striking pattern of brain stem necrosis occurs following acute and total failure of blood supply (cardiac arrest encephalopathy)[16]. There is symmetrical, bilateral necrosis of the nuclei running throughout the entire length of the brain stem (Fig. 5.16). It is usually associated with lesions elsewhere, particularly in the deep cerebral nuclei.

Malformations (see Chapter 11)

HII is one of the recognized causes of malformation of the brain. For this to occur the insult must occur during the first two trimesters when the brain structures are developing. Malformations of the cortex, such as polymicrogyria, may be seen in watershed territories or on the edges of infarcts arising before 28 weeks[22]. Insults occurring before 20 weeks interfere with neuronal migration leading to cortical malformation as well as heterotopic neuronal masses in the white matter due to failed migration.

Infections (see Chapter 10)

Viral infections of the developing brain are well recognized. Their effects include neuronal necrosis, gliosis and calcification, which can be very dense and diffuse. Infections in the first two trimesters may cause malformations such as polymicrogryia. The pattern of damage is related to the gestational age at the time of infection as well as the specific agent.

Cytomegalovirus

Cytomegalovirus is the most common viral infection in the developing brain, involving endothelial cells as well as neurons and glial cells. The virus frequently causes poly-microgyria due to its effects on the vascular endothelium[15]. There is frequently a dense band of calcification in the periventricular tissues.

Herpes simplex

Herpes simplex is rare *in utero* but may be acquired at birth or in the neonatal period. The effects on the brain are devastating with widespread cystic damage and parenchymal hemorrhage. The appearances on scan may be mistaken for extensive HII following trauma or shaking (Fig. 10.8).

Bacterial infections

Bacterial infections are uncommon *in utero*, but Listeria is occasionally seen. It causes granulomatous vascular lesions with small focal infarctions (see Fig. 10.17).

Candida

Candida is the commonest cerebral infection in the neonate. The typical case shows widespread lesions up to half a centimeter in diameter and sometimes cystic, so-called small microabscesses, throughout the cerebral parenchyma, not in a vascular distribution (Fig. 5.17). The organism is readily demonstrated with histological stains as are the presence of microabscesses.

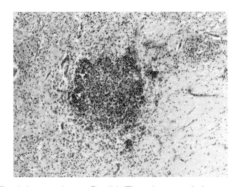

Fig. 5.17 Focal damage due to Candida. There is a rounded mass of cells, reactive glia and macrophages, in the deep white matter. (H&E × 45.)

Summary

- Postmortem examination is necessary to define pathological processes in the developing brain.
- An understanding of normal and abnormal brain development is essential to the interpretation of brain scans.
- The brain undergoes a sequence of reactive cellular changes following injury, the nature and severity of which depend on age at insult.
- The patterns of damage show some dependency on age: white matter damage is characteristic of the immature brain while the cortex is vulnerable in the term infant.
- Damage in the first two trimesters may cause malformation.

References

1. Back SA, Gan X, Li Y *et al.* (1998) Maturation-dependent vulnerability of oligodendrocytes to oxidative stress-induced death caused by glutathione depletion. *J Neurosci* **18(16)**, 6241–6253.
2. Barkovich AJ and Sargent SK (1995) Profound asphyxia in the premature infant: imaging findings. *Am J Neuroradiol* **16**, 1837–1846.
3. Blair E (1996) Obstetric antecedents of cerebral palsy. *Fetal and Maternal Medicine Review* **8**, 199–215.
4. Cohen M and Roessman U (1994) *In utero* brain damage: relationship of gestational age to pathological consequences. *Dev Med Child Neurol* **36**, 263–270.
5. Dammann O and Leviton A (1997) Maternal intrauterine infection, cytokines, and brain damage in the preterm newborn. *Pediatr Res* **42(1)**, 1–8.
6. Dammann O and Leviton A (1998) Infection remote from the brain, neonatal white matter damage, and cerebral palsy in the preterm infant. *Semin Pediatr Neurol* **5(3)**, 190–201.
7. Darrow VC, Alvord EC, Mack LA *et al.* (1988) Histologic evolution of the reactions to haemorrhage in the premature human infant's brain. *Am J Pathol* **130**, 44–58.
8. Feess-Higgins A and Larroche J-C (1987) *Development of Human Foetal Brain: An Anatomical Atlas.* Paris, Masson.
9. Felderhoff-Mueser U, Rutherford MA, Squier WV *et al.* (1999) Relation between magnetic resonance images and histopathological findings of the brain in extremely preterm infants. *AJNR Am J Neuroradiol* **20(7)**, 1349–1357.
10. Gilles FH, Leviton A and Dooling EC (1983) *The Developing Human Brain, Growth and Epidemiologic Neuropathology.* Boston, John Wright.
11. Grafe M (1994) The correlation of prenatal brain damage with placental pathology. *J Neuropath Exp Neurol* **53**, 407–415.
12. Hansen A, Leviton A, Paneth N *et al.* (1998) The correlation between placental pathology and intraventricular hemorrhage in the preterm infant. *Pediatr Res* **43(1)**, 15–19.
13. Kuban KCK and Gilles FH (1985) Human telancephalic angiogenesis. *Ann Neurol* **17**, 539–548.
14. Maalouf E, Battin M, Counsell S *et al.* (1997) Arthrogryposis multiplex congenita and bilateral midbrain infarction following maternal overdose of coproxamol. *Europ J Paed Neurol* **5/6**, 1–4.
15. Marques Dias MJ, Harmant van Rijckevorsel G, Landrieu P *et al.* (1984) Prenatal cytomegalovirus disease and cerebral microgyria: evidence for perfusion failure, not disturbance of histogenesis, as the major cause of micropolygyria in CMV fetal encephalopathies of circulatory origin. *Biol Neonate* **50**, 61–74.
16. Pasternak JF (1993) Hypoxic–ischemic brain damage in the term infant. *Pediatr Clin N Am* **4**, 1061–1072.
17. Pryds O and Edwards AD (1996) Cerebral blood flow in the newborn infant. *Arch Dis Child* **74**, F63–F69.
18. Roessmann U and Gambetti P (1986) Pathological reaction of astrocytes in perinatal brain injury. *Acta Neuropathol (Berl)* **70**, 302–307.
19. Rutherford M, Pennock J, Schwieso J *et al.* (1996) Hypoxic–ischaemic encephalopathy: early and late magnetic resonance imaging findings in relation to outcome. *Arch Dis Child Health* **75**, F145–F151.
20. Squier MV and Keeling JW (1991) The incidence of prenatal brain injury. *Neuropathol Appl Neurobiol* **17**, 29–38.
21. Volpe JJ (1989) Intraventricular haemorrhage in the premature infant – current concepts. Part 1. *Ann Neurol* **25**, 3–11.
22. Williams RS, Ferrante RJ and Caviness VS (1976) The cellular pathology of microgyria. *Acta Neuropathol (Berl)* **36**, 269–283.
23. Yoon BH, Romero R, Kim CJ *et al.* (1997) High expression of tumor necrosis factor-alpha and interleukin-6 in periventricular leukomalacia. *Am J Obstet Gynecol* **177(2)**, 406–411.

Part IV

Disorders in the newborn infant

The asphyxiated term infant

Mary A Rutherford

6

Contents

Hypoxic–ischemic encephalopathy

Infants who have been asphyxiated during delivery may develop signs of hypoxic–ischemic encephalopathy (HIE). This term is used to describe mature neonates (gestation >37 weeks) who show signs of fetal distress prior to delivery, who have abnormal Apgar scores and require resuscitation at birth and who show specific neurological abnormalities during the first 24 h after delivery. Signs of fetal distress include abnormal cardiotocograph recordings such as decreased variability, late decelerations (type II dips), and a baseline bradycardia <100/min with or without meconium-stained liquor. A fetal scalp pH of less than 7.2 is also indicative of fetal hypoxia, although values of <7.0 are usually found. Abnormal neurological signs in HIE include feeding difficulties, irritability, abnormalities of tone, convulsions and a decreased conscious level. The severity of HIE may be graded as stage I, II or III according to Sarnat and Sarnat[38]. Classification is difficult in ventilated infants and those receiving anticonvulsant medication. Even when all the criteria for HIE are fulfilled it may still be difficult to attribute an infant's clinical signs as solely due to hypoxia/ischemia. A pre-existing neurological condition may predispose an infant to an abnormal delivery and/or a hypoxic–ischaemic insult and a screen for infection, metabolic disorders and congenital malformations is always warranted. Although preterm infants are at high risk of asphyxia, the HIE staging should be reserved for term infants. Despite improvements in perinatal care in the developed world, asphyxia remains a major cause of mortality, resulting in up to 25% of perinatal mortality and morbidity and giving rise to between 8 and 15% of all cases of cerebral palsy.

Imaging

Infants with signs of HIE may be scanned with three different techniques during the neonatal period: cranial ultrasound, computerized tomography (CT) and magnetic resonance imaging (MRI). Cranial ultrasound has the advantage of being mobile and easily used on the neonatal unit. It is ideal for doing daily or twice daily scans to follow the evolution of changes within the brain. As with all techniques, expertise is needed not only to obtain the correct scan views but more importantly to interpret the results correctly. This is most easily done at the time of scanning, although video replay provides a suitable method of retrospective review. It is exceedingly difficult to interpret paper reprints, particularly when they have been taken by a different operator. Cranial ultrasound is valuable for identifying cerebral edema and parenchymal or intraventricular hemorrhage. Areas of parenchymal infarction may take several days to be visualized as an echo density. Using a 5 MHz transducer to increase penetration, echo densities within the basal ganglia are easily visualized and are predictive of outcome[17,33] although they may take several days to become apparent. Using a 10 Mhz transducer allows identification of areas of cortical highlighting and subcortical white matter infarction[16]. Cranial ultrasound is very good at identifying cystic lesions within the parenchyma. Using the posterior fontanelle improves the ability of cranial ultrasound to detect lesions following HIE[14]. Cranial ultrasound will always provide a method for screening and monitoring the evolution of lesions but is not as good as MRI at determining the exact site, and extent of lesions. The combination of cranial ultrasound and MRI is ideal for assessing the newborn brain.

CT has the advantage that it is available in many hospitals and is relatively cheap. However, machines, as with MRI, are usually at a distance from the neonatal unit and CT scanning involves exposure to a significant amount of radiation. It is not therefore suitable for serial scanning. CT is good for identifying acute hemorrhage and this has been the one advantage over MRI. However, the ability of the MR to detect acute hemorrhage has improved with gradient echo sequences and it is now less justifiable to use CT to image neurologically abnormal infants. CT has been used to study infants with HIE[1] but there are very few recent studies. Decreased attenuation in the white matter during the second week from delivery has been associated with an abnormal outcome. A more recent study documented the presence of cortical abnormalities consistent with highlighting on MRI (see below) in infants with HIE[12]. In our experience CT is often unable to detect significant basal ganglia and thalamic lesions.

MRI is a relatively new technique but is becoming more widely available. In addition, a few MR suites are now being installed either within or adjacent to neonatal units. MR provides superb definition of the brain compared to both ultrasound and CT. It does not involve the use of radiation and is therefore suitable for serial scanning. It is multiplanar, which results in improved detection of lesions and better estimation of their exact site and size. MR data are readily quantifiable. A combination of ultrasound and MRI is ideal for assessing the neurologically abnormal neonate. Careful comparative studies between these techniques, ideally with additional histology, should result in MRI improving the abilities of cranial ultrasound to detect lesions rather than replacing it as an imaging technique.

MRI pulse sequences

Commercial scanners contain sequences that are appropriate for studying the adult brain but some sequences will need to be adapted for neonatal brain imaging (see Chapters 1 and 2). The choice of sequences used for an examination is limited by their availability and the duration of the scan. Infants may be clinically unstable, or sedation may wear off. For neonatal imaging we routinely used a T1 weighted spin echo (SE 860/20), a conventional T2 weighted spin echo (SE 2700/120) and an inversion recovery (IR 3800/30/950) sequence. In addition, we now perform a T2 weighted fast spin echo (SE 3000/208) sequence. Diffusion weighted imaging has been time consuming in the past but fast imaging has made this a practical addition to MRI examinations. Image resolution using fast diffusion weighted images may not be sufficient to produce adequate anatomical detail for mapping of white matter tracts but it is useful for the early identification of white matter infarction. There is little information about the role of contrast enhancement in infants with HIE. The appearances of the normal neonatal brain following contrast have been described[8] (see Chapter 4). Contrast may 'enhance' cortical abnormalities in HIE but there may also be confusion with the presence of contrast within cortical veins and in our experience the abnormality was always detectable prior to contrast administration. The use of contrast enhancement is essential if infection is suspected and as the diagnosis of HIE is not always clear cut there is an argument for using contrast routinely. Fluid attenuated inversion recovery (FLAIR) sequences have proved useful for the identification of both subarachnoid and intraventricular hemorrhage in adult patients but have not been systematically studied in the neonate[26]. The FLAIR sequence is useful after the first year of life for identifying abnormally increased T2 consistent with glial tissue (Fig. 6.11, cases 6.4 and 6.7). Proton density images may be useful in the first few days after delivery as abnormalities within the basal ganglia and thalami appear early[6]. This sequence may also provide early information on 'cortical edema'[6] or loss of gray/white matter differentiation. To date we have not found it more useful than early T1 and T2 weighted images. Adult fast imaging has shown the role of diffusion/perfusion sequences for identifying early ischemia. The role of perfusion weighted imaging in the neonate has yet to be established.

Patterns of injury

MRI has been widely used to investigate the asphyxiated infant[2,3,6,9,19,34-36]. The abnormalities identified on imaging will vary according to the magnet and sequences used and the postnatal age of the infant at the time of the scan. The pattern of injury seen on MRI is related to the type and severity of the insult. Severe acute asphyxia is associated with lesions in the basal ganglia, thalami, brain stem, hippocampus and the corticospinal tracts around the central fissure[3,23,27,28,30,31]. This has been termed central cortico–subcortical involvement. This is the most common pattern of injury following acute fetal distress during labor and delivery.

Infants with a chronic, possibly repetitive insult are more likely to show abnormalities within the cortex and white matter. This may have a classical parasagittal distribution, involving the territory between major arteries[41]. Infants with white matter lesions may fulfill all the criteria for HIE but often the clinical condition of the infant and the amount of damage seen on imaging appear to be out of keeping with the documented perinatal fetal distress. Repeated antenatal insults in these infants are thought to prime the white matter by diverting blood to metabolically more active parts of the developing brain such as the basal ganglia and thalami. A comparatively small perinatal insult may therefore result in extensive damage to the white matter and cortex (cases 6.6 and 6.7). Some infants may sustain severe white matter and severe basal ganglia and thalamic injury. This may result from a more severe perinatal insult occurring in combination with a chronic or repetitive insult that primes the white matter (case 6.8).

Major white matter infarction may also be seen in infants who have other predisposing factors such as hypoglycemia[7,20,25,39,42]. Some of these infants may also show other systemic abnormalities, for example conjugated hyperbilirubinemia, suggestive of an underlying metabolic disorder. Infants with primarily white matter damage may have a hemorrhagic component to their lesions (see Chapter 9). We have found an incidence of large parenchymal hemorrhagic lesions in infants with apparent HIE of approximately 5%. The outcome in these atypical infants may depend on any underlying pathology, for example a metabolic or thrombotic disorder, which should be sought. Caution needs to be exercised in predicting outcome from imaging alone. In our experience

Table 6.1 Early findings that may be identified during the first week after birth
Brain swelling
Loss of the normal signal in the posterior limb of the internal capsule
Abnormal signal intensities in the basal ganglia and thalami
Brain stem lesions
Loss of gray/white matter differentiation
Cortical highlighting (T1 weighted sequences)

these infants develop mild motor signs but may have a significant cognitive deficit.

During the first week after delivery there are six main areas of abnormality that may be identified on MRI in infants who fulfill all the criteria for HIE. Whilst one particular pattern may predominate, in most infants there are a combination of abnormalities. The early MRI findings are listed in Table 6.1.

Early MRI findings

BRAIN SWELLING

Abnormalities consistent with swelling of the brain may appear during the first 24–48 h following an asphyxial episode, mirroring the changes identified on ultrasound. These signs are best identified on T1 weighted spin echo sequences. Five signs of brain swelling may be demonstrated: (1) loss of extracerebral space; (2) loss of sulcal markings; (3) closure of the Sylvian fissures; (4) narrow interhemispheric fissure; and (5) slit-like anterior horns of the lateral ventricles (Fig. 6.1). There may be loss of the normal

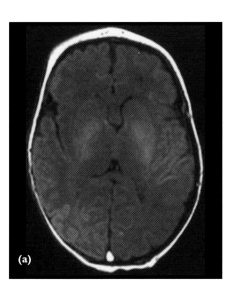
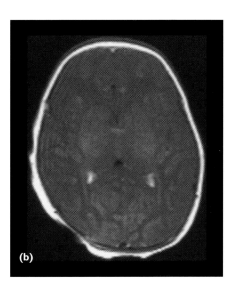

Fig. 6.1 Brain swelling. T1 weighted spin echo sequence (SE 860/20) of two different term-born infants aged 2 days. **(a)** Normal brain with no obvious swelling. The ventricles of a normal term-born infant are usually narrow. **(b)** Severe brain swelling showing slit-like ventricles, complete 'closure' of the interhemispheric fissure and no visible extracerebral space or sulci.

anatomical detail. Infants with severely swollen brains will have all signs. More severe swelling may be associated with white matter and cortical lesions. Mild degrees of brain swelling may be seen in infants who have not had documented asphyxia and infants with severe acute insults may have no obvious swelling.

Evolution

Brain swelling, even if initially severe, is usually no longer evident by the second week.[34]

Pathology

Swelling is likely to represent brain edema, but it is not easy to differentiate between vasogenic or cytotoxic edema on conventional scans alone. Brain swelling on T1 weighted images may be associated with some loss of gray/white matter differentiation; if this is severe and also present on the inversion recovery and T2 weighted images then it is likely to be cytotoxic edema. Diffusion weighted imaging during the first week after delivery will also identify areas of cytotoxic edema with impending tissue breakdown. On diffusion weighted images areas of infarction are seen as abnormal high signal intensity consistent with restricted diffusion of water.

Clinical outcome

The presence of brain swelling makes assessment of the brain more difficult. However, if the underlying brain is normal in appearance at the end of the first week once the swelling has disappeared, the clinical outlook is good, although follow-up

scans may show patchy increased T2 in the periventricular white matter (case 6.1). These periventricular changes may just represent immature unmyelinated white matter, so-called terminal zones, but are usually more marked than in normal children and are not always confined to the posterior periventricular white matter. We are currently looking at the neurodevelopmental outcome at school age in infants with stage I and II HIE who were developmentally normal at 2 years of age in order to identify more subtle minor motor difficulties or cognitive impairments.

THE POSTERIOR LIMB OF THE INTERNAL CAPSULE

The normal term infant will have evidence of myelination in approximately one-third to one-half of the posterior limb of the internal capsule (PLIC) on a T1 weighted sequence. Some myelin within the posterior limb should be visible from 37 weeks' gestation or slightly earlier in ex-preterm infants. This can be seen as high signal intensity on T1 weighted spin echo or inversion recovery sequences and low signal intensity on T2 weighted spin echo sequences (Fig. 6.2). The inversion recovery sequence is the best for demonstrating myelination within the internal capsule in the neonatal period. Using a fast spin echo T2 weighted image myelin may be clearly seen as low signal intensity within a higher signal intensity posterior limb but the low signal intensity seen on conventional T2 weighted imaging may be more subtle. The normal appearances of the posterior limb of the internal capsule using diffusion weighted imaging are also shown in Figure 4.7.

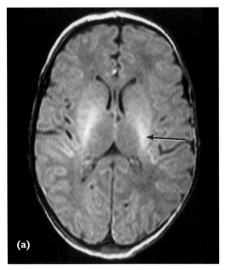 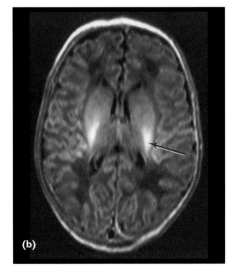 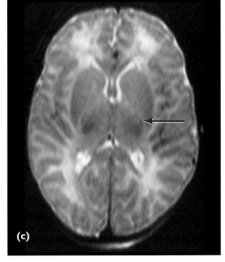

Fig. 6.2 Normal appearances of the posterior limb of the internal capsule. **(a)** T1 weighted spin echo sequence (SE 860/20). **(b)** Inversion recovery sequence (IR 3800/30/950). **(c)** T2 weighted spin echo sequence (SE 2700/120). Myelination within the posterior limb of the internal capsule is marked with an arrow. The most obvious signal from myelin is seen in the inversion recovery image **(b)**. The low signal from myelin on the T2 weighted image **(c)** is the least obvious.

Loss of the normal signal intensity within the posterior limb of the internal capsule

A complete loss or a change in the normal signal intensity from myelin may be seen following perinatal asphyxia. This may may take 1–2 days to evolve and there may therefore be apparently normal signal intensity from myelin on the first scan if done very early (Fig. 6.3). The signal intensity from myelin may be diminished or asymmetrical, 'equivocal', prior to its loss. In association with the loss of normal signal intensity from within the limb there may be abnormal signal intensities running parallel to the posterior limb in the lentiform nucleus. These should not be confused with the normal signal from myelin (Fig. 6.18, case 6.3). There may also be abnormal low signal intensity on T1 weighted images or abnormally high signal intensity on T2 weighted images in the unmyelinated more anterior portion of the internal capsule (Fig. 6.3) Occasionally the internal capsule may look grossly abnormal on T1 weighted imaging but surprisingly normal on T2 weighted images. A combination of sequences is always recommended. This sign will always be easier to detect towards the end of the first week and in the presence of abnormal signal intensity either side of the posterior limb in the lentiform nucleus and thalami.

Evolution

The normal signal intensity from myelin may return after some weeks or months, although it is often irregular in outline. The rate of return depends on the severity of injury to the basal ganglia and thalami. In the presence of gross atrophy of the basal ganglia and thalami the tracts appear to be irreversibly damaged and if and when myelination appears it is very irregular and discontinuous (Fig. 6.3).

Pathology

The increased T1 within the PLIC is consistent with edema or infarction. The finding of an increased signal on diffusion weighted imaging in all three planes of sensitization (Fig. 6.4) is indicative of cytotoxic edema with loss of anisotropy. Infants who have had abnormal signal intensity within the posterior limb and who have died in the acute stages of HIE show histological signs of edema in this region (Fig. 6.4)[18].

Outcome

The loss of a signal intensity within a structure is easier to detect than an exaggeration which is highly dependent on the sequence and the windowing used to obtain the image.

In our experience all term infants with HIE who show abnormal signal intensity within the PLIC have an abnormal neurodevelopmental outcome (sensitivity 0.91, specificity 1.0, positive predictive value 1.0) (cases 6.3–6.7)[36]. It is important to have a correct estimate of gestation as the absence of myelin on MRI is a normal finding below 37 weeks' gestation. In addition, infants with a primary metabolic disorder may have delayed myelination which would include an absence of myelin within the posterior limb at term (see Chapter 17). Certain metabolic disorders, for example non-ketotic hyperglycemia, which present in the neonatal period may mimic HIE and a metabolic screen in any asphyxiated infant is always warranted.

THE BASAL GANGLIA AND THALAMI

The basal ganglia include the head of the caudate nucleus, the globus pallidum and the putamen, which together form the lentiform nucleus (Fig. 6.5).

Using T1 weighted imaging there is high signal within the PLIC and some high signal within the ventro-lateral nuclei of the thalami. Some high signal may be seen in the globus pallidum at term and this may be exaggerated in infants with asphyxia.

Using T2 weighted imaging the ventro-lateral nuclei of the thalami are seen as low signal intensity. Myelin within the posterior limb is seen as a small area of low signal intensity within a high signal intensity capsule. There may be a thin region of low signal intensity along the lateral borders of the lentiform nucleus.

Abnormal signal within the basal ganglia and thalami

Abnormalities within the basal ganglia and thalami are a frequent finding following severe acute asphyxia. This is thought to be due to the increased metabolic rate of this region which is actively myelinating at term[11]. In addition, the structures contain a high proportion of excitatory amino acid receptors. Abnormal signal intensity is most frequently seen within the posterior part of the lentiform nucleus and in the region of the ventro-lateral nuclei of the thalami (Figs 6.5 and 6.18). In severe injury there may be diffuse abnormality throughout the structures. We grade these basal ganglia and thalamic lesions as mild, moderate, and severe. Mild lesions are focal and seen in the presence of a normal signal intensity within the PLIC. They are typically inferior in position. Moderate lesions are focal involving the posterior and lateral lentiform nucleus and lateral thalamus with an equivocal or abnormal signal intensity within the PLIC. Severe lesions are more widespread involving all areas including the caudate head with very severe diffuse lesions and extending into the mid-brain and mesencephalon. They are always associated with an abnormal signal intensity within

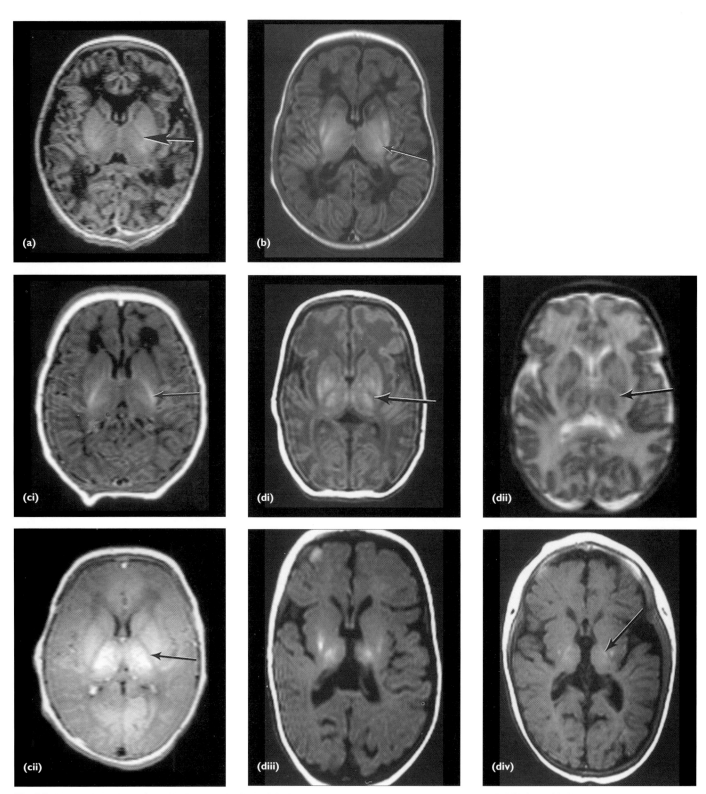

Fig. 6.3 Abnormal signal intensity within the posterior limb of the internal capsule. Inversion recovery sequence (IR 3800/30/950). **(a)** Complete loss of the normal SI at 1 day of age in an infant with stage III HIE who died. **(b)** Partial loss of the normal signal intensity at 4 days of age in an infant with HIE II who developed a mild quadriplegia. The signal intensity on the left is diminished (*arrow*). **(c)** Delayed loss of signal intensity **(i)** image obtained at 2 days, showing a normal high signal intensity within the posterior limb, and **(ii)** image at 4 days (with contrast) in an infant with stage III HIE who subsequently died. **(d)** T1 weighted spin echo sequence (SE 860/20) **(i)** and T2 weighted fast spin echo sequence (FSE 3000/208) **(ii)**. Absent signal intensity in an infant with stage II HIE at 15 days of age. The T2 weighted images show the posterior limb of the internal capsule as a broad band of high signal intensity (*arrow*). There is no normal low signal intensity within this, consistent with the presence of normal myelin. There are obvious abnormal signal intensities in the thalamus and lentiform nucleus either side of the abnormal internal capsule. **(iii)** The same infant at 2 months of age. The signal intensity within the internal capsule is still absent. The abnormal signal intensities within the thalamus and lentiform nucleus are still present. **(iv)** The same infant at 5 months of age. There is some signal intensity within the internal capsule. This is thin and not appropriate for 5 months. The abnormal signal intensities within the thalamus and internal capsule are much less obvious.

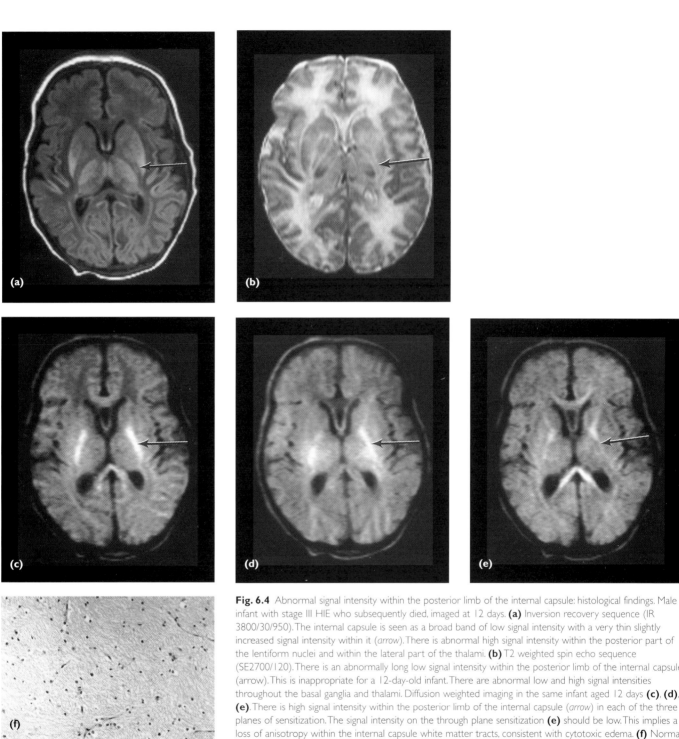

Fig. 6.4 Abnormal signal intensity within the posterior limb of the internal capsule: histological findings. Male infant with stage III HIE who subsequently died, imaged at 12 days. **(a)** Inversion recovery sequence (IR 3800/30/950). The internal capsule is seen as a broad band of low signal intensity with a very thin slightly increased signal intensity within it (*arrow*). There is abnormal high signal intensity within the posterior part of the lentiform nuclei and within the lateral part of the thalami. **(b)** T2 weighted spin echo sequence (SE2700/120). There is an abnormally long low signal intensity within the posterior limb of the internal capsule (arrow). This is inappropriate for a 12-day-old infant. There are abnormal low and high signal intensities throughout the basal ganglia and thalami. Diffusion weighted imaging in the same infant aged 12 days **(c)**, **(d)**, **(e)**. There is high signal intensity within the posterior limb of the internal capsule (*arrow*) in each of the three planes of sensitization. The signal intensity on the through plane sensitization **(e)** should be low. This implies a loss of anisotropy within the internal capsule white matter tracts, consistent with cytotoxic edema. **(f)** Normal histological appearances of the posterior limb of the internal capsule (H&E). **(g)** Abnormal appearances in the infant with stage III HIE, who died at 2 weeks of age. There are abnormal edematous areas throughout the section. An increased water content within the internal capsule would lower its signal intensity on a T1 weighted image and increase its signal intensity on a T2 weighted image, as seen on the conventional imaging in **(a)** and **(b)**. The diffusion weighted imaging changes are consistent with this edema being cytotoxic.

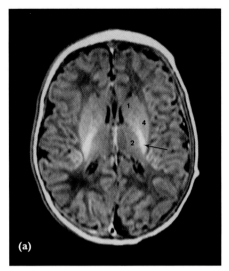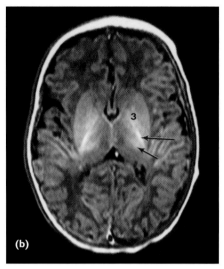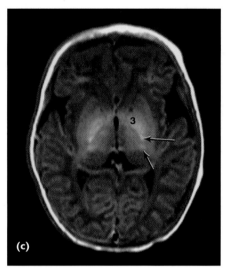

Fig. 6.5 Magnified view of the normal basal ganglia and thalami. Inversion recovery sequence (IR 3800/30/950). **(a)** Upper basal ganglia level; **(b)** mid-basal ganglia level; **(c)** low basal ganglia and thalamic level. Normal appearance of the basal ganglia and thalami at term. Posterior limb of the internal capsule (*long arrow*); ventro-lateral nucleus of the thalamus (*short arrow*); 1, caudate head; 2, thalami; 3, globus pallidum; 4, putamen. Note that there is a diffuse slightly increased signal in the globus pallidum, most marked inferiorly. This is very dependent on the windowing used.

the PLIC. The exact signal intensity and site of lesions within the basal ganglia may vary between individual infants (Fig. 6.6). Whilst areas of abnormal high signal intensity on T1 weighted images are usually seen as low signal intensity on T2 weighted images (Fig. 6.6) in some cases the signal intensity on T2 weighted imaging is more heterogeneous (Fig. 6.6). The reasons for this are not clear and may only be explained by very detailed imaging and pathological comparisons.

Abnormalities within the corticospinal tracts around the central fissure, the hippocampus (Fig. 6.19, case 6.4) and brain stem (Fig. 6.8) often accompany abnormalities within the basal ganglia and thalami[27,28,30].

Evolution

Abnormal signal intensity with the basal ganglia and thalami gradually increases over the first week of life. By 2 weeks it is at its most obvious. In mild or moderate abnormalities of the basal ganglia the abnormal signal intensity becomes gradually less obvious and between 3 and 9 months there may be no detectable abnormalities. The lentiform nuclei and thalami may be slightly atrophied but this may not be obvious on visual analysis of the images alone. From 9 months there may be abnormal increased signal intensity within the thalami and posterior putamen. On T1 weighted images there may be additional low signal intensity in the posterior putamen but abnormal low signal intensity in the thalami may only be very subtle. The disappearance of clinically significant lesions is very important. Infants may still develop severe motor

impairment despite the apparently normal imaging appearance at around 6 months of age (Fig. 6.7).

In more severe injury to the basal ganglia and thalami, from 2 weeks onwards, there is focal or diffuse atrophy with or without the formation of cysts. The high signal intensity on T1 weighted imaging gradually decreases over the first year of life when the basal ganglia and thalami may show varying degrees of atrophy (cases 6.3–6.5). Infants with multifocal or diffuse lesions within the basal ganglia and thalami also have progressive white matter atrophy. The white matter may have an initial streaky appearance. It is unclear whether this atrophy is due to the initial insult or secondary to the severe damage to the basal ganglia. The atrophy may result from the severence of preformed thalamo-cortical projections which then fail to reconnect and develop. The ability of the basal ganglia and thalami to produce or receive new connections may also be impaired.

Associated abnormalities within the hippocampus are usually not evident until the second week of life when a generalized high signal intensity is seen on T1 weighted images (Fig. 6.19, case 6.4). This is associated with later atrophy and dilation of the temporal horn of the lateral ventricles (Fig. 6.19, case 6.4).

Pathology (see Chapter 5)

Lesions with a short T1 and short T2 are generally assumed to be hemorrhagic but we have not demonstrated macroscopic hemorrhage in infants who have died following severe basal ganglia and thalamic injury. There is, however, diffuse

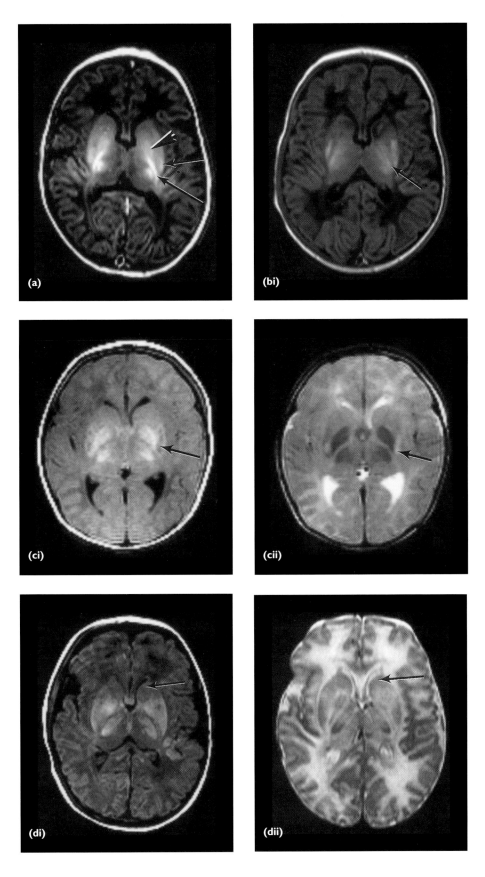

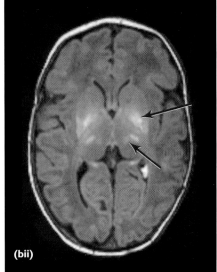

Fig. 6.6 Abnormal signal intensity within the basal ganglia and thalami. The abnormal appearances vary between infants, time from insult and with the windowing of the images but can be divided into three groups of increasing severity. Inversion recovery sequence (IR 3800/30/950). **(a)** Mild abnormalities with normal SI in the PLIC (*long arrow*). There is abnormal increased signal intensity in the ventro-lateral thalamic nuclei and in the lateral putamen (*short arrow*). There is obvious but probably normal high signal intensity within the globus pallidum (*black and white arrowhead*). This image has been quite tightly windowed. **(b)** Moderate, focal lesions with equivocal **(i)** or abnormal **(ii)** SI in the PLIC; **(i)** shows a normal signal intensity within the PLIC on the right but a rather thin signal intensity on the left which is associated with a parallel low signal intensity. Both images show abnormal high signal intensity within the lateral putamen and the lateral thalamic nuclei. In **(ii)** there is additional high signal more medially in the globus pallidum (*long arrow*) and a discrete rounded high signal intensity in the medial thalamus (*short arrow*). **(c)** Severe, widespread lesions with abnormal SI within the PLIC. **(i)** T1 weighted spin echo sequence (SE 860/20) and **(ii)** T2 weighted spin echo sequence (SE 2700/120). There is marked high signal within the putamen, globus pallidum and lateral thalamus. There are additional low signal intensity cyst-like lesions (*arrow*) in the lateral putamen. **(i)** There is abnormal low signal intensity within the globus pallidum posterior putamen and lateral thalamus. There is abnormal high signal intensity within the lateral putamen, consistent with cyst-like lesions (*arrow*) **(ii)**. **(d)** Severe, widespread lesions with abnormal SI within the PLIC. There is abnormal high signal intensity in the lateral putamen, globus pallidum and lateral thalami. **(i)** There is low signal intensity in the caudate heads (*arrow*). **(ii)** The abnormal low signal intensity is less obvious than in **(c)**. There is a mix of low and high signal intensities in the putamen and lentiform. The caudate heads have an abnormal low signal intensity (*arrow*).

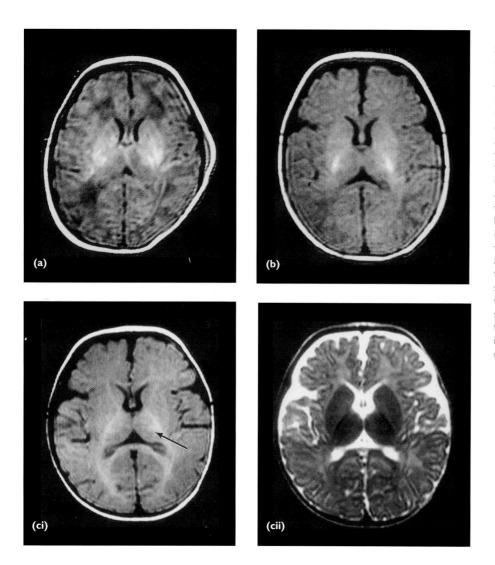

Fig. 6.7 'Disappearing' abnormalities in the basal ganglia and thalami. T1 weighted spin echo sequence (SE 860/20) of a term infant with stage II HIE. Some motion artifact **(a)** At 4 days of age there are abnormal high signal intensities within the lentiform and thalami. The signal intensity within the PLIC is difficult to differentiate on either side and is definitely abnormal on the right. **(b)** At 2 months of age there are no residual abnormal signal intensities within the lentiform or thalami. Myelination within the posterior limb of the internal capsule is incomplete and therefore delayed for 2 months of age. **(c) (i)** At 6 months of age there is myelin within the posterior and anterior limbs. There may be a small area of abnormally increased signal intensity in the lateral thalami, in the region of the ventro-lateral nucleus (*arrow*) but no other abnormalities. There is no obvious cyst formation in the posterior putamen. **(c) (ii)** T2 weighted fast spin echo. There are no abnormal signal intensities within the basal ganglia and thalami. The brain looks slightly atrophic but atrophy of the basal ganglia and thalami is not obvious by visual analysis alone. This infant has a significant motor impairment at 1 year of age.

necrosis in these infants. Capillary proliferation occurs within hours of ischemic injury and this may give rise to the short T1 and short T2 lesions seen on MRI. In addition, the combination of very short T1 and very short T2 may be due to neuronal mineralization (Fig. 6.15). Other possible explanations for the abnormal signal intensity are iron deposition[15], the presence of lipids as a by-product of membrane break down, or at a later state of abnormal myelin. Histology of the basal ganglia and thalami in children with a history of birth asphyxia, who die later in infancy or childhood, may show signs of 'status marmoratus' due to abnormally myelinated fibers[24]. The MR appearances of histologically proven 'status marmoratus' have not been described, perhaps, in part, because of the difficulties in obtaining consent for postmortem in older infants and children (case 6.5).

The bilateral abnormalities seen in term infants with severe HIE need to be distinguished from primary thalamic hemorrhage which may rarely be bilateral (see Chapter 9).

Clinical outcome

Lesions within the basal ganglia and thalami can be scored. The severity of the score is directly related to the outcome of the infant[6,33,35]. Infants with persistent abnormal signal intensity all have some abnormalities at follow-up. The outcome with mild lesions with preservation of the signal from myelin in the PLIC is not clear, although these infants may show mildly abnormal tone during the first year and later develop a tremor in early childhood. More marked movement disorders may develop in adolescents with a history of perinatal asphyxia but imaging data were not available for these cases[37]. Moderate focal lesions that evolve to small cyst formation in the posterior part of the putamen and areas of increased T2 in the region of the ventro-lateral nuclei of the thalami are associated with the development of a fairly pure athetoid quadriplegia with normal head growth and intellectual preservation (case 6.3)[32]. More extensive severe multifocal abnormalities are associated with a mixed spastic/athetoid quadriplegia with a secondary microcephaly, some intellectual deficit and often persistent convulsions (case 6.4). Diffuse abnormalities resulting in severe atrophy throughout the basal ganglia and thalami are associated with the development of a spastic quadriplegia, secondary microcephaly, severe intellectual deficit and persistent convulsions, which are often difficult to control. There are additional marked feeding difficulties which usually necessitate the insertion of a gastrostomy (Fig. 6.20, case 6.5). These infants may have involvement of the mid-brain, with a diffuse increased signal on T1 weighted imaging, but this is not always easy to detect. In some infants obvious infarction of the dorsal brain stem can be identified. These infants may survive for a surprisingly long time (Fig. 6.8b).

BRAIN STEM LESIONS

Infants that develop stage III hypoxic–ischemic encephalopathy usually have severe basal ganglia lesions with extension into the mid-brain, pons and medulla. The site of lesions within the brain stem is usually dorsal. These findings explain the clinical state of an unrousable infant with no gag reflex, no facial expression and no normal eye movements. These infants are usually, but not always, unable to breathe independently. The brain stem lesions may be seen as low signal intensity on T1 weighted images and high signal intensity on T2 weighted images. These changes are consistent with infarction (Fig. 6.8). Sometimes a diffuse abnormal signal intensity is seen, high on T1 and

low on T2 weighted images. Brain stem lesions are usually associated lesions in the basal ganglia and thalami, in the hippocampus and in the corticospinal tracts around the central fissure.

THE CORTEX

The newborn cortex has a relatively short T1 and T2 compared to adjacent white matter. This difference lasts for approximately 3 months. A gradual lengthening of the T1 and T2 probably reflects the density of white matter processes and synapses increasing with age. This occurs with a simultaneous decrease in the T1 and T2 of the adjacent subcortical white matter (see Chapter 4).

Cortical highlighting

Following perinatal asphyxia areas of cortex may show abnormal highlighting with a further shortening of both T1 and T2. We have termed it highlighting as it is easiest to identify on T1 weighted images where it is demonstrated as areas of abnormal high signal intensity. The abnormal cortex may have a low signal intensity on T2 weighted sequences but this is usually much less obvious (Fig. 6.9b). The cortical highlighting is most frequently seen around the central fissure where it can be the only abnormality on imaging in mild asphyxia (Fig. 6.9a). The cortex around the interhemispheric fissure (Fig. 6.9a,c) and the insula (Fig. 6.9b) may also be involved and in extreme cases almost the entire cortex may be

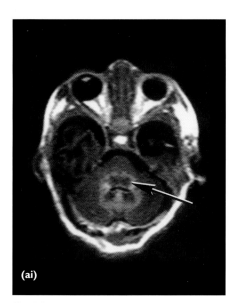
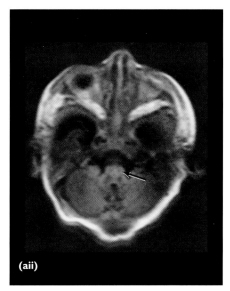
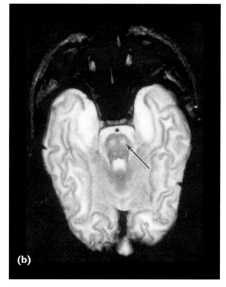

Fig. 6.8 Brain stem lesions. Term infant with stage III HIE. **(a)** Inversion recovery sequence (IR 3500/30/950). There are bilateral abnormal low signal intensity lesions within the pons (*arrow*) **(i)** and in the medulla **(ii)**. **(b)** Term infant with stage III HIE who required no ventilatory support and subsequently survived for 1 year. T2 weighted sequence. There are bilateral high signal intensity areas consistent with infarction in the brain stem (*arrow*).

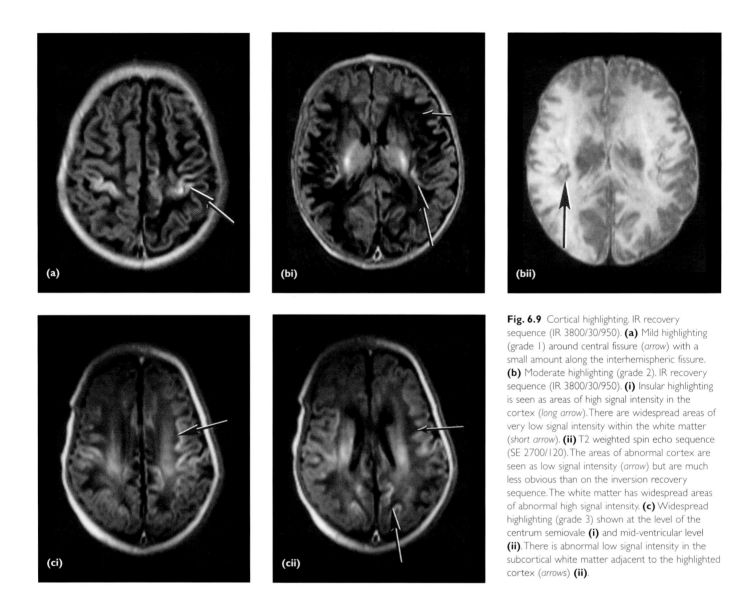

Fig. 6.9 Cortical highlighting. IR recovery sequence (IR 3800/30/950). **(a)** Mild highlighting (grade 1) around central fissure (*arrow*) with a small amount along the interhemispheric fissure. **(b)** Moderate highlighting (grade 2). IR recovery sequence (IR 3800/30/950). **(i)** Insular highlighting is seen as areas of high signal intensity in the cortex (*long arrow*). There are widespread areas of very low signal intensity within the white matter (*short arrow*). **(ii)** T2 weighted spin echo sequence (SE 2700/120). The areas of abnormal cortex are seen as low signal intensity (*arrow*) but are much less obvious than on the inversion recovery sequence. The white matter has widespread areas of abnormal high signal intensity. **(c)** Widespread highlighting (grade 3) shown at the level of the centrum semiovale **(i)** and mid-ventricular level **(ii)**. There is abnormal low signal intensity in the subcortical white matter adjacent to the highlighted cortex (*arrows*) **(ii)**.

abnormally highlighted (Fig. 6.22, case 6.7). The depths of the sulci are more frequently affected (Fig. 6.9).

Evolution

The abnormal signal may take several days to develop, reaching its maximum during the second week after the asphyxial insult and lasting for several weeks. During the second week abnormal signal intensity may develop in the subcortical white matter adjacent to areas of highlighted cortex (Fig. 6.9). This is consistent with ischemic damage to the white matter, which then proceeds to break down and atrophy. Early changes in the subcortical white matter can be detected with diffusion weighted imaging (Fig. 6.10).

Barkovich describes the appearances of 'cortical edema' on proton density images in the first few days following delivery at a time when the heavily T2 weighted images may be normal[6]. This finding is consistent with a loss of gray/white matter differentiation. The value of the proton density image will depend on how much gray/white matter contrast the sequence produces in the normal neonatal brain. This may differ between systems and sequences.

Pathology

The abnormalities within the cortex on conventional imaging may represent ischemia of one or all cortical layers giving rise to laminar necrosis. The deep layers of the cortex are known to be more vulnerable to hypoxic–ischemic injury. It is unclear why necrosis of the cortex should give rise to a decrease in T1 and T2 but these changes probably reflect capillary proliferation at the cortical/white matter boundary

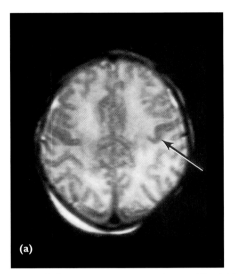 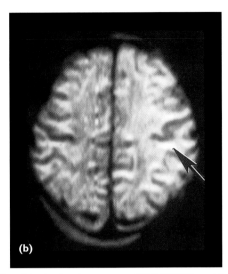 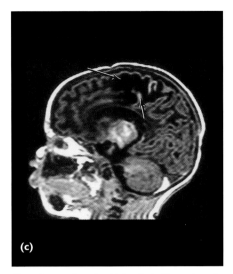

Fig. 6.10 Subcortical white matter abnormalities. **(a)** T2 weighted spin echo sequence (SE 2700/120) aged 2 days. There is some low signal intensity in the cortex of the central fissure (*arrow*). **(b)** Diffusion weighted imaging on the same day. There is marked increased signal intensity within the subcortical white matter (*arrow*). **(c)** T1 weighted spin echo sequence (SE 860/20). Sagittal plane. At 1 month of age there are widespread areas of abnormal low subcortical signal intensity consistent with infarction (long arrow) there are some residual areas of cortical highlighting (*short arrow*) and the cortex is very thin superiorly. There is abnormal signal intensity within the basal ganglia and thalami. There is a residual subdural hemorrhage behind the cerebellum.

(see Chapter 5). Capillary proliferation occurs after approximately 3 days following infarction, the timing fits with the first appearances of cortical highlighting on MRI. The subcortical white matter changes are consistent with infarction resulting from the primary injury. This may be as a result of a direct insult to the white matter or may be secondary to the damage in the deep layers of the cortex. The low signal intensity representing breakdown of the tissue takes at least 1 week to appear on conventional imaging.

Outcome

Cortical highlighting is usually associated with other lesions in the brain and therefore it is difficult to identify specific neurodevelopmental sequelae. Minor degrees of highlighting may be associated with a normal outcome although long-term follow-up is necessary to identify the presence of more subtle cognitive deficits. Widespread highlighting has been associated with the development of a spastic diplegia, microcephaly and moderate intellectual deficit, but without continuing convulsions (case 6.7). These findings may in part be secondary to the associated white matter abnormalities. Later imaging of the cortex is difficult although cortical structures clearly remain even after extensive highlighting. Abnormal signal intensity presumed to be secondary to laminar necrosis of the cortex has been reported in older children with cerebral palsy[40] but we have been unable to identify this sort of detail with conventional imaging.

GRAY/WHITE MATTER DIFFERENTIATION

The normal-term brain shows good differentiation between cortical gray and adjacent white matter (Fig. 6.2). This is apparent for the first 3 months of life by which time the T1 and T2 of the white matter have decreased and the T1 and T2 of the cortex have increased and the differentiation is less obvious.

Loss of gray/white matter differentiation

Focal infarction in isolation is not a typical finding in HIE but may accompany other lesions. Infarction in infants with HIE is usually bilateral and in a parasagittal distribution, with more marked changes posteriorly. The loss of differentiation results from a change in the normal signal intensity within the cortex and the white matter. The cortex loses its typical short T1 short T2 properties. Barkovich attributes this to cortical edema and reports that this sign may be detected earliest using a proton density image[6]. Whilst the T1 and T2 values of the cortex lengthen with infarction so do those in the white matter. Some loss of differentiation may be seen on T1 weighted spin echo images in the presence of brain swelling but this may normalize to reveal an intact brain. If there is additional loss of differentiation on an inversion recovery, or on T2 weighted sequence, then this represents impending infarction. Regions with loss of differentiation may be easily identified with diffusion weighted imaging which shows a pattern consistent with restricted diffusion for the first week of life, becoming less obvious as conventional imaging becomes more abnormal (Fig. 6.11).

During the second week the gray/white matter differentiation returns but is exaggerated due to a shortening of the T1 and T2 in the cortex, perhaps secondary to capillary proliferation, and an increase in T1 and T2 in the white matter (Fig. 6.11).

Pathology

The loss of differentiation is a result of cytotoxic edema resulting from severe ischemia, as seen in areas of focal infarction (see Chapter 7). Diffusion weighted imaging confirms the presence of infarction[10,29]. The exaggeration of the cortical signal during the second week of life with a shortening of the T1 and T2 may also represent capillary proliferation.

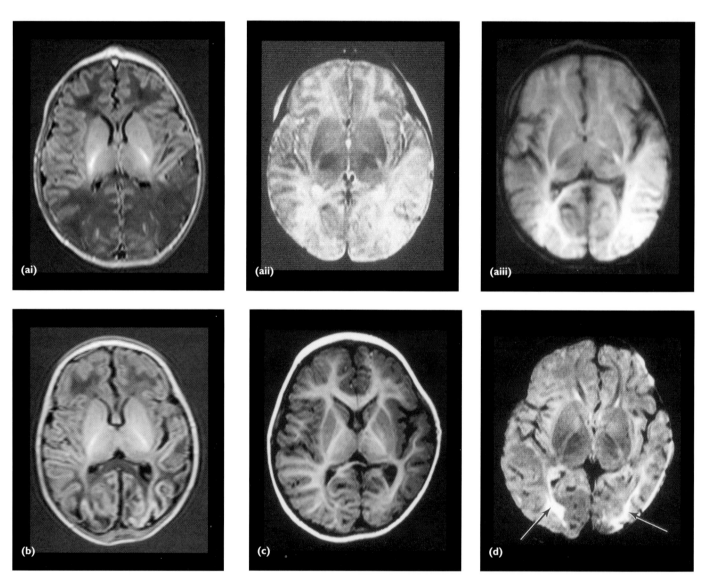

Fig. 6.11 Loss of gray/white matter differentiation. **(a)** Female infant with stage II HIE. Imaged at 3 days of age. **(i)** T1 weighted spin echo sequence (SE 860/20). There is a complete loss of the normal gray/white matter differentiation in the posterior parietal and occipital lobes. This is consistent with extensive infarction in both parietal lobes. The basal ganglia and thalami appear normal and there is normal high signal from myelin in the posterior limb of the basal ganglia. **(ii)** T2 weighted spin echo sequence (SE 2700/120). There is loss of the normal low signal from the cortex and some increase in the signal intensity within the white matter in both temporal and occipital poles. **(iii)** Diffusion weighted imaging. There is abnormal high signal intensity within the temporal and occipital lobes. This is consistent with restricted diffusion of water. **(b)** Inversion recovery sequence (IR 3800/30/950). Imaged at 2 weeks. There is now exaggerated differentiation between the cortex, which is abnormally highlighted, and the white matter which has abnormal low signal intensity. **(c)** Inversion recovery sequence (IR 3600/30/850). Imaged at 1 year of age. There is atrophy of both temporal lobes with decreased myelin, which is more marked on the left. **(d)** FLAIR (fluid attenuated IR 6500/160/2100) sequence at 2 years of age. There is abnormal high signal intensity (*arrows*) consistent with glial tissue in both temporal and occipital lobes. At age 2 years this infant was microcephalic but with only minimal asymmetry of tone. At 4 years she had a short attention span and poor concentration which made assessment difficult but her general development was only at the 3-year level.

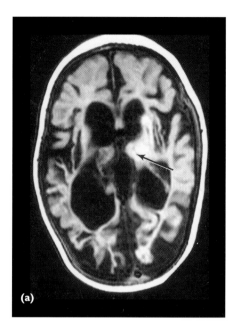 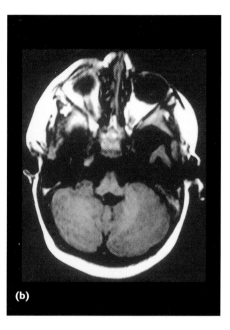

Fig. 6.12 Cerebellar preservation. Infant with stage II HIE, case 6.8, imaged at 7 months. Inversion recovery sequence (IR 3400/30/800). Transverse plane. **(a)** Low ventricular level. There is widespread cystic breakdown of the hemispheres and marked atrophy of the basal ganglia and thalami (*arrow*). **(b)** Cerebellar level. The cerebellum is apparently preserved although mild atrophy may be difficult to detect.

Neurodevelopmental outcome

The clinical outcome in infants that show loss of gray/white matter differentiation preceding infarction depends on the extent and site of the infarction, the presence of other lesions and additional underlying diagnoses. In the absence of basal ganglia lesions the motor outcome may be surprisingly good even with extensive white matter loss (Fig. 6.11). Marked cystic breakdown within the white matter may be accompanied by severe basal ganglia lesions. The outcome in these infants is very poor (Fig. 6.23, case 6.8).

THE CEREBELLUM

Conventional MRI is able to detect abnormalities in the regions of the brain described but may not detect changes in other areas of the brain which have nonetheless been damaged.

The cerebellum appears to be relatively resistant to hypoxic–ischemic damage. In infants with widespread destruction of all other areas of the brain the cerebellum may remain intact and look relatively normal (Fig. 6.12). Certain regions of the cerebellum, for example the dentate nucleus, are reported in animal studies as being sensitive to asphyxial damage. Changes in the dentate nucleus are difficult to identify with MRI. The visualization of these structures is angle dependent in the transverse plane. Abnormalities probably represent an exaggeration of the normal low and high signal intensity. In a study comparing MRI to histological appearances following severe birth asphyxia we were unable to detect any abnormal signal intensity within the dentate nucleus although at histology the dentate was classified as abnormal in every infant[18] (Fig. 6.13).

We have used a computer quantification program to measure cerebellar hemisphere volume and vermis volume. Both parameters were reduced in infants with severe basal ganglia

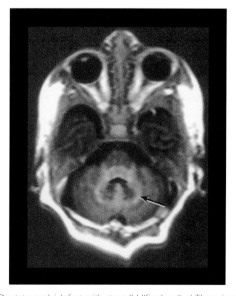

Fig. 6.13 Dentate nuclei. Infant with stage II HIE who died. There is an exaggeration of the normal high signal around the dentate nuclei (*arrow*). This is subjective and dependent on the windowing of the images. The cerebellum was histologically abnormal with neuronal necrosis within the dentate nuclei and Purkinje cells.

and thalamic lesions, along with their total brain volume; however, the reduction in vermal volume was more marked[22]. It is not clear whether this atrophy results from initial undetected lesions in the cerebellum or whether it represents a secondary atrophy or degeneration.

The majority of infants with HIE survive. In those that die it may not have been possible to get detailed imaging prior to death. There is therefore very little correlation between ultrasound or MRI and histology[16,18]. The use of pathological terms to describe MR findings is common practice but may hinder our understanding and cause confusion between different clinical and research groups.

Pattern recognition, scoring systems and prediction of outcome in term infants with HIE

Many authors have described scoring systems for the pattern of injury detected on early MRI following birth asphyxia[6,21,33,35]. These scoring systems are useful for classifying lesions for research studies. Many of them, however, are too complicated for routine clinical use. MRI has a vital role in the prediction of outcome but correct interpretation of imaging findings is not easy. MRI should never be used as a sole technique for prediction of outcome and the subsequent altering of clinical management. In addition, the prediction of an abnormal outcome is only the first step. The definition of abnormal outcome differs between studies and is often not very specific. MRI in the neonatal period is able, unlike other neurological investigations, to give precise details on the type

of abnormal outcome. Some abnormal outcomes may not be severe enough to warrant the possible complications inherent in any early intervention, for example hypothermia, when these become more widely available. MRI provides invaluable information on the patterns and evolution of injury following HIE. This information will prove vital for monitoring the effects, both desired and not, of any future interventions. Interestingly, in a small pilot group of term infants with severe HIE who were treated with hypothermia we had an incidence of hemorrhagic/ thrombotic cerebral complications of approximately 20%, compared to approximately 5% in our long-term cohort of untreated infants. This may reflect bias from our patient selection with the treated group representing the severe end of the spectrum of infants with HIE, but warrants further investigation.

The preterm asphyxiated brain

Ischemic lesions within the preterm brain are discussed elsewhere (see Chapter 8). The pattern of injury seen in the preterm brain will, as in the term infant, depend on the nature of the insult and probably to a lesser extent to the gestational age of the fetus or infant. Severe acute insults which often correspond to a well-documented clinical event, for example attempted maternal suicide, result in injury to the basal ganglia and thalami (Fig. 6.14). The specific regions within the basal ganglia and thalami may be different from the term asphyxiated brain[4,5]. In addition, cortical highlighting is not obvious around the central sulcus in the preterm brain, perhaps reflecting less metabolic activity and

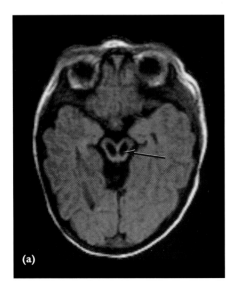 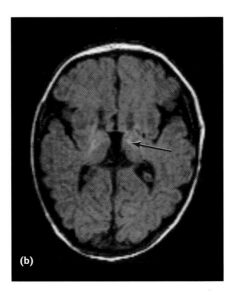

Fig. 6.14 Antenatal brain stem infarction. Female infant born at 41 weeks' gestation with arthrogryposis multiplex congenita. Her mother took an overdose of co-proxamol at 22 weeks' gestation. This was associated with maternal convulsions and a period of hypotension. She also abused cocaine and alcohol during the pregnancy. T1 weighted spin echo sequence (SE 860/20). Imaged at 8 days of age. **(a)** There are bilateral infarcts within the mesencephalon (*arrow*). **(b)** The basal ganglia and thalami are atrophied and the normal anatomy distorted; there is also abnormal linear increased signal intensity within the thalami (*arrow*).

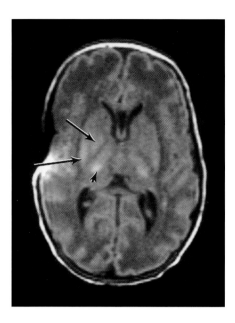

Fig. 6.15 Acute hypoxic–ischemic injury in a preterm infant. Male infant born at 28 weeks' gestation who had a severe collapse at 30 weeks. Imaged postmortem at 32 weeks. T1 weighted spin echo sequence (SE 2700/20). There is bilateral abnormal increased signal intensity within the putamen (*long arrow*), globus pallidum (*short arrow*) and thalami (*arrowhead*). The posterior limb of the internal capsule is seen as very low signal intensity. There is an artifact of uncertain origin over the right insula cortex. The thalamic lesions, which were very low signal intensity on T2 weighted images, were found to be mineralized on histology.

therefore less vulnerability. These severe events may occur following delivery (Fig. 6.15) but with good neonatal intensive care are relatively rare. The more common injury seen in the preterm brain is to white matter probably because of the type of insult to which preterm infants are exposed, for example sepsis and chronic hypoxia[13] and because the developing white matter is particularly vulnerable. The type of insult may, however, be a major determinant of the eventual injury as term-born infants with a history of a chronic or repetitive injury or possible sepsis will also show mainly white matter damage.

CASE 6.1. NO FOCAL LESIONS (FIG. 6.16)

This female infant was born by ventouse delivery at 40 weeks' gestation, following an uneventful pregnancy. Prior to delivery there was prolonged rupture of membranes and maternal pyrexia, with a fetal tachycardia and fresh meconium-stained liquor. The infant had Apgar scores of 3 at 1 min and 7 at 5 min. The cord pH was 6.7. She had a single documented clinical convulsion but an EEG showed good background activity. She was classified as having stage II HIE.

■ *Normal MR images at the end of the first week are associated with a normal neurodevelopmental outcome at school entry.*

Neurodevelopmental follow-up

Her development was within normal limits at 4.5 years of age.

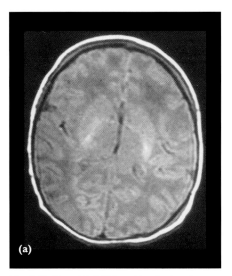 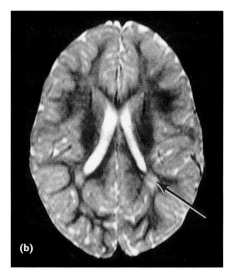 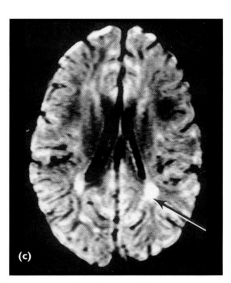

Fig. 6.16 Case 6.1. **(a)** T1 weighted spin echo sequence (SE 860/20). Aged 2 days. There is moderate brain swelling but preservation of the gray/white matter differentiation. There is a normal signal from myelin in the posterior limb of the internal capsule. **(b)** Aged 18 months. T2 weighted spin echo sequence (SE 2700/120). There is mild dilatation of the ventricles right more than left. There is a small amount of increased signal intensity in the periventricular white matter bilaterally, which is most marked posteriorly (*arrow*). This is in the region of the terminal zones and may just represent unmyelinated white matter, although it does have a high signal intensity on the FLAIR (fluid attenuated IR 6500/160/2100) sequence (*arrow*)**(c)**.

CASE 6.2. MILD BASAL GANGLIA AND THALAMIC LESIONS (FIG. 6.17)

This female infant was born at 40 weeks' gestation by normal vaginal delivery with a birth weight of 3.45 kg. There was fetal distress with type II dips for approximately 20 min prior to delivery. Apgar scores were 1 at 1 min and she required intubation for poor respiratory effort. She had clinical convulsions on day 2 that required phenobarbital. She was classified as stage II HIE.

■ *Mild basal ganglia and thalamic abnormalities may be associated with late-onset motor abnormalities, for example tremor or possibly dystonia.*

Neurodevelopmental follow-up

She is now 5 years old and is developmentally normal. She has an obvious tremor that interferes with her fine motor function.

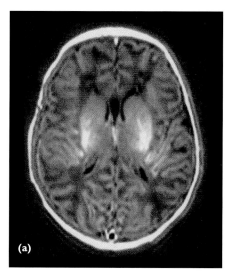 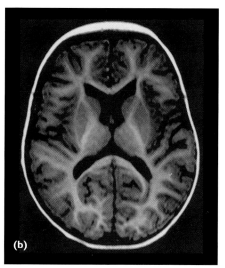 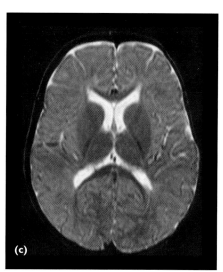

Fig. 6.17 Case 6.2. **(a)** Inversion recovery sequence (IR 3800/30/950). Imaged at 5 days of age. There is abnormal high signal intensity within the thalami and putamen. There is excessive high signal in the region of the posterior limb of the internal capsule. This may be due, in part, to overtight windowing of the image. **(b)** Inversion recovery sequence (IR 3600/30/850), and **(c)** T2 weighted spin echo sequence (SE 2700/120). Aged 9 months. The basal ganglia and thalami are of normal appearance on both image sequences.

CASE 6.3. MODERATE BASAL GANGLIA AND THALAMIC LESIONS (FIG. 6.18)

This female infant was born at 41 weeks' gestation by forceps delivery with a birth weight of 3.2 kg. Her mother was a primigravida and the pregnancy was uneventful, except for transient proteinuria at 34 weeks' gestation. Apgar scores were 3 at 1 min and 3 at 5 min. The umbilical cord pH was 7.13. She required ventilation for 5 h. Abnormal movements were noted at 1 h of age. She was classified as having stage II HIE.

■ *Moderate focal basal ganglia lesions are associated with the development of athetoid quadriplegia. There is usually good head growth and normal intelligence.*

Neurodevelopmental follow-up

At 4 years of age she has an athetoid cerebral palsy. She is able to take some steps using a walking aid. She is dysarthric but is of above average intelligence.

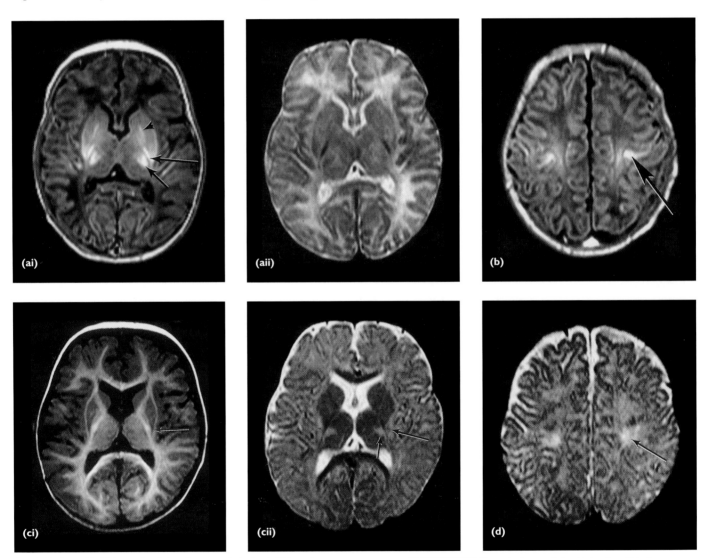

Fig. 6.18 Case 6.3. **(a)** Imaged at 5 days. Low ventricular level. **(i)** Inversion recovery sequence (IR 3800/30/950). There is abnormal signal intensity within the lentiform, posteriorly and anteriorly (*arrowhead*) and in the region of the ventro-lateral thalamic nuclei (*short arrow*). The signal intensity from myelin is present (*long arrow*) but associated with a parallel low signal intensity. **(ii)** T2 weighted spin echo sequence (SE 2700/120). The low signal representing myelin in the posterior limb of the internal capsule is slightly excessive for a conventional T2 weighted spin echo. It is difficult to see the abnormal signal intensities within the lentiform nuclei and thalami. **(b)** Centrum semiovale. Inversion recovery sequence (IR 3800/30/950). There is cortical highlighting, most obvious around the central fissure (*arrow*). **(c)** Imaged at 1 year of age. Low ventricular level. **(i)** Inversion recovery sequence (IR 3400/30/800). There are small low signal intensity lesions in the posterior putamen (*arrow*) consistent with cysts. **(ii)** T2 weighted spin echo sequence (SE 2700/120). There are areas of abnormal high signal intensity in the posterior putamen (*long arrow*) and in the lateral thalamus (*short arrow*). The lateral border of the putamen is flattened indicating atrophy. **(d)** Centrum semiovale. T2 weighted spin echo sequence (SE 2700/120). There is high signal intensity around the central fissure at the site of the previous cortical highlighting in **(b)**.

CASE 6.4 SEVERE BASAL GANGLIA AND THALAMIC LESIONS (FIG. 6.19)

This male infant was born at 42 weeks' gestation by forceps delivery with a birth weight of 4 kg. His mother was a primigravida and her pregnancy was uneventful. There was meconium-stained liquor following spontaneous rupture of membranes. Some decelerations were noted on the cardiotocogram (CTG). Apgar scores were 0 at 1 min, and 1 at 10 min. Abnormal movements were noted at 1.5 h of age. He was classified as having stage II HIE. He was ventilated for 3 days.

Neurodevelopmental follow-up

He had severe feeding difficulties that required nasogastric tube feeding until approximately 8 months of age. At 4 years of age he is microcephalic and has a mixed quadriplegia with athetoid movements of his face and arms and marked spasticity in his legs. He has no speech but communicates with hand and eye movements. He is unable to sit independently. He has a moderate intellectual deficit. He has developed epilepsy and requires anticonvulsants.

■ *Severe basal ganglia and thalamic lesions are associated with the development of a secondary microcephaly, in the absence of cystic white matter breakdown. The more extensive the basal ganglia and thalamic lesions, the more likely the development of a spastic cerebral palsy. Feeding difficulties are also more likely but may improve with age. Intelligence is unlikely to be normal. Convulsions may re-occur during infancy or childhood.*

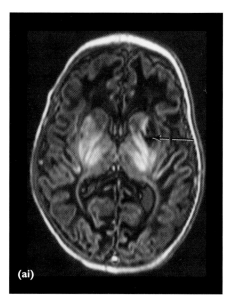 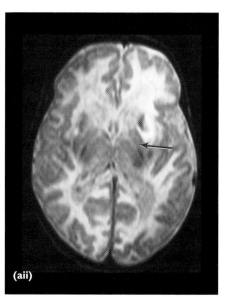 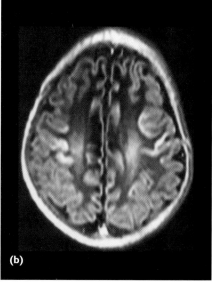

Fig. 6.19 Case 6.4. Aged 13 days. **(a)** Low ventricular level. **(i)** Inversion recovery sequence (IR 3800/30/950). There is abnormal signal intensity throughout the basal ganglia and thalami. There is a cyst in the anterior lentiform nucleus and caudate head on the left (*arrow*). There is some high signal in the region of the internal capsule but this is too long for normal myelination and is accompanied by a parallel low signal intensity. There is cortical highlighting within the insula with abnormal low signal intensity in the adjacent subcortical white matter. **(ii)** T2 weighted spin echo sequence (SE 2700/120). There are marked abnormal low and high signal intensities throughout the lentiform nuclei. The cyst is seen as high signal intensity on the left. The abnormal signal in the thalami is less obvious than on the T1 weighted images and the signal from myelin in the posterior limb of the internal capsule is relatively normal posteriorly but can be seen to extend anteriorly particularly on the left (*arrow*). This would be too excessive for normal myelination. **(b)** Centrum semiovale. Inversion recovery sequence (IR 3800/30/950). There is extensive cortical highlighting higher up the brain at the level of the centrum semiovale and most marked around the central fissure. There is widespread low signal intensity in the white matter. **(c)** Hippocampal level. There is abnormal high signal intensity in the medial temporal lobe in the region of the hippocampus (*arrow*). **(d)** Aged 13 months. Low ventricular level. **(i)** Inversion recovery sequence (IR 3400/30/800). There is marked atrophy of the hemispheres and the basal ganglia and thalami. There is now high signal intensity consistent with myelin in the posterior limb of the internal capsule. In addition there is myelin throughout the brain but this is deficient for this age and very thin. The cyst remains on the left. **(ii)** T2 weighted spin echo sequence (SE 2700/120). There is abnormal high signal intensity along the lateral border of the atrophied lentiform nuclei. There is additional abnormal high signal intensity within the thalami. There is some low signal intensity consistent with myelin in the posterior limb of the internal capsule and in the anterior and posterior corpus callosum. **(iii)** FLAIR sequence (fluid attenuated IR 6500/160/2100). Areas of increased signal

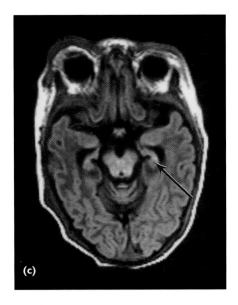

intensity consistent with gliosis are more prominent than on the T2 weighted images. **(e)** Centrum semiovale. **(i)** T2 weighted spin echo sequence (SE 2700/120). There is abnormal high signal intensity in a 'bats wing' pattern in the centrum semiovale and the site of the previous cortical highlighting and abnormal low signal in the subcortical white matter (see **b**). **(ii)** FLAIR sequence (fluid attenuated IR 6500/160/2100). The high signal intensity consistent with gliosis is more marked than on the T2 weighted images. **(f)** Hippocampal level. FLAIR sequence (fluid attenuated IR 6500/160/2100). There is atrophy with dilation of the temporal horns of the lateral ventricles. There is abnormal increased signal intensity consistent with gliosis (*arrow*).

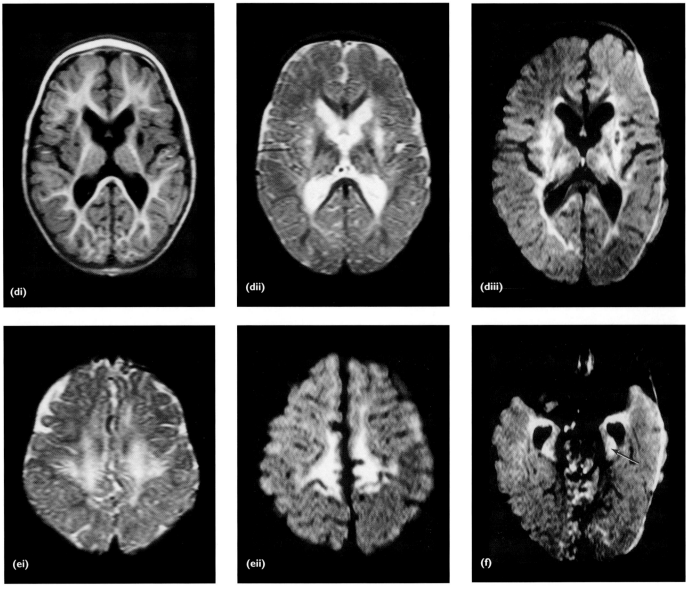

CASE 6.5. VERY SEVERE DIFFUSE BASAL GANGLIA AND THALAMIC LESIONS (FIG. 6.20)

This female infant was born at 39+ weeks' gestation by emergency cesarian section following a failed forceps and failed ventouse delivery. Her mother was a primigravida and her pregnancy was uneventful. There was marked fetal distress and a cord prolapse during a forceps delivery. She was eventually delivered by cesarian section. Apgar scores were 2 at 1 min and 5 at 5 min. The birth weight was 3.8 kg. The infant was ventilated for 12 h. She developed convulsions at 18 h and was reventilated until day 4. An EEG showed a supressed background with seizure activity. She was classified as having stage II HIE.

Neurodevelopmental outcome

This little girl developed a spastic quadriplegia with extensor posturing and severe microcephaly. She had persistent difficulties with sucking and swallowing and required the insertion of a gastrostomy tube. She had frequent convulsions which were difficult to control. She died from respiratory complications at 3 years of age.

■ *Very severe diffuse basal ganglia and thalamic lesions are associated with a very poor neurodevelopmental outcome or early death. There are usually severe feeding difficulties and on-going convulsions. Involvement of the mid-brain and brain stem may be obvious on MR imaging.*

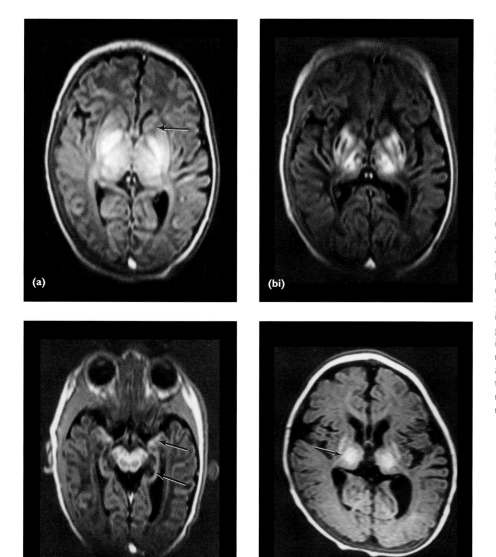

Fig. 6.20 Case 6.5. **(a)** Aged 10 days. Inversion recovery sequence (IR 3800/30/950). There is abnormal signal intensity throughout the thalami, the putamen and the globus pallidum. There is a low signal intensity running along the posterior limb of the internal capsule. There is a very low signal intensity in the anterior limb of the internal capsule (*arrow*). There are widespread areas of cortical highlighting and the white matter has an abnormal low signal intensity. There has been resolution of previously documented brain swelling. **(b)** Aged 3 weeks. Transverse plane. Inversion recovery sequence (IR 3800/30/950). **(i)** Low ventricular level. The abnormal high and low signal intensity within the basal ganglia and thalami are at their most obvious. The low signal probably represents cyst formation. **(ii)** Hippocampal level. There is abnormal high signal intensity within the medial temporal lobe (*arrows*). There is abnormal high and low signal intensity within the brainstem. **(c)** Aged 6 months. Inversion recovery sequence (IR 3600/30/700). There is marked plagiocephaly. There is severe atrophy of the white matter and basal ganglia and thalami. There is some high signal in the internal capsule consistent with myelin but this is not normal in appearance (*arrow*). There is abnormal high signal intensity throughout the thalamus and in the atrophied putamen. This may represent status marmoratus. Myelination is markedly deficient throughout the brain.

CASE 6.6. WHITE MATTER INFARCTION (FIG. 6.21)

This male infant was delivered at 39+ weeks by emergency cesarian section. This was his mother's second pregnancy. She noticed intermittent decreased fetal movements from 36 weeks. She presented at 39 weeks with decreased movements and tightenings. Meconium-stained liquor was noted following rupture of the membranes. An emergency cesarian section was performed following a fetal scalp blood sample with a pH 7.02 and decreased variability on the CTG. Apgar scores were 1 at 1 min and 3 at 5 min. His birth weight was 3.19 kg. The infant was ventilated from 8 h of age for recurrent apnea. Clinically obvious convulsions were noted from 12 h of age. He was classified as having grade II HIE. He was extubated at 48 h. Numerous skin pustules were noted but a septic screen was negative.

Neurodevelopmental outcome

He developed a secondary microcephaly, a strabismus and a visual field deficit. He has a dystonic posture of his right arm with poor hand function. At 6 years of age he walks independently. He has not had any further convulsions. He attends a mainstream school but has considerable learning difficulties.

■ *Infants with HIE who have predominantly white matter lesions usually have a more complicated antenatal course, suggesting a chronic or repetitive injury or possible sepsis. The degree of associated basal ganglia involvement probably reflects the severity of any acute perinatal asphyxia. Motor impairment is usually less severe than intellectual impairment.*

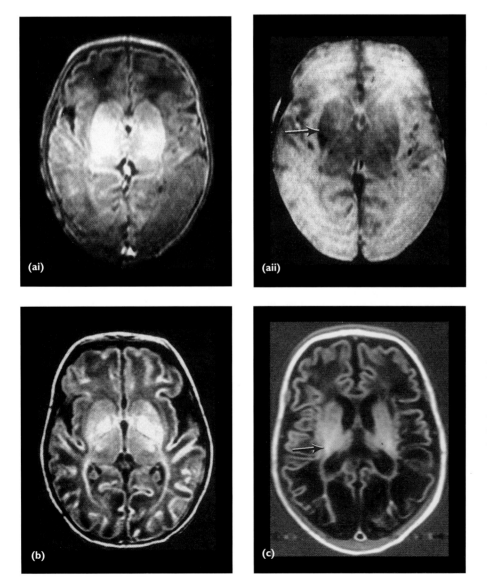

Fig. 6.21 Case 6.6. **(a)** Aged 4 days. **(i)** T1 weighted spin echo sequence (SE 860/200). There is brain swelling with widespread loss of gray/white matter differentiation in the parietal and occipital lobes. There is some diffuse high signal within the basal ganglia. There are a few areas of cortical highlighting. There is a diffuse high signal intensity within the basal ganglia and thalami, partly due to tight windowing of the images. There is abnormal low signal in frontal lobes. **(ii)** T2 weighted spin echo sequence (SE 2700/120). There is almost complete loss of gray/white matter differentiation. There is some low signal intensity in both lentiform nuclei more marked in the lateral putamen on the right (*arrow*). There is no low signal from myelin within the posterior limb of the internal capsule. **(b)** Aged 10 days. Inversion recovery sequence (IR 3800/30/950). There is now an exaggeration of the normal gray/white matter differentiation. There is widespread highlighting of the cortex with low signal within white matter consistent with infarction. There is bilateral high signal in lentiform, globus and lateral thalami. This may be partly due to very tight windowing. Windowing images which have either very high or very low signal intensity within the brain can be very difficult. It is difficult to detect any high signal from myelin within the posterior limb of the internal capsule, although the level of the image is slightly low. **(c)** Aged 5 weeks. Inversion recovery sequence (IR 3800/30/950). There is extensive cyst formation throughout the white matter. The cortex appears thin. There is a small amount of high signal intensity at the base of the posterior limb consistent with myelination (*arrow*). **(d)** Aged 3 months. Inversion recovery sequence (IR 3800/30/950). **(i)** Low ventricular level. There is marked cystic change with atrophy of the white matter. The posterior limb is myelinated, although slightly asymmetrical. There is some myelin appearing at the anterior limb on the left. The anterior limb should be fully myelinated at 3 months. **(ii)** Centrum semiovale. There is extensive infarction of the posterior parietal lobes. **(e)** Aged 7

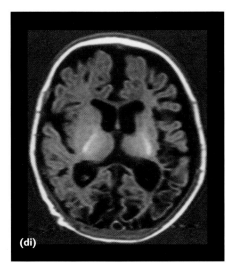 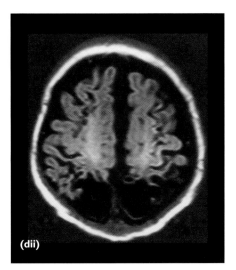 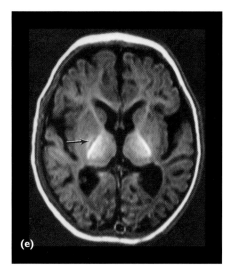

months. Inversion recovery sequence (IR 3800/30/950). There is widespread atrophy of the brain with decreased myelination. There is myelin in the frontal lobes which usually appears at around 6 months. Myelin has progressed in the anterior limb of the internal capsules. The basal ganglia and thalami are relatively preserved. There is some abnormal high signal intensity in the right lentiform nucleus (*arrow*).

CASE 6.7. WIDESPREAD CORTICAL INJURY (FIG. 6.22)

This female infant was born by emergency cesarian section at 39 weeks' gestation. Her mother had had two previous miscarriages. During this pregnancy she had a threatened abortion at 9 weeks. An antepartum hemorrhage at 24 weeks was attributed to a low-lying placenta. She had several further bleeds until 32 weeks. She was induced at 39 weeks at which time she had a further larger bleed. There were CTG decelerations to 77, a baseline of only 105 beats/min and the trace showed poor variability. The baseline dropped to 70 beats/min just prior to delivery. Her birth weight was 4.2 kg. Apgar scores were 0 at 1 minute, 2 at 5 min and 3 at 10 min. She developed convulsions at 24 h of age. She was classified as having stage II HIE.

Neurodevelopmental outcome

This little girl developed a secondary microcephaly and a mild spastic diplegia. She walks with a rollator. She has an IQ of approximately 50.

■ *Cortical and white matter injury are associated with mild motor impairment usually in the form of a spastic diplegia. Intellectual impairment is more severe. Late MR images may resemble classic periventricular leukomalacia (PVL) and may be wrongly attributed to an antenatal insult, as in the preterm population. Whilst the injury in these term-born infants may be secondary to a chronic or repetitive antenatal insult the structural lesions themselves are perinatal in onset. It is possible that if these infants could be identified, an elective cesarian section prior to term may modify or even prevent the injury to the brain.*

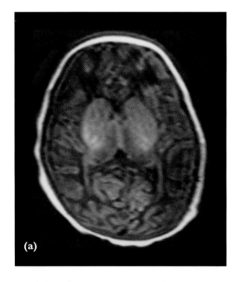

(a)

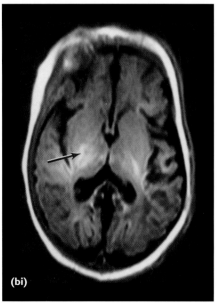

(bi)

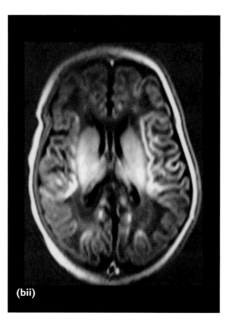

(bii)

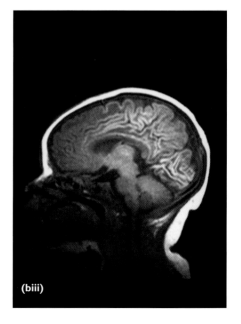

(biii)

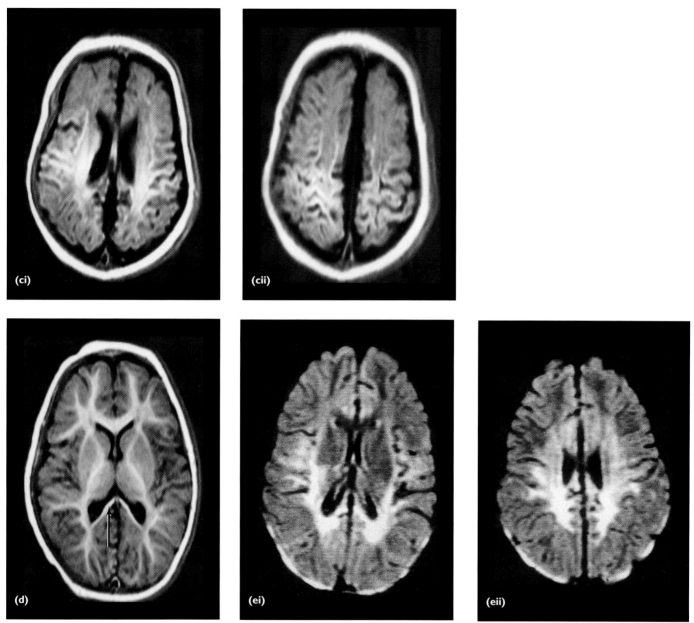

Fig. 6.22 Case 6.7. **(a)** Aged 3 days. T1 weighted spin echo sequence (SE 860/20). There is marked brain swelling with some loss of gray/white matter differentiation. There are multiple artifacts through the image secondary to intravenous lines. **(b)** Aged 18 days. Inversion recovery sequence (IR 3800/30/950). Sagittal plane. **(i)** Low ventricular level. There is widespread cortical highlighting. There is asymmetry of posterior limb and some high signal in right lentiform (*arrow*). **(ii)** Mid-ventricular level. There is widespread cortical highlighting and abnormal low signal intensity in the subcortical white matter. The extent of these abnormalities is well shown on the sagittal image **(iii)**. **(c)** Aged 6 weeks. Inversion recovery sequence (IR 3800/30/950). **(i)** Mid-ventricular level. **(ii)** Centrum semiovale. There is marked atrophy of white matter with ventricular dilation. There is extensive high signal intensity within the cortex and white matter. This is more pronounced and diffuse than the original cortical highlighting. **(d)** Aged 1 year. Low ventricular level. Inversion recovery sequence (IR 3400/30/800). There is generalized atrophy of the hemispheres with a decreased amount but a normal pattern myelination. The corpus callosum is very thin posteriorly (*arrow*). The ventricles are not dilated. Without knowledge of the head circumference it is difficult to assess the degree of brain atrophy on these images. **(e)** FLAIR sequence (fluid attenuated IR 6500/160/2100). **(i)** Mid-ventricular level. **(ii)** High ventricular level. There is extensive abnormal increased T2 at the site of the previous cortical and white matter abnormalities. Despite this apparent gliosis the ventricular outline remains rounded, unlike those in more typical periventricular leukomalacia.

CASE 6.8. WIDESPREAD WHITE MATTER CYSTIC BREAKDOWN AND SEVERE BASAL GANGLIA AND THALAMIC LESIONS (FIG. 6.23)

This female infant was born by normal vaginal delivery following an uneventful pregnancy. There was some fresh meconium-stained liquor following an artificial rupture of the membranes. There were some decelerations noted on the CTG. She unexpectedly required extensive resuscitation. She developed convulsions on day 1. She was classified as stage II HIE.

Neurodevelopmental outcome

At 5 years of age she was microcephalic and had a severe spastic quadriplegia. She was fed by gastrostomy. She had seizures which required anticonvulsant medication. She showed some awareness of her surroundings but developmental progress was severely delayed.

■ *In some infants there is extensive cystic breakdown of the white matter and severe basal ganglia lesions. This may result from a combination of chronic repetitive injury which primes the white matter followed by a severe perinatal insult which is the final 'insult' for the white matter but sufficiently severe as to cause significant basal ganglia and thalamic lesions. These children have a very poor outcome but may show more awareness than those with severe basal ganglia lesions without white matter cysts. Both groups of children will develop a secondary microcephaly.*

■ *Occasionally, infants sustain very severe damage to the brain perinatally with very little evidence of fetal distress. Further investigation to identify predisposing factors is warranted to help predict prognosis and for genetic counselling.*

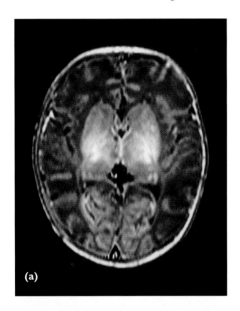

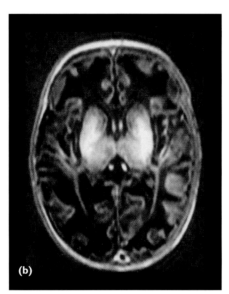

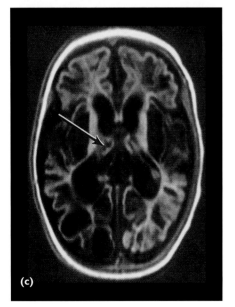

Fig. 6.23 Case 6.8. **(a)** Aged 3 days. Inversion recovery sequence (IR 3800/30/950). There is diffuse abnormal signal intensity within the basal ganglia and thalamus. It is difficult to identify the normal posterior limb of the internal capsule. There is generalized loss of gray/white matter differentiation. **(b)** Aged 6 weeks. Inversion recovery sequence (IR 3800/30/950). There is more excessive abnormal high signal intensity throughout the basal ganglia and thalami. The internal capsule is not distinguishable. There is widespread low signal intensity in the white matter consistent with infarction. The cortex appears very thin and highlighted. **(c)** Aged 4 months. Inversion recovery sequence (IR 3800/30/950). There is complete cystic breakdown of the white matter with marked atrophy of the basal ganglia and thalami (*arrow*).

Summary

- Obtain a detailed antenatal and perinatal history from both parents and professionals.

- Ensure the diagnosis of hypoxic–ischemic encephalopathy is correct. Exclude other additional causes of encephalopathy or any predisposing factors.

- Metabolic disorders may masquerade as HIE or co-exist. A metabolic screen in any infant with apparent HIE is always warranted.

- Time the imaging carefully. MR imaging within the first few days may give valuable information to plan management but be prepared to repeat if a day 1 or 2 scan is normal in an abnormal infant with HIE II or III. Image during the second week for maximum information about the pattern of injury and therefore the clinical outcome.

- Choose your sequences to detect the suspected lesions. The clinical history, neurological examination and cranial ultrasound may be useful guides.

- Severe acute injury, for example placental abruption, is usually associated with abnormalities in the basal ganglia and thalami and the posterior limb of the internal capsule. There may be additional lesions in the brain stem in severe cases. Associated hippocampal lesions are best seen during the second week.

- Marked white matter and cortical changes suggest a more chronic possibly repetitive injury, for example hypoxia – ischemia, infection, hypoglycemia. These infants often fulfill all the accepted criteria for HIE although the perinatal insult may be mild.

- Early clinical signs may give information about the pattern of injury. Infants who are breast or bottle feeding normally within 2 weeks are unlikely to have a severe lesion within the basal ganglia and thalami. They may still have a moderate or mild basal ganglia and thalamic lesion or severe white matter involvement.

- An abnormal signal within the posterior limb of the internal capsule is a good early predictor of abnormal outcome. Early diffusion weighted imaging should detect white matter infarction.

- The nature of the abnormal outcome can be determined by the extent of basal ganglia injury. In the absence of lesions within the basal ganglia and thalami the site and extent of white matter injury is important; however, if the signal intensity within the posterior limb is normal the motor outcome is likely to be normal or only mildly abnormal.

References

1. Adsett DB, Fitz CR and Hill A (1985) Hypoxic–ischaemic cerebral injury in the term newborn: correlation of CT findings with neurological outcome. *Dev Med Child Neurol* **27**, 155–160.
2. Baenziger O, Martin E, Steinlin M *et al.* (1993) Early pattern recognition in severe perinatal asphyxia: a prospective MRI study. *Neuroradiology* **35**, 437–442.
3. Barkovich AJ (1992) MR and CT evaluation of profound neonatal and infantile asphyxia. *Am J Neuroradiol* **13**, 959–972.
4. Barkovich AJ and Sargent SK (1995) Profound asphyxia in the premature infant: imaging findings. *Am J Neuroradiol* **16**, 1837–1846.
5. Barkovich AJ and Truwit CL (1990) Brain damage from perinatal asphyxia: correlation of MR findings with gestational age. *Am J Neuroradiol* **11**, 1087–1096.
6. Barkovich AJ, Hajnal BL, Vigneron D *et al.* (1998a) Prediction of neuromotor outcome in perinatal asphyxia: evaluation of MR scoring systems. *Am J Neuroradiol* **19**, 143–149.
7. Barkovich AJ, Ali FA, Rowley HA *et al.* (1998b) Imaging patterns of neonatal hypoglycemia. *Am J Neuroradiol* **19**, 523–528.
8. Barkovich AJ, Latal-Hajnal B, Partridge JC *et al.* (1997) MR contrast enhancement of the normal neonatal brain. *Am J Neuroradiol* **18**, 1713–1717.
9. Byrne P, Welch R, Johnson MA (1990) Serial magnetic resonance imaging in neonatal hypoxic–ischaemic encephalopathy. *J Pediatr* **117**, 694–700.
10. Cowan FM, Pennock JM, Hanrahan JD *et al.* (1994) Early detection of cerebral infarction and hypoxic ischemic encephalopathy in neonates using diffusion weighted magnetic resonance imaging. *Neuropediatrics* **25**, 172–175.
11. Chugani HT and Phelps ME (1986) Maturational changes in cerebral function in infants determined by 18 FDG positron emission tomography. *Science* **231**, 840–843.
12. Cullen A, Donoghue V and King MD (1998) High attenuation gyri on CT in postasphyxial encephalopathy. *Ir J Med Sci* **167**, 193–195.
13. Dammann O and Leviton A (1997) Maternal intrauterine infection, cytokines, and brain damage in the preterm newborn. *Pediatr Res* **42**, 1–8.
14. De Vries LS, Eken P, Beek E *et al.* (1996) The posterior fontanelle: a neglected acoustic window. *Neuropediatrics* **27**, 101–104.
15. Dietrich RB and Bradley WG Jr (1988) Iron accumulation in the basal ganglia following severe ischemic-anoxic insults in children. *Radiology* **168**, 203–206.
16. Eken P, Jansen GH, Groenendaal F *et al.* (1994) Intracranial lesions in the fullterm infant with hypoxic–ischaemic encephalopathy: ultrasound and autopsy correlation. *Neuropediatrics* **25**, 301–307.
17. Eken P, Toet MC, Groenendaal F *et al.* (1995) Predictive value of early neuroimaging, pulsed Doppler and neurophysiology in full term infants with hypoxic–ischaemic encephalopathy. *Arch Dis Child Fetal Neonatal Ed* **73**, F75–80.

18. Jouvet P, Cowan FM, Cox P *et al.* (1999) Reproducibility and accuracy of MR imaging of the brain after severe birth asphyxia. *Am J Neuroradiol* **20**, 1343–1348.

19. Keenay SE, Adcock EW and McArdle CB (1991) prospective observations of 100 high risk neonates by high-field (1.5 Tesla) magnetic resonance imaging of the central nervous system II. Lesions associated with hypoxic–ischaemic encephalopathy. *Pediatrics* **87**, 431–438.

20. Kinnala A, Rikalainen H, Lapinleimu H (1999) Cerebral magnetic resonance imaging and ultrasonography findings after neonatal hypoglycemia. *Pediatrics* **103**, 724–729.

21. Kuenzle C, Baenziger O, Martin E *et al.* (1994) Prognostic value of early MR imaging in term infants with severe perinatal asphyxia. *Neuropediatrics* **4**, 191–200.

22. Le Strange E, Saeed N, Counsell S *et al.* (2000) Magnetic resonance image quantification following hypoxic–ischemic injury to the neonatal brain ISMRM Denver Colorado Abstract 1928.

23. Leech RW and Alvord EC (1977) Anoxic–ischemic encephalopathy in the human neonatal period. The significance of brain stem involvement. *Arch Neurol* **34**, 109–113.

24. Malamud N (1950) Status marmoratus: a form of cerebral palsy following birth injury or inflammation of the central nervous system. *J Pediatrics* **37**, 610–619.

25. Murakami Y, Yamashita Y, Matsuishi T (1999) Cranial MRI of neurologically impaired children suffering from neonatal hypoglycaemia. *Pediatr Radiol* **29**, 23–27.

26. Okuda T, Korogi Y, Ikushima I (1998) Use of fluid-attenuated inversion recovery (FLAIR) pulse sequences in perinatal hypoxic–ischaemic encephalopathy. *Br J Radiol* **71**, 282–290.

27. Pasternak JF and Goery MT (1998) The syndrome of acute near-total intrauterine asphyxia in the term infant. *Pediatr Neurol* **18**, 391–398.

28. Pasternak JF, Predey TA and Mikhael MA (1991) Neonatal asphyxia: vulnerability of basal ganglia, thalamus and brainstem. *Pediatr Neurol* **7**, 147–149.

29. Pennock JM, Cowan FM, Schweiso JE *et al.* (1994) Clinical role of diffusion weighted imaging: neonatal studies. *Magma* **2**, 273–278.

30. Rademaker RP, van der Knaap MS, Verbeeten B Jr *et al.* (1995) Central cortico-subcortical involvement: a distinct pattern of brain damage caused by perinatal and postnatal asphyxia in term infants. *J Comput Assist Tomogr* **19**, 252–263.

31. Roland EH, Hill A, Norman MG *et al.* (1988) Selective brainstem injury in an asphyxiated newborn. *Ann Neurol* **23**, 89–92.

32. Rutherford MA, Pennock JM, Murdoch-Eaton DM *et al.* (1992) Athetoid cerebral palsy and cysts in the putamen after hypoxic–ischaemic encephalopathy. *Arch Dis Child* **67**, 846–850.

33. Rutherford MA, Pennock JM and Dubowitz LMS (1994) Cranial ultrasound and magnetic resonance imaging in hypoxic–ischaemic encephalopathy: a comparison with outcome. *Dev Med Child Neurol* **36**, 813–825.

34. Rutherford MA, Pennock JM, Schwieso JE *et al.* (1995) Hypoxic–ischaemic encephalopathy: early magnetic resonance imaging findings and their evolution. *Neuropediatrics* **26**, 183–191.

35. Rutherford MA, Pennock JM, Schwieso JE *et al.* (1996) Hypoxic–ischaemic encephalopathy: early and late MRI findings and clinical outcome. *Arch Dis Child* **75**, 141–151.

36. Rutherford MA, Pennock J, Counsell S *et al.* (1998) Abnormal magnetic resonance signal in the internal capsule predicts poor developmental outcome in infants with hypoxic–ischaemic encephalopathy. *Pediatrics* **102**, 323–328.

37. Saint-Hilaire MH, Burke RE, Bressman SB *et al.* (1991) Delayed-onset dystonia due to perinatal or early childhood asphyxia. *Neurology* **41**, 216–222.

38. Sarnat HB and Sarnat MS (1976) Neonatal encephalopathy following fetal distress: a clinical and electrophysiological study. *Arch Neurol* **33**, 696–705.

39. Traill Z, Squier M and Anslow P (1998) Brain imaging in neonatal hypoglycaemia. *Arch Dis Child Fetal Neonatal Ed* **79**, F145–147.

40. van der Knaap MS, Smit LS, Nauta JP *et al.* (1993) Cortical laminar abnormalities: occurrence and clinical significance. *Neuropediatrics* **24**, 143–148.

41. Volpe JJ, Herscovitch P, Perlman JM *et al.* (1985) Positron emission tomography in the asphyxiated term newborn: parasagittal impairment of cerebral blood flow. *Ann Neurol* **17**, 287–296.

42. Yokochi K (1998) Clinical profiles of subjects with subcortical leukomalacia and border-zone infarction revealed by MR. *Acta Pediatr* **87**, 879–883.

Cerebral infarction in the full-term infant

Eugenio Mercuri, Lilly Dubowitz and Mary A Rutherford

7

Contents

Introduction

Neonatal cerebral infarction or stroke may be defined as 'a severe disorganization of gray and/or white matter architecture caused by embolic, thrombotic or ischemic events'. The increase in neonatal imaging in infants with abnormal neurological signs has highlighted the wide spectrum of these lesions[2,4,6,8,9,11,13,16,19,23,26,28,29]. Infarcts may be divided into two main types: those occurring within the territory of a major artery and those occurring in the borderzone or watershed areas.

Arterial infarction

AETIOLOGY

The most commonly reported type of neonatal cerebral infarction in the full-term infant are ischemic lesions in the territory of a major cerebral artery. The middle cerebral artery is most commonly affected and, as found in adult stroke, the left middle cerebral artery is three to four times more frequently involved than the right[15]. Infants with involvement of the anterior or posterior cerebral artery may be asymptomatic and therefore underdiagnosed. In addition, lesions in these regions can be difficult to detect with cranial ultrasound[19,23].

Before the advent of neuroimaging, infarction was thought to be a rare condition, recognized only at post-mortem examination in infants with congenital heart disease or other life-threatening conditions such as disseminated intravascular coagulation or sepsis.

Following the introduction of neonatal cranial ultrasound and CT scanning in the late 1970s, cerebral infarcts were also identified in infants who survived, most of them being associated with severe perinatal asphyxia[2]. Large infarcts were also observed in young children who had no obvious perinatal problems and it was thought that in these cases the infarcts must have occurred antenatally. More recently, early and serial imaging in the newborn has allowed us to recognize that infarcts are more frequent than assumed, and has also provided information about the spectrum of these lesions and their possible etiology[4,6,8,9,11,13,16,19,23,26,28,29].

The etiology of most arterial infarcts remains unclear as only a minority are associated with the clinical conditions reported in earlier studies. Severe adverse antenatal and perinatal factors are relatively rare, and whilst many of these infants have some signs of fetal distress, their Apgar scores are usually normal at 5 min[19]. The onset of convulsions in the first days of life is usually the first clinical sign leading to diagnostic investigation. In recent years, the etiological role of hematological factors in cerebral infarction has been studied, with some reports of an increased incidence of heterozygosity for factor V Leiden. In our own cohort of 24 infants with arterial infarction, five infants were heterozygous for factor V Leiden all of whom developed a hemiplegia, compared to only one of the 19 infants without factor V Leiden[24].

CLINICAL FINDINGS

Infants with focal infarction do not usually have an encephalopathy; they are alert and responsive to visual and auditory stimuli. Convulsions are often the first and only clinical sign, which will draw attention to the presence of the lesion in the first days of life. The convulsions are usually unilateral at the onset but may become generalized during the seizure. Some infants may show abnormal tone in the limbs usually contralateral but occasionally ipsilateral to the lesion[7]. These abnormal neonatal signs, if present, are often transient and do not predict later outcome[23]. In some cases abnormal clinical signs during the neonatal period are either absent or so subtle that they escape detection (Fig. 7.2). The neurodevelopmental outcome in infants with perinatal infarction is variable, ranging from normality to the presence of a hemiplegia. Early continu-ous EEG may demonstrate seizure activity but assessment of the background activity is most important for predicting motor outcome[23,32]. Infants with or without a later hemiplegia may be at risk for non-motor impairments that become obvious in early childhood (see case histories).

MRI FINDINGS

The spectrum of lesions is wide, ranging from small abnor-malities in the basal ganglia (Fig. 7.1a) to very extensive ones, which involve most of the hemisphere (Fig. 7.1b). There may also be combinations of lesions within the same infant (Fig. 7.1c). The exact site of an infarct may be diffi-cult to define. Infarcts in the posterior territory of the mid-dle cerebral artery may be confused with infarcts arising from

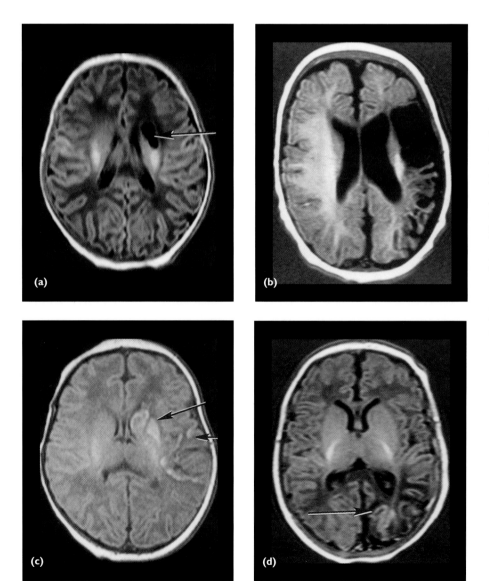

Fig. 7.1 **(a)** Inversion recovery sequence (IR 3800/30/950). Infant aged 3 weeks. There is a small infarct involving the head of the caudate nucleus and the lentiform on the left (*arrow*). **(b)** Inversion recovery sequence (IR 3800/30/800). Infant aged 12 months. There is extensive infarction and atrophy of the left hemisphere. There is reduced high signal intensity from myelination on the left. The ventricles are dilated. **(c)** T1 weighted spin echo sequence (SE 860/20). Infant aged 7 days. There is abnormal signal intensity within the caudate head and lentiform on the left (*long arrow*). There is additional highlighting of the Sylvian cortex and low signal within the adjacent subcortical white matter (*short arrow*). **(d)** Inversion recovery sequence (IR 3800/30/950). Infant aged 9 days. There is an infarct involving the left parieto/temporal/occipital region. The involvement of the medial aspect of the occipital lobe (*arrow*) indicates posterior cerebral artery territory. This lesion may represent an asymmetrical watershed lesion. Careful examination of all levels of imaging to identify involvement of other watershed areas is indicated.

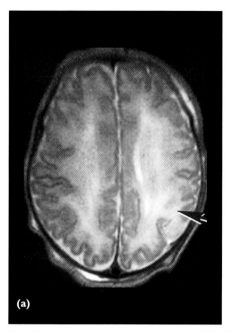 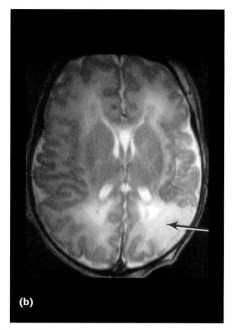 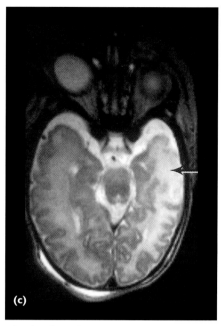

Fig. 7.2 (a),(b),(c) Fast spin echo sequence (FSE 3000/208). Infant aged 3 days. This infant was enrolled as a control patient for an imaging study. He had no presenting signs. The infarct in the territory of the MCA was picked up incidentally. There is loss of gray/white matter differentiation with abnormal high signal intensity (arrows) involving the parietal (**a**), occipital (**b**) and temporal (**c**) lobes. The signal intensity changes are consistent with a perinatal insult.

the posterior cerebral artery or from asymmetrical watershed lesions (see below) (Fig. 7.1d). Confusion may arise because of individual variation in the arterial distribution to the brain. In addition, as the brain grows and the infarct evolves, the site of abnormality on MRI may appear to shift, further complicating the issue (case 7.3).

The following classification for middle cerebral artery infarcts according to the branch involved has been suggested by de Vries *et al.*[6]:

■ main branch
■ cortical branch
■ lenticulostriate branches.

Although all these lesions can occur in both preterm and full-term infants, the involvement of the main branch or of one of the cortical branches is more frequently observed in the full-term infant and lesions in the lenticulostriate branch in the preterm infant (see Chapter 8).

Main branch/cortical branch

In the neonate these lesions are mainly ischemic without a hemorrhagic component, unlike the infarcts which occur in older children and in adults. The initial lesion is seen as a loss of gray/white matter differentiation with mainly low signal intensity on T1 and high signal intensity on T2 weighted images (Fig. 7.2)

Infarcts associated with occlusion of the main branch of the middle cerebral artery (MCA) may involve the white matter and cortex within the frontal, parietal, temporal and occipital lobes (Fig. 7.2) There may be additional involvement of the ipsilateral internal capsule and the basal ganglia/thalamus (Fig. 7.3). An infarct in the territory of a cerebral artery may also occur in association with other ischemic or hemorrhagic lesions in the ipsilateral or contralateral hemisphere (Fig. 7.4). The main infarction can be associated with a contralateral infarction (case 7.7), with more discrete ischemic lesions (Fig. 7.5) or punctate hemorrhagic lesions (Fig. 7.6) in the white matter. Infants with bilateral MCA territory lesions may develop the perisylvian syndrome (case 7.7).

The site and extent of the changes relating to occlusion of a cortical branch is quite variable. In our recent series of 20 infants with cortical branch infarcts, only four infants had additional lesions within the basal ganglia/thalamus and the internal capsule[23].

Using serial imaging it is possible to observe the evolution of infarcted areas over the first few weeks and months of life.

Evolution first week

Changes during the first few days of life may be difficult to identify with conventional imaging alone (Fig. 7.7). Conventional imaging during the first week will show a loss

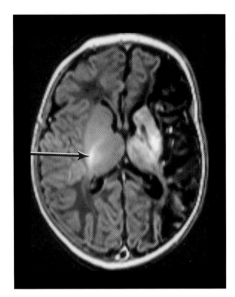

Fig. 7.3 Inversion recovery sequence (IR 3800/30/950). Infant aged 14 days. There is a large infarct involving the left hemisphere. There are additional abnormal high and low signal intensities within the basal ganglia and thalamus and the internal capsule on the left. The normal signal from myelin in the posterior limb of the internal capsule is only seen on the right (*arrow*).

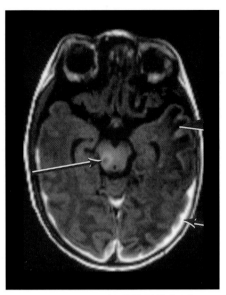

Fig. 7.4 Inversion recovery sequence (IR 3800/30/950). Infant aged 6 days. There is a small area of infarction in the temporal pole on the left (*arrowhead*). The infarct was more extensive on superior slices. There is a small hemorrhagic lesion in the right mesencephalon (*long arrow*). There is subdural hemorrhage around the surface of the brain (*short arrow*).

of gray/white matter differentiation with a generally low signal intensity in the region of the infarct on T1 weighted images. On T2 weighted images there is a loss of differentiation and generally increased signal intensity (Fig. 7.8). Changes are usually easier to identify on T2 weighted scans (Fig. 7.8). Diffusion weighted imaging during the first week 'highlights' infarcted areas and this then aids detection on the conventional images (Figs 7.7 and 7.8). The abnormalities on diffusion weighted imaging become less obvious by the end of the first week by which time the abnormalities are more obvious on the conventional T1 and T2 weighted images (Fig. 7.8). Animal studies have reported that changes on diffusion are more evident a few hours after an acute ischemic insult and tend to be less evident a few days after, thus the sequence of findings in infants with infarcts suggest that the acute event occurred around the perinatal period[5].

Evolution second to sixth week

During the second week following an infarction there may be an exaggeration of gray/white matter differentiation with areas of cortex becoming highlighted and white matter becoming even lower signal intensity using T1 weighted imaging (Fig. 7.8). From 2 weeks onwards there may be breakdown of infarcted tissue. The extracerebral space may widen. A porencephalic cyst may form although there is usually some tissue visible within it, especially if windowed appropriately prior to image processing (case 7.1). On T1

weighted sequences high signal areas may appear around the penumbra of the infarct. The histological correlation for this lesion is not clear but it may represent capillary proliferation or possibly the presence of lipid-laden macrophages.

Evolution 6 weeks to 1 year

Over the next few months as the brain grows the infarct may appear to decrease in size and in some infants the original lesion may be difficult to identify (case 7.3). The affected hemisphere, however, usually looks smaller than the non-affected one and shows a generalized decrease in myelination most obvious around the site of the infarct. This clearly relates to the original size of the lesion and its evolution. Using a specifically designed computer program we have been able to accurately match and subtract serially acquired volume acquisition images in infants with focal infarcts[27]. Using this technique we have been able to identify the early changes in signal intensity and tissue breakdown. Matching and then subtracting the serially acquired images has then shown us that there may be excessive growth in and around the infarct over the next few months (Fig. 7.9). These changes are not detectable on visual analysis of the conventional images. This excessive growth may lead to the virtual disappearance of smaller infarcts. Regions of unexpected excessive growth may correspond to previously unrecognized regions of white matter damage (Fig. 7.15). Conventional imaging shows that regions of excessive

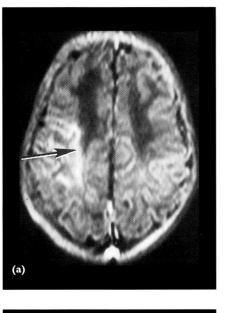

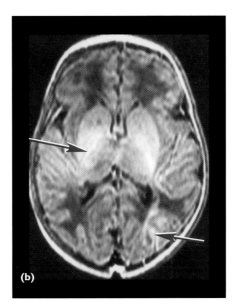

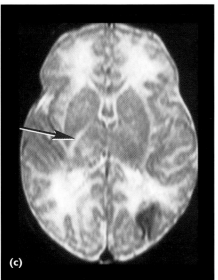

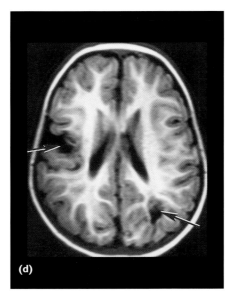

Fig. 7.5 Inversion recovery sequence (IR 3800/30/950). **(a, b)** Infant aged 6 days. There is abnormal high signal intensity within the cortex of the right Sylvian fissure. **(a)** (*arrow*) There is an asymmetry of the signal intensity from myelin in the posterior limb of the internal capsule with decreased signal intensity on the right (*long arrow*). There is an additional abnormal low signal intensity within the right thalamus and lentiform nucleus. There is an additional area of abnormal high signal intensity within the left occipital lobe **(b)** (*arrow*). T2 weighted sequence (SE 3000/120). Same infant aged 6 days. **(c)** The abnormalities within the cortex are seen as low signal intensity and are more obvious. The abnormalities within the lentiform and thalamus are seen as high signal intensity. The posterior limb of the internal capsule has abnormally high signal intensity throughout (*arrow*). Inversion recovery sequence (IR 3400/30/800) **(d)** at 20 months of age. There are two discrete areas of infarction (*arrows*) and mild dilation of the ventricles.

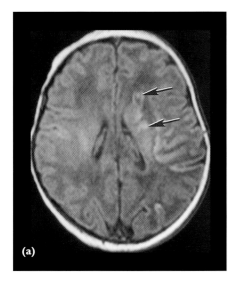

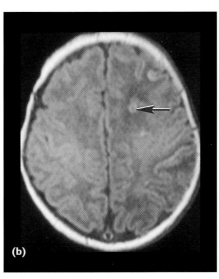

Fig. 7.6 T1 weighted spin echo sequence (SE860/20). **(a)**, **(b)** Infant aged 7 days (as in Fig. 7.1c). There are small high signal intensity hemorrhagic lesions in the white matter and basal ganglia (*arrows*).

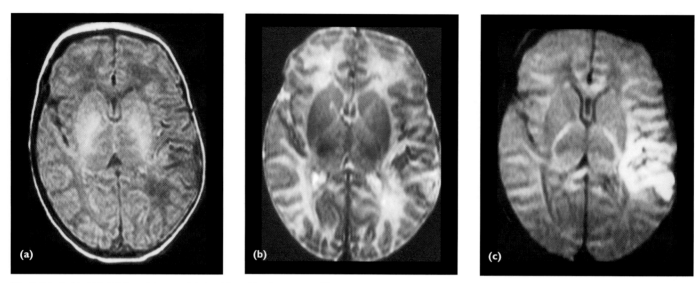

Fig. 7.7 Left-sided MCA infarct. Infant aged 4 days. T1 weighted spin echo (SE 860/20) **(a)**, T2 weighted spin echo sequence **(b)**, and diffusion weighted image **(c)** anterio-posterior sensitization. The abnormalities on conventional imaging are subtle. The diffusion changes consistent with restriction of water.

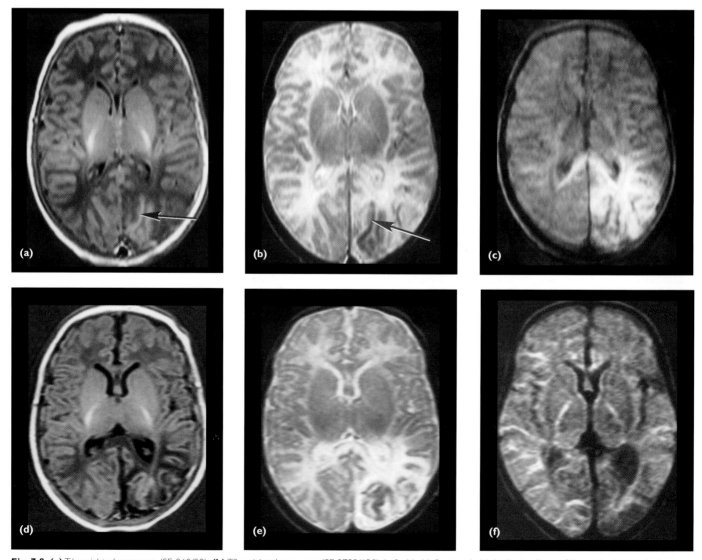

Fig. 7.8 (a) T1 weighted sequence (SE 860/20). **(b)** T2 weighted sequence (SE 2700/120). Left-sided infarct, probably in the territory of the posterior cerebral artery (*arrows*). **(c)** Diffusion weighted imaging. Infant aged 4 days. The abnormalities are more striking on the diffusion weighted images. **(d)** T1 weighted sequence (SE 860/20). **(e)** T2 weighted sequence (SE 2700/120). **(f)** Diffusion weighted imaging. Same infant aged 9 days. The abnormalities are more obvious on the conventional spin echo sequence images. The diffusion abnormalities are no longer evident.

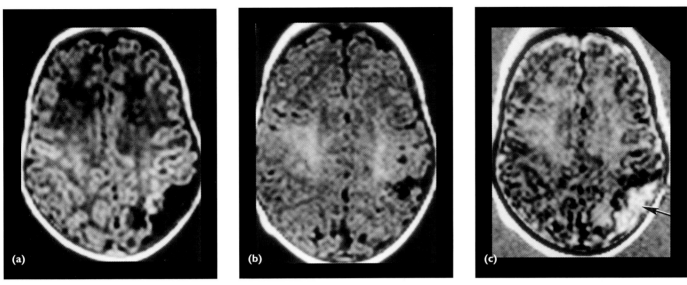

Fig. 7.9 TI weighted volume acquisition images taken at 4 weeks **(a)** and 3 months **(b)**. There is a region of infarction in the left posterior parietal lobe, which has decreased in size. After registering **(a)** and **(b)** there is high signal intensity consistent with new brain growth (*arrow*) within the original infarcted area **(c)**.

growth appear to have normal imaging characteristics and that in general infants with focal infarction have relatively small amounts of glial tissue on later imaging. The period of excess growth seems to start around 6 weeks and end by approximately 1 year of age.

Wallerian degeneration

In the acute stages of MCA infarction there may be abnormal signal intensity within the brain stem, presumably resulting from the phenomenon of diaschisis (case 7.7). Diaschisis is the term applied to acute metabolic changes that occur in connected but distant areas of the brain in response to a focal injury. This has been traditionally used to describe changes in the cerebellum following infarction of the forebrain.

In both perinatal main and cortical branch infarction changes in the size of brain stem due to secondary atrophy, Wallerian degeneration, become evident after 6–8 weeks and may become progressively more obvious (Fig. 7.10). Infants that show earlier asymmetry may have had an antenatal insult in addition to their perinatal infarct (Fig. 7.11). Early serial imaging may help to distinguish separate insults (case 7.1). Secondary degeneration may also give rise to atrophy of the ipsilateral thalamus, in the absence of initial involvement. Both ipsilateral and contralateral cerebellar atrophy have been demonstrated following focal infarction. This is thought to arise from the phenomenon of diaschisis. However, in a series of 10 term infants with perinatal focal infarction we have shown that cerebellar hemisphere growth

was symmetrical and comparable to controls over the first year of life[14].

Lenticulostriate branch

These lesions are more frequently observed in preterm infants[6] but can occasionally be seen in full-term infants (see Chapter 8). Unlike infarcts in the territory of cortical

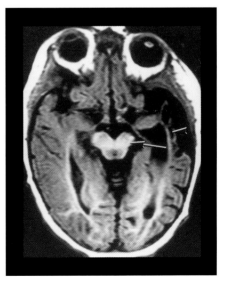

Fig. 7.10 Inversion recovery sequence (IR 3800/30/950). Infant aged 12 months. Left MCA infarction with involvement of the anterior temporal lobe (*arrowhead*). There is asymmetry of the mesencephalon with atrophy consistent with Wallerian degeneration on the left (*arrow*).

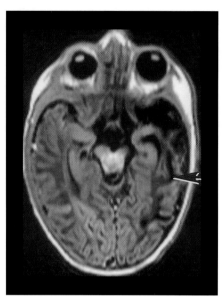

Fig. 7.11 Inversion recovery sequence (IR 3800/30/950). Infant aged 2 weeks. There is obvious asymmetry of the brain stem, with atrophy of the left in this infant who presented with seizures on day 2. The infarct seen in the left anterior lobe (*arrow*) looks about 1–2 weeks old. The brain stem asymmetry may originate from a previous lesion that is no longer identifiable.

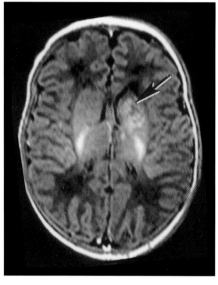

Fig. 7.12 Inversion recovery sequence (IR 3800/30/950). Infant aged 6 days. There is a hemorrhagic infarct in the left caudate head (*arrow*).

branches, they often have a hemorrhagic component. The lesions generally involve the lentiform and, sometimes, the caudate and/or the thalamus and the internal capsule (Fig. 7.12). Infants may also show a combination of cortical branch and basal ganglia lesions (Fig. 7.3). Small cystic lesions within the basal ganglia found incidentally on imaging are likely to represent small old infarcts (case 7.1).

Borderzone infarcts

ETIOLOGY

Perinatally acquired infarcts may also occur not in the distribution of one main artery but in the borderzone or watershed regions between arterial territories, so-called parasagittal lesions[31]. These lesions which, so far, have only been described in full-term infants, are thought to be due to an acute decrease in cerebral blood flow[31]. The affected areas will therefore be those that are most susceptible to hypotension and a fall in perfusion, such as the regions in the posterior lobes which represent the end fields among all the three main cerebral arteries.

Adverse antenatal factors are not frequent but in our experience these lesions, unlike the arterial infarcts, are usually associated with perinatal distress and/or mild signs of hypoxic–ischemic encephalopathy. These infants may show CTG abnormalities, meconium-staining liquor and instrumental deliveries are frequent. They may require some respiratory assistance such as facial O_2 or bagging but not intubation. The Apgar scores are often low at 1 min but recover quickly within 5 or 10 min (case 7.5). This pattern of injury may also be seen in infants with hypoglycemia[1].

CLINICAL FINDINGS

Infants with parasagittal lesions may develop seizures in the first 48 h although this may not be the first presenting sign. On neurological examination these infants are hypotonic; this is partly due to the fact that they are often assessed after the onset of seizures and the administration of anticonvulsants. The neonatal EEG may be normal, show epileptic discharges but a normal background or, in some cases, show a discontinuous background activity[23].

MRI FINDINGS

The lesions are generally bilateral, involving the posterior convexity (Fig. 7.13, case 7.5) and, in some cases, the anterior lobes. These lesions are quite symmetrical but in some, the lesion can be more predominant on one side, involving the anterior and posterior lobes and giving only a minimal involvement of the contralateral hemisphere (Fig. 7.14). The lesions are ischemic and seen as low signal intensity on T1 and high signal intensity on T2, but may have hemorrhagic components. The evolution of these lesions is similar to that observed in more focal cerebral infarcts with similar changes of excessive growth demonstrable on serial registration (Fig. 7.15). Occasionally, areas of infarction are seen adjacent to

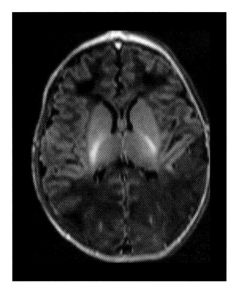

Fig. 7.13 Inversion recovery sequence (IR 3800/30/950). Term infant presenting with seizures following delivery on to the floor at home. Imaged at 5 days. There is bilateral loss of gray/white matter differentiation in the posterior parietal and temporal lobes. The basal ganglia are normal and the internal capsule is appropriately myelinated. This infant became microcephalic, has mild developmental delay but a normal motor outcome.

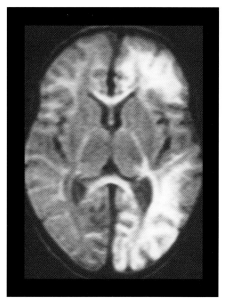

Fig. 7.14 Asymmetrical borderzone infarction. Diffusion weighted image, infant aged 6 days, showing abnormal restriction giving high signal intensity in the left frontal, parietal, temporal and occipital lobes. There is no obvious involvement of the right hemisphere at this level.

subdural hemorrhage (case 7.6). The exact association between these two lesions is unclear. It is possible that the subdural hemorrhage interferes with venous drainage resulting in venous infarction of the adjacent parenchyma. It has also been suggested that the infarction results from arterial spasm.

Neurodevelopmental outcome in arterial and borderzone infarcts: prognostic factors

MOTOR OUTCOME

Until a few years ago most of the studies on neonatal infarcts, with a few exceptions, reported a very high incidence of abnormal motor outcome, mainly hemiplegia[3,10,12,13,16–18,25,28,30,33]. Because of these early studies, parents of infants with cerebral infarction have been counselled about the high risk of their children developing cerebral palsy. With the increase in the detection of infarcts in infants without birth asphyxia, however, it has become evident that the incidence of abnormal motor outcome is lower than assumed[8,23].

We have reviewed a series of 24 children all of whom had early neonatal MRI[23]. The infants were followed longitudinally for at least 2 years in order to establish the best prognostic indicators in the neonatal period. Hemiplegia was present in only 20% of the children investigated. The presence of adverse antenatal and perinatal factors was not significantly associated with abnormal outcome.

We were unable to find any significant association between the neonatal neurological examination and outcome as abnormal signs in the neonatal period were found in infants with and without a normal outcome.

Neonatal MRI findings were better predictors of outcome. The presence of hemiplegia, however, did not seem to relate to the type of infarction, as the incidence was similar in both arterial and borderzone infarcts. In contrast, the extent of the lesion, and in particular the concomitant involvement of hemisphere, basal ganglia and internal capsule, was significantly associated with outcome. While infants who had involvement of one or two of these three components tended to have a normal motor outcome, infants with involvement of all three sites, developed an abnormal motor outcome (cases 7.4 and 7.7).

We have also shown that neonatal EEG can be equally predictive of late outcome. While all the infants who had normal background activity had a normal motor outcome[23], irrespective of the presence or absence of epileptic discharges, all the infants with abnormal background activity, *unilateral or bilateral*, developed hemiplegia.

Our recent studies[24] on the association between perinatal infarction and thrombotic disorders have shown a strong association between factor V Leiden and the development of

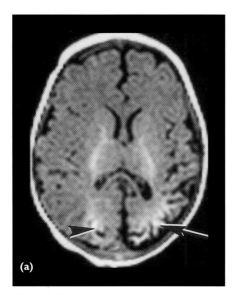
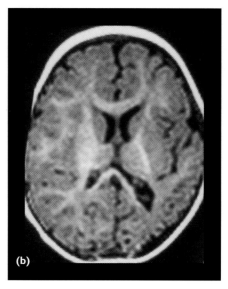
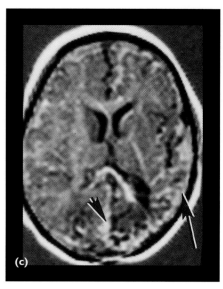

Fig. 7.15 Registration and subtraction of images. T1 weighted volume acquisition. **(a)** Aged 2 months, note the highlighting around the edge of the infarcted tissue on the left *(arrowhead)*. There is an additional small area of infarction on the right *(arrow)*. **(b)** Aged 6 months. There is atrophy and decreased myelin throughout the left hemisphere. **(c)** Subtraction image. There is high signal intensity around the atrophied left hemisphere consistent with new brain growth *(arrow)*. There is high signal intensity along the medial aspect of the right occipital lobe with a resultant decreased width of the interhemispheric fissure. This may represent an area of previously unrecognized white matter injury.

hemiplegia. Further studies are warranted to look at this relationship in more detail and to investigate the potential role of other prothrombotic factors such as the G20210A mutation in the prothrombin gene and the C677T mutation in the methylenetetrahydrofolate reductase gene.

VISUAL OUTCOME

The association between cerebral infarction and visual abnormalities has been well documented in children and adults suffering from stroke[20,34]. In these cases there appears to be a good correlation between the severity of MRI abnormalities and the severity of visual impairment. Lesions affecting the striate occipital cortex and the optic radiations are generally associated with contralateral hemianopia and lesions affecting the parietal lobe with abnormal visual attention and, in the most severe cases, with contralateral visual neglect.

Using a battery of tests, which were specifically designed to evaluate visual function in the first year of life, we have been able to demonstrate that infants with infarction have normal acuity and ocular movements but may show narrow-er visual fields and abnormal visual attention, as tested by fixation shift[21,22]. It is of interest, however, that in contrast to adults, not all the children who had involvement of the structures of the visual pathway on MRI developed abnormal visual function. Only 50% of the infants with involvement of the optic radiation had abnormal fields and only 50% of the infants with parietal lobe lesions had an abnormal fixation shift in the first year of life. These findings suggest that the immature brain can to some extent compensate for early lesions affecting the visual pathway.

NEUROCOGNITIVE OUTCOME

The plasticity of the neonatal brain may allow normal motor function in the presence of large areas of infarction; however, this may cause a 'crowding out' effect and occur at the expense of neurocognitive functions that develop later in childhood (see case histories). Long-term prospective follow-up studies to assess language, behaviour and neurocognitive functions in infants with and without a motor impairment will further define the extent and quality of compensation following perinatal infarction.

CASE 7.1

This male infant was born at 39 weeks' gestation (birth weight 3.132 kg).

Antenatal

His mother was a caucasian primigravida with known endometriosis. She was admitted to hospital at 34 weeks with abdominal pain, which settled spontaneously. Fetal movement and heart rate monitoring were satisfactory.

Labor and delivery

The onset of labor was spontaneous at 39.6 weeks. Five hours before delivery there were variable decelerations to 70 beats/min on the cardiotocogram (CTG) for which she was given facial oxygen. Three hours before delivery, grade 1 meconium was noted, a fetal blood sample at that time showed a pH of 7.32. The variable decelerations continued and a

■ *Neurodevelopmental outcome is not always predictable.*

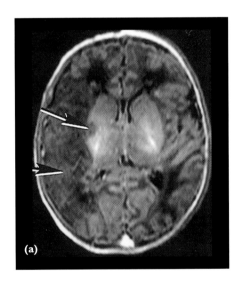
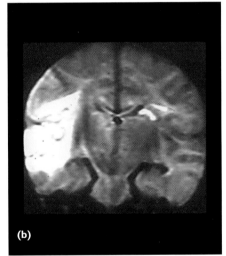
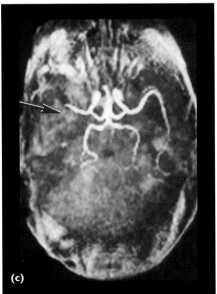
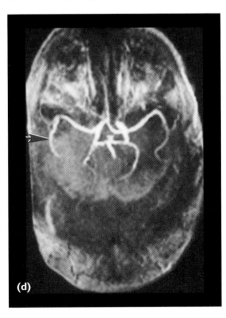

Fig. 7.16A Early imaging, Cranial ultrasound showed a right-sided echo density and a small left-sided hemorrhagic lesion on day 5. Inversion recovery sequence (IR 3800/30/950) **(a)** at 5 days of age shows a large area with loss of gray/white matter differentiation on the right (*arrowhead*) and a small cyst on the lateral edge of the right lentiform nucleus (*arrow*). The areas of abnormality are well shown on the diffusion weighted imaging in the coronal plane. There is some additional increased signal intensity on the left. **(b)**. Early angiography (day 5) shows poor filling in the MCA on the right (*arrow*) **(c)**. This has improved 1 week later (day 11) (*arrow*) **(d)**.

cesarian section was performed for failure to progress and fetal distress. The cord pH was 7.15. Apgar scores were 9 at 1 min and 10 at 5 min but thick meconium was present. Suction revealed that this was all above the cords.

Maternal pathology

At the time of the cesarian section lesions were noted in both ovaries with adhesions to the parametrium. On microscopy, these were shown to contain hemorrhagic decidua with thrombotic vessels. Coagulation and thrombophilic screening were normal.

Postnatal course

The infant was transferred to the postnatal ward but became jittery at 24 h, which was more marked on the left. Episodes of desaturations were noted at 36 h and an EEG confirmed neonatal convulsions. The EEG on day 3 showed continuous background activity with seizure activity mainly on the right.

Neurological evaluation

Neonatal neurological examination on day 3 showed asymmetrical limb tone fisting and nystagmus. On day 9 the asymmetrical limb tone persisted; his head control and visual alertness were poor. At 1 month he still had poor head control and asymmetrical arm tone. At 3 months there was no asymmetry of tone but he tended to first with both hands more so on the right. At 9 months he had a tight right popliteal angle but no other asymmetries were present. At 4 years he had mild general hypotonia with very mildly increased tone in the lower limb on the right the ipsilateral side of the main infarct. He had a strong preference for his left hand and although he had a pincer grasp on the right, this was cruder than on the left. On Griffiths developmental scales he scored at a 4-year level on all subscales except for performance where he performed at a 3-year 8-month level. He has had no further convulsions. Visual function is normal.

Thrombotic screen

Coagulation and thrombophilic screening was normal.

Comment

This infant had a substantial infarct on the right, yet developed a right-sided hemiplegia, presumably related to the very small lesion seen in the left hemisphere and associated with abnormalities in the left internal capsule.

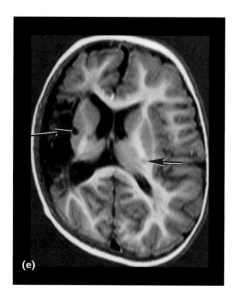

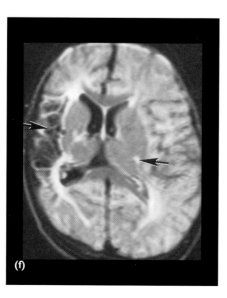

Fig. 7.16B Late imaging. Inversion recovery sequence (IR 3400/30/800). **(e)** Aged 1 year. There is a large infarct on the right. The separate cystic lesion is seen on the lateral border of the lentiform nucleus (*long arrow*). There is abnormal signal intensity within the internal capsule on left (*short arrow*) FLAIR (IR 6500/160/600) sequence. **(f)** Abnormal signal intensity within the internal capsule is seen as high signal intensity (*long arrow*). This may be related to the left-sided lesion seen on early diffusion images. Strands of tissue within the infarct are more easily visible (*short arrow*).

(e)

(f)

CASE 7.2

This female infant was born at 40 weeks' gestation (birth weight 3.956 g).

■ *Good motor outcome with frontal lesions.*

Antenatal

Her mother was a caucasian primigravida. There were no adverse antenatal factors and she went into spontaneous labor.

Labor and delivery

A baseline fetal tachycardia of 160–170 beats/min and early decelerations to 80 beats/min were noted 5 h before delivery, the fetal scalp pH was 7.31. There was a delay in second stage, maternal pyrexia and further fetal bradycardia and so she was delivered by Simpson's Forceps, which required three pulls. Apgar scores were 8 at 1 min and 10 at 5 min.

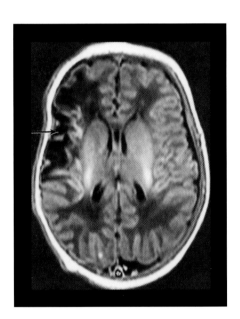

Fig. 7.17A Early imaging. Inversion recovery sequence (IR 3800/30/950). Infant aged 10 days. There is a region of low signal intensity within the right frontal white matter (*arrow*). There is associated highlighting of the cortex. The signal intensity from myelin within the posterior limb of the internal capsule is symmetrical and normal.

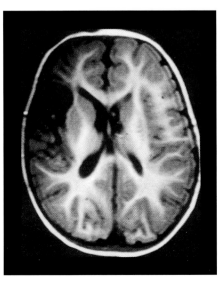

Fig. 7.17B Late imaging. Inversion recovery sequence (IR 3600/30/800) at 10 months of age shows an infarct in the right frontal lobe.

Postnatal course

The infant went to the postnatal ward with her mother. An infection screen was negative. She remained well until the second day when she developed left-sided twitching in her arm and leg. An EEG showed spikes and sharp waves before phenobarbital was given but subsequently normalized.

Early imaging

Cranial ultrasound showed increased echogenicity in the region of the right Sylvian fissure on day 3. MRI at 10 days showed an infarct in the right frontal lobe.

Neurological evaluation

Neonatal neurological examination on day 9 showed mildly asymmetrical limb tone and some truncal hypotonia. At 8 weeks of age she still had mildly reduced tone but no asymmetries. At 3 months some fisting and a tighter popliteal angle was noted on the ipsilateral side of the lesion but by 6 months she was completely normal. At 3 years 6 months she was neurologically completely normal but had a very strong right-hand preference. Her Griffiths subscales ranged from 3 y 6 m–4 y 4 m with the lowest score in language and the highest in the performance scale. At 5 y 6 m she had a normal neurological examination. A normal Movement ABC. Her scores on the WIPPS were 100 for performance and 85 for language. Her visual function was also normal. She has had no further convulsions.

Thrombotic screen

Coagulation and thrombophilic screening was normal.

Comment

Mild asymmetries during the first few months of life are not predictive of motor outcome. Her borderline language abilities at 5.5 years suggest other developmental abilities may be impaired.

CASE 7.3

This male infant was born at 40 weeks' gestation (birth weight 2.8 kg).

Antenatal

His mother was an Indian primigravida. Her antepartum course was uneventful.

Labor and delivery

There was a spontaneous onset of labour which progressed well until 2 h before delivery when a fetal tachycardia (165–170 beats/min) with some loss of variability were observed. These persisted for 1 h and then fetal decelerations with slow recovery were noted. One hour later an emergency cesarian section was performed for failure to progress and fetal distress. Apgar scores were 9 at 1 min and 10 at 10 min.

Postnatal course

The infant was sent to the postnatal ward with the mother where he remained well until 14 h of age when he developed marked twitching in the right arm and leg which became generalized 2 h later. Cranial ultrasound was normal at 24 h but on day 4 showed increased echogenicity in the region of the left Sylvian fissure.

Neurological evaluation

Neonatal neurological examination at 14 h revealed a jittery infant with normal tone, good fixation and no other abnormal movements. On day 6 he had mildly asymmetrical arm tone but was otherwise normal. When seen at 4 weeks he had completely normal tone but was

■ *Perinatally acquired infarcts may be difficult to identify later in childhood.*

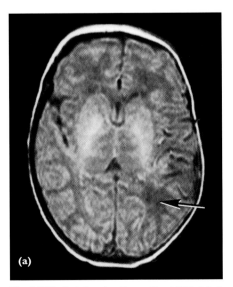 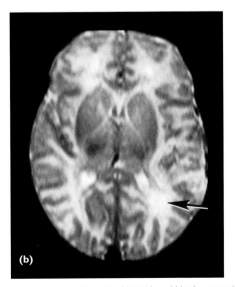 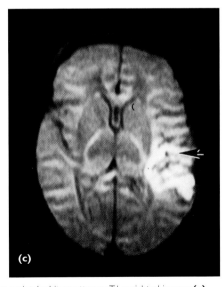

Fig. 7.18A Early imaging. Conventional MRI at 2 days shows only minimal low signal intensity within the posterior parietal white matter on T1 weighted images **(a)** (*arrow*) and minimal high signal on T2 weighted images **(b)** (*arrow*). There is no obvious loss of gray/white matter differentiation. On the diffusion weighted image there is obvious abnormal high signal intensity, more anteriorly **(c)**. The appearances of the internal capsule are normal on all images.

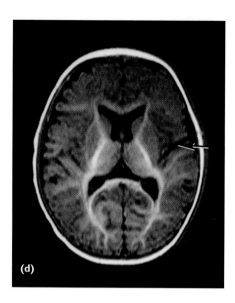

Fig. 7.18B Late imaging. **(d)** Inversion recovery sequence (IR 3400/30/800) at 6 months of age shows only a small closed 'cleft' (*arrow*) in the region of the infarct as seen on diffusion weighted imaging.

(d)

visually inattentive. The child remained completely normal with symmetrical postures, tone and movement. At 4 years 6 months he has equal fine manipulation in both hands, his sub-scores on the Griffiths scale range from 4 to 5 years with the lowest score on the performance scale. He has had no further convulsions. His visual function is normal.

Thrombotic screen

He showed an increased factor VIII.

Comment

Perinatally acquired MCA infarcts may evolve to resemble clefts that could be wrongly classified as congenital in origin.

CASE 7.4

This male infant was born at 39 weeks' gestation (birth weight 3.58 kg).

Antenatal

His mother was a caucasian primigravida mother who had two previous first trimester abortions. She also had ulcerative colitis and was treated with steroids throughout the pregnancy.

Labor and delivery

She was induced at 39 weeks' gestation for raised blood pressure. Labor was reported as normal. The Apgar score was 7 at 1 min, the infant being limp and dusky but he picked up rapidly on facial O_2 and the Apgar was 10 at 5 min. The cord pH was 7.07.

Postnatal course

The infant was transferred to the postnatal ward with the mother and remained well until 24 h of age when he was noted to feed poorly and had three episodes of stiffening which were interpreted as convulsions. An EEG on day 6 showed an asymmetrical background with sharp waves and spikes on the left but no seizure activity.

Early imaging

Cranial ultrasound showed an area of increased echogenicity in the area of the Sylvian fissure on day 4.

■ *Early MRI, EEG and the presence of factor V Leiden may all independently predict later hemiplegia.*

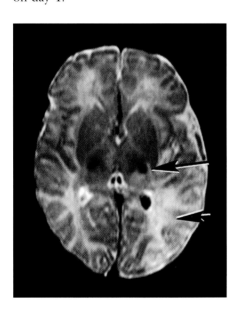

Fig. 7.19A Early imaging. T2 weighted sequence (SE 2700/120) imaging on day 4 showed a loss of gray/white matter differentiation in the left temporo-parietal region (*arrowhead*). The signal from myelin in the posterior limb of the internal capsule is asymmeterical. There is a small area of abnormal increased signal intensity in the thalamus extending into the posterior part of the posterior limb of the internal capsule (*arrow*). There is low signal intensity within the choroid plexus of the posterior horn of the left lateral ventricle, consistent with hemorrhage.

Neurological evaluation

Neurological examination on day 5 showed some asymmetry of tone and poor head control. The hypotonia was still present on day 19 but there was no asymmetry. At 7 weeks of age he was still mildly hypotonic, had intermittent fisting but had no asymmetries. At 6 months he had dystonic posturing of the right arm and increased tone in the right shoulder girdle. At 9 months, in addition to the previous findings, he started to show a marked hand preference and had asymmetry in his popliteal angle but had symmetrical vertical kicking. At 16 months the dystonic arm posturing was more marked, he had a tighter shoulder girdle but no limitation of pronation and supination on the right. He had a left-hand preference with a better grasp on the left, but his gait was normal. At 4 years he shows signs of a mild right hemiplegia. He has asymmetry of upper limb with abnormal tone in the shoulder girdle and limitation of pronation and supination but he has some independent finger movement and is able to put coins in a moneybox. The lower limb is also only mildly affected with some asymmetry of tone but no functional impairment. His Griffiths subscales range from 3 years on the perceptual scale to 4 years 4 months on practical reasoning. He has had no further convulsions. He shows a mild asymmetry in visual fields with the right narrower than the left.

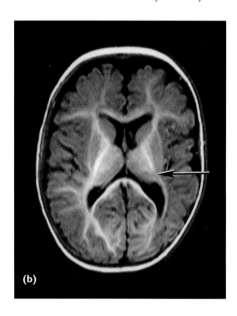

Fig. 7.19B Late imaging. Inversion recovery sequence (IR 3000/30/860) at 6 months of age shows atrophy of the left hemisphere. There is a small interruption in the myelin in the posterior limb of the internal capsule on the left (*arrow*).

(b)

Thrombotic screen

This infant was heterozygous for factor V Leiden.

Comment

This child's hemiplegia could have been predicted from his early EEG with asymmetrical background activity, the initial pattern of injury on MR and possibly from his factor V Leiden heterozygosity. He has obvious perceptual problems in addition to his hemiplegia.

CASE 7.5

This female infant was born at 41 weeks' gestation (birth weight 2.94 kg).

Antenatal

This was the third pregnancy of a caucasian woman with a previous history of infertility. She had one first trimester abortion and one living child with congenital heart defects. This pregnancy was uneventful until 3 days before delivery when she presented with severe abdominal pain. There was no bleeding and there was no evidence that she was in labor on vaginal examination. The CTG was normal. Three days later she was admitted in labor.

Labor and delivery

Late deceleration with loss of variability were noted, a fetal blood sample showed a pH of 7.1 and an emergency cesarian section was planned. This, however, was delayed by a further 2 h as there was difficulty in getting an epidural sited. At delivery, meconium grade 2–3 was present. The Apgar score was 5 at 1 min, the infant was treated with suction and facial oxygen, and the Apgar score was 9 at 5 min.

Postnatal course

At 2 h apneas and staring episodes were noted but no abnormal movements were recorded. The EEG showed abnormal background activity and continuous seizure activity with different seizure patterns occurring simultaneously in both hemispheres. Cranial ultrasound on day 1 showed bilateral echogenicities, which were more marked on the right. These were less marked on day 2.

■ *Infants with borderzone parasagittal injury may present with more of an encephalopathy.*

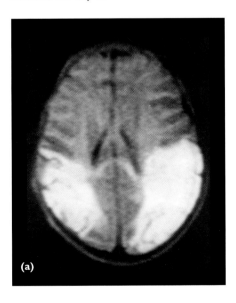

(a)

Fig. 7.20A Early imaging. **(a)** Diffusion weighted imaging at a high ventricular level on day 4 shows abnormal high signal intensity in the parietal lobes bilaterally consistent with parasagittal borderzone infarction.

Neurological examination

Neonatal neurological examination on day 2 showed an infant with poor alertness, abnormal eye movements, hypotonia but no asymmetry. On day 4 she had adducted thumbs but normal tone and normal alertness. At 6 weeks she was generally hypotonic, had abnormal finger postures but had good visual alertness. At 3 months slight asymmetry of tone was noted but otherwise she appeared normal. At 10 months she had intermittent fisting of the right hand with a strong left-hand preference and mild asymmetry of lower limb tone. Her Griffiths sub-scores were between 10.5 and 11.5 months. The findings at 2 years were similar but this time some difference in hand function was also noted. However, at 3 years although she had marked left-hand preference the fine manipulative function of her right hand was excellent. The asymmetries in the upper and lower limb tone persisted. Although she had a tendency to tiptoe she was able to walk with a heel-toe gait and actively dorsiflex her foot. On the Griffiths scale her performance varied from 2.8 months to 3.6 months. Her poorest scale was her eye/hand co-ordination because of her very poor drawing ability. Although she coped well with puzzles she showed some other perceptual difficulties. Her visual function is normal. She has had no further convulsions.

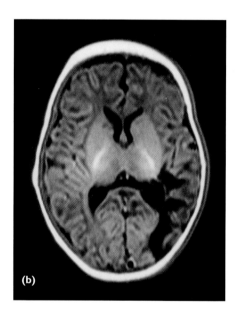

(b)

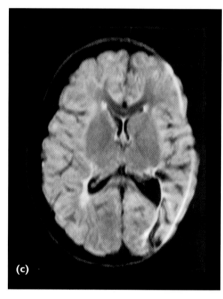

(c)

Fig. 7.20B Late imaging. **(b)** Inversion recovery sequence (IR 3600/30/900) image at a low ventricular level at 3 months. There is normal signal intensity from myelin in both posterior limbs of the internal capsule. Myelination is slightly delayed, as there is no myelin in the anterior limb. There is a porencephalic cyst in the left parietal lobe. **(c)** FLAIR sequence (IR 6500/160/600) at 20 months. There is no longer a porencephalic cyst. There is marked atrophy of the left parietal lobe with some increased signal intensity consistent with glial tissue. Both occipital poles appear atrophied. There is a small amount of increased T2 in the posterior periventricular white matter on the right.

Thrombotic status

Factor V Leiden was not measured in this child but was normal in both parents. She also has an increased factor VIII.

CASE 7.6

This male infant was born at 39 weeks' gestation (birth weight 3.35 kg).

- *Arterial infarction may be associated with additional hemorrhagic lesions.*

Antenatal

His mother was a caucasian primigravida. The pregnancy was uneventful until the day before delivery when she had rather severe abdominal pain.

Labor and delivery

She went into spontaneous labor. There were some CTG decelerations with quick recovery 6 h before delivery, but after that the quality of the fetal monitoring was poor. The infant was delivered by spontaneous vaginal delivery. The Apgar score was 3 at 1 min. The infant picked up quickly with suction and facial O_2. The cord pH was 7.06.

Postnatal course

The infant went to the postnatal ward with the mother and was apparently well till a few hours later when he was noted to be 'floppy and sleepy' and the blood glucose stick was reported as 1.4. On day 2 he was still very floppy but the blood glucose stick was now in the normal range. He would not suck on the breast but took a bottle well. He was noted to be more floppy on the right and a jittery episode lasting 15 s was reported. EEG and CFM showed discontinuous background activity with epileptic discharges. Cranial ultrasound on day 2 showed increased echogenicity on the left compatible with infarction.

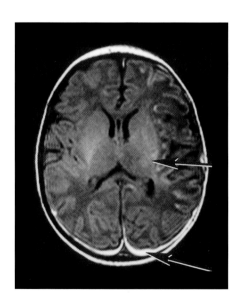

Fig. 7.21A Early imaging. T1 weighted spin echo sequence (SE 860/20) on day 6 showed multiple areas of cortical highlighting in the left hemisphere with abnormal low signal intensity in the adjacent white matter. There was subdural hemorrhage (*long arrow*) and a hemorrhagic lesion in the right brain stem (Fig. 7.4). The signal intensity within the posterior limb of the internal capsule is asymmetrical, being abnormal on the left (*short arrow*). There is a small area of abnormal high signal intensity in the posterior part of the lentiform nucleus adjacent to the posterior limb on the left.

Neurological evaluation

Neonatal neurological examination on day 3 revealed an extended posture, diminished axial and limb tone but no asymmetries. On day 8 the posture was normal, tone was still diminished and was now asymmetrical with reduced tone on the left. At 7 weeks he followed better to the left, still had some hypotonia but no other asymmetries. At 3 months his tone was symmetrical, he had better isolated movements on the right side, but better sensation on the left. At 7.5 months the movements in his arms were symmetrical; however, he kicked better with his left leg. Tone in the right arm was increased, there was a tendency to tiptoe on the right and the popliteal angle was also tighter on that side. At 2 years of age his gross and fine motor function was age appropriate, but he had some asymmetry of tone in the upper and lower limb. His hand function was also considerably poorer in the right hand although he had some independent finger movement. His Griffiths subscores were between 22 and 22.5 months. His visual function was normal. He has had no further convulsions.

Thrombotic screen

This infant was factor V Leiden heterozygous, as was his father.

Comment

The presence of heterozygous factor V Leiden is associated with an abnormal neuromotor outcome. There is also some association with the presence of additional hemorrhagic lesions.

CASE 7.7

This male infant was born at 39 weeks' gestation (birth weight 3.049 kg).

Antenatal

His mother was a caucasian primigravida. Her pregnancy was uneventful till 36 weeks' gestation when she was admitted to hospital with severe abdominal pain. There was no evidence of any bleeding and all investigation regarding the cause of these symptoms were negative, however, a tachycardia of 160 beats/min was recorded several times on the CTG while she was an in-patient.

■ *Bilateral middle cerebral artery infarction.*

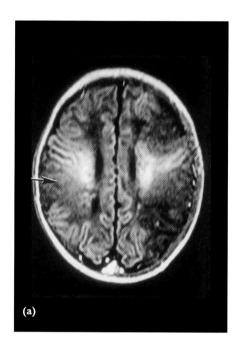

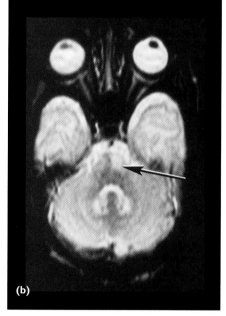

Fig. 7.22A Early imaging. Inversion recovery sequence (IR 3800/30/950) at a high ventricular level on day 6 showed loss of gray/white matter differentiation throughout most of the left hemisphere and in the parietal lobe on the right (*arrow*) **(a)**. T2 weighted sequence (SE 2700/120) imaging through the mesencephalon shows abnormal increased signal intensity (*arrow*) consistent with acute degeneration or diaschisis **(b)**.

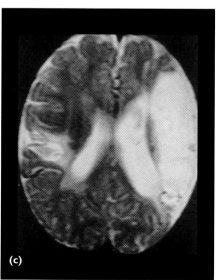

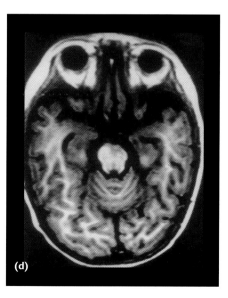

Fig. 7.22B Late imaging. T2 weighted (SE 2700/120) image **(c)** at 12 months shows bilateral areas infarction involving the perisylvian cortex. This is more marked on the left than the right. Inversion recovery (IR 3400/30/800). **(d)** There is asymmetry of the brain stem with atrophy on the left.

Labor and delivery

The onset of labor was spontaneous. Four hours before delivery decelerations to 90 beats/min and lasting for 45 s were recorded but the fetal scalp pH was 7.3. One hour before delivery persistent decelerations to 70 beats/min were recorded. The fetal blood sample was 7.2. The infant was delivered by easy forceps delivery following manual rotation. Meconium grade 2 was noted at delivery. The Apgar scores were 9 at 1 min and 10 at 5 min.

Postnatal course

The infant went with the mother to the postnatal ward. At 8 h he had some dusky episodes and was transferred to the NICU. During the next few hours further apneic attacks were noted some of which were accompanied by jerky movements of his arms and legs. These were confirmed as convulsions by EEG. EEG showed bilateral but asymmetrical abnormal background activity.

Neurological evaluation

Neurological examination on day 8 showed he had generally decreased tone but no asymmetries. He had good auditory and visual orientation. At 6 weeks he still had no asymmetry but he had generally increased tone in both arms. When seen at 3 months his movements and tone were symmetrical but at 7 months he was noted to keep his right arm in a dystonic posture with intermittent fisting of the hand. He had a marked left-hand preference while sitting, but when lying in the prone he used both hands equally. When held in vertical suspension his kick was very asymmetrical. During the next 18 months his hemiplegia became more pronounced with further increase in tone both in his upper and lower limb. In spite of his deterioration in hand function he made good use of his right hand in bimanual manipulative tasks. He walked with a hyperextended knee but had no circumduction and at times even managed a heel-toe gait. His main problem became his poor articulation and excessive drooling but he did not appear to have major cognitive difficulties. At 4 years 6 months he was a bright little boy with a moderate hemiplegia, who in spite of his difficulties was able to participate in various sport activities including tennis and skiing. His visual function was normal. He has had no further convulsions.

Thrombotic status

Coagulation profiles of the parents were normal but they have not been tested for factor V Leiden.

Comment

This child's marked problems with articulation and swallowing are consistent with a perisylvian syndrome. Infants with perinatally acquired bilateral MCA infarction can present with the perisylvian syndrome.

Summary

IMAGING

* Arterial infarcts can be clinically silent.

* Infants with convulsions need to be imaged even if they have normal Apgar scores and no other clinical signs.

* Early first week cranial ultrasound may be normal in infants with focal infarction.

* Perform MRI at the end of the first week of life for most information about the site and extent of infarction.

* Diffusion weighted imaging can help to identify the lesions in the first days of life.

* Excessive growth occurs in and around infarcts from 6 weeks postinfarction.

* Some infarcts may be difficult to detect later in the first year.

PROGNOSIS

* The prognosis of infants with cerebral infarction can be determined by the extent of the lesions on MRI. The concomitant involvement of hemisphere, internal capsule and basal ganglia is likely to be associated with abnormal motor outcome.

* EEG can also be a useful prognostic indicator. An abnormal background activity is likely to be associated with abnormal motor outcome.

* Perinatal infarction may be associated with an abnormal prothrombotic state. Factor V Leiden is associated with the later development of hemiplegia in infants with perinatal infarction.

* Infants with focal infarction may show subtle neurodevelopmental deficits later in childhood despite a normal gross motor outcome.

References

1. Barkovich AJ, Ali FA, Rowley HA et al. (1998) Imaging patterns of neonatal hypoglycemia. Am J Neuroradiol 19, 523–528.
2. Barmada MA, Moossy AJ and Shuman RM (1979) Cerebral infarcts with arterial occlusion in neonates. Ann Neurol 6, 495–502.
3. Bouza H, Dubowitz LMS, Rutherford M et al. (1994) Prediction of outcome in children with congenital hemiplegia: a magnetic resonance imaging study. Neuropediatrics 25, 60–66.
4. Clancy R, Malin S, Laraque D et al. (1985) Focal motor seizures heralding stroke in full term neonates. AJDC 139, 601–606.
5. Cowan FM, Pennock JM, Hanrahan JD et al. (1994) Early detection of cerebral infarction and hypoxic ischemic encephalopathy in neonates using diffusion-weighted magnetic resonance imaging. Neuropediatrics 25, 172–175.
6. De Vries L, Groenendal F, Eken P et al. (1997) Infarcts in the vascular distribution of the middle cerebral artery in preterm and fullterm infants. Neuropediatrics 28, 88–96.
7. Dubowitz L, Dubowitz V and Mercuri E (1999) The Neurological Assessment of the Preterm and Full-Term Newborn Infant, 2nd edn. Clinics in Developmental Medicine 148, London, McKeith Press.
8. Estan J and Hope P (1997) Unilateral neonatal cerebral infarction in full term infants. Arch Dis Child 76, F88–F93.
9. Filipeck PA, Krishnammorthy KS, Davis KR et al. (1987) Focal cerebral infarction in the newborn: a distinct entity. Pediatr Neurol 3, 141–147.
10. Fujimoto S, Yokochi K, Togari H et al. (1988) Outcome of neonatal strokes. AJDC 142, 1086–1088.
11. Hill AD, Martin J, Danemann A et al. (1983) Focal ischaemic cerebral injury in the newborn: diagnosis by ultrasound and correlation with computed tomographic scans. Pediatrics 71, 790–793.
12. Koelfen W, Freund M, Konig S et al. (1993) Results of parenchymal and angiographic magnetic resonance imaging and neuropsychological testing of children after stroke as neonates. Eur J Pediatr 152, 1030–1035.
13. Koelfen W, Freund M and Varnholt V (1995) Neonatal stroke involving the middle cerebral artery in term infants: clinical presentation, EEG and imaging studies, and outcome. Dev Med Child Neurol 37, 204–212.
14. Saeed N, Le Strange E, Rutherford M (1999) Cerebellum segmentation employing texture analysis and knowledge based image processing. 1SMRM. Abstract 2190.
15. Larroche JCL and Amiel CE (1966). Thrombose de l'artere sylvienne a la period neonatale. Arch Fr Pediatr 23, 257–274.
16. Levy SR, Abrams IF, Marshall PC et al. (1985) Seizures and cerebral infarction in the full term newborn. Ann Neurol 17, 366–370.
17. Mannino FL and Trauner DA (1983) Stroke in neonates. J Pediatr 102, 605–610.
18. Mantovani JF and Gerber GJ (1984) Idiopathic neonatal cerebral infarction. AJDC 138, 359–362.
19. Mercuri E, Cowan F, Rutherford M et al. (1995) Ischaemic and haemorrhagic brain lesions in newborns with seizures and normal Apgar scores. Arch Dis Child 73, F67–F74.
20. Mercuri E, Spano M, Bruccini F et al. (1996) Visual outcome in children with congenital hemiplegia: correlation with MRI findings. Neuropediatrics 27, 184–188.
21. Mercuri E, Atkinson J, Braddick O et al. (1996) Visual function in perinatal cerebral infarction. Arch Dis Child 75, F76–81.
22. Mercuri E, Atkinson J, Braddick O et al. (1997) The aetiology of delayed visual maturation: short review and personal findings. Eur J Paed Neurol 1, 31–34.
23. Mercuri E, Rutherford M, Cowan F et al. (1999) Early prognostic indicators of outcome in infants with neonatal cerebral infarction: a clinical EEG and MRI study. Pediatrics 103, 39–46.

24. Mercuri E, Cowan F, Gupte G *et al.* Coagulation status in infants with neonatal cerebral infarction. *Pediatrics* (in press).
25. Perlman JM, Rollins NK and Evans D (1994) Neonatal stroke: clinical characteristics and cerebral blood flow velocity measurements. *Pediatr Neurol* **11**, 281–284.
26. Rollins NK, Morriss MC, Evans D *et al.* (1993) The role of early MR in the evaluation of the term infant with seizures. *Am J Neurol Radiol* **15**, 239–248.
27. Rutherford MA, Pennock JM, Dubowitz LMS *et al.* (1997) Does the brain regenerate after perinatal infarction? *Eur J Paed Neurol* **1**, 13–18.
28. Sran SK and Baumann RJ (1988) Outcome of neonatal strokes. *Am J Dis Child* **142**, 1086–1088.
29. Suzuki S and Wada Y (1992) Neonatal cerebral infarction: symptoms, CT findings and prognosis. *Brain Dev* **14**, 48–52.
30. Traunner DA and Mannino FL (1986) Neurodevelopmental outcome after neonatal cerebrovascular incident. *J Pediatr* **108**, 459–461.
31. Volpe JJ (1994) *Neurology of the Newborn*, 2nd edn. Philadelphia, Saunders.
32. Wertheim D, Mercuri EM, Faundez JC *et al.* (1994) Prognostic value of continuous EEG in full term infants with hypoxic ischaemic encephalopathy. *Arch Dis Child* **71**, F97–F102.
33. Wulfeck BB, Trauner DA and Tallal PA (1991) Neurological, cognitive and linguistic features of infants after early stroke. *Pediatr Neurol* **7**, 266–269.
34. Zeki S (1993) *A Vision of the Brain*. Oxford, Blackwell Scientific Publications.

Ischemic lesions in the preterm brain

Linda S de Vries, Floris Groenendaal and Linda C Meiners

8

Contents

Introduction

Only a small number of preterm infants develop severe ischemic lesions in the neonatal period, compared to a larger group of infants who develop severe intraventricular hemorrhages with or without parenchymal involvement. Even though extensive white matter damage is not common, it almost invariably leads to cerebral palsy later in infancy. Early recognition is of importance, enabling us to start appropriate guidance of both the child as well as the family. While extensive cysts in the periventricular white matter can be easily recognized with cranial ultrasound, smaller cysts or just increased periventricular echogenicity can be more difficult to identify. Several studies are in progress to assess the additional value of early neonatal MRI in these conditions.

Focal infarction, usually in the region of the middle cerebral artery is even less common and rarely reported in the literature. Both types of ischemic lesion are discussed and illustrated with images obtained with ultrasound as well as with MRI.

Periventricular leukomalacia (PVL)

White matter damage following hypoxia–ischemia was observed by pathologists as early as 1867, when Virchow first described yellowish white areas in the periventricular white matter[36]. The term periventricular leukomalacia (PVL) was first coined in 1962 by Banker and Larroche, as white (leukos) spots and softening (malacia) were seen in the periventricular white matter[3]. These early pathology studies were mostly restricted to infants with a gestational age of 34 weeks or more. Medical and technical developments of the last decades have allowed survival of infants with a gestational age of 23 weeks or above. Postmortem studies of these more immature infants show a more diffuse pattern of white matter damage, differing from the classical PVL as described by Banker and Larroche[3]. For the younger group some authors prefer the term 'white matter damage', to PVL. Autopsy findings very much depend on the duration between the insult and the time of death[25]. A large number of astrocytes and macrophages are often noted in the affected area after several days. Liquefaction of the center of the necrotic area can occur after 10–20 days. Liquefaction can result in small cavities, usually not in communication with the lateral ventricle. In the majority of the cases, however, only gliosis and calcification develop in the affected area, without cavitation. Eventually the cystic lesions disappear and ex-vacuo dilatation of the adjacent ventricle may then develop.

Although PVL is traditionally considered as an ischemic lesion and whilst many infants develop PVL following a well-documented clinical event, in many others the lesions are detected incidentally with cranial ultrasound. In the latter group it may not be possible to identify any episodes of severe hypoxia–ischemia, although in some infants there may be a history of sepsis or clinical evidence of infection (Fig. 8.7). It is clear that factors other than ischemia play an important role in white matter damage. The increased vulnerability of the immature oligodendrocyte to glutamate has been shown using cultured oligodendroglia[1]. The proinflammatory cytokines have been associated with the development of white matter damage and may even play a role before delivery. An association of raised IL-1β, IL-6 and TNF-α studied in the amniotic fluid, as well as in the cord blood, and white matter disease is now well established, with data coming from both animal experiments as well as from clinical studies[38]. Cytotoxic cytokines can, however, also be released *during* ischemia[28]. PVL may also be associated with postnatal events. All infants with clinical deterioration, for example secondary to sepsis, should have regular ultrasound examinations over the following weeks. Complications occurring after delivery may also be related to mechanical ventilation. Vasoconstriction due to hypocarbia is a common risk factor and care should be taken to avoid this, especially when using high frequency ventilation.

CRANIAL ULTRASOUND

Since 1983 many groups have shown that cystic PVL can be diagnosed using cranial ultrasound[32]. Correlation with autopsy findings varies in the different studies published during the last decade. The sensitivity was very high in the infants who died once cystic lesions had developed. A high number of false negatives was found, by some, in infants with non-cavitating PVL, as small areas of PVL and diffuse gliosis often went unnoticed on cranial ultrasound[15]. Other groups, however, were able to show a good correlation in these non-cystic cases[32]. Serial ultrasound scans for a long enough period of time (several weeks) are essential when trying to diagnose PVL. An area of echodensity appears between 24 and 48 h following a known insult but cysts do not evolve for a further 2–4 weeks. Although there is not one accepted classification system for PVL, the following one may be used[8]:

- Grade I: areas of increased echogenicity, usually seen within 24–48 h after an insult and persisting beyond day 7 but not evolving into cysts.
- Grade II: localized small cysts, often located in the fronto-parietal periventricular white matter.
- Grade III: extensive cystic lesions, often particularly prominent in the parieto-occipital periventricular white matter. The cysts usually do not communicate with the lateral ventricle. They collapse after several weeks and are no longer visible on cranial ultrasound once the child is 2–3 months old. At this stage, irregular *ex-vacuo* ventricular dilatation can be noted, due to atrophy of the periventricular white matter[8].
- Grade IV: extensive cystic lesions extending into the deep (subcortical) white matter.

COMPUTED TOMOGRAPHY

Computed tomography (CT) is of limited value in the diagnosis of PVL. In the acute stage, non-hemorrhagic PVL cannot be recognized as the high water content of the immature brain results in insufficient contrast between normal brain tissue and areas affected by hypoxia–ischemia. At a later stage, the specific shape of the lateral ventricles, the decrease in white matter and the prominent deep sulci can be appreciated on CT[4].

MRI

The first MRI studies describing infants with an ultrasound diagnosis of PVL stem from the mid-1980s. At that time MRI investigations were usually performed during the first or second year of life, once the child had developed signs of cerebral palsy[2,12,13]. Subsequently, studies were published of MRI findings in infants with spastic diplegia, without knowledge of previous ultrasound data[20]. Baker *et al.*[2] were the first to describe the classical triad of MRI findings from infancy onwards, consisting of (i) ventriculomegaly with irregular outline of the body and trigone of the lateral ventricle; (ii) reduced amount of white matter, especially at the level of the trigone, frequently also extending throughout the centrum semiovale and (iii) deep prominent sulci, abutting the ventricle. These findings can be identified on both T1 and T2 weighted imaging. MRI has the advantage that an increased signal intensity on T2 weighted imaging highlights areas of presumed gliosis. Once myelination has occurred, the fluid attenuated inversion recovery (FLAIR) sequence is particularly useful for demonstrating periventricular and cortical gliosis. The attenuated (low) signal of CSF with the high signal of most parenchymal pathology, enhances the detection of lesions adjacent to CSF spaces.

Baker *et al.*[2] emphasized the possible presence of an area of normally increased signal intensity on T2 weighted images, dorsal and superior to the trigone of the lateral ventricles, not to be mistaken for areas of gliosis. These areas are referred to as 'terminal zones', representing association tracts, which contain less myelinated axons, throughout the first decade. This lower myelination density leads to higher signal on T2 weighted images. These areas are separated from the lateral ventricle by a thin rim of normal myelin. This feature distinguishes them from the abnormal signal seen in cases with PVL, abutting the ventricular wall. Furthermore, no loss of white matter is seen in the terminal zones and the ventricles should be of a normal size and shape. The differentiation is best made on coronal slices.

One of the first *neonatal* MRI studies did not compare ultrasound and MRI findings, but studied whether progress in myelination at 44 weeks postmenstrual age was affected by the occurrence of an intraventricular hemorrhage or cystic-PVL (c-PVL)[34]. Infants with c-PVL had a significantly delayed myelination, using T1 weighted axial images, compared with both infants without ultrasound abnormalities as well as those with intraventricular hemorrhages of different degrees. They subsequently reported that there was a significant correlation between the delayed myelination and neurodevelopmental outcome at 1 year[14].

More recently neonatal MRI studies in neonates with PVL have been performed in several centers, both very early, in the non-cystic stage, and also later, once the cysts have developed[30,35]. A recent study by Maalouf et al.[22] showed that a large number of infants with a gestational age (GA) below 30 weeks (22/29) have diffuse and excessive high signal intensity in the white matter (DEHSI) on T2 weighted images at term age. This was commonly associated with imaging signs suggestive of cerebral atrophy, ventricular dilation and widening of the extracerebral space, and they therefore suggested this to be a sign of white matter disease. These white matter appearances may be non-specific but look very similar to the white matter signal intensity in non-cystic areas in infants with PVL (see Fig. 3.24) and may represent a mild form of diffuse white matter damage.

In addition to conventional sequences, sequences such as diffusion weighted imaging (DWI) and quantitative 3-D volumetric imaging[17,18] have been used to assess the preterm neonatal brain. Inder et al. reported on a case that developed extensive c-PVL[17]. DWI, performed on day 5 in the absence of ultrasound abnormalities, showed diffuse abnormalities throughout the white matter on DWI. A repeat MRI confirmed the development of cystic lesions. The association between PVL and the development of apparently undamaged regions of the brain has been shown in a more recent study by the same group. They were able to show a reduction in the gray matter volume using 3-D volumetric imaging at term age in those with PVL compared with normal controls and preterm infants without PVL[18].

COMPARISON STUDIES

MRI and postmortem

In a correlation study by Schouman-Claeys et al.[29], MRI data were compared with autopsy findings in eight preterm infants, with a GA ≤33 weeks, who died between 3 and 7 weeks of age. Death occurred 3–11 days following the MRI scan. Four types of abnormalities with different signal intensities were recognized on MRI, using coronal T1 weighted images. In type A the zones had a signal intensity similar to that of CSF. These correlated with cavities at postmortem in all cases (Fig. 8.1). In type B the zones were of moderately low signal with less clearly demarcated boundaries than in type A. These areas corresponded with translucent sparsely cellular patches or small cavities. In type C the zones were of very high signal intensity and sometimes heterogeneous. These areas correlated with hemorrhagic cavities (Figs 8.2 and 8.3). In type D the zones had a moderately high signal

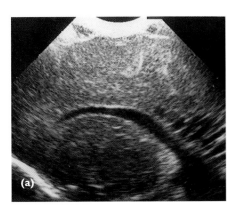
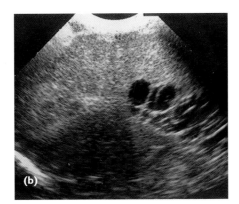
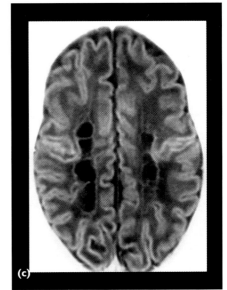

Fig. 8.1 (a), (b) Cranial ultrasound, parasagittal views showing extensive cystic lesions at 3 weeks of age. The cysts are separate from the lateral ventricle. **(c)** MRI performed at 40 weeks PMA. At the level of the central semiovale (CSO) the cysts can be seen as well-delineated hypointense areas, extending throughout the parietal white matter on this inversion recovery image (type A).

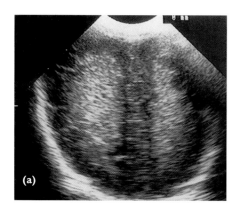 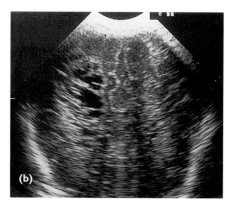

Fig. 8.2 Ultrasound performed at 3 and 6 weeks of age in an infant, born at 29 weeks. Coronal views angled backwards, showing patchy areas of increased echogenicity in the parieto-occipital white matter **(a)**. Some cysts are seen, more on the right than on the left side. A repeat ultrasound at 40 weeks PMA shows extensive cysts throughout the periventricular white matter, more on the right than on the left **(b)**.

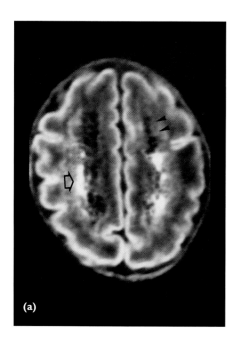 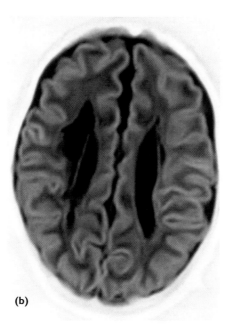

Fig. 8.3 (a) Transverse MR inversion recovery image of the same infant at 3 weeks of age, at the level of the CSO, shows areas of increased signal, suggestive of hemorrhage (*open arrowhead*) (type C) and areas of low signal suggestive of cavitation (type B). **(b)** A repeat MR, IR, performed at 40 weeks PMA, shows extensive areas of cavitation (type A). The septi are not seen as clearly as on ultrasound.

appearing as streaks or punctate areas. These areas correlated with hypercellular lesions with or without siderophages (Figs 8.4 and 8.5). The extent of periventricular lesions was underestimated on MRI and small thalamic lesions were overlooked in three cases. On the whole, a precise evaluation of PVL was possible using T1 weighted MR images.

MRI AND ULTRASOUND

Neonatal period

Several comparison studies have been reported, performed in the neonatal period as well as later in infancy[19,24,25,30,35]. Keeney *et al.*[19] enrolled 100 high-risk newborns, admitted to

their neonatal intensive care unit, into a prospective MRI study. Twelve cases were identified as having PVL and 10 of these 12 cases had already been detected using ultrasound. Four of the 12 cases were also examined with CT, and PVL was detected in only one of them. In all 12 cases MRI showed hemorrhagic lesions, when scanned before the end of the 4th week of life. When the MRI was done between 4 and 8 weeks of age, cysts were seen. By 8 weeks of age resolution of cysts was noted with or without the appearance of ventricular dilatation.

Van Wezel-Meijler *et al.*[35] studied 25 infants with 'flares' (defined as areas of increased echogenicity, present for 1–6 days, (*n* = 15) or PVL grade 1 (*n* = 10) on ultrasound. Echogenicity was defined as echogenic or less echogenic

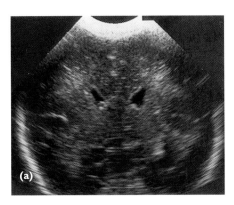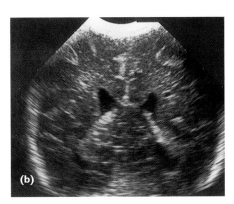

Fig. 8.4 Cranial ultrasound, coronal views, performed 2 days and 21 days following an episode of severe hypocarbia, showing areas of mild echogenicity at the external angle of the lateral ventricle **(a)** evolving into localized cysts **(b)**.

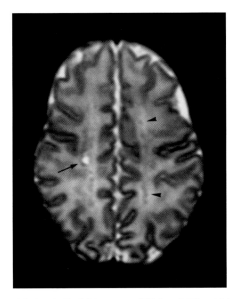

Fig. 8.5 Same infant as in Fig. 8.4, transverse MRI, heavily T2 weighted spin-echo image at 40 weeks PMA, showing one small area of high signal intensity on the right at the level of the CSO, compatible with a small cyst (*arrow*). Many small areas of low signal intensity can be seen throughout the white matter, suggestive of hypercellular lesions (*arrowheads*) (type D). (With permission Roelants *et al.* 2001 Neuropediatrics[27].)

than the choroid plexus, but not inhomogeneous. The broader zones of signal intensity changes within the white matter on MRI corresponded with periventricular echo densities seen on ultrasound. Sie *et al.* have also studied infants with inhomogeneous ('patchy') flares with or without cystic evolution[30]. They were able to show that hemorrhagic PVL was more common (60%) than reported previously in post-mortem studies (25%) and that the cysts were noted to be more numerous and sometimes seen earlier on MRI than on ultrasound.

In our own population we have been able to study 35 cases with different grades of PVL. The infants were studied in the neonatal period using a Philips imaging system operating at 1.5 Tesla (Table 8.1). Proton MR spectroscopy was

performed during the same session. Most infants studied so far had cystic PVL (3 grade I, 10 grade II and 22 grade III). The scan was performed within the first 4 weeks of life in 15 infants (3 grade I, 3 grade II, 9 grade III), at 6 weeks of age in 1 with grade III and at 40 weeks' postmenstrual age in 19 infants (7 grade II and 12 grade III). The MRI was performed twice during the neonatal period in two infants. Punctate high signal changes on inverse recovery (IR) were seen in all our grade I (Fig. 8.6), 1 of the grade II and 5 of the grade III cases and all of these had their examination within the first 4 weeks. This finding was not present in any of the infants who had their first scan at 40 weeks postmenstrual age (PMA). Two infants, however, showed linear streaks of low signal on T2 weighted sequence at the level of the centrum semiovale (CSO) (Fig. 8.5). In five of our cases with localized cysts on ultrasound (grade II), the cysts could no longer be visualized at the time of the MRI examination (40 weeks) by either technique. In these patients only mild ventricular dilatation was noted, sometimes associated with a rim of short T1 outlining the lateral ventricle, suggestive of a glial cell reaction. In three infants abnormalities were found on MRI which were not seen using ultrasound. In one infant an unexpected area of infarction was identified in the striatum. In another case (Fig. 8.7) small cysts were also seen in the temporal lobes and in the third case, a lesion was also found in the cerebellum. In general, there was good agreement between ultrasound and MRI,

Table 8.1 Pulse sequence parameters in the neonatal period

Pulse sequence	TR (ms)	TI (ms)	TE (ms)
T1 weighted CSE	514	–	15
T2 weighted TSE	4211	–	150
IR	3347	600	30

TE, echo time; TR, repetition time; TI, time to inversion; IR, inverse recovery; CSE, conventional spin echo; TSE, turbo spin echo.

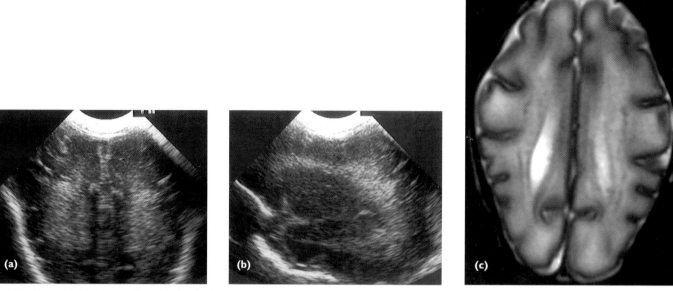

Fig. 8.6 Preterm infant, born at 28 weeks, who developed grade I PVL on cranial ultrasound, as can be seen on coronal **(a)** and parasagittal **(b)** view. MRI, heavily T2 weighted spin-echo image **(c)** at 32 weeks' PMA, shows increased signal intensity of the periventricular white matter, bordered by a rim of low signal intensity.

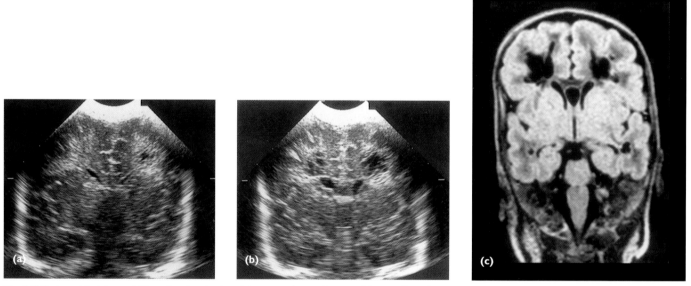

Fig. 8.7 Preterm infant, born at 29 weeks, who developed therapy-resistant seizures at 36 weeks PMA. Enterovirus was cultured from nose and throat. Ultrasound, coronal views, showed areas of increased echogenicity 48 h after the onset of the seizures. Also note the increased echogenicity in the right thalamus **(a)**. Evolution into cysts, extending into the deep white matter is seen 10 days later **(b)**. MRI was performed at this stage (38 weeks PMA) **(c)**. Coronal FLAIR, shows extensive areas of low signal intensity compatible with CSF. The septation of the cystic zone cannot be recognized on MRI, as on ultrasound. Additional cysts in both temporal lobes were, however, noted on MRI and not seen on ultrasound. (**c**: with permission Roelants *et al.* 2001 Neuropediatrics[27].)

when performed around 40 weeks' PMA. However, using MRI cysts were seen earlier, appeared more extensive (Fig. 8.8) and appeared to be associated with petechial hemorrhages when the infants were studied at an early stage (2–4 weeks after the insult). In our most recent case DWI was performed at 6 weeks of age, when the cysts were already present on both ultrasound and on conventional T1 and T2 weighted sequences. Extensive areas of high signal intensity were seen on DWI adjacent to the cystic lesions possibly preceding further cystic degeneration (Fig. 8.9).

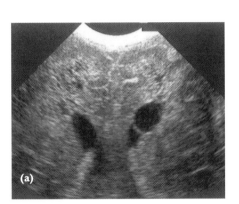
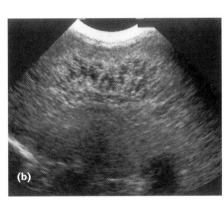
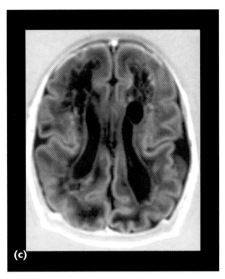

Fig. 8.8 Hydropic preterm infant, born at 32 weeks. Following a period of severe and prolonged hypotension, marked echogenicity was noted and extensive cysts subsequently developed. Coronal **(a)** and parasagittal **(b)** views at 2 weeks of age, using a 10 MHz transducer. A large subendymal pseudocyst is seen on the left as well as the bilateral onset of the development of diffuse cystic degeneration in the periventricular and deep white matter. **(c)** MRI of the same infant, inversion recovery sequence, performed on the same day, shows petechial hemorrhages within the white matter, as well as extensive areas of low signal intensity throughout the periventricular and deep white matter. (With permission Roelants *et al.* 2001 Neuropediatrics[27].)

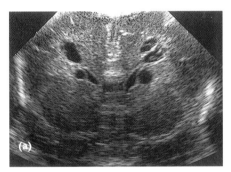
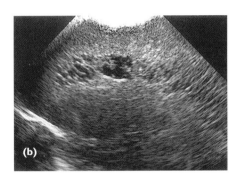

Fig. 8.9 Coronal **(a)** and parasagittal **(b)** views at 6 weeks of age, using a 10 MHz transducer. Following weekly ultrasound examinations, extensive cysts have developed, not preceded by severe echogenicity. Also note the subependymal pseudocysts. MRI, performed on the same day shows areas of high signal intensity on a heavily T2 weighted spin-echo image **(c)** and high signal intensity areas adjacent to these cystic areas on DWI **(d)**.

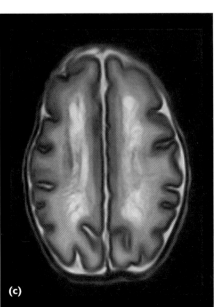
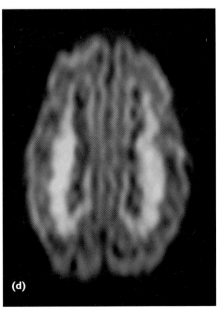

Antenatal onset

Cranial ultrasound noted cystic lesions, present on day 1, in only three cases. In two of them their monozygous co-twin had died 2–3 weeks previously (Fig. 8.10) and in the third case the mother had been physically assaulted 4 weeks prior to delivery. The fourth case had areas of increased periventricular echogenicity, associated with an intraventricular hemorrhage, present on the first ultrasound scan following acute loss of fetal movements 2 days prior to an emergency cesarian section.

So far only 16 of the 29 surviving infants who had a neonatal MRI have had a repeat scan during the second year of life. A good correlation was found between areas of gliosis in infancy and the cystic lesions seen during the neonatal period.

Infancy

MRI compared with neonatal ultrasound

Comparison of MRI, performed during infancy, with previous ultrasound data, was first carried out in the late 1980s. De Vries et al.[7] performed sequential MRI studies, between 36 weeks PMA and 36 months in 13 cases with extensive c-PVL or subcortical leukomalacia. Both imaging data as well as neurodevelopmental outcome differed between those with cysts restricted to the periventricular white matter and those where the cysts extended into the deep white matter. In the latter group cysts usually persisted on late MRI scans

and little or no myelination was found. From the clinical point of view this group also showed more severe motor and mental impairment as well as cerebral visual impairment. They subsequently studied 15 infants, who developed cerebral palsy, following persistent echo densities (grade I, n = 5), localized c-PVL (grade II, n = 4) or extensive c-PVL (grade III, n = 6)[9]. There was good correlation between the degree of PVL diagnosed using ultrasound and the extent of the MRI changes noted in infancy. Periventricular high signal intensity (PVHI) on T2 weighted images was present in all cases but was most extensive in the grade III cases. In the grade II cases, with only a few small cysts on ultrasound, PVHI on T2 weighted images and associated ventricular dilatation, was more extensive than expected. Irregular ventricular enlargement was only seen in those with c-PVL.

MRI and neurodevelopmental outcome

In order to correlate abnormalities on MRI with neurodevelopmental outcome, many groups have performed MRI in infancy in children with spastic diplegia or quadriplegia. When assessing MRI, attention has been paid to the following characteristics[33]: thinning of the corpus callosum, irregular ventricular shape, ventricular enlargement, diminished peritrigonal white matter, delay in myelination, PVHI on T2 weighted images and the presence of cortical damage. In general, there appears to be a good agreement between the severity of MRI abnormalities and the severity of motor and

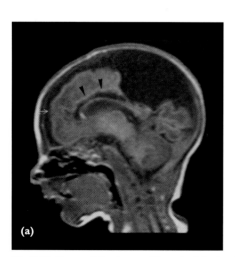
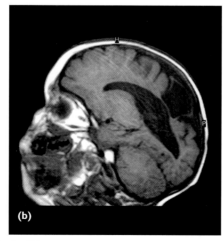
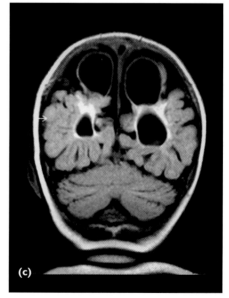

Fig. 8.10 Preterm infant born at 32 weeks, following death of his monozygous co-twin. **(a)** Parasagittal T1 weighted image shows a large parietal cystic defect. Also note the small rim of low signal intensity runs alongside the wall of the lateral ventricle (*arrowheads*). These abnormalities were present in both hemispheres. **(b)** A repeat parasagittal T1 weighted image at 15 months corrected age shows a reduction in the size of the cystic defect, although the angulation is different. **(c)** A coronal FLAIR shows large bilateral parietal cysts as well as extensive gliosis around the lateral ventricles.

cognitive sequelae[6,31,33,37]. All studies have shown that the extent of PVHI, the degree of white matter reduction and ventricular enlargement correlated with the degree of motor impairment. Some authors found a correlation between the degree of these abnormalities and cognitive development[6]. This was, however, not confirmed by others (Fig. 8.11)[37].

Iai et al.[16] further emphasized that the ratio of the thickness of the splenium divided by the length of the corpus callosum correlates with severity of motor impairment (Fig. 8.11).

MRI and cerebral visual impairment

A number of studies have shown a correlation between cerebral visual impairment (CVI) and the presence of MR abnormalities of the posterior visual pathways in infants with PVL[5,11,21]. CVI is regarded as visual impairment due to a disturbance to the posterior pathways, that is the optic radiation and/or the primary visual cortex. Cioni et al.[5] studied 30 infants with grade I and II (n = 18) or grade III (n = 12) PVL. They found that half of the cases with grade III PVL had severe loss of visual acuity, reduced visual field and abnormal ocular motility, but none was completely blind.

Table 8.2 Pulse sequence parameters in infancy

Pulse sequence	TR (ms)	TI (ms)	TE (ms)
T1 weighted CSE	544	–	16
T2 weighted TSE	3072	–	50/150
IR	2818	600	20
FLAIR	7565	2000	120

TE, echo time; TR, repetition time; TI, time to inversion; IR, inverse recovery; FLAIR, fluid attenuated inverse recovery; CSE, conventional spin echo; TSE, turbo spin echo.

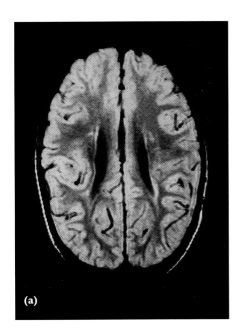

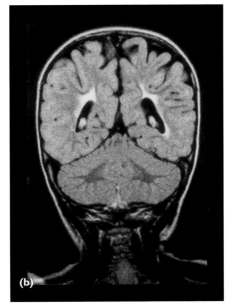

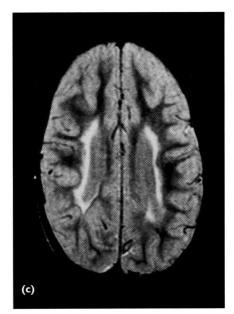

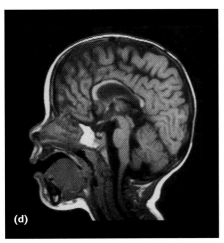

Fig. 8.11 (a) MRI performed at 2.5 years of age in an infant with a grade I PVL on ultrasound. T2 TSE (3000/50), axial slice at mid-ventricular level. Small areas of PVHI and slight reduction in peritrigonal white matter are seen, more extensive on the left. **(b)** MRI performed at 22 months of age, in an infant with PVL grade II on neonatal ultrasound. FLAIR sequence, coronal slice. Extensive PVHI involving the optic radiation is noted on both sides. The left ventricle is mildly dilated and slightly irregular in shape. **(c)** MRI performed at 24 months of age in an infant with PVL grade III on neonatal ultrasound (same infant as Fig. 8.1). T2 TSE (3000/50), axial slice at the mid-ventricular level, shows extensive areas of PVHI and irregularly dilated ventricles. **(d)** MRI performed at 15 months of age in an infant with PVL III on neonatal ultrasound. Mid-sagittal T1 weighted image, showing marked thinning of especially the dorsal part of the corpus callosum.

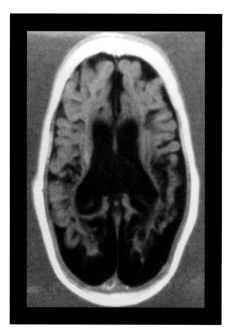

Fig. 8.12 Transverse MRI, IR, performed at 16 months in an infant born at 37 weeks. Severe encephalopathy was present following a twin-to-twin transfusion syndrome. There is mild *ex-vacuo* dilatation, severe delay in myelination, and extensive damage to the occipital white matter and cortex.

On MRI, abnormalities in the optic radiation were found in 50%. In 17% the visual cortex was also affected. They suggested that lesions at the level of the optic radiation, rather than lesions in the visual cortex itself, are the anatomical substrates for CVI in *preterm* infants.

Eken *et al.*[11] prospectively studied a cohort of 65 high-risk preterm and full-term newborns, admitted to our neonatal intensive care unit. Nine developed severe CVI and were functioning as blind children. All had a GA ≥35 weeks and all showed extensive cysts on ultrasound extending into the subcortical white matter. They showed severe abnormalities on MRI, involving both the optic radiation as well as the visual cortex (Fig. 8.12).

Infarction

Focal infarction is often referred to as 'neonatal stroke'. It has mainly been reported in full-term infants, who tend to present with hemiconvulsions during the first few days of life (see Chapter 7). Data on preterm infants are scarce. Paneth *et al.*[26] reported that 17% of their postmortem cases, belonging to a cohort of preterm infants born in the New Jersey counties between 1984 and 1987, had lesions in the thalami or basal ganglia.

We have studied 23 infants with a GA <37 weeks with focal infarction. Seventeen of these have been described previously[10]. In 19 of these 23 cases an MRI was performed, either in the neonatal period (*n* = 17) or later in infancy (*n* = 2). Abnormalities on ultrasound were hardly ever seen during the first few days of life. A gradual increase in echogenicity was first noted by the end of the first week. In two of the 23 cases the infarction was first noted in the cystic phase, having been missed during their echogenic phase, either due to a very anterior or a very peripheral location of the lesion. The lesions sometimes remained echogenic up till term age, but usually became cystic on ultrasound. Two infants had an associated IVH with posthemorrhagic ventricular dilatation and three other cases also showed c-PVL.

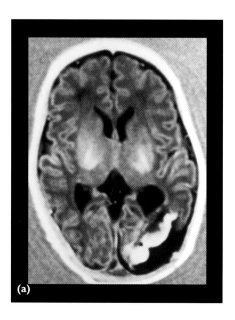

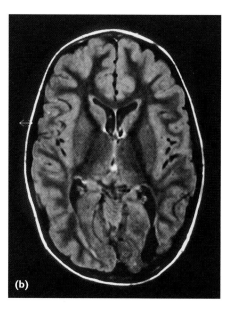

Fig. 8.13 (a) Transverse MRI, IR, performed at 40 weeks' PMA in an infant born at 36 weeks' GA, with a hemorrhagic occipital parenchymal lobe infarction, associated with coagulopathy. He did not develop any asymmetry in tone but had a global delay with a DQ of 71 at 24 months of age. **(b)** Transverse MRI, FLAIR sequence, performed at the age of 56 years, showing the residual damage following the infarction. Mild gliosis is seen in the occipital white matter on the right side.

(a)

(b)

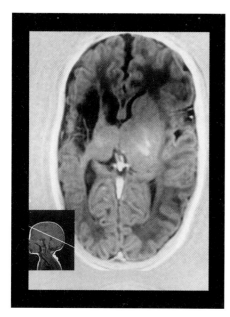

Fig. 8.14 MRI in a preterm infant with a GA of 32 weeks. Routine US performed at 2 weeks of age shows cystic changes in the distribution of the right middle cerebral artery. MRI, IR, axial slice, performed at 40 weeks PMA, shows an area of cavitation and *ex-vacuo* dilatation of the right ventricle. Also note the absence of myelination of the posterior limb of the right internal capsule. He developed a moderate hemiplegia and has a DQ of 91 at 24 months of age.

Neonatal MRIs were performed around 40 weeks' PMA, once cystic evolution had taken place on ultrasound. In all but one of the infants, the lesion had been identified on ultrasound and this was the reason for performing the MRI. Three infants had involvement of the main branch of the middle cerebral artery, one had an infarct in the distribution of the posterior cerebral artery and one of the anterior cerebral artery. Nine showed involvement of one or more lenti-culostriate branches, two had cortical branch involvement and one showed a watershed infarction between areas supplied by the middle and anterior cerebral artery.

MRI

Infarction was seen as an area of low signal intensity on IR and increased signal intensity on T2 weighted spin echo sequences. An additional finding of a previous hemorrhage within the area of infarction was present in only two cases (Fig. 8.13). The posterior limb of the internal capsule of the affected hemisphere may also be involved (Fig. 8.14). This presents as a decrease in signal on IR images and an increase in signal on T2 weighted images.

ANTENATAL ONSET

In five of the 23 cases the infarction was considered to be of antenatal onset. Three were part of a twin-to-twin trans-fusion syndrome, one was one of triplets and the last case suffered severe arrythmia before delivery (Fig. 8.15). One of the twins had involvement of the main branch and in the other three the lenticulostriate branches were involved.

NEURODEVELOPMENTAL OUTCOME

The three infants with main branch involvement of the middle cerebral artery developed a hemiplegia in contrast to the two cases with either a posterior or anterior infarction. Among those with smaller infarcts, eight out of 18 have so far developed adverse neurological sequelae, due to associated c-PVL in two, and due to the lacunar infarcts in the other six cases.

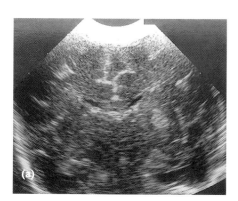
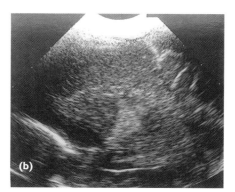
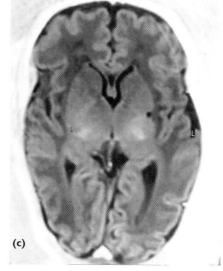

Fig. 8.15 **(a, b)** Ultrasound at 2 weeks of age in a preterm infant born at 33 weeks GA, following antenatal supraventricular tachycardia, showing an echodensity in the left lentiform nucleus. **(c)** MRI, IR sequence, performed at 38 weeks PMA, showing a small cyst in the left putamen. (With permission Govaert and de Vries, *Clin Dev Med* 1998 and *Neuropediatrics*, 1997.)

Case histories

CASE 8.1

Female infant, born following an emergency cesarian section at 31 weeks' gestation, because of decelerations on the CTG.

Her first cranial ultrasound scan, performed on day 1, showed areas of increased echogenicity. Periventricular cysts started to develop from day 13 onwards. On day 9 an area of increased echogenicity was also noted in the right caudate nucleus.

The first MRI was performed at 40 weeks' postmenstrual age. The inversion recovery images show areas of low signal intensity, similar to that of CSF, mainly in the frontal white matter, at a low ventricular level (Fig. 8.16). At the level of the CSO a few more areas with low signal are noted, suggestive of cavitation (type A) (*arrow*) (Fig. 8.17). More posteriorly a streaky line of high signal is noted, suggestive of a glial cell reaction or mineralization (type D) (*arrowheads*).

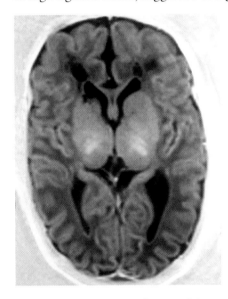

Fig. 8.16

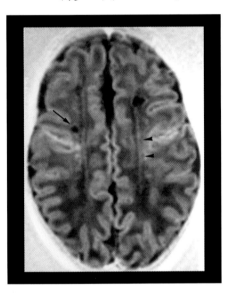

Fig. 8.17

A second MRI was done at 24 months of age. A coronal FLAIR still shows the small cavity at the level of the right caudate nucleus and areas of high signal intensity at the level of the corticospinal tracts (Fig. 8.18). An axial proton density SE sequence shows high signal intensity throughout the CSO extending into the parietal white matter (Fig. 8.19). Also note the linear area of low SI at the same site as the neonatal IR, suggestive of mineralization (*arrowheads*).

This girl is now 2 years old. She has developed a spastic diplegia and also shows some dystonic hand movements. She is not yet able to speak and has a developmental quotient (DQ) of 70 uncorrected and 80 corrected for her prematurity (excluding the motor subscale).

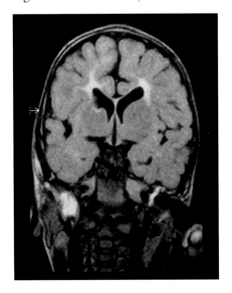

Fig. 8.18

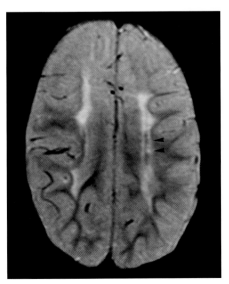

Fig. 8.19

CASE 8.2

Female infant born following an emergency cesarian section at 33 weeks, because of signs of fetal distress on the CTG and a reverse flow on Doppler studies of the umbilical cord. Mother suffered a 'flu-like episode' 5 weeks prior to delivery.

She had a good start (Apgar 7 at 1 min and 9 at 5 min). She weighed 1.5 kg (p 10–50), had a length of 42 cm (p 3–10) and a head circumference of 30 cm (p 10–50). Routine lab results showed a low platelet count of $35 \times 10^9/l$. She was diagnosed to have a congenital cytomegalovirus (CMV) infection.

Her first ultrasound scan after referral on day 9 did not show any areas of periventricular calcification or lenticulostriate vasculopathy. However, she had areas of increased echogenicity throughout the left hemisphere (Fig. 8.20a). She was scanned again 4 weeks later and by then she had developed some cysts in these previously echogenic areas (Fig. 8.20b).

An MRI was performed at 40 weeks' postmenstrual age and the area of focal infarction in the region of the middle cerebral artery was confirmed (Fig. 8.21). Note the line of high signal surrounding the area of infarction, suggestive of hemorrhage or a glial cell reaction. Also note the absence of the posterior limb of the internal capsule on the affected side.

Although occipital cysts can be found in cases with congenital CMV infection, the cystic lesion in this infant is unlikely to be due to the late onset CMV infection in this case. Considering the timing of the CMV infection, and the timing of the cystic evolution on ultrasound, the infarcts were more likely to result from prolonged fetal distress before and around the time of delivery.

She is now 30 months old. She has mild sensorineural hearing loss. She shows a mild asymmetry in tone and has a DQ of 87 uncorrected and 92 corrected for her prematurity. Her head circumference is below the 3rd centile (43 cm) with weight and length on the 50th centile.

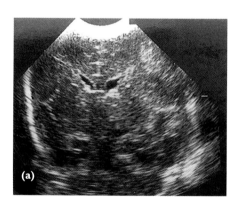
(a)

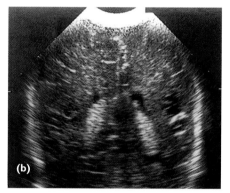
(b)

Fig. 8.20

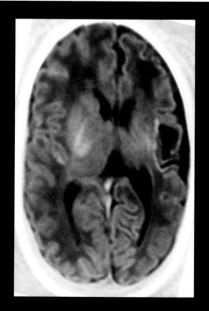

Fig. 8.21

Summary

■ Cerebral ischemic lesions in the preterm infant can be diagnosed using MRI in the neonatal period.

■ MRI changes of the white matter, following hypoxia–ischemia have been studied both in the early neonatal period as well as in the first decade of life.

■ So far it is uncertain whether MRI provides additional information compared to repeated neonatal ultrasound in the neonatal period, although there is increasing amount of data to suggest this. Especially when using non-conventional sequences such as DWI in the echogenic stage of PVL subsequent evolution into cystic lesions may be predicted.

■ It is possible that quantitative 3-D volumetric MRI to measure structures such as the cortex can help in the prediction of future cognitive defects.

■ MRI is also a very useful technique to detect focal ischemic lesions in the preterm brain. Different patterns of 'neonatal stroke' have been identified.

■ Future studies of cerebral ischemic lesions in the preterm infant may help in defining the physiological mechanisms underlying these lesions. These studies may eventually lead to interventions to reduce brain damage.

References

1. Back SA, Gan X, Li Y *et al.* (1998) Maturation-dependent vulnerability of oligodendrocytes to oxidative stress-induced death caused by glutathione depletion. *J Neurosc* **18**, 6241–6253.
2. Baker LL, Stevenson DK and Enzmann DR (1988) End-stage periventricular leukomalacia: MR evaluation. *Radiology* **168**, 809–815.
3. Banker BQ and Larroche J-L (1962) Periventricular leukomalacia in infancy: a form of neonatal anoxic encephalopathy. *Arch Neurol* **7**, 386–410.
4. Chow PP, Horgan JG and Taylor KJW (1985) Neonatal periventricular leukomalacia: real-time sonographic diagnosis with CT correlation. *Am J Neuroradiol* **6**, 383–388.
5. Cioni G, Fazzi B, Ipata AE *et al.* (1996) Correlation between cerebral visual impairment and magnetic resonance imaging in children with neonatal encephalopathy. *Dev Med Child Neurol* **38**, 120–132.
6. Cioni G, Di Paco MC, Bertuccelli B *et al.* (1997) MRI findings and sensorimotor development in infants with bilateral spastic cerebral palsy. *Brain Dev* **19**, 245–253.
7. De Vries LS, Connell JA, Dubowitz LMS *et al.* (1987) Electrophysiological, neurological and MRI abnormalities in infants with extensive cystic leukomalacia. *Neuropediatrics* **18**, 61–66.
8. De Vries LS, Eken P and Dubowitz LMS (1992) The spectrum of leukomalacia using cranial ultrasound. *Beh Brain Res* **49**, 1–6.
9. De Vries LS, Eken P, Groenendaal F, *et al.* (1993) Correlation between the degree of periventricular leukomalacia diagnosed using cranial ultrasound and MRI later in infancy in children with cerebral palsy. *Neuropediatrics* **24**, 263–268.
10. De Vries LS, Groenendaal F, Eken P *et al.* (1997) Infarcts in the vascular distribution of the middle cerebral artery in preterm and fullterm infants. *Neuropediatrics* **28**, 88–96.
11. Eken P, de Vries LS, van Nieuwenhuizen O *et al.* (1996) Early predictors of cerebral visual impairment in infants with cystic leukomalacia. *Neuropediatrics* **27**, 16–25.
12. Feldman HM, Scher MS and Kemp SS (1990) Neurodevelopmental outcome of children with evidence of periventricular leukomalacia on late MRI. *Pediatr Neurol* **6**, 296–302.
13. Flodmark O, Lupton B, Li D *et al.* (1989) MR imaging of periventricular leukomalacia in childhood. *Am J Neuroradiol* **10**, 111–118.
14. Guit GL, van de Bor M, den Ouden L *et al.* (1990) Prediction of neurodevelopmental outcome in the preterm infant: MR staged myelination compared with US. *Radiology* **175**, 107–109.
15. Hope PL, Gould SJ, Howard S *et al.* (1988) Ultrasound diagnosis of pathologically verified lesions in the brains of very preterm infants.

Dev Med Child Neurol **30**, 457–471.
16. Iai M, Tanabe Y, Goto M *et al.* (1994) A comparative magnetic resonance imaging study of the corpus callosum in neurologically normal children and children with spastic diplegia. *Acta Paediatr* **83**, 1086–1090.
17. Inder T, Huppi P, Zientara GP *et al.* (1999) Early detection of periventricular leukomalacia by diffusion-weighted magnetic resonance imaging techniques. *J Pediatr* **134**, 631–634.
18. Inder TE, Hüppi PS, Warfield S *et al.* (1999) Periventricular white matter injury in the premature infant is followed by reduced cerebral cortical gray matter volume at term. *Ann Neurol* **46**, 755–760.
19. Keeney SE, Adcock EW and McArdle CB (1991) Prospective observations of 100 high-risk neonates by high field (1.5 Tesla) magnetic resonance imaging of the central nervous system; II: Hypoxic–ischaemic encephalopathy. *Pediatrics* **87**, 431–438.
20. Koeda T, Suganama I, Kohno Y *et al.* (1990) MR imaging of spastic diplegia. Comparative study between preterm and term infants. *Neuroradiology* **32**, 187–190.
21. Lanzi G, Fazzi E, Uggetti C *et al.* (1998) Cerebral visual impairment in periventricular leukomalacia. *Neuropediatrics* **29**, 145–150.
22. Maalouf EF, Duggan PJ, Rutherford MA *et al.* (1999) Magnetic resonance imaging of the brain in a cohort of extremely preterm infants. *J Pediatr* **135**, 351–357.
23. Maalouf EF, Duggan PJ, Counsell SJ *et al.* Comparison of findings on cranial ultrasound and magnetic resonance imaging in preterm infants. Pediatrics 2001; 107:719–727.
24. Millet V, Bartoli JM, Lacroze V *et al.* (1998) Predictive significance of magnetic resonance imaging at 4 months of adjusted age after a perinatal insult. *Biol Neonate* **73**, 207–219.
25. Paneth N, Rudelli R, Monte W *et al.* (1990) White matter necrosis in very low birth weight infants: neuropathologic and ultrasonographic findings in infants surviving six days or longer. *J Pediatr* **116**, 975–984.
26. Paneth N, Rudelli R, Kazam E *et al.* (1994) Associated pathologic lesions: cerebellar haemorrhage, pontosubicular necrosis, basal ganglia necrosis. In: *Brain Damage in the Preterm Infant. Clin Dev Med* **131**, London, MacKeith Press, pp. 163–170.
27. Roelants-van Rijn AM, Groenendaal F, Beek FJ *et al.* Neuropediatrics: in press. Parenchymal brain injury in the preterm infant: comparison of cranial ultrasound, MRI and neurodevelopmental outcome.
28. Savman K, Blennow M, Gustafson K *et al.* (1998) Cytokine response in cerebrospinal fluid after birth asphyxia. *Pediatr Res* **43**, 746–751.

29. Schouman-Claeys E, Henry-Feugeas MC, Roset F *et al.* (1993) Periventricular leukomalacia: correlation between MR imaging and autopsy findings during the first 2 months of life. *Radiology* **189**, 59–64.

30. Sie LTL, van der Knaap MS, van Wezel-Meijler G *et al.* (2000) Early MR features of hypoxic ischaemic brain injury in neonates with periventricular densities on sonograms. *Am J Neuroradiol* **21**, 852–861.

31. Sugita K, Takeuchi A, Iai M *et al.* (1989) Neurologic sequelae and MRI in low-birth weight patients. *Paediatr Neurol* **5**, 365–369.

32. Trounce JQ, Fagan D and Levene MI (1986) Intraventricular haemorrhage and periventricular leukomalacia: ultrasound and autopsy correlation. *Arch Dis Child* **61**, 1203–1207.

33. Truwit CL, Barkovich AJ, Koch TK *et al.* (1992) Cerebral Palsy: MR findings in 40 patients. *Am J Neuroradiol* **13**, 67–78.

34. van de Bor M, Guit GL, Schreuder AM *et al.* (1989) Early detection of delayed myelination in preterm infants. *Pediatrics* **84**, 407–411.

35. van Wezel-Meijler G, van der Knaap MS, Sie LTL *et al.* (1998) Magnetic resonance imaging of the brain in premature infants during the neonatal period. Normal phenomena and reflection of mild ultrasound abnormalities. *Neuropediatrics* **29**, 89–96.

36. Virchow R (1867) Zur pathologischen Anatomie des Gehirns I: congenitale encephalitis und myelitis. *Arch Pathol Anat* **38**, 129–142.

37. Yokochi K, Aiba K, Horie M *et al.* (1991) Magnetic resonance imaging in children with spastic diplegia: correlation with the severity of their motor and mental abnormality. *Dev Med Child Neurol* **33**, 18–25.

38. Yoon BH, Jun JK, Romero R *et al.* (1997) Amniotic fluid inflammatory cytokines (interleukin-6, interleukin-1beta and tumor necrosis factor-alpha), neonatal brain white matter lesions and cerebral palsy. *Am J Obstetr Gyn* **177**, 19–26.

Hemorrhagic lesions of the newborn brain

9

Mary A Rutherford

MRI appearances of hemorrhage

The MRI appearances of blood are dependent on the oxidation state of hemoglobin and its environment. The appearances of hemorrhage vary with time in adult patients allowing the lesion to be aged (Table 9.1) but imaging studies on the evolution of hemorrhagic lesions in neonates are limited[22]. The signal intensity of a hemorrhagic lesion also depends on the field strength of the magnet and the sequence used to obtain the image; as a rule the evolution of hemorrhage appears faster at lower field strengths.

In our experience the evolution of cerebral hemorrhage in the immature brain is similar to that in the adult, although we have relatively few examples of perinatally acquired parenchymal hemorrhage before 3 days of age. The evolution of small parenchymal hemorrhagic lesions is not so typ-

Table 9.1 Evolution of signal intensity from hemorrhage (adult data, idealized)

Age of parenchymal hemorrhage	T1 weighted image	T2 weighted image	Hemoglobin state
Hyperacute (<3 h)	Nil	Nil	Oxyhemoglobin
Acute (3 h–3 days)	Isointense	Low SI	Intracellular deoxyhemoglobin
Early subacute (3–10 days)	High SI	Low SI	Intracellular methemoglobin
Late subacute (10 days–3 weeks)	High SI	High SI	Extracellular methemoglobin
Chronic (3 weeks plus)	Nil/low SI	Low SI	Hemosiderin

SI, signal intensity.

Table 9.2 Evolution of signal intensity in parenchymal hemorrhage (neonatal data)

Age of hemorrhage	T1 weighted image	T2 weighted image
2 days	Nil/high SI rim	Low SI
3–10 days	High SI/nil	Low SI (with ↑high SI periphery)
10 days–21 days	High SI	High SI
3–6 weeks	High SI	High SI (with ↑low SI periphery)
6 weeks–10 months	Nil/min high SI	Low SI/nil
10–22 months	Nil	Min low SI/nil

SI, signal intensity.

Table 9.3 Evolution of signal intensity in extracerebral hemorrhage (neonatal data)

Age of hemorrhage	T1 weighted image	T2 weighted image
<3 days	High SI	Low SI/nil
3 days	High SI	High SI
3–10 days	High SI	Low SI (some high SI)*
10–21 days	High SI	Low SI (some high SI)*
3–6 weeks	Min high SI/nil	Low SI
6 weeks–10 months	Nil	Low SI/nil

*In larger lesions; SI, signal intensity.

ical as they may not show a persistent long T2 component. Tables 9.2 and 9.3 summarize our serially acquired MRI findings in 49 infants with perinatal hemorrhage in one or more sites of the brain. Twenty-nine of these infants were term (105 sets of images) and 15 were preterm 23–36 weeks' gestation (49 sets of images).

Extracerebral hemorrhage appears to behave slightly differently from parenchymal hemorrhage. Large intraventricular hemorrhages with clot within the ventricular system may have a long T2 component seen between 3 days and 3 weeks but this is not seen in smaller hemorrhages. Similarly, extracerebral hemorrhage generally only has a long T2 component if large. The experience in older infants with non-accidental injury is different again and may be related to the larger size of lesions or possibly to the presence of repeated injury (see Chapter 13). Parenchymal hemorrhages in the neonate behave slightly differently depending on their size and this may reflect different etiology. In our experience smaller hemorrhages within the parenchyma are easier to see on T1 weighted images than on conventional T2 weighted images (Figs 9.3 and 9.16). Small punctate hemorrhages may have a rim of long T1, long T2 around them on initial imaging consistent with either edema or ischemia. It may be difficult to decide whether the peripheral part of any hemorrhagic lesion represents evolving hemorrhage, edema or

ischemia. Small hemorrhagic lesions do not appear to show a long T2 component. At follow-up, the previous small hemorrhagic lesions are seen as areas of long T1, long T2 regions consistent with gliosis. These are often bigger than the original hemorrhage (Fig. 9.16). This suggests that the hemorrhage may have been secondary within a larger area of primary ischemia with ischemic tissue producing the long T1, long T2 rim around the hemorrhagic lesion.

Figure 9.1 illustrates the evolution of signal intensity within a large parenchymal hemorrhage in the neonatal brain.

Etiology

The etiology of hemorrhagic lesions differs according to the site of hemorrhage and the gestational age of the infant.

Hemorrhagic lesions are associated with perinatal trauma, asphyxia and infection as well as congenital and acquired clotting disorders, but may occur spontaneously without a cause being found[20]. Occasionally, hemorrhages arise from a vascular anomaly (see Chapter 12) and rarely from a malignancy. Clinically, hemorrhagic lesions may be asymptomatic or they may be associated with signs of birth trauma, signs of birth asphyxia or bleeding from other sites. Asphyxiated infants often have prolonged and difficult deliveries and may develop disseminated intravascular coagulation. In an individual infant there may be several precipitating factors which result in a hemorrhagic lesion.

Hemorrhage may occur as the principal lesion or may complicate venous or arterial infarction, for example parenchymal venous infarction in the preterm infant (Fig. 9.26). It is therefore appropriate to perform a hemorrhagic and thrombotic screen in any term neonate presenting with intracranial hemorrhage. In addition, details of vitamin K administration need to be confirmed[8] and the mother's blood examined for platelet antibodies to exclude alloimmune thrombocytopenia (Fig. 9.2). These hematological investigations should also be performed in the preterm neonate presenting with anything other than an uncomplicated germinal layer/intraventricular hemorrhage.

Approximately 5% of term infants with signs of hypoxic–ischemic encephalopathy (HIE) have marked parenchymal hemorrhagic lesions. These infants may also have hypoglycemia and jaundice suggestive of an underlying metabolic disorder (Fig. 9.19) although a specific diagnosis may not be found. There is an unclear association between hypoglycemia and hemorrhage. The typical pattern of injury associated with hypoglycemia is an ischemic parasagittal lesion, usually in the posterior parietal lobes (see Chapter 6). It is possible that when hemorrhage is seen in infants with

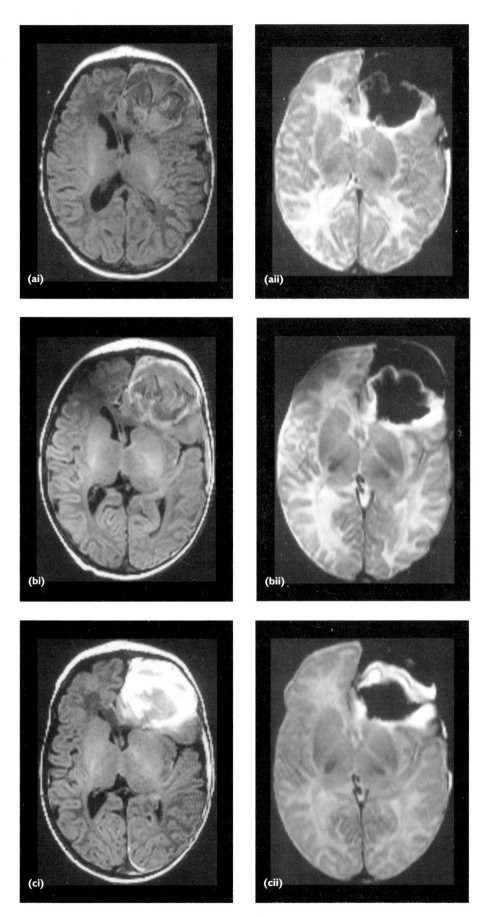

Fig. 9.1 This female infant was delivered at term by normal vaginal delivery. Her Apgar scores were 7 at 1 min and 9 at 5 min. She was discharged home at 24 h. Her mother noted abnormal movements consistent with fits from day 2. T1 weighted (SE 860/20) and T2 weighted (SE 2700/120) spin echo and inversion recovery sequences (IR 3400/30/800) in the transverse plane. **(a)** At 3 days there is a large area of abnormal signal intensity in the left frontal lobe on T1 weighted images **(i)**. This is isointense with a higher signal intensity rim. The area is mainly low signal intensity with a thin high signal intensity peripheral component on T2 weighted images **(ii)**. **(b)** At 4 days the high signal rim around the hemorrhage is more obvious on both T1 weighted **(i)** and T2 weighted **(ii)** images. **(c)** At 9 days the hematoma is now mostly high signal on the T1 weighted image **(i)** with an isointense center. There is now a larger rim of high signal intensity on the T2 weighted images **(ii)** corresponding to the presence of extracellular methemaglobin.

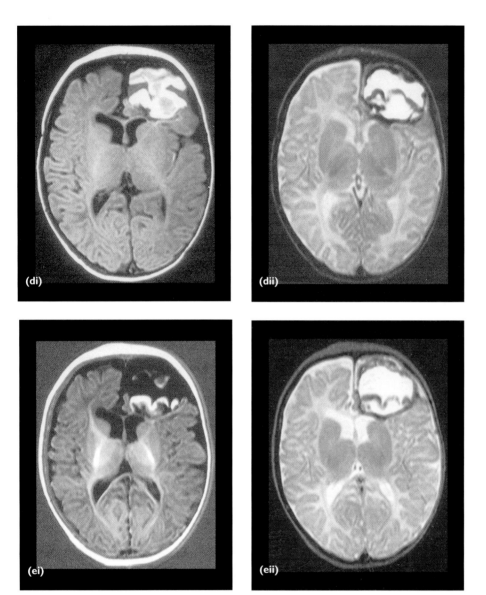

Fig. 9.1 continued (d) At 7 weeks the hematoma is smaller but remains high signal on T1 weighted images **(i)**. It is mostly high signal on T2 weighted images **(ii)** with a low signal rim and central features. **(e)** At 3 months the hematoma is largely resolved to leave a cyst. There is a residual high signal intensity on inversion recovery (IR) images **(i)**. There is also a rim of low signal intensity on T2 weighted images **(ii)** due to the presence of hemosiderin in the walls of the cyst. Her neurodevelopmental outcome was good. At the age of 3 years 2 months she scored between 3 and 3.5 years on Griffiths developmental assessment. She had a right-hand preference but only mild asymmetry in tone in the popliteal angles.

hypoglycemia that these lesions represent hemorrhagic infarcts (Fig. 9.3)

Hemorrhagic lesions that occur prior to delivery also have variable etiology including trauma, congenital clotting disorders, alloimmune thrombocytopenia, infection and drug abuse[2,19]. Hemorrhagic lesions may be detected on antenatal ultrasound scan or occasionally with fetal MRI, or they may present as relatively mature lesions shortly after birth. In infants with marked ventricular dilation at birth, signs of short T2 along the ventricular outline may be the only clue to a previous hemorrhage (Fig. 9.4).

In the neonate who has already been discharged from hospital, non-accidental injury needs to be considered as a cause of cerebral hemorrhage (see Chapter 13) in addition to late hemorrhagic disease of the newborn[18].

Sites of hemorrhage

Hemorrhage may occur at any of the levels within the cranium as shown in Fig. 9.5.

The meninges consist of the dura mater, the subarachnoid layer and the pia mater. The outer part of the dura mater is attached to the bone forming the periosteum. Hemorrhage between the outer dura layer and the skull is termed extradural. The inner layers fold down into the brain to form the falx cerebri, tentorium cerebelli and the falx cerebelli. The dura encircles the sinuses, namely the superior and inferior sagittal, the straight and the right and left transverse sinus. The space between the inner dura layer and the arachnoid layer is minimal and is the site of subdural hemorrhage. The subarachnoid space, however, contains CSF, arteries and

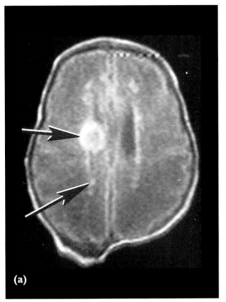 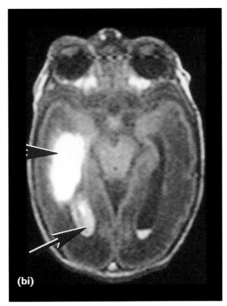 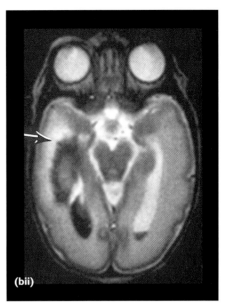

Fig. 9.2 This male infant was delivered at 30 weeks' gestation by emergency cesarian section for maternal pre-eclampsia and fetal distress. He was hypoglycemic from birth and also noted to be thrombocytopenic. A diagnosis of alloimmune thrombocytopenia was made following examination of maternal blood. Cranial hemorrhage was noted on routine ultrasound examination on day 1. MRI at 6 days of age showed several hemorrhagic areas. **(a)** High ventricular level. T1 weighted (SE 860/20) sequence. There is a large area of high signal intensity on the right consistent with a germinal layer hemorrhage (*short arrow*). There are multiple areas of abnormal high signal intensity along the ventricular margin, consistent with hemorrhagic venous infarction (*long arrow*). The hemorrhagic lesions were seen as low signal intensity on T2 weighted images. **(b)** Level of the mesencephalon. **(i)** T1 weighted (SE 860/20) sequence. There is a large abnormal high signal intensity which is probably extending from the right temporal horn of the lateral ventricle into the parenchyma (*arrowhead*). This is consistent with a germinal layer hemorrhage with hemorrhagic venous infarction. The germinal layer hemorrhage probably originates from residual germinal matrix at the roof of the temporal horn. There is an intraventricular hemorrhage (*arrow*). **(ii)** T2 weighted (SE 2700/120) sequence. The venous infarct is seen as low signal intensity. The white matter adjacent to the hemorrhagic lesion has an abnormal high signal intensity (*arrow*). This could be due to edema or ischemia.

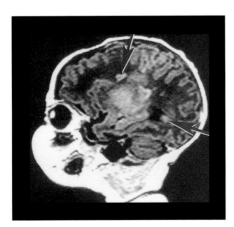 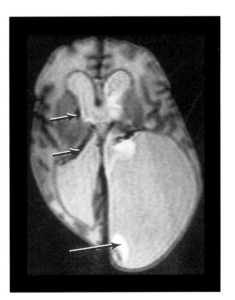

Fig. 9.3 This male infant was born at term by emergency cesarian section for fetal distress. Apgar scores were 6 at 1 min and 9 at 5 min and the cord pH was 7.3. He presented at 2 days of age with convulsions and was noted to be hypoglycemic. MRI was performed at 5 days. During infancy this infant had 2 further convulsions associated with hypoglycemia. No specific diagnosis has been made. T1 weighted (SE 860/20) sequence. Sagittal plane. There are small areas of abnormal high signal intensity within the white matter consistent with acute hemorrhage (*arrows*). The hemorrhage was seen as low signal intensity on T2 weighted images.

Fig. 9.4 This 3-day-old male infant presented with a large head following delivery at term. T2 weighted (SE 2700/120) sequence. There is massive dilation of the ventricles with several areas of low signal intensity consistent with previous hemorrhage (*short arrows*). There are additional areas of high signal intensity consistent with old clot (*long arrow*).

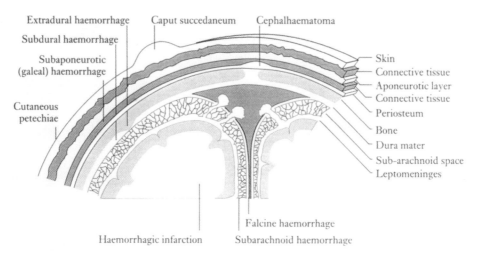

Fig. 9.5 The coverings of the brain. (Reproduced from 'Vascular lesions of mature infants' in *Neonatal Cerebral Ultrasound* by Janet Rennie, Cambridge University Press, 1997, with permission.)

veins. In the region of the sagittal sinus the arachnoid layer forms granulations that pierce the dura. These return CSF to the blood in the superior sagittal sinus. The pia mater is thin, rich in capillaries and closely adherent to the brain.

Extracranial hemorrhage

CAPUT SUCCEDANEUM

This very common lesion involves the presence of edema beneath the skin, which may be accompanied by hemorrhage. These collections cross suture lines and usually resolve within a few days. MRI is not necessary in these infants unless a large blood loss is suspected or an underlying lesion is sought. Caput is very common after vaginal delivery (Fig. 9.6) but may be particularly severe following a vacuum extraction.

SUBGALEAL OR SUBAPONEUROTIC HEMORRHAGE

These collections usually increase in size in the first few days after delivery as a consequence of birth trauma, particularly following vacuum extraction (Fig. 9.7)[7]. Blood may track down into the cervical regions underneath the attachments of the occipito-frontalis muscle and blood loss may consequently be massive. Subgaleal hemorrhage may also occur following non-accidental injury.

CEPHALHEMATOMA

A cephalhematoma is a subperiostial hemorrhage and is therefore confined by cranial sutures (Fig. 9.8). Cephalhematomas occur in approximately 1% of live births and are more common with forceps delivery. They may

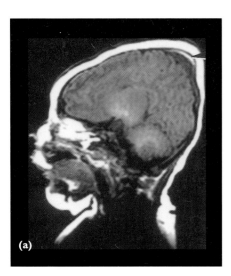

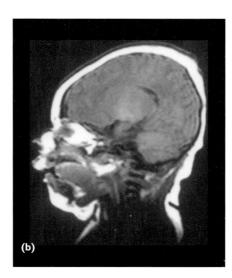

Fig. 9.6 Term infant born by normal vaginal delivery with shoulder dystocia. **(a)** T1 weighted (SE 860/20) sequence in the sagittal plane aged 1 day showing caput succedaneum with a small area of high signal intensity consistent with hemorrhage (*arrow*). **(b)** The caput had disappeared on follow-up scan at 7 days and the head has changed shape.

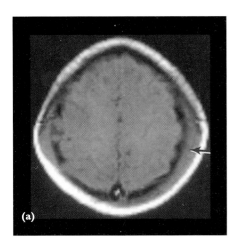

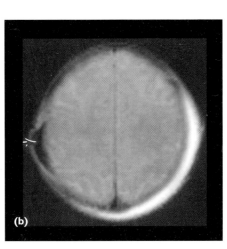

Fig. 9.7 Subgaleal hemorrhage. This female infant was born at term by vacuum extraction for fetal distress. The cord pH was 6.7 and Apgar scores were 0 at 1, 5 and 10 min. She developed stage III HIE and died at 2 days of age. **(a)** T1 weighted (SE 860/20) sequence. Transverse plane at 1 day of age. There is an extensive isointense extracerebral collection around the surface of the skull (*arrow*) **(b)** T2 weighted (SE 2700/120) sequence. The extracerebral collection has a high signal intensity. There is an additional more circumscribed area, which is low signal intensity (*arrowhead*).

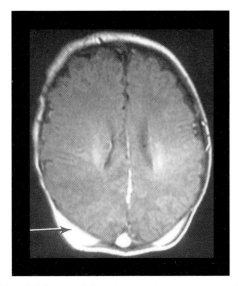

Fig. 9.8 This male infant was delivered at term by emergency cesarian section for fetal distress. He developed stage II HIE and was imaged at 7 days. T1 weighted (SE 860/20) sequence. There are bilateral areas of high signal intensity consistent with cephalhematoma (*arrow*). The cephalhematoma was seen as a low signal intensity on T2 weighted images.

increase in size following the delivery and may then take several weeks to resolve. They are not of clinical significance but may be associated with other lesions within the brain. Some cephalhematomas may calcify.

Subdural hemorrhage

The incidence of subdural hemorrhage is likely to be underestimated, as small collections may be asymptomatic[10]. Subdural hemorrhages are associated with prolonged, difficult and or traumatic deliveries either instrumental or by breech presentation. Major lesions are now relatively uncommon with improved obstetric care and the trend for fetuses

presenting by the breech to be delivered by cesarian section. In a recent large series of neonatal subdural hemorrhage over 31% of the infants had a spontaneous vaginal delivery[9]. Subdural hemorrhage may also occur secondary to congenital clotting disorders[4]. Subdural hemorrhage is the most common lesion following non-accidental injury and it is therefore important to have a thorough knowledge about the clinical history and the evolution of perinatally acquired subdural hemorrhage.

ETIOLOGY OF SUBDURAL HEMORRHAGE

Prolonged and difficult labor gives rise to excessive vertical molding and fronto-occipital elongation causing stretching of the dura mater, the falx and the tentorium, which may then lead to tearing and consequent venous disruption. Subdural hemorrhage may arise from the bridging veins from the cortex to the superior sagittal sinus or from superficial cortical veins without actual tearing of the dura. As the major sinuses are contained within the dural folds, dural tears may cause extensive bleeding. It is possible that some large subdural hemorrhages are also due to arterial bleeding. Large posterior fossa hemorrhages may arise following over-extension of the neck during a breech delivery. The resulting occipital osteodiastasis causes direct trauma to the contents of the posterior fossa including cerebellar hemorrhage. Rarely, posterior fossa hemorrhage may be secondary to a tumor.

SITES OF SUBDURAL HEMORRHAGE

Tentorial

Major lethal tears of the tentorium are usually infratentorial. They may result in rupture of the vein of Galen, and straight or transverse sinuses. Clots may extend into the posterior fossa and, when large, may result in compression of the brain stem

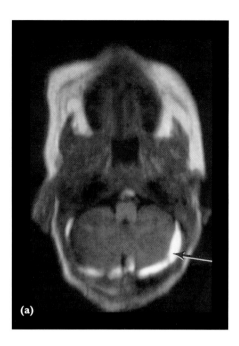 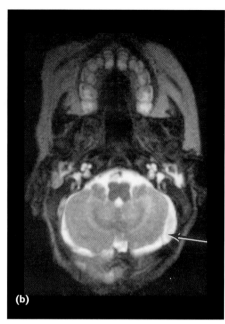

Fig. 9.9 This term infant was delivered by vacuum extraction. Apgar scores were 3 at 1 min and 7 at 5 min. He developed convulsions on day 1. He was imaged at 14 days. **(a)** T1 weighted (SE 860/20) sequence. There is high signal in the posterior fossa consistent with subdural hemorrhage (*arrow*). **(b)** T2 weighted (2700/120) sequence. The hemorrhage is high signal intensity consistent with a perinatal lesion in this infant. Differentiation from transverse sinus thrombosis may be difficult.

and death. With the advent of modern imaging less severe tentorial tears are now being recognized more often. Blood may stay confined to the free edge of the tentorium but extension can result in either supratentorial or infratentorial (often retrocerebellar) subdural hemorrhage. Hemorrhage from a tentorial tear may also extend into the ventricular system, the cerebral parenchyma or the cerebellar parenchyma. Posterior fossa hemorrhage may also result from rupture of small infratentorial veins with an intact tentorium. Small subdural hemorrhages in the posterior fossa are common in infants imaged following birth asphyxia and are usually of no clinical significance. Infratentorial subdural hemorrhage may be difficult to distinguish from transverse sinus thrombosis (Fig. 9.9). The two may co-exist or a subdural hemorrhage may compress the sinus predisposing to thrombosis.

Falx

Ruptures of the falx are much less common than those in the tentorium. They usually result in hemorrhage from the inferior sagittal sinus and give rise to a clot in the longitudinal cerebral fissure overlying the corpus callosum.

Convexity

Rupture of superficial cortical veins gives rise to a convexity subdural hemorrhage, which may be accompanied by subarachnoid hemorrhage. Convexity hemorrhage is less common than posterior fossa hemorrhage but the two may co-exist. When perinatal in origin these convexity hemorrhages are mainly unilateral. Larger convexity hemorrhages

may be associated with more marked changes within the brain parenchyma. Infarction of the brain may occur either from arterial occlusion[6] or possibly from impaired venous drainage (Fig. 9.10). Large parenchymal hemorrhages may also occur. These may occur as separate lesions because of a hemorrhagic tendency or occur secondarily in associated areas of infarction (Fig. 9.19).

Large subdural hemorrhages may result in impairment of CSF flow and associated ventricular dilation or widening of the extracerebral space (external hydrocephalus). The impairment may be secondary to occlusion of the foramina by a mass effect of the subdural or from interference with the reabsorption of CSF (Fig. 9.19). The evolution of subdural hemorrhage may result in the formation of a subdural effusion, which may remain at the site of a previous subdural for many months. Effusions are also associated with rebleeding although we have not seen this phenomenon following a perinatally acquired subdural hemorrhage.

Subarachnoid hemorrhage

The exact incidence of subarachnoid hemorrhage is uncertain although it is a relatively common and usually benign form of hemorrhage. Diagnosis based on the presence of red blood cells in a CSF tap probably overestimates the incidence. It is more common in preterm infants. On MRI subarachnoid hemorrhage may give rise to diffuse high signal around the central fissure. This has to be distinguished from changes due to normal myelination in the corticospinal tracts around the central sulcus and to the abnormal short T1

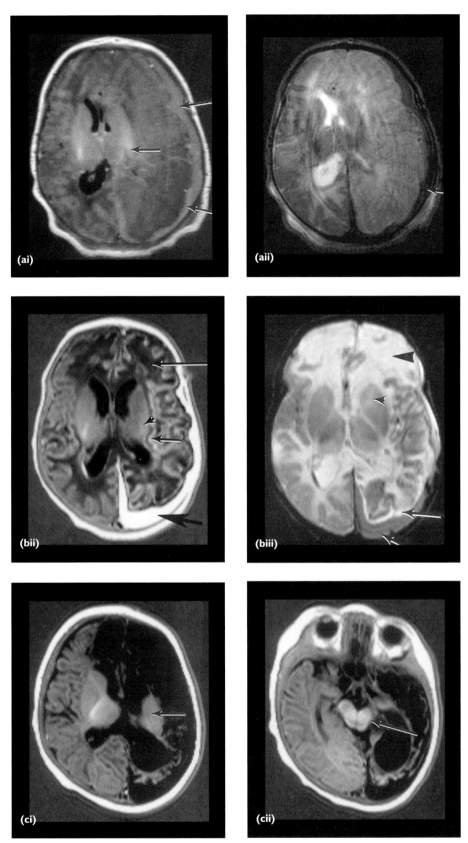

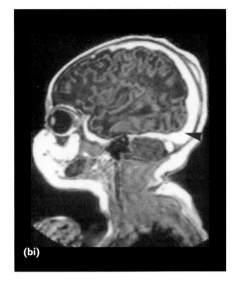

throughout the left hemisphere and possibly in the frontal lobe on the right. There is some high signal intensity within the posterior limb (*central arrow*) on the left but it is distorted. **(ii)** T2 weighted (SE 2700/120) sequence. The subdural is seen as low signal intensity (*arrow*). **(b)** Aged 10 days **(i) (ii)**. Inversion recovery (IR 3800/30/950) sequence. The extensive subdural hemorrhage is now seen as high signal intensity in both transverse and sagittal planes (*black short arrow/arrowhead*). There is widespread abnormal low signal intensity within the white matter (*long arrow*) with highlighting of the cortex (*short arrow*) consistent with infarction. The cortical highlighting is likely to be secondary to capillary proliferation. There is no high signal intensity from myelin in the posterior limb on the left (*small arrowhead*). **(iii)** T2 weighted (SE 2700/120) sequence the subdural is isointense with lower signal bands within it (*short arrow*). There is an inner layer of high signal intensity (*long arrow*). There is complete loss of gray/white matter differentiation in the frontal lobes and some loss posteriorly on the left (*large black arrowhead*). There is abnormal high signal intensity in the caudate heads, left more than right (*small arrowhead*). The low signal intensity from myelin is clearly seen in the right but not the left posterior limb of the internal capsule. **(c)** Inversion recovery (IR 3400/30/800) sequence aged 12 weeks. **(i)** Low ventricular level. There is a widened extracerebral space with left hemispheric infarction and left basal ganglia infarction. There is some residual thalamic tissue on the left (*arrow*) but no myelin in the internal capsule. There is additional loss of the right frontal lobe. There is ventricular dilation, which is more marked on the left. **(ii)** Level of the mesencephalon. There is almost total infarction of the left temporal lobe and asymmetry of the brain stem consistent with Wallerian degeneration (*arrow*). At 18 months this infant had a marked right-sided hemiplegia and generalized developmental delay, performing between 8 and 14 months on the Griffiths developmental scales. She also had a strabismus. Her head circumference had crossed from the 10th centile to the 50th centile despite this extensive tissue loss.

Fig. 9.10 This female infant was born at 39 weeks' gestation by vacuum extraction. There was prolonged rupture of membranes and shoulder dystocia at delivery. The Apgar scores were 8 at 1 min and 10 at 5 min, the cord pH was 7.24. She developed a tense fontanelle and generalized convulsions starting at 20 h of age. **(a)** Aged 2 days **(i)**. Inversion recovery (IR 3800/30/950) sequence. There is a large isointense subdural hemorrhage (*lateral arrows*) on the left producing a mass effect. There is loss of gray/white matter contrast

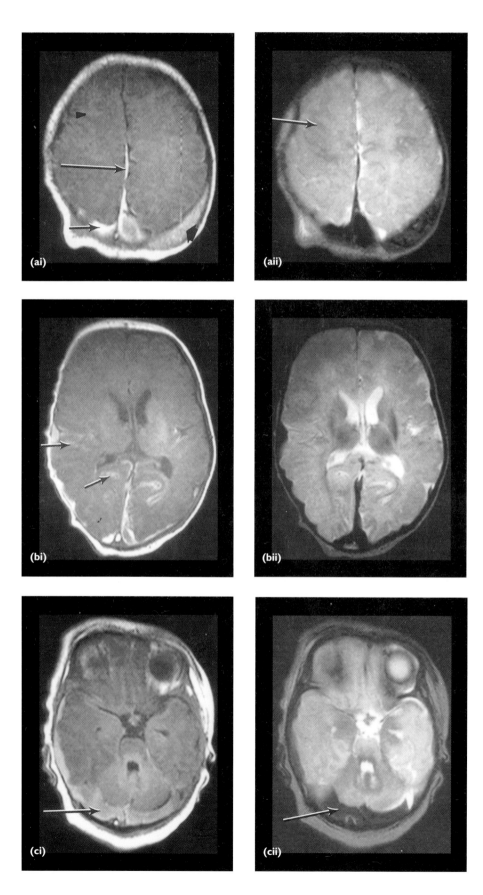

Fig. 9.11 This female infant was born at term by vacuum extraction. Both placental and cord abruption were noted at the delivery. Her Apgar scores were 0 at 1 min and 0 at 5 min. She developed stage II HIE. She was imaged at 5 days. **(a)** Centrum semiovale. **(i)** T1 weighted spin echo (SE 860/20) sequence. There is high signal intensity along the interhemispheric fissure (*long arrow*) and around the posterior part of each hemisphere (*short arrow*) consistent with extensive subdural hemorrhage. There is a localized slightly high signal intensity on the left consistent with a cephalhematoma (*large black arrowhead*). There is some slightly high signal intensity outlining the cortical markings consistent with cortical highlighting (*small arrowhead*). **(ii)** T2 weighted (SE 2700/120) sequence. The cephalhematoma and subdural hemorrhage have a low signal intensity. The 'cortical highlighting' is seen more easily than on the T1 weighted image. It has a low signal intensity (*arrow*). **(b)** Low ventricular level. **(i)** T1 weighted spin echo (SE 860/20) sequence. There is high signal intensity lining the sulci consistent with subarachnoid hemorrhage (*arrows*). This appears different to the superior levels of cortical highlighting shown in **(a)**. There is marked loss of gray/white matter differentiation throughout the brain. **(ii)** T2 weighted (SE 2700/120) sequence. The subarachnoid hemorrhage has a low signal intensity. **(c)** Posterior fossa. **(i)** T1 weighted spin echo (SE 860/20) sequence. There is bilateral subdural hemorrhage which is slightly high signal intensity (*arrow*). **(ii)** T2 weighted (SE 2700/120) sequence. The subdural is low signal intensity (*arrow*).

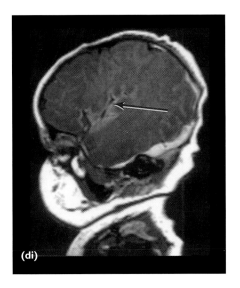

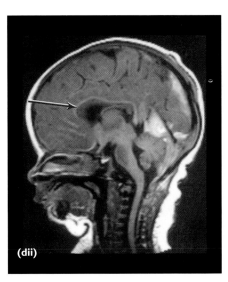

Fig. 9.11 *continued* **(d)** T1 weighted spin echo (SE 860/20) sequence. Parasagittal plane. **(i)** Lateral view. There is extensive high signal around the Sylvian fissure (*arrow*). **(ii)** Sagittal plane. There is high signal along the superior aspect of the corpus callosum (*arrow*). This child is currently 1 year old. She has severe microcephaly and generalized developmental delay.

referred to as 'cortical highlighting' as seen in infants with HIE (see Chapter 6). Abnormal signal intensity from subarachnoid hemorrhage follows the contours of the brain and should outline sulci (Figs 9.11 and 9.20). More extensive subarachnoid hemorrhage may be difficult to distinguish from subdural hemorrhage and the two may co-exist.

Thrombosis of sagittal sinus

ANATOMY

The venous drainage of the brain involves two major systems (Fig. 9.12). The external system of the superior sagittal sinus and the internal system of the inferior sagittal sinus join with the deep cerebral veins to form the great vein of Galen (great cerebral vein) and the straight sinus. The two sagittal sinuses join to drain into the straight sinus. The straight sinus drains into the right and left transverse sinus.

ETIOLOGY

Thrombosis of the sinuses may be secondary to trauma, an increased hematocrit, sepsis (see Chapter 10), dehydration or to cardiac failure[11]. Thrombosis at multiple sites has also been reported in infants with inherited thrombotic disorders such as factor V Leiden[17]. Several factors may combine in one individual (Fig. 9.13). Flow within the sinuses is relatively slow in the neonate, perhaps predisposing them to thrombosis.

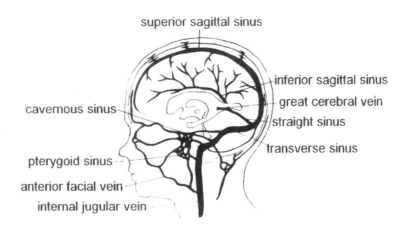

Fig. 9.12 The sinuses of the brain. (Adapted with permission from Volpe, *Neurology of the Newborn* 3rd edn. Saunders.)

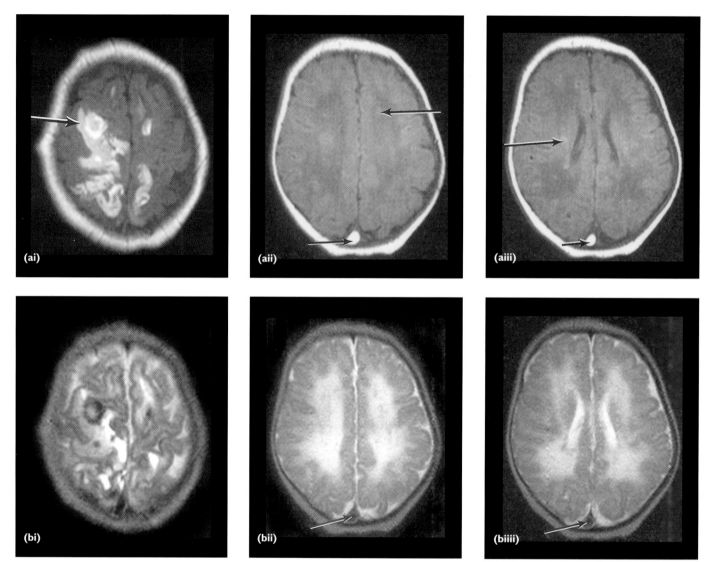

Fig. 9.13 This male infant with Down's syndrome was born at 39 weeks' gestation by cesarian section for fetal distress. Apgar scores were 8 at 1 min and 9 at 5 min. He presented with generalized convulsions on day 2. He was found to be both thrombocytopenic and polycythemic. **(a)** T1 weighted spin echo (SE 860/20) sequence aged 8 days. **(i)** There are bilateral hemorrhagic lesions of the cortex superiorly (*arrow*) with **(ii)** smaller white matter hemorrhagic lesions (*long arrow*) seen on lower slices and **(iii)** persistent high signal within the superior sagittal sinus consistent with sagittal sinus thrombosis (*short arrow*). **(b)** T2 weighted spin echo (SE 2700/120) sequence aged 8 days. **(i)** The superior cortical hemorrhagic lesions are seen as a mixture of high, isointense and low signal intensity and **(ii)**, **(iii)** the superior sagittal sinus is seen as low signal intensity (*arrow*) consistent with either thrombosis or very fast flow. The parenchymal white matter lesions are difficult to identify. At 2.5 years he showed a global developmental delay consistent with Down's syndrome, scoring between 14.5 and 17 months on Griffiths developmental assessment. He had a right-hand preference but no focal neurological signs.

IMAGING APPEARANCES

The differential diagnosis of sinus thrombosis includes changes due to normal or slow flow and subdural hemorrhage. Abnormally slow flow within the sinuses, secondary to congestive cardiac failure, may cause a 'functional' thrombosis (Fig. 9.15). Thin image slices are needed to eliminate changes secondary to blood flow and it is helpful to obtain images in several planes, a sagittal image being most useful to confirm the diagnosis of sagittal or straight sinus thrombosis. On T1 weighted transverse images normal flow in the sagittal sinus will be high or low signal intensity depending on the direction and velocity of flow in relation to the slice. Thrombosis is a possibility if the signal intensity within the sinus is high on all slices (Fig. 9.13). On T2 weighted imaging, low signal intensity within the sagittal sinus may represent fast flow or thrombosis. Injection of

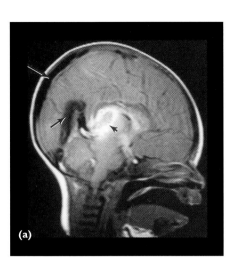
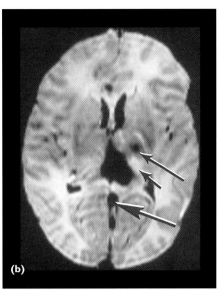

Fig. 9.14 This male infant was born by normal vaginal delivery at term. Apgar scores were 2 at 1 min and 5 at 5 min and the cord pH was 6.7. The EEG was isoelectric. Cranial ultrasound showed bilateral IVH with ventricular dilation, subdural hemorrhage and a possible vein of Galen aneurysm. The infant was weaned off the ventilator but required nasogastric feeding until his death at 2 months of age. **(a)** T1 weighted spin echo (SE 860/20) sequence sagittal plane aged 5 days. There is a large hemorrhagic lesion in the posterior thalamus (*arrowhead*) extending into the retrothalamic cistern. The vein of Galen and straight sinus are seen as low signal intensity, suggestive of thrombosis. They are distended and abnormally tortuous (*short arrow*). This may represent a primary vascular malformation. There is abnormal low signal intensity within the superior sagittal sinus (*long arrow*). This is also suggestive of thrombosis. **(b)** T2 weighted spin echo (SE 2700/120) sequence. There is low signal intensity in the lateral and third ventricle consistent with hemorrhage and in the straight sinus consistent with thrombosis (*large arrow*). There is abnormal high signal intensity within the thalami, more marked on the left (*short small arrow*). There is also abnormal low signal intensity in the left thalamus, more anteriorly (*long small arrow*). There is abnormal high signal intensity within the left posterior limb of the internal capsule. Postmortem at 2 months of age showed old thrombus within the torcula, occluding the junction with the left transverse and superior sagittal sinus. There was no evidence of an aneurysm of the vein of Galen and no comment on the straight sinus.

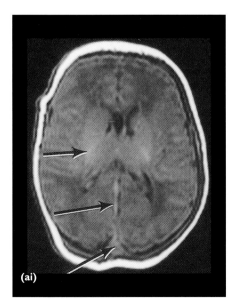
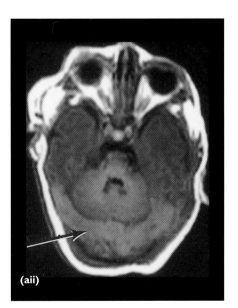
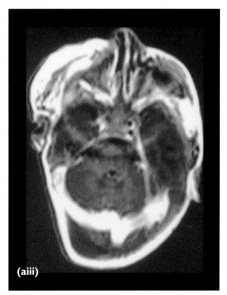

Fig. 9.15 This term infant was born by emergency cesarian section for fetal distress. The cord pH was 6.8 and Apgar scores were 0 at 1 min. He was noted to be hypoglycemic on day 1 but this was easily corrected. Abnormal clotting with thrombocytopenia was also noted on day 1 and he required five platelet transfusions. He developed congestive cardiac failure and was grossly edematous at the time of imaging. Liver function was also persistently abnormal. **(a)** T1 weighted (SE 860/20) sequence. **(i)**, **(ii)** There is isointense signal within the sagittal and transverse sinus and high signal in the straight sinus consistent with thrombosis (*long arrows*). There is some loss of gray/white matter differentiation. There is normal high signal intensity from myelin in the posterior limb of the internal capsule (*short arrow*). **(iii)**, **(iv)** T1 weighted (SE 860/20) sequence with contrast enhancement. The sagittal, straight and transverse sinuses enhance with contrast suggesting that the thrombosis is only partial or that the appearances are consistent with very slow flow secondary to the congestive cardiac failure.

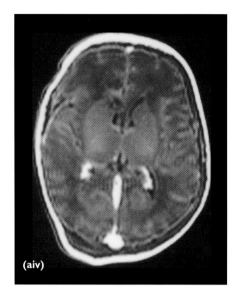

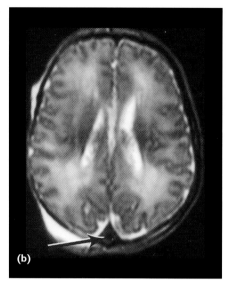

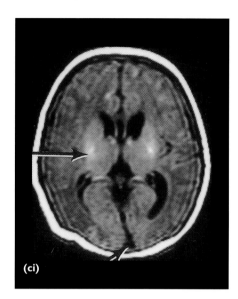

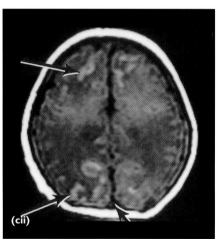

Fig. 9.15 *continued* **(b)** T2 weighted (SE 2700/120) sequence in the transverse plane at 19 h. There is low signal intensity in the sagittal sinus (*arrow*); this was seen on every slice and is consistent with either thrombus or high flow. **(c)** T1 weighted (SE 860/20) sequence **(i)**, **(ii)** at 5 days of age. There is now some low signal within the sagittal sinus (*short arrows*) but there are multiple areas of abnormal signal intensity in the cortex and subcortical white matter consistent with hemorrhagic infarction (*long arrows*). **(ii)** The basal ganglia, thalami and internal capsules (*arrow*) **(i)** are of normal appearance. The evolution of these images is consistent with a diagnosis of partial thrombosis secondary to congestive cardiac failure, which has resulted in multiple areas of cortical and subcortical infarction. The normal appearance of the internal capsules is an encouraging sign for future motor development but neurocognitive function is unlikely to be normal.

contrast may help confirm the diagnosis as may repeat imaging. Enhancement suggests flow within the sinus and therefore excludes complete thrombosis. Phase-encoded angiography is specific for flow and may be of considerable value in demonstrating obstruction. The diagnosis may be very difficult. If there is additional subdural hemorrhage this may compress the sinus and make image interpretation more difficult. This compression can in itself result in partial or complete thrombosis.

COMPLICATIONS

Thrombosis of the sinuses impedes venous drainage from the brain and may result in venous infarction within the region of brain that drains into the sinus. This involves the thalami in thrombosis of the straight sinus and vein of Galen

(Fig. 9.14) or the cortex and subcortical white matter with thrombosis of the sagittal sinus (Fig. 9.15). Infarction is characteristically bilateral and hemorrhagic. It typically involves the cortex and subcortical white matter.

Parenchymal hemorrhage

Parenchymal hemorrhages may be focal or multifocal and of any size. They may be clinically symptomatic or found incidentally. Predisposing factors include birth asphyxia, instrumental delivery and infection. More unusual causes are primary clotting abnormalities or congenital vascular abnormalities (Fig. 9.20) (see Chapter 12).

Multifocal small hemorrhages may be found in term infants presenting with convulsions during the first few days

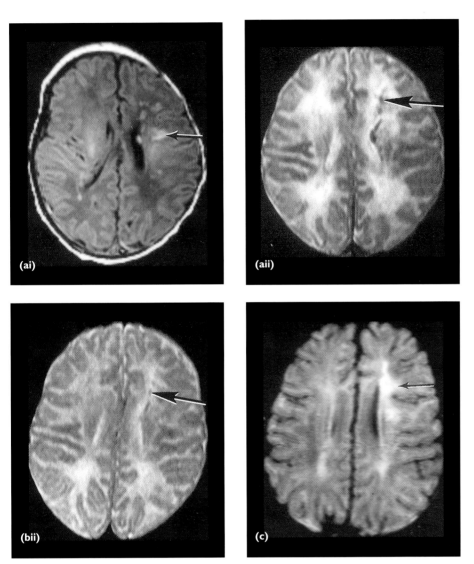

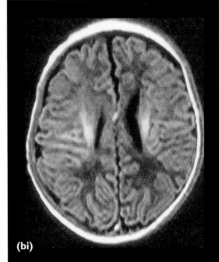

Fig. 9.16 This male infant was born at term by normal vaginal delivery. Apgar scores were 9 at 1 min and 10 at 5 min. He presented with right-sided followed by generalized seizures on day 3. A full clotting and thrombophilia screen were normal **(a)** Inversion recovery (IR 3800/30/950) sequence **(i)** T2 weighted spin echo (SE 2700/120) sequence **(ii)** aged 8 days. There are multiple small hemorrhagic lesions in both hemispheres (*arrows*). There is mild dilation of the left lateral ventricle. **(b)** At 6 weeks of age the hemorrhagic lesions were no longer visible on T1 weighted scans **(i)** but were still evident, although reduced, as low signal intensity, on the T2 weighted images (*arrow*) **(ii)**. **(c)** Fluid attenuated inversion recovery (FLAIR) (IR 6500/160/2100) sequence at 15 months. There are areas of increased T2 consistent with gliosis (*arrow*). His last assessment at 5.5 years revealed mild ankle asymmetry only. His general development was very good for his age but he showed some perceptual difficulties.

of life. These infants may have had some fetal distress but do not fulfill all the criteria for HIE[12] (see Chapter 6). They are usually sent to the postnatal ward following delivery and subsequently noted to be twitching (Fig. 9.16). Seizures are usually short lived.

Hemorrhagic lesions in the parenchyma can occur at any gestation (Fig. 9.17) prior to, during or following delivery. Parenchymal hemorrhagic lesions may co-exist with hemorrhage elsewhere in the cranium (Fig. 9.18).

Some infants presenting with HIE develop large intracranial hemorrhages. These infants may have had little documented fetal distress or show fetal distress in the absence of labor. In addition to their neurological complications they show metabolic derangement including abnormal clotting, hypoglycemia and conjugated hyperbilirubinemia (Fig. 9.19). The pattern of injury, mainly white matter, and

the neurodevelopmental outcome are atypical for HIE. Basal ganglia involvement may be minimal or asymmetrical and later cognitive problems are more marked than motor impairment. Underlying metabolic disorders should always be sought, although they may not be identified.

Arterio-venous malformations

These are dealt with in a separate chapter (see Chapter 12). Figure 9.20 shows an example of multiple hemangiomas in the brain of a neonate. They were associated with acute perinatal hemorrhage and were initially indistinguishable from primary hemorrhage without an obvious vascular malformation.

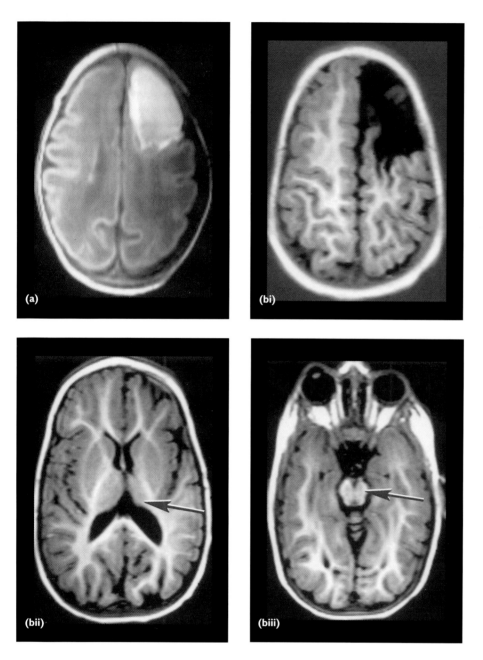

Fig. 9.17 This preterm infant was born at 29 weeks' gestation. Cranial ultrasound demonstrated bilateral intraventricular hemorrhage with a left-sided parenchymal echo density, thought initially to be a venous infarct. **(a)** Inversion recovery (IR 3800/30/ 950) sequence at 3 weeks. There is high signal in the left frontoparietal lobe consistent with hemorrhage of between 3 days and 6 weeks. This was completely separate from the ventricles. **(b)** Inversion recovery (IR 3400/30/800) sequence at 9 months showing **(i)** atrophy of the left frontal lobe **(ii)** atrophy of the thalamus (*arrow*) and **(iii)** asymmetry of the brain stem (*arrow*). This child is now 7 years old and has a right-sided hemiplegia.

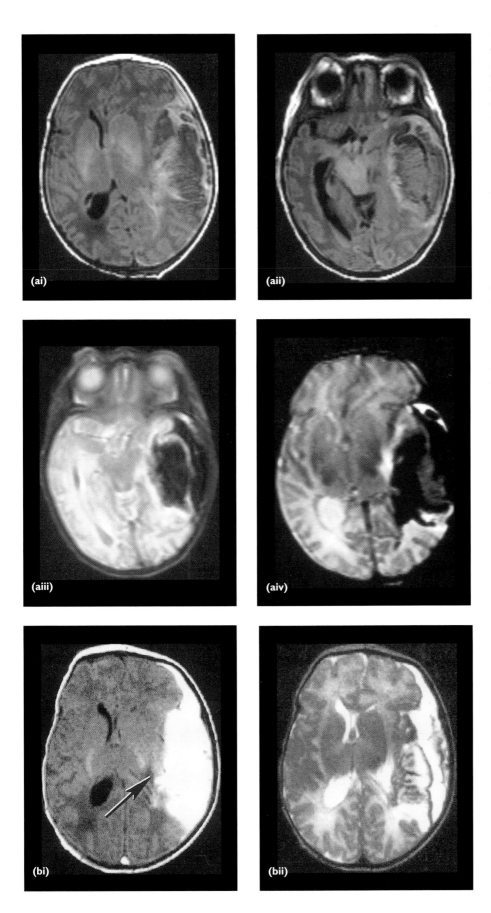

(ai)

(aii)

(aiii)

(aiv)

(bi)

(bii)

Fig. 9.18 This female infant was born at term by vaginal delivery following manual rotation of the head immediately prior to delivery. The Apgar scores were normal and no resuscitation was required. She went home at 6 h of age but was noted to be excessively sleepy. She subsequently developed convulsions and apneas that required ventilation for 3 days. A hemorrhagic screen was normal. **(a)** Inversion recovery (IR 3800/30/950) sequence **(i)**, **(ii)** and T2 weighted spin echo (SE 2700/120) sequence **(iii)**, **(iv)** at 3 days of age. Transverse plane at low ventricular and mesencephalon level. There is a large hemorrhage within the left temporal and parietal lobes with mid-line shift, brainstem deviation and tentorial herniation (not shown). The hemorrhage is mainly isointense on T1 and low signal intensity on T2 weighted images. There is additional subdural hemorrhage in the left Sylvian fissure, although it is quite difficult to separate the two lesions. There is mild dilation of the right lateral ventricle which appears to contain hemorrhage. This dilation is presumably secondary to obstruction. **(b)** Inversion recovery (IR 3800/30/950) sequence and T2 weighted spin echo (SE 2700/120) sequence. Two weeks of age. The hemorrhagic lesion in the temporal and parietal lobes is now all high signal on the T1 weighted image **(i)** and on the T2 weighted image **(ii)**. It is possible to differentiate the subdural from the parenchymal hemorrhage on T2 weighted image but not on the T1 weighted image. It is possible to see myelin in both posterior limbs although there is an area of abnormal signal intensity at the base of the internal capsule (*arrow*), seen most clearly as low signal intensity in **(i)**. There is residual brain swelling, mid-line shift and brain stem deviation and there is mild right-sided ventricular dilatation.

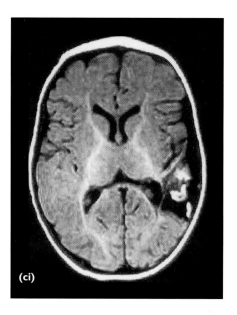

(ci)

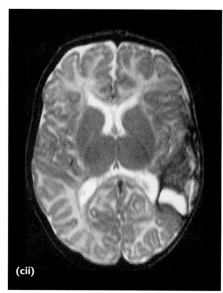

(cii)

Fig. 9.18 *continued* (c) At 4 months, there is now an established left temporal lobe infarct. There is persistent high signal on T1 and low signal on T2 weighted imaging, the latter being compatible with the presence of hemosiderin. The signal from myelin in the posterior limb is also asymmetrical but only on the T2 weighted image where although it is longer, it is rather thin. At 1 year of age she had a strong preference for her left hand with some asymmetry in tone. Her general development was at the lower end of the normal range. She had had no further convulsions. The source of the parenchymal hemorrhage in this infant may have been a secondary hemorrhagic infarct from impaired venous drainage or interruption of arterial supply by the subdural hemorrhage. It is also possible that it arose independently as a separate hemorrhagic lesion although this seems less likely.

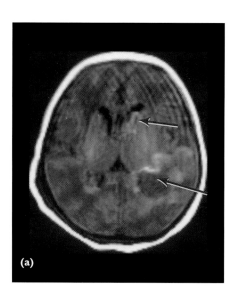

(a)

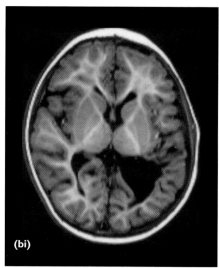

(bi)

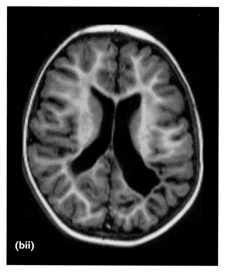

(bii)

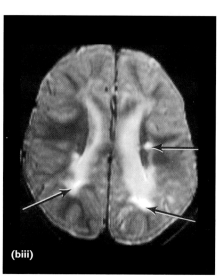

(biii)

Fig. 9.19 This male infant was born by emergency cesarian section at term for severe fetal distress. The cord pH was 6.7. His Apgar scores were 0 at 1 min and 1 at 5 min and birthweight was 3920 g. He developed convulsions and was staged as HIE II. He had persistent hypoglycemia. He developed a severe neonatal hepatitis with prolonged conjugated jaundice. Ultrasound showed bilateral intraventricular hemorrhage with a lesion in the left temporoparietal lobe. **(a)** T1 weighted spin echo (SE 860/20) sequence at 3 days of age. There is a hemorrhagic lesion in the left temporal region (*long arrow*) and in the left caudate head (*short arrow*). These are isointense with a high signal intensity rim. This image is motion artifacted. **(b)** Inversion recovery (IR 3400/30/800/) sequence at 2 years of age. **(i)** Low ventricular level. There is a porencephalic dilation of the left posterior ventricular horn at the site of the perinatal hemorrhage. There is a paucity of myelin. **(ii)** Mid-ventricular level. There is bilateral ventricular dilation with angulation of both ventricles posteriorly. These images could easily be mistaken as being secondary to periventricular leukomalacia. **(iii)** T2 weighted spin echo (SE 2700/120) sequence. There is high signal consistent with gliosis in the periventricular white matter, most marked posteriorly (*arrows*).

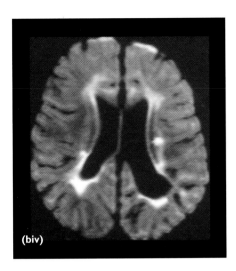

Fig. 9.19 *continued* (iv) Fluid attenuated inversion recovery (FLAIR) (IR 6500/160/2100) sequence. This sequence accentuates the gliotic changes. The late imaging findings in this child are typical of periventricular leukomalacia but are not due to antenatal injury to the preterm brain. They are the result of a well-documented perinatal process. At 4 years of age he had signs of a mild diplegia but was mobile. There was some upper limb involvement with clumsy movements of his arms and hands. He was hyperactive with severe cognitive deficits.

(biv)

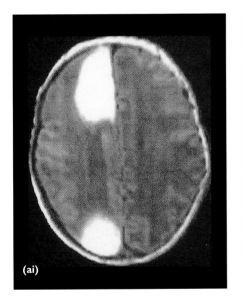

(ai)

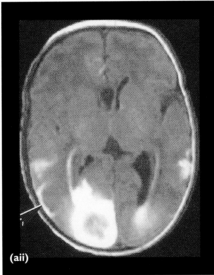

(aii)

Fig. 9.20 This male infant was born by emergency cesarian section for fetal distress at 36 weeks' gestation. Cardiotocogram (CTG) showed decelerations prior to delivery and there were decreased fetal movements for 24 h. Apgar scores were 4 at 1 min and 7 at 5 min. The cord pH was 7.04 and the birthweight was 1.96 kg. He developed respiratory distress and was ventilated for 1 day. Routine ultrasound demonstrated a well-localized echo density in the right frontoparietal region. He developed convulsions and was given phenobarbital. **(a)** T1 weighted spin echo (SE 860/20) **(i)**, **(ii)** and T2 weighted spin echo (SE2700/120) **(iii)**, **(iv)** aged 7 days. There are multiple hemorrhagic lesions, many appear to lie on the meningeal surface and project inwards. There is a large subarachnoid hemorrhage (*arrowhead*) which is exerting a mass effect. At 3 months of age this infant developed skin hemangiomas and further imaging demonstrated a hemorrhagic lesion on the lung. A diagnosis of multiple hemangiomatosis was made. The skin lesions have regressed.

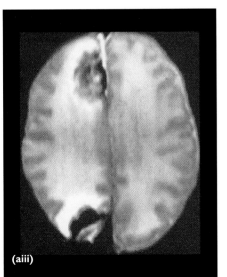

(aiii)

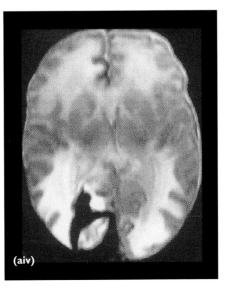

(aiv)

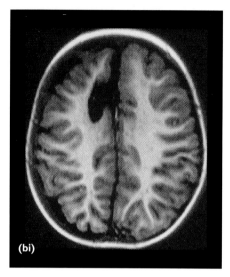
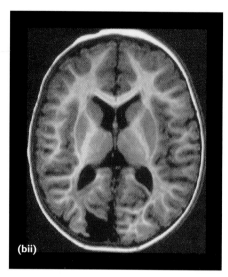
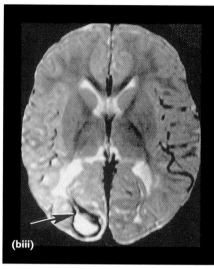

Fig. 9.20 *continued* **(b)** Inversion recovery (IR 3400/30/800) **(i) (ii)** and T2 weighted spin echo (SE 2700/120) **(iii)** sequence at 2 years. There are defects in the brain at the sites of the previous hemorrhagic lesions. There is low signal intensity lining (*arrow*) one of these defects and consistent with hemosiderin, on the T2 weighted image **(iii)**. At 5 years of age he showed some dystonic components to fine hand and finger movement and had some mild asymmetry of tone around the ankle. He had some visual difficulties and was hyperactive. He read well for his age.

Thalamic hemorrhage

Thalamic hemorrhage is usually unilateral and associated with intraventricular hemorrhage[1]. Primary thalamic hemorrhage needs to be distinguished from the bilateral thalamic abnormalities seen in HIE. Infants with thalamic hemorrhage do not usually present with 'full blown' HIE (Fig. 9.21).

Although the bilateral lesions seen following HIE are high signal intensity on T1 weighted images and low signal intensity on T2 weighted images, pathological comparisons in this condition do not identify hemorrhage in the thalami. The signal intensities seen may, however, be due to capillary proliferation in regions of infarction. In addition, following asphyxia, the abnormal signal intensity within the thalami is bilateral

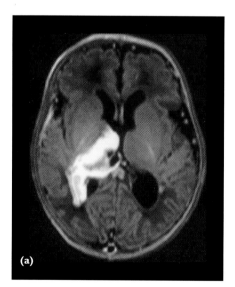
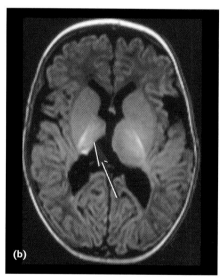
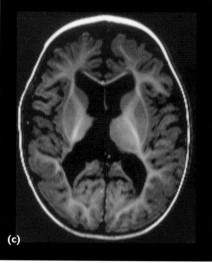

Fig. 9.21 This male infant was born by normal vaginal delivery at term. Apgar scores were 8 at 1 min and 9 at 5 min. His birthweight was 3.01 kg. He developed seizures at 12 h of age. Cranial ultrasound showed a large IVH with right parenchymal and thalamic involvement. His EEG was abnormal with discontinuous background. **(a)** Inversion recovery sequence (IR 3800/30/950) aged 8 days. There is hemorrhage involving the right thalamus and the right lateral ventricle. There is bilateral ventricular dilation. **(b)** Inversion recovery sequence (IR 3800/30/950) imaged 18 days. There has been resolution of the hemorrhage. There is atrophy of the left thalamus (*arrow*). The ventricles remain dilated and are now irregular in outline. Myelin is visible in both posterior limbs of the internal capsule. **(c)** Inversion recovery (IR 3600/80/300) sequence aged 9 months. There is thalamic atrophy on the right. The ventricles remain dilated and irregular in outline. Myelination is reduced generally. These appearances could be mistaken for being secondary to periventricular leukomalacia. At 19 months he was hypotonic and had a homonomous hemianopia but no other focal neurological signs. He was not pulling himself to stand and moved by bottom shuffling. He had general developmental delay more marked with performance items. He had an abnormal EEG and was on carbemezapine.

and usually more focal, effecting the lateral thalamic nuclei and sometimes the medial nuclei.

Basal ganglia hemorrhage

Hemorrhage into the caudate is usually seen as a secondary extension from germinal layer hemorrhage in the preterm infant. It may also occur as an isolated event in the term infant (Fig. 9.22), although differentiation from a hemorrhagic infarction involving a deep branch of the middle cerebral artery is not easy (see Chapter 7).

Cerebellar hemorrhage

Cerebellar hemorrhage has been reported in 10–25% of very preterm infants on postmortem studies[14]. It may be related to the standard of care and positioning of the infant and has been associated with increased pressure from mask ventilation[15]. Using MRI we have identified hemorrhagic lesions within the cerebellum in approximately 3% of a cohort of infants born at less than 30 weeks' gestation. Cerebellar hemorrhage may escape detection using ultrasound through the anterior fontanelle and result in cerebellar atrophy later on[13]. This atrophy could similarly be secondary to undiagnosed infarction (Fig. 9.29). Routine ultrasonography through the posterior fontanelle in premature infants may improve detection. Improved detection may confirm that cerebellar hemorrhage in preterm infants is often clinically silent and may not always be associated with significant morbidity.

In the term infant cerebellar hemorrhage may be primary, secondary to venous infarction or may complicate massive intraventricular or subarachnoid hemorrhage. Laceration of the cerebellum may occur secondary to trauma such as occipital osteodiastasis in breech deliveries. The vermis is reported to be the initial site of the lesion in the majority of term infants.

Symptoms often occur in the first day in the term infant following a difficult delivery but presentation may not occur until later in the neonatal period (Fig. 9.23). There may be brain stem disturbances, with abnormalities in eye movements. Increasing head circumference may be secondary to ventricular dilation (Fig. 9.23). The outcome with severe cerebellar hemorrhage is poor with a high mortality in preterm infants. It is associated with a lower mortality in term infants but there is a high incidence of motor and intellectual problems with prominent cerebellar signs[21].

The decision as to whether surgical treatment is necessary is difficult and it is likely that surgery is best reserved for those children with brain stem signs[16].

Intraventricular hemorrhage

INCIDENCE AND ETIOLOGY

Intraventricular hemorrhage (IVH) in the preterm brain usually arises from the germinal matrix (GM) whilst intraventricular hemorrhage in the term infant originates from the choroid plexus. Germinal matrix/intraventricular hemorrhage (GMH/IVH) occurs in between 30 and 40% of infants weighing less than 1500 g or approximately 30 weeks' gestation. The incidence increases with decreasing gestation. There has been a decreased incidence in severe IVH and its complications with the increasing use of surfactant therapy.

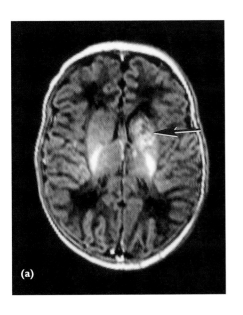
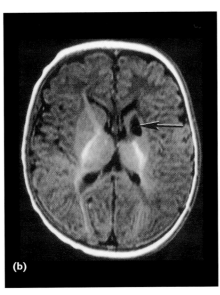

Fig. 9.22 This female infant was born at 41 weeks' gestation by emergency cesarian section. Apgar scores were 8 at 1 min, and 9 at 5 min. She developed seizures. EEG showed asymmetrical seizure activity and cranial ultrasound showed an echo density in the left basal ganglia. **(a)** Inversion recovery (IR 3800/30/950) sequence aged 10 days. There is an isolated hemorrhagic lesion in the left caudate head, this may be a hemorrhagic infarction. **(b)** Follow-up imaging at 3 months showed a cystic infarct of the left caudate head (*arrow*). At 18 months this child showed no asymmetry on neurological examination. Her developmental scales were between 16.5 and 20 months, the lowest score being for performance with some difficulty with the puzzle tasks. The child has developed normally and had no signs of a hemiplegia at 3 years.

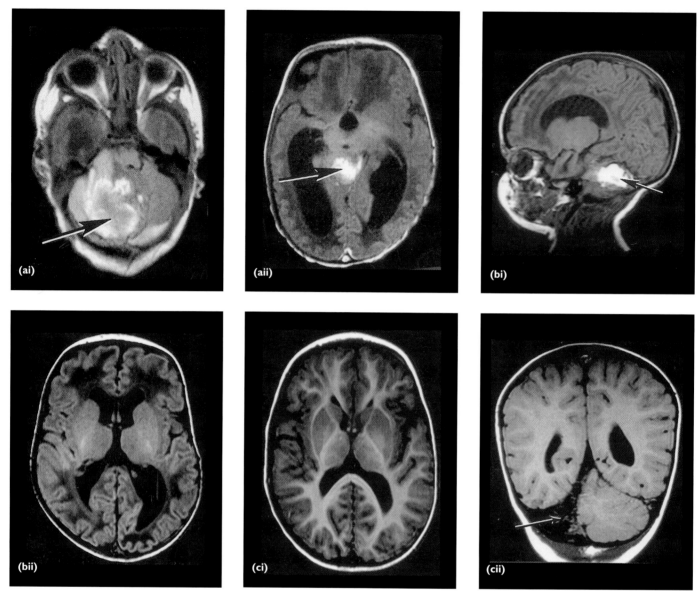

Fig. 9.23 This male infant was born by spontaneous vaginal delivery at term. The cord pH was 7.16 but the Apgar scores were normal. He presented at 1 week of age with an increasing head circumference. Cranial ultrasound showed dilated lateral and third ventricles with increased echo density within the cerebellum. **(a)** T1 weighted spin echo (SE 860/20) sequence aged 7 days. **(i)** There is a mixed signal intensity hemorrhagic lesion involving the right hemisphere and vermis of the cerebellum (*arrow*). **(ii)** High signal intensity is seen in the vermis (*arrow*). There is marked dilation of the lateral ventricles and the third ventricle. The aqueduct is also slightly dilated. There is abnormal low signal intensity within the white matter, presumably due to edema from the raised intraventricular pressure. **(b)** T1 weighted spin echo (SE 860/20) sequence. Sagittal **(i)** and transverse **(ii)** plane aged 23 days. The hemorrhage is resolving (*arrow*) **(i)**. The ventricles remain dilated and the white matter still shows abnormal low signal intensity **(ii)**. **(c)** Inversion recovery (IR 3400/30/800) **(i)** and T1 weighted (SE 860/20) **(ii)** sequence in the coronal plane aged 15 months. Myelination has proceeded normally. The ventricles are now only mildly dilated **(i)**. There is infarction of the posterior part of the right cerebellar hemisphere (*arrow*) **(ii)**. Developmental follow-up at 15 months of age is within normal limits with minimal delay in speech. On neurological examination he is hypotonic. His head growth remains along the 50th centile. A hemorrhagic screen was normal.

APPEARANCES

MRI provides excellent visualization of the GM and is able to identifying regions of matrix in the roof of the temporal horn, which are not visualized with ultrasound (Fig. 9.24). MRI can be used to document the involution of the GM with increasing gestation (Fig. 9.24). Imaging through the transverse plane may explain its superiority in detection over ultrasound where images are routinely obtained only in the coronal and sagittal planes. In a cohort of infants of less than 30 weeks' gestation we have found an incidence of

GMH/IVH of approximately 40% on initial MRI (see Chapter 3).

GMH may occur at different sites and can be differentiated from normal GM by its size and shape (Fig. 9.24). IVH secondary to GMH is most often identified in the posterior horns of the lateral ventricle (Fig. 9.24). When extensive, however, it can be seen tracking through the ventricular system (Fig. 9.26aii). Low signal intensity on T2 weighted images due to the presence of hemosiderin may be seen weeks or even months after a GMH/IVH. In addition, on T1 weighted images, a high signal lining the ventricle may be seen months after a hemorrhage. This may represent enhancement of ependymal lining but the etiology is unclear.

IVH can be graded with CT and with cranial ultrasound but this has not been formally done with MRI. A grading system using MRI may need to add more grades in order to describe the different sites involved.

In term infants the germinal layer has largely involuted and intraventricular hemorrhage in the term infant usually originates from the choroid plexus (Fig. 9.25). The site of origin may be difficult to identify in the presence of a large IVH.

Complications of GLH/IVH

VENOUS INFARCTION

Venous infarction arises as a consequence of thrombosis in the terminal veins of the hemorrhagic germinal layer. Infarcts are usually associated with a large GMH/IVH but

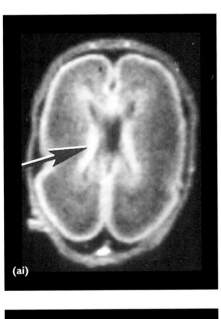
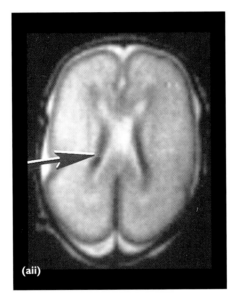
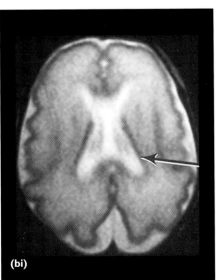
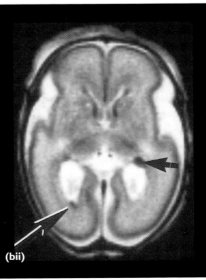

Fig. 9.24 Germinal matrix normal appearances. **(a)** Twenty-four week gestation infant aged 4 days. T1 weighted (SE 860/20) sequence **(i)** and T2 weighted fast spin echo (FSE 3000/208) sequence **(ii)** at mid-ventricular level showing normal appearances of the germinal layer overlying the caudate as symmetrical regions of low signal intensity on T2 and high signal intensity on the T1 weighted image (*arrows*). **(b)** Twenty-eight week gestation infant T2 weighted fast spin echo (FSE 2700/120) sequence. Mid-ventricular level. **(i)** The germinal matrix is involuting and is seen as a narrower area of low signal intensity (*arrow*). **(ii)** Low ventricular level. The germinal layer can be seen in the anterior horn of the lateral ventricle and in the roof of the temporal horn. There is a small matrix hemorrhage in the roof of the temporal horn on the left (*black arrowhead*) and blood in the posterior horn on the right (*arrow*).

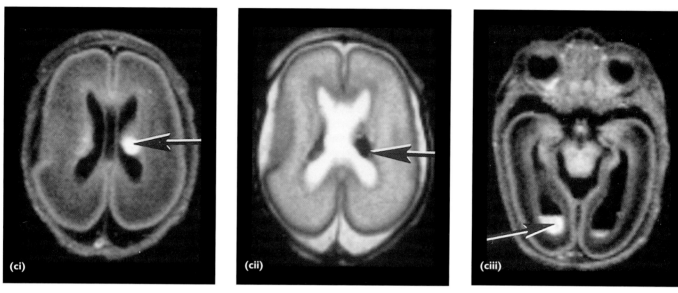

Fig. 9.24 *continued* **(c)** Twenty-four week gestation infant imaged at 1 day of age. T1 weighted (SE 860/20) **(i)** and T2 weighted fast spin echo (FSE 3000/208) sequence **(ii)** at mid-ventricular level. There is asymmetry of the germinal matrix consistent with hemorrhage (*arrows*). T1 weighted (SE 860/20) sequence **(iii)**. There is bilateral intraventricular hemorrhage (*arrow*). The infant was imaged in the supine position and there is a fluid–fluid level consistent with hemorrhage.

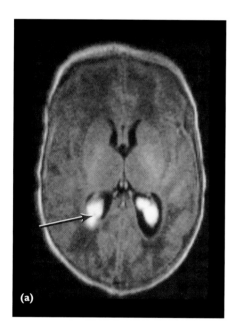

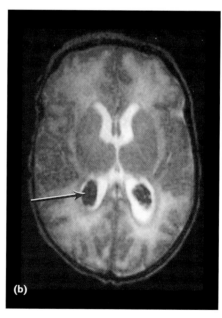

Fig. 9.25 This male infant was born at term following maternal pre-eclampsia and as a result of an IVF pregnancy. Postnatally, he was noted to have a persistent acidosis and high lactate. An initial hemorrhagic screen was negative. Imaged at 7 days of age. **(a)** T1 weighted spin echo (SE 860/20) sequence and **(b)** T2 weighted spin echo (SE 2700/120) sequence at 7 days of age. There is abnormal signal intensity within the choroid consistent with hemorrhage (*arrows*).

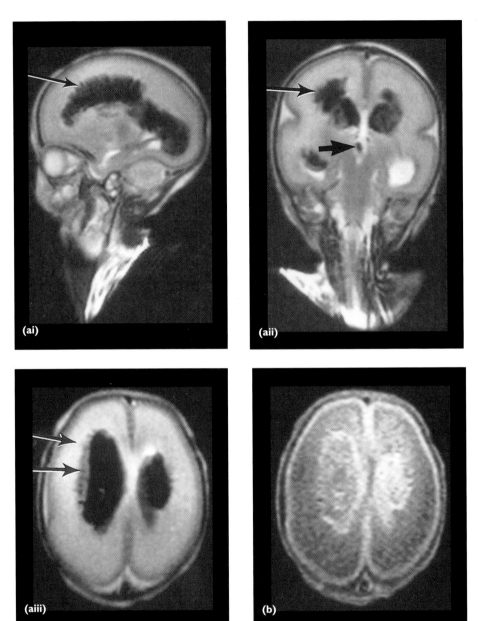

(ai)

(aii)

(aiii)

(b)

Fig. 9.26 This preterm infant was delivered at 26 weeks. He died at 3 weeks of age and an MRI was performed postmortem. **(a)** T2 weighted fast spin echo (FSE 3000/208) sequence in **(i)** sagittal, **(ii)** coronal and **(iii)** transverse planes. There is bilateral GMH/IVH. There is abnormal linear signal intensity fanning out from the ventricles consistent with hemorrhagic venous infarction (*arrows*). There is high SI in the adjacent WM consistent with ischemia (*top arrow*). **(iii)** Blood in the third ventricle can be identified on the coronal images (*black arrowhead*). **(b)** T1 weighted spin echo (SE 860/20) sequence in transverse plane. The hemorrhage and hemorrhagic infarction are seen as predominantly high signal intensity.

may occur with isolated GMH. MRI has improved the detection of lesions that appear to be secondary to venous infarction. Areas of hemorrhagic infarction may occur at any of the sites of germinal matrix that can be identified by MRI[5] (Figs 9.26, 9.27 and 9.28). Occasionally, T2 weighted MR images may show multiple linear abnormalities in the white matter of the centrum semiovale associated with hemorrhage in the germinal matrix. These linear abnormalities may represent distended or blocked draining veins.

In surviving infants venous infarction usually evolves to produce a porencephalic cyst (Fig. 9.29). These infants have a high incidence of later hemiplegia. In a study by De Vries looking at preterm infants with unilateral lesions there was a strong association between abnormal signal intensity within the posterior limb of the internal capsule on the affected side and the later development of a hemiplegia[3].

As described previously, GMH/IVH may occur antenatally as can the various complications.

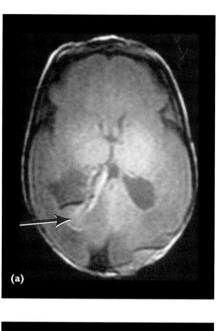

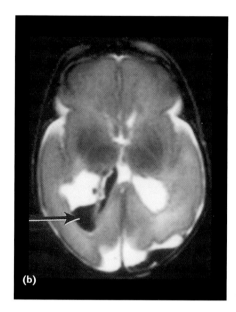

Fig. 9.27 This male infant was the first born of triplets at 24 weeks +5 days' gestation. He had normal imaging throughout life but had a clinical deterioration at 6 weeks of age associated with an incarcerated inguinal hernia. Imaging was performed immediately after death. T1 weighted spin echo (SE 20/860) **(a)** and T2 weighted fast spin echo (FSE 3000/208) **(b)** sequence. There is a hemorrhagic lesion in the right temporal lobe. There is additional hemorrhage within the right posterior horn (*arrows*) These findings are consistent with venous infarction. Histology confirmed the presence of germinal matrix and intraventricular hemorrhage. The periventricular white matter showed pyknotic cells and axon retraction balls consistent with recent infarction.

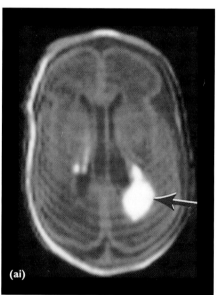

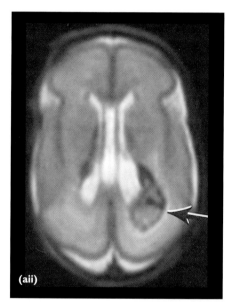

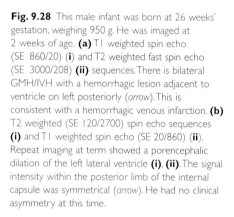

Fig. 9.28 This male infant was born at 26 weeks' gestation, weighing 950 g. He was imaged at 2 weeks of age. **(a)** T1 weighted spin echo (SE 860/20) **(i)** and T2 weighted fast spin echo (SE 3000/208) **(ii)** sequences. There is bilateral GMH/IVH with a hemorrhagic lesion adjacent to ventricle on left posteriorly (*arrow*). This is consistent with a hemorrhagic venous infarction. **(b)** T2 weighted (SE 120/2700) spin echo sequences **(i)** and T1 weighted spin echo (SE 20/860) **(ii)**. Repeat imaging at term showed a porencephalic dilation of the left lateral ventricle **(i)**, **(ii)**. The signal intensity within the posterior limb of the internal capsule was symmetrical (*arrow*). He had no clinical asymmetry at this time.

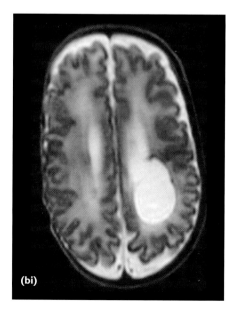

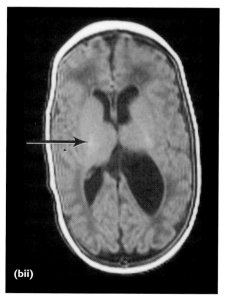

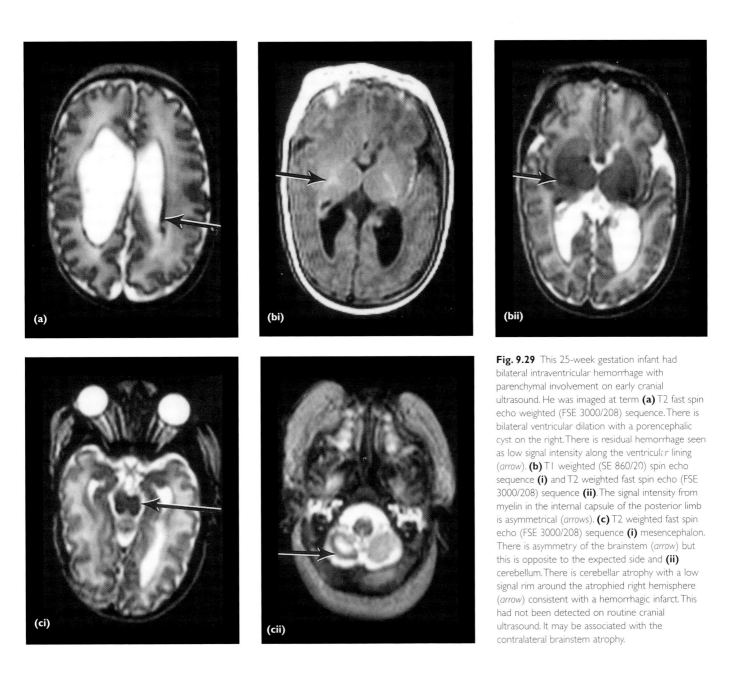

Fig. 9.29 This 25-week gestation infant had bilateral intraventricular hemorrhage with parenchymal involvement on early cranial ultrasound. He was imaged at term **(a)** T2 fast spin echo weighted (FSE 3000/208) sequence. There is bilateral ventricular dilation with a porencephalic cyst on the right. There is residual hemorrhage seen as low signal intensity along the ventricular lining (*arrow*). **(b)** T1 weighted (SE 860/20) spin echo sequence **(i)** and T2 weighted fast spin echo (FSE 3000/208) sequence **(ii)**. The signal intensity from myelin in the internal capsule of the posterior limb is asymmetrical (*arrows*). **(c)** T2 weighted fast spin echo (FSE 3000/208) sequence **(i)** mesencephalon. There is asymmetry of the brainstem (*arrow*) but this is opposite to the expected side and **(ii)** cerebellum. There is cerebellar atrophy with a low signal rim around the atrophied right hemisphere (*arrow*) consistent with a hemorrhagic infarct. This had not been detected on routine cranial ultrasound. It may be associated with the contralateral brainstem atrophy.

Ventricular dilation

Posthemorrhagic ventricular dilation is due to interference with the normal flow of CSF (Fig. 9.30). The incidence of ventricular dilation increases with the severity of GMH/IVH. Cranial ultrasound is an ideal tool for monitoring ventricular dilation in the presence of an open fontanelle. Many units will have guidelines for measurements of the frontal horns, although dilation tends to be maximal in the occipital or posterior horns (colpocephaly) which are not routinely measured. More detailed imaging with MRI is usually required prior to shunt surgery and for monitoring the progress or shunt complications after closure of the fontanelle. Most modern shunts are MR compatible and good quality images can be produced. It is very important to check the MR compatibility of any intraventricular device (see Chapter 1). Metallic components may move when placed in the magnetic field. They may also cause an enormous susceptibility artifact, which may render images uninterpretable.

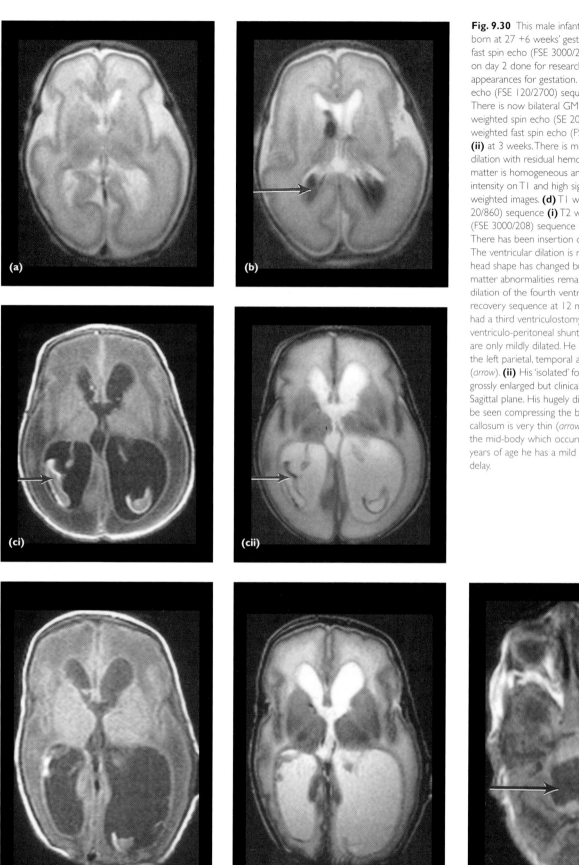

Fig. 9.30 This male infant was the second of twins born at 27 +6 weeks' gestation. **(a)** T2 weighted fast spin echo (FSE 3000/208) sequence performed on day 2 done for research purposes shows normal appearances for gestation. **(b)** T2 weighted fast spin echo (FSE 120/2700) sequence at 7 days of age. There is now bilateral GMH/IVH (*arrow*). **(c)** T1 weighted spin echo (SE 20/860) sequence **(i)** T2 weighted fast spin echo (FSE 120/2700) sequence **(ii)** at 3 weeks. There is marked bilateral ventricular dilation with residual hemorrhage (*arrow*). The white matter is homogeneous and is uniformly low signal intensity on T1 and high signal intensity on the T2 weighted images. **(d)** T1 weighted spin echo (SE 20/860) sequence **(i)** T2 weighted fast spin echo (FSE 3000/208) sequence **(ii)** imaged at 6 weeks. There has been insertion of a reservoir on the left. The ventricular dilation is marked but static. The head shape has changed but the diffuse white matter abnormalities remain. **(iii)** There is marked dilation of the fourth ventricle (*arrow*). **(e)** Inversion recovery sequence at 12 months of age. He has had a third ventriculostomy and two revisions of a ventriculo-peritoneal shunt. **(i)** His lateral venticles are only mildly dilated. He has marked atrophy of the left parietal, temporal and occipital lobes (*arrow*). **(ii)** His 'isolated' fourth ventricle remains grossly enlarged but clinically asymptomatic. **(iii)** Sagittal plane. His hugely dilated fourth ventricle can be seen compressing the brainstem. The corpus callosum is very thin (*arrow*) with an interruption in the mid-body which occurred postsurgery. At 2 years of age he has a mild global developmental delay.

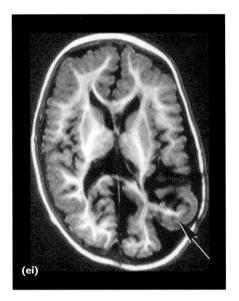
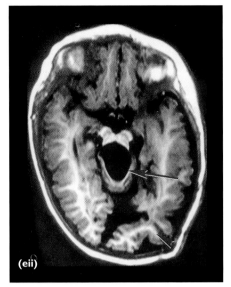
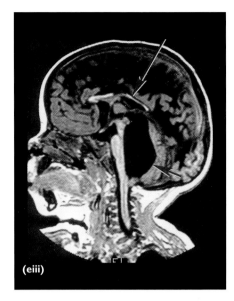

Summary

- Hemorrhage is often present at more than one site.
- MRI can be used to time the onset of lesions.
- Evolution of the signal intensity of hemorrhage depends on the site and size of the lesion.
- Hemorrhage may be primary or secondary and occur within an arterial or venous infarct.

- There is a strong association between traumatic delivery, especially vacuum extraction and hemorrhagic lesions.
- A coagulation and thrombotic profile should be performed in all infants with significant hemorrhage.
- Neurodevelopmental outcome varies with the site of hemorrhage, the presence of additional lesions and the underlying cause.

References

1. De Vries LS, Smet M, Goemans N *et al.* (1992) Unilateral thalamic haemorrhage in the pre-term and full-term newborn. *Neuropediatrics* **23**, 153–156.
2. De Vries LS, Eken P, Groenendaal F *et al.* (1998) Antenatal onset of haemorrhagic and/or ischaemic lesions in preterm infants: prevalence and associated obstetric variables. *Arch Dis Child Fetal Neonatal Ed* **78**, F51–56.
3. De Vries LS, Groenendaal F, van Haastert IC *et al.* (1999) Asymmetrical myelination of the posterior limb of the internal capsule in infants with periventricular haemorrhagic infarction: an early predictor of hemiplegia. *Neuropediatrics* **30**, 314–319.
4. Ehrenforth S, Klarmann D, Zabel B *et al.* (1998) Severe factor V deficiency presenting as subdural haematoma in the newborn. *Eur J Pediatr* **157**, 1032.
5. Felderhoff-Mueser U, Rutherford M, Squier W *et al.* (1999) Relation between magnetic resonance images and histopathological findings of the brain in extremely sick preterm infants. *Am J Neuroradiol* **20**, 1349–1357.
6. Goevart P (1993) *Cranial Haemorrhage in the Term Newborn Infant.* London, MacKeith Press.
7. Goevart P, Moens K and Leroy J (1992) Vacuum extraction, bone injury and neonatal subgaleal bleeding. *Eur J Paediatrics* **151**, 532–535.
8. Greer FR (1995) Vitamin K deficiency and hemorrhage in infancy. *Clin Perinatol* **22**, 759–777.
9. Hayashi T, Hashimoto T, Fukada S *et al.* (1987) Neonatal subdural haematoma secondary to birth injury. *Child Nerv Syst* **3**, 23–29.
10. Jayawant S, Rawlinson A, Gibbon F *et al.* (1998) Subdural haemorrhages in infants: population based study. *BMJ* **317**, 1558–1561.
11. Kuharik MA and Edwards MK (1987) Cerebral venous distention associated with cardiac failure in infants. *Am J Neuroradiol* **8**, 657–659.
12. Mercuri E, Cowan F, Rutherford M *et al.* (1995) Ischaemic and haemorrhagic brain lesions in newborns with seizures and normal Apgar scores. *Arch Dis Child Fetal Neonatal Ed* **73**, F67–74.
13. Mercuri E, He J, Curati WL *et al.* (1997) Cerebellar infarction and atrophy in infants and children with a history of premature birth. *Pediatr Radiol* **27**, 139–143.
14. Merrill JD, Piecuch RE, Fell SC *et al.* (1998) A new pattern of cerebellar hemorrhages in preterm infants. *Pediatrics* **102**, E62.
15. Pape KE, Armstrong DL and Fitzhardinge PM (1976) Central nervous system pathology associated with mask ventilation in the very low birthweight infant: a new etiology for intracerebellar hemorrhages. *Pediatrics* **58**, 473–483.
16. Perrin RG, Rutka JT, Drake JM *et al.* (1997) Management and outcomes of posterior fossa subdural hematomas in neonates. *Neurosurgery* **40**, 1190–1199.
17. Pohl M, Zimmerhackl LB, Heinen F *et al.* (1998) Bilateral renal vein thrombosis and venous sinus thrombosis in a neonate with factor V mutation (FV Leiden). *J Pediatr* **132**, 159–161.

18. Rutty GN, Smith CM and Malia RG (1999) Late-form hemorrhagic disease of the newborn: a fatal case report with illustration of investigations that may assist in avoiding the mistaken diagnosis of child abuse. *J Forensic Med Pathol* **20**, 48–51.

19. Sherer DM, Anyaegbunam A and Onyeije C (1998) Antepartum fetal intracranial hemorrhage, predisposing factors and prenatal sonography: a review. *Am J Perinatol* **15**, 431–441.

20. Thorp JA, Poskin MF, McKenzie DR *et al.* (1997) Perinatal factors predicting severe intracranial hemorrhage. *Am J Perinatol* **14**, 631–636.

21. Williamson WD, Percy AK, Fishman MA *et al.* (1985) Cerebellar hemorrhage in the term neonate: developmental and neurologic outcome. *Pediatr Neurol* **1**, 356–360.

22. Zuerrer M, Martin E and Boltshauser E (1991) MR imaging of intracranial hemorrhage in neonates and infants at 2.35 Tesla. *Neuroradiology* **33**, 223–229.

Neonatal brain infection

Susan Blaser, Venita Jay, Laurence E Becker and E Lee Ford-Jones

10

Contents

Introduction

Neonatal CNS infections, whether acquired *in utero* (congenital), intrapartum or postnatally remain an important cause of acute and long-term neurological morbidity. Pathologic features and associated imaging patterns depend upon the stage of development of the CNS, the affinity of a specific infective agent for a specific CNS cell type, and the ability of the host to respond to that insult. With the discovery of cytokines and adhesion molecules, and the demonstration of lymphocyte recruitment across the blood–brain barrier (BBB), the CNS is now known to be able to mount and propagate an inflammatory response to infections. This immune response has been invoked in neonatal brain damage even when the maternal infection, which may have had its onset before pregnancy, does not directly involve the fetal brain. The effects of infection on the rapidly developing brain, which continually evolves in its susceptibility to damage, in association with an evolving immune system lead to complex patterns of pathology and imaging features dissimilar to those seen in an older child ill with a similar infectious agent.

Certain factors aid in the diagnosis and differentiation of the congenital and neonatal infections. The etiologic agent may be known if the mother was exposed to an infectious agent or had a symptomatic infection. Conclusive diagnosis is dependent upon comprehensive clinical evaluation, ophthalmologic examination, microbiological testing of the infant and mother, and serial follow-up serology of the infant. Additionally, the actual clinical presentations of infection in the neonate are different for viruses, bacteria and parasites. Infants with bacterial infections are likely to present with sepsis, while those with cytomegalovirus (CMV) or toxoplasmosis infections may be clinically asymptomatic at birth despite their obvious intracranial involvement on imaging or ophthalmologic examination. Neonates with viral infections may present with active hepatitis, skin vesicles or petechiae.

The mechanism of infection and damage is also different amongst the infectious agents, leading to more specific imaging and pathologic appearances. Viruses, for example, tend to produce a selective necrosis of specific cell types, whereas bacteria and fungi are less selective. Also, different patterns of calcifications on CT or pathologic specimens are typical for the various STORCH (syphilis, toxoplasmosis, rubella, CMV, human immunodeficiency virus (HIV) and herpes simplex) infections, and the timing of insult during fetal life may lead to either teratogenic or encephaloclastic effects. Clinical and imaging differentiation amongst these disorders and amongst their respective infective agents is, therefore, frequently possible[3,8,20,21,73,83].

Imaging protocols

MRI should include conventional T1 and T2 weighted imaging in at least two planes in any infant with suspected infection. The sagittal plane is useful for detecting thrombosis in the sinuses. Axial images should always include full posterior fossa views to visualize the transverse sinuses. The use of contrast is mandatory for detecting early changes within the meninges or parenchyma and for establishing the full extent of any abnormalities. The role of diffusion weighted imaging in patients with infection is now being recognized. Time allowing, a fluid attenuated inversion recovery (FLAIR) sequence may give additional postcontrast information.

Neonatal CNS bacterial and fungal infections

Predisposing factors for bacterial infections in the newborn include maternal sepsis or chorioamnionitis, maternal cervical colonization of agents such as group B streptococcus, prolonged rupture of membranes prior to delivery, complications of labor and delivery, and deficiencies of cell-mediated or humoral immunity in the infant. Nosocomial and iatrogenic etiologies include exposure to reservoirs of pathogens within the neonatal intensive care unit, and invasive procedures such as endotracheal intubation, central vascular access, or CSF diversion. Group B streptococcus and *Escherichia coli* (*E. coli*) are the most common bacteria causing significant disease in the neonate. Infection from enteric organisms is more frequent during the first 2 weeks of life particularly with the use of intrapartum group B streptococcus prophylaxis, while those from streptococcus and staphylococcus species become more prevalent during the second 2 weeks of life. There is a particular propensity for *E. coli* to infect the neonate as the 19-S macroglobulin fraction which contains maternal antibodies to coliform bacteria does not cross the placenta, leading to a lack of passively acquired immunity to Gram-negative organisms. Other important agents in the neonatal period are *Listeria monocytogenes* and other members of the Enterobacteriaceae group, *Citrobacter* sp. and *Enterobacter* sp. *Staphylococcus aureus* and *Epidermidis* infections are particularly common in surgical neonates and those with indwelling shunts or central venous lines. By 2 months of age, with loss of passive immunity, there is a rise in CNS infections from *Hemophilus*, *Pneumococcus* and *Meningococcus*.

Hematogenous spread of bacteria from omphalitis, urinary tract infection or pneumonia leads to co-existence of peritonitis, arthritis, and in some cases, meningitis. Entry into the CNS requires the bacteria to cross an epithelial–mucosal barrier, such as upper respiratory tract, intestinal mucosa, or umbilical stump, to reach the blood stream. The actual site and mechanism of egress of bacteria from the blood stream into the CSF is not fully defined in every case.

Pathways include extension through structures without intact BBB such as the choroid plexus, factors released by the organism which allow intracellular transport and direct vessel wall invasion, and vascular compromise with direct invasion of adjacent necrotic brain tissue. Non-hematogenous pathways leading to CSF infection include direct extension, for example from an overlying scalp infection, or direct inoculation via ventricular shunt or puncture. Neonates with bacterial CNS infections frequently present with apnea, lethargy and other signs of fulminant systemic illness or shock rather than signs of meningeal irritation (Fig. 10.2). Bulging fontanel and seizures are non-specific features seen in association with any cause of increased intracranial pressure in this age group, even when there is no intracranial involvement by the infecting agent. Premature infants, due to the deficiencies in neonatal host defense mechanisms and to higher permeability of leptomeninges, are even more susceptible than full-term neonates to bacterial infections, including meningitis. They also have a much higher mortality. Mortality rates for infants with group B streptococcus, for example, range from 70% for prematures weighing under 1 kg to 10% or less in infants weighing over 2.5 kg[4,40,48,57,70,85].

Complications of bacterial meningitis are extremely common in infants under 6 months of age. Follow-up imaging is therefore suggested in neonates to exclude the presence of complications requiring surgical intervention or change in therapy. These complications include cerebritis, infarction (Fig. 10.1), brain abscess, subdural effusion or empyema, sinus thrombosis, ventriculitis and hydrocephalus. In uncom-

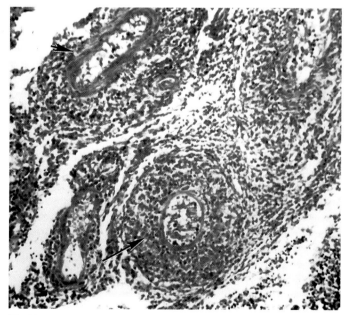

Fig. 10.1 Tubercular infection with vasculitis. Several vessels are shown in this field with transmural inflammatory infiltrate (*arrow*). Arteritis (*arrowhead*) is a common complication in tubercular meningitis. Vasculitis of arteries and veins may lead to thrombosis and hemorrhagic infarction. (H&E stain, low power view.)

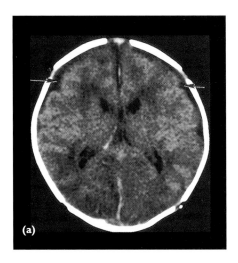
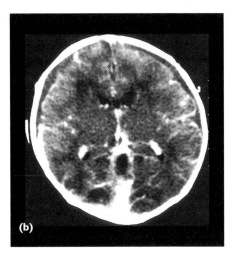

plicated bacterial meningitis, organisms and purulent enhancing inflammatory cell exudate fill the sulci over the hemispheres and extend along the perivascular spaces. Engorgement of surface vessels occurs and leaky blood–meningeal barrier from perivascular inflammation leads to meningeal and cisternal enhancement. The presence and extent of this enhancement is more consistently documented on MR than CT, but can be demonstrated on both imaging modalities (Figs 10.2 and 10.3). Initially, the exudate consists of granulocytes, later monocytes increase and there is progressive organization of the exudate with fibroblast proliferation. Subdural effusions, empyemas, leptomeningeal scarring and fibrosis, and arachnoiditis with loculated CSF further complicate neonatal meningitis,

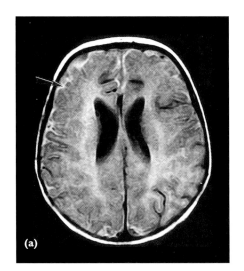
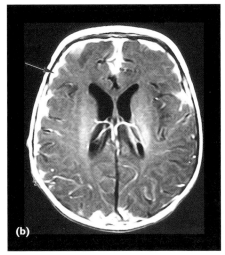
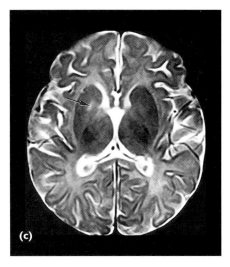

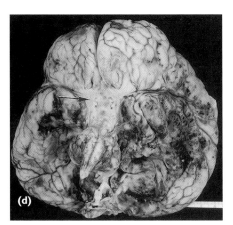

Fig. 10.3 *E. coli* meningitis with lenticulostriate infarction. FLAIR **(a)** axial image in a full-term neonate shows increased signal filling the sulci (*arrow*). This inflammatory exudate enhances (*arrow*) on T1W (500/20) axial image following administration of gadolinium-DTPA **(b)**. Focal increased signal of infarction (*arrow*) is present in the right basal ganglia on T2W (3000/120) image **(c)**. Thick basal purulent exudate (*arrow*) obscuring vessels is seen on autopsy specimen **(d)** in another infant who died from *E. coli* meningitis.

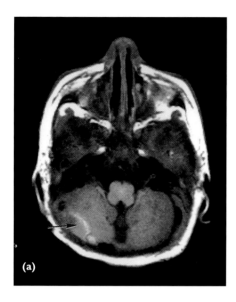 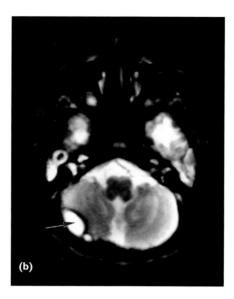

Fig. 10.4 *E. Coli* empyema T1 (600/14) **(a)** and T2 weighted (3000/120) **(b)** axial images in a 3-week-old with complex congenital heart disease and *E. coli* meningitis demonstrate a focal epidural collection effacing the right cerebellar hemisphere (*arrow*). Note the subtle low signal on T2W image of the surrounding brain tissue, likely due to local vascular congestion. This collection was unsuspected before imaging and was surgically proven to be an empyema.

although these collections have been reported to be less common in neonates than in infants older than 2 months of age. Sterile subdural effusions are present in up to half of children presenting with meningitis within the first year of life. A very small percentage of these, approximately 2%, will develop into empyemas. Subdural effusions and empyemas may require surgical sampling for differentiation, although useful imaging features suggesting empyema formation are enhancing rinds and signal intensity which fails to match CSF. Empyemas are more likely to contain proteinaceous fluid, with signal intensity on T2W images greater than CSF. Subjacent brain signal is also more likely to be abnormal in the presence of empyemas than in the presence of an effusion. Brain signal subjacent to empyema or infected collections is variable, with increased signal on T2W imaging reflecting edema or ischemia[25,34,82,85]. Decreased signal intensity on T2W imaging of the adjacent cortex and subcortical white matter likely reflects the increased vascular perfusion and loss of vessel autoregulation in the underlying brain (Fig. 10.4).

Ventricular enlargement may result from occlusion of the foramina of Monro, the aqueduct of Sylvius, and the 4th ventricular outlets by fibrinous inflammatory exudate which occurs even in the absence of ventriculitis. Ventriculitis, however, is a common and early component of neonatal meningitis, as the choroid plexus is a common site of bacterial entry into the CNS. Intraventricular exudate covers the choroid plexus, disrupts the ependymal lining and leads to subependymal venous thrombosis and eventual subependymal necrosis. Imaging features of ventriculitis should be sought in all patients with meningitis, but may be subtle in early cases. Pus-fluid levels and ependymal thickening may be seen on all imaging modalities, including sonography. A periventricular band of increased echogenicity has been reported to be a suggestive feature on brain sonography.

This band may also be seen with chemical ventriculitis following intraventricular hemorrhage, in association with interstitial edema related to obstructive hydrocephalus, or with periventricular calcifications in STORCH infections. Ependymal enhancement and thickening on MR and CT may also be seen following intraventricular hemorrhage. Intraventricular cyst formation and bridging ependymal strands lead to ventricular isolation and difficult to treat loculations in survivors in the convalescent and chronic stages[8,22,34,63,84] (Fig. 10.5).

Brain tissue involvement, or cerebritis, follows extension of exudate along the perivascular spaces. Cerebritis is commonly present at autopsy in cases of meningitis; however, the features of gyriform signal change and enhancement are not always present during the early stages of brain involvement. These foci of signal change and enhancement may resolve with therapy, or progress. As the infection progresses, exudate covering the surface veins leads to thrombophlebitis and cortical venous occlusion in adults. Venous occlusions in neonatal meningitis are usually secondary to fibrinous thrombi within the congested veins, rather than extension from the major venous sinuses and occur earlier in the course of disease in infants than they do in adults (Fig. 10.6). Meningitis-related infarctions are usually venous, although occasionally there is arterial infarction from basal leptomeningeal arterial involvement (Figs 10.1 and 10.3). Infarcts from either route occur in approximately 30% of neonates with meningitis and are frequently large and hemorrhagic. Cortical and white matter infarctions occur, and white matter involvement is significantly more common in the neonate than in the adult. Subependymal and periventricular venous occlusion and infarction contribute to the damage. Residual gliosis, encephalomalacia and porencephaly are present on follow-up imaging[15,25,34].

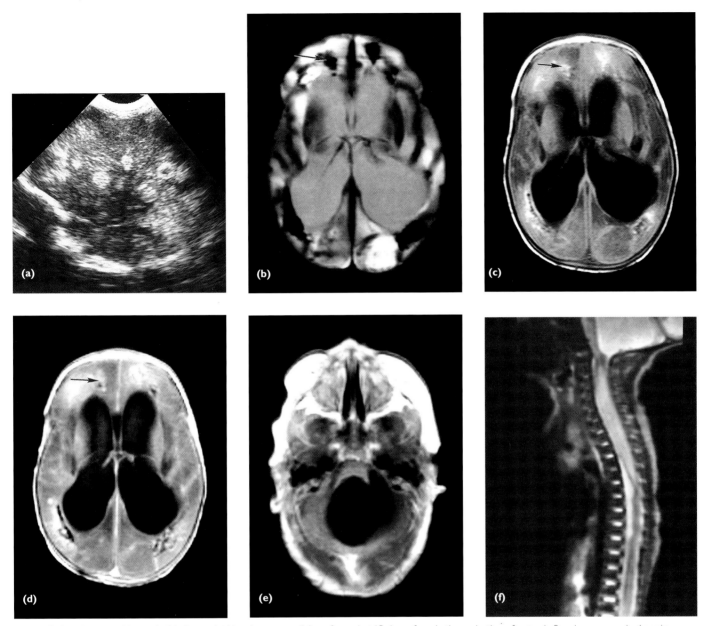

Fig. 10.5 *Pseudomonas* with ventriculitis. Parasagittal head sonogram **(a)** performed at 15 days of age in the evaluation of systemic *Pseudomonas* sepsis, dropping hemoglobin, and low platelet count in a 31 week gestational age twin demonstrates multiple echogenic foci within brain substance. T2 (3000/120) **(b)**, and unenhanced and enhanced T1W (600/22) axial images **(c,d,e)** from an MR performed at 30 days of life show loculated, isolated ventricles, multifocal brain hemorrhage (*arrow*), and adherent choroid plexus glomus. Spinal empyemas were also identified **(f)**. Subsequent MR at 2 years of age (not shown) confirmed extensive periventricular brain substance destruction and calcification in a shunted and severely developmentally delayed child.

Brain abscesses may result from a hematogenous source, from direct inoculation, or by local spread particularly into infarcted brain. Unlike the adult, most brain abscesses in the newborn result as a complication of bacterial meningitis. Five to 10% of neonates with meningitis will go on to develop abscesses, with the exception of those infected with *Citrobacter* sp. in whom 75% will develop abscesses. When the organisms are of low virulence, early and late stages of cerebritis may be seen, with minimal BBB disruption and contrast enhancement. In the older infant, rapid develop-

ment of enhancement occurs, related to the acute inflammatory reaction. Enhancement may be diffuse prior to the development of a collagen capsule and a necrotic center. Imaging features of well-developed abscesses in the older infant include peripheral edema and central necrosis with abscess fluid hyperintense to CSF on short TR (repetition time) scans and hyperintense to gray matter on long TR scans. Concentric zones of varying intensity are common, as are abscess capsules with signal hyperintense relative to brain on short TR and hypointense relative to white matter on

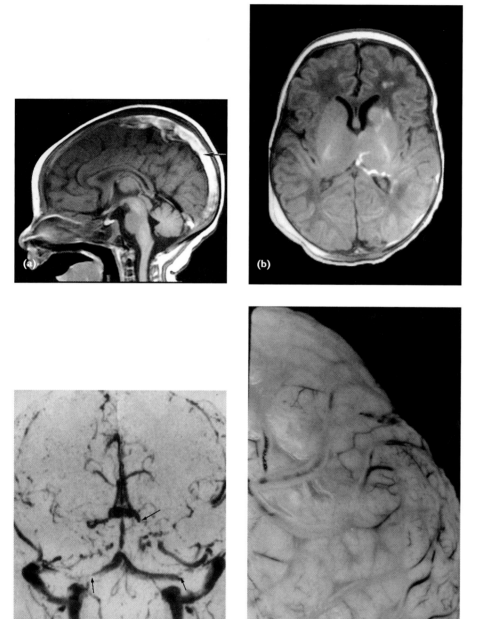

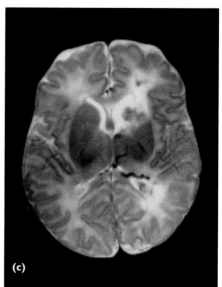

Fig. 10.6 Sinovenous thrombosis in a neonate presenting with sepsis. Unenhanced sagittal **(a)** and axial **(b)** T1W and T2W **(c)** and 2D TOF MR venography **(d)** views demonstrate superior sagittal sinus **(a)** (*arrow*), left internal cerebral and medial atrial venous thrombosis and associated hemorrhagic frontal white matter and basal ganglia infarction. The venogram **(d)** shows no filling of the left internal cerebral vein (*top arrow*) and poor filling of the tranverse sinuses (*bottom arrows*). Close up of meningeal surface in a case of acute bacterial meningitis. Note purulent exudate filling the sulci and covering the superficial veins in another patient, some of which appear to be thrombosed **(e).**

long TR scans. The capsular signal intensity is likely due to the presence of free radicals from macrophages. Immunocompromised patients and neonates, whose immune system is immature, often fail to mount a significant inflammatory response and subsequently have misleading or poorly developed imaging findings. Neonatal abscesses are often large and lack well-defined capsular formation. Mortality is significantly higher in the youngest infants[29,45,85] (Figs 10.7 and 10.8) although focal frontal cerebral abscesses may be clinically silent in the preterm infant and the long-term outcome surprisingly good (Fig. 10.8).

SPECIFIC ORGANISMS

Group B streptococcus (GBS)

GBS is a partially preventable, but unfortunately common etiologic agent of neonatal meningitis. Systemic group B streptococcal infections occur in up to 10% of neonates in whom there is maternal colonization of the cervix, leading to a rate of 1–5 per 1000 live births. Meningitis co-exists in approximately 5–10% of those. Myelitis has been reported. Prematurity, prolonged rupture of membranes, and maternal chorioamnionitis are known to increase the risk of neonatal

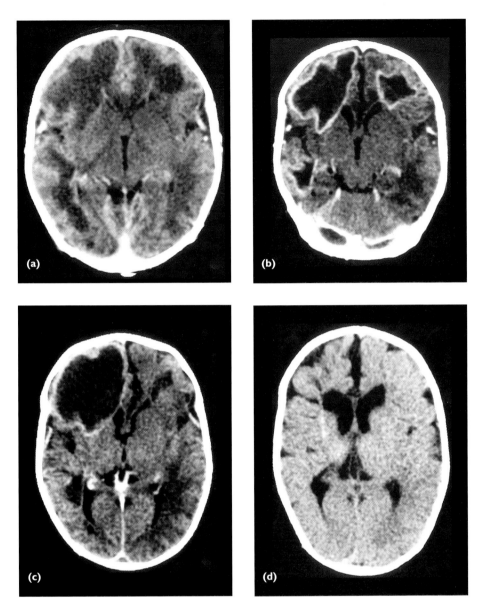

Fig. 10.7 *Citrobacter* – serial CT imaging in a full-term infant developing sepsis at day 8 *Citrobacter* meningitis with sterile 'abscess', due to brain infarction. Initially cerebritis with frontal lobar swelling is seen at 11 days **(a)**. Large areas of white matter necrosis with rim enhancement **(b)** are subsequently seen at 19 days. Proven abscess **(c)** eventually shows mass effect and 'rounding' is shown at 28 days. Follow-up CT **(d)** at 4 months of age at presentation in status epilepticus demonstrates atrophy, focal scarring, and faint calcification.

infection. Infections may appear within the first 24 h, or up to 3 months of age. Neonates are more likely than the older infants to have a shock-like presentation and fulminant course, and very low birth weight infants have a mortality approximating 70%. Those with later-onset disease have a more insidious presentation with meningitis and osteomyelitis. Necrologic sequelae in survivors of GBS meningitis include hydrocephalus, developmental delay and seizures (Fig. 10.2)[4,32,69].

Listeria monocytogenes

Listeria monocytogenes, a Gram-positive bacteria, has a tendency to infect the very young and the very old. Food contamination, particularly from unpasteurized cheese, is responsible for many adult cases. *Listeria* causes purulent leptomeningitis with one important differentiating factor from the other causes of neonatal meningitis: the fetus and the placenta may become infected, with the result being spontaneous abortion or preterm labor. Chronic involvement of the female genital tract leads to habitual abortion. A typical clinical picture in early-onset neonatal *Listeria* infections includes a maternal flu-like illness, preterm labor with intact membranes, meconium staining, perinatal asphyxia, neonatal respiratory distress, a maculopapulovesicular skin eruption, a monocytic predominance in the endotracheal aspirate, meningitis and intraventricular hemorrhage. CNS involvement is more common in infants with a late onset of infection. Involvement of the meninges and brain consists of miliary granulomas and micro-abscesses. The predilection

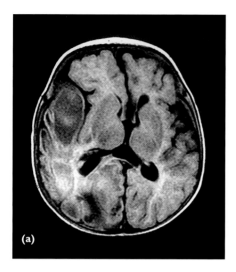

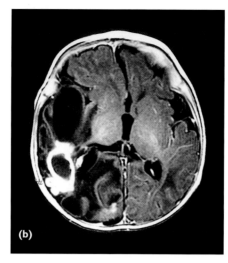

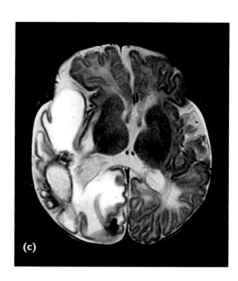

Fig. 10.8 *Citrobacter diversus* – MR in a 5-week-old infant. FLAIR **(a)**, enhanced T1W **(b)**, and T2W (3000/120) **(c)** axial MR images in a 5-week-old neonatal intensive care unit 'graduate' demonstrates multiple necrotic and infected cavities with rim enhancement, daughter cysts, and fluid with varying signal intensity in keeping with blood and pus. Pathologic specimen **(d)** in another patient with *Citrobacter* demonstrates large white matter abscess.

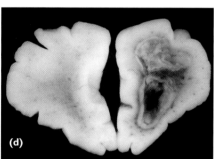

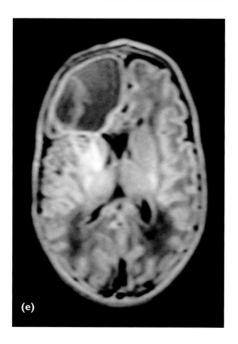

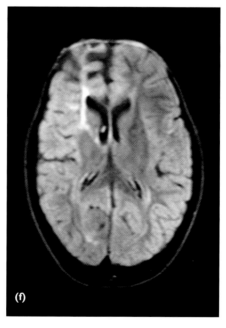

Fig. 10.8 *Enterobacter sakazakki.* T1 (860/20) weighted sequence in a 34-week premature infant aged 4 days **(e)**, and 6 years **(f)**. The large frontal abscess was clinically silent. At 6 years there is atrophy and gliosis of the right frontal lobe. Development is normal although he suffers from focal convulsions of recent onset. (With permission Dr Mary Rutherford.)

for purulent meningoencephalitis or involvement of the pons and medulla oblongata in adult *Listeria* infection is not seen in the fetus and neonate. Hydrocephalus, cystic encephalomalacia, and periventricular cavitation and calcification may be present in survivors[2,4,34] (Fig. 10.8).

Citrobacter diversus

Citrobacter diversus is a Gram-negative enteric bacterium, also with a predilection for the old and the very young. In the debilitated elderly patient, it infects the urinary tract and respiratory system. In the infant, it causes neonatal sepsis and

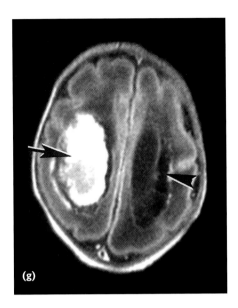
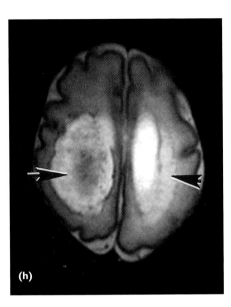

Fig. 10.8 *Listeria monocytogenes.* T1 (860/20) **(g)** and T2W fast spin echo (3000/208) **(h)** axial images in a 3-week-old infant born prematurely at 32 weeks following a symptomatic *Listeria monocytogenes* infection in the mother. There is a large intraventricular hemorrhage with adjacent infarction on the right (*arrow*). There are extensive periventricular cystic lesions on the left (*arrowhead*). (With permission Dr Mary Rutherford.)

meningitis. *Citrobacter* sp. rarely infect the infant older than 8 weeks of age, while the premature infant is particularly prone to infection. Poor intracellular survival in the host with an intact, mature immune system is felt to be responsible for the low virulence associated with *C. diversus* beyond the neonatal period. Acquired vertically or in nursery outbreaks, it is more important as a pathogen for its severity of sequelae than its actual prevalence. *Citrobacter* accounts for less than 5% of cases of meningitis in the neonate, but leads to brain abscesses in 75% or more of infants with meningitis. Neurological sequelae are present in the majority of the survivors of *Citrobacter* meningitis. Relapse and recurrent ventriculitis with prolonged persistence in the CNS has been described. Spinal cord abscesses have also been reported. Imaging features are characteristic with multiple, large, ring-enhancing lesions of white matter necrosis, cavitated infarcts and abscess formation. Pathologic features consist of meningeal vascular congestion, ventriculitis with focal ependymal disruption, periventricular and wide-spread white matter necrosis[27,38,81,85] (Figs 10.7 and 10.8).

Fungal meningitis

Fungal meningitis may be acquired *intra utero* from an ascending chorionic infection, during birth from an infected maternal genital tract, or postnatally. *Candida*, a saprophyte of healthy persons, is the most frequent of these fungal agents. Debilitation, immunocompromised state, in-dwelling central lines and antibiotic therapy predispose to candidiasis. Premature infants are particularly susceptible. Systemic candidiasis is reported to occur in 3–5% of very low-birth-weight neonates, with CNS involvement in up to 64% of these. CNS involvement is often difficult to prove

antemortem, as concentration within the CSF may be low and the growth rate in culture medium slow. The hallmark of the pathological changes are micro-abscesses. Micro-abscesses may be demonstrated at postmortem in infants with apparently normal MRI. Small macro-abscesses are the most common imaging finding in the very low-birth-weight neonate, with small echogenic rim-like micro-abscesses symmetrically scattered in the subcortical, periventricular and basal ganglia regions. Discrete punctate or rim-enhancing disseminated small macro-abscesses are very well shown on enhanced T1W images. Confluence of macro-abscesses, ventricular dilatation and ventriculitis may also be demonstrated. Differentiation from the lesions of periventricular leukomalacia is based on the pattern and timing of involvement, with the lesions of candidiasis occurring later, and more frequently involving the deep gray structures. Parenchymal involvement is more typical, but ventricular involvement also occurs. Intraventricular strands and debris, thickened irregular choroid plexus, and thickened, irregular ventricular walls are seen. Follow-up imaging demonstrates regression of lesions, although calcified granulomas occur. Invasion of the brain and spinal cord leads to necrotizing encephalitis and encephalomyelitis. Pathologic specimens demonstrate widespread necrotizing encephalitis, granulocytic infiltrates, reactive glial proliferation and large abscesses or military micro-abscesses. Acute *Candida* foci, with infiltrating neutrophils, yeasts and pseudohyphae, may be widespread, involving deep white and gray matter and the subependymal germinal layer. Particular involvement is present in the watershed zones. The smaller chronic foci tend to localize within the cortex, basal ganglia, brain stem nuclei and leptomeninges. In the older infant, *Candida* tends to cause a purulent leptomeningitis and ventriculitis similar to bacterial agents. Hydrocephalus and CSF loculation are common complications (Fig. 10.9). *Aspergillus*, extremely rare in the young infant, will cause similar pathological, and therefore imaging, features. *Mucormycosis*, also extremely rare, leads to infarction due to direct vascular invasion and thrombosis, in addition to the necrosis from parenchymal invasion seen with other fungal infections[8,30,34,51,54,86].

Infant botulism

Infant botulism is a disease of the slightly older infant, although neonatal cases have been described. Infants under 1 year of age are at risk due to the composition of the intesti-

nal flora. *Clostridium botulinum* spores ingested with contaminated honey colonize the intestinal tract, bind to intestinal epithelium, germinate, and produce a neurotoxin which is subsequently absorbed. Skeletal muscle is paralyzed from presynaptic blockade of acetylcholine release. Infants present with difficulties eating, intestinal and gastric dilatation, ocular and bulbar paralysis, descending muscle paralysis and apnea. Intracranial manifestations are felt to relate to associated hypoxia. MR features have not been described, although we have seen demyelination of the corpus callosum and enhancing cauda equina nerve roots in a 6-month-old infant who presented with feeding difficulties, ptosis and a history of honey ingestion[78].

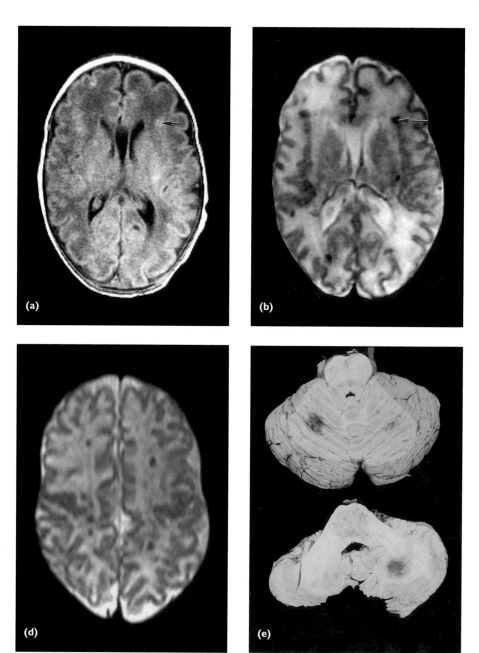

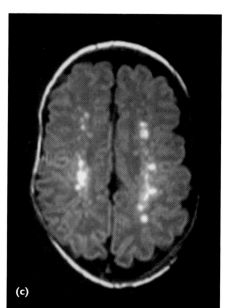

Fig. 10.9 *Candida* abscesses in a 15-day-old premature infant. T1 (500/20) **(a)** and T2W (3000/120) **(b)** axial images in a premature infant with systemic candidiasis demonstrate multiple foci of small macro-abscesses (*arrow*). T1 (860/20) **(c)** and T2 (2700/120) **(d)** weighted images in a second preterm infant born at 26 weeks and imaged at 41 weeks, 12 weeks after an episode of candidal septicemia. There are multiple lesions within the white matter consistent with calcification of *Candida* macro-abscesses. Coronal pathologic sections of the cerebellum and brain stem **(e)** in another patient demonstrate multiple foci of cerebritis.

Tuberculosis

Tuberculosis may occur in the very young infant, but is extremely rare in the neonate. Connatal tuberculosis has been described in the case of active maternal tuberculosis, although it was more common in the pre-antituberculous chemotherapeutic era. Infection occurs via the placenta, aspiration of amniotic fluid during delivery, or following postnatal respiratory exposure. Miliary dissemination is seen, although basal leptomeningitis with brain infarction due to occlusion of the basal perforators is more common (Fig. 10.1). Hydrocephalus, tubercules demonstrating massive caseation and poor peripheral lymphohistiocytic reaction, and late leptomeningeal calcification are complications[34,56].

CONGENITAL INFECTIONS (STORCH)

Considerable progress has been made in preventing or treating congenital infection with immunizations and intrauterine diagnosis and therapy. However, these infections, usually including syphilis, toxoplasmosis, rubella, CMV, HIV and herpes simplex virus (HSV) have not been eliminated. CMV remains the most common, affecting 1 in 100 live births in the US. HIV, *Treponema pallidum* and *Toxoplasma gondii* follow with a rising incidence of vertically transmitted HIV. Herpes simplex virus and varicella zoster affect 1 in 5000, and 1 in 10 000 respectively, while the incidence of rubella has decreased to 1 in 100 000. Routes of transmission vary somewhat, with HIV and rubella most commonly transmitted *in utero*, HSV transmitted during birth, and CMV transmitted *in utero*, intrapartum and postpartum. Additional congenital infections include chicken pox, hepatitis, enterovirus, parvovirus, lymphocytic choriomeningitis virus, Q fever, malaria and tuberculosis[31,43].

Diagnosis of congenital infections, whether they reach the fetus via a hematogenous transplacental route or by ascent through the birth canal, remains challenging. The requisite maternal infections are usually asymptomatic and some infants may be clinically normal at birth, only clinically manifesting occult ocular, audiologic and CNS complications later on. Intrauterine growth retardation, hydrocephalus or microcephaly, echogenic bowel, pseudomeconium ileus, hepatic or brain calcifications, hydrops fetalis, ascites, and pleural or pericardial effusions should suggest intrauterine infection. Specific testing is required. Polymerase chain reaction (PCR) testing on amniotic fluid, for example, is available in suspected cases of *Toxoplasmosis gondii* infections. Neonatal features may suggest the presence of a congenital infection, although many are not specific. Systemic involvement includes intrauterine growth retardation in rubella, toxoplasmosis and CMV. Hepatosplenomegaly is reported in CMV, rubella, toxoplas-mosis, HSV, syphilis, enterovirus and parvovirus B19. Likewise, progressive hearing loss occurs in rubella, CMV, toxoplasmosis and syphilis. Anemia can occur with many of the congenital infections, although it is a particular feature of parvovirus B19 due to the propensity of the virus for the fetal red cell. Other clinical features may be more specific, for example congenital heart disease in rubella, and limb paralysis and cicatrices in varicella. Cutaneous lesions are also useful markers. Petechiae, purpura, jaundice and dermal erythropoieses are seen in toxoplasmosis, rubella and CMV, while symptomatic infants with herpes simplex virus infections may show single or grouped cutaneous vesicles, conjunctivitis and oral ulcers[28,31].

Pathologic and radiologic features differ somewhat amongst the congenital infections, although calcifications and necrosis are hallmarks. Plain films features, such as 'celery-stalking' of long bones may occur in syphilis and rubella, while patterns of CNS calcification may also give useful clues. Infants with CMV, for example, frequently have periventricular injury with subsequent necrosis and calcifications. Toxoplasmosis leads to more diffuse calcifications, although basal ganglia and periventricular calcifications are common. Calcifications are also seen in parvovirus and in lymphocytic choriomeningitis virus infections. Branching echogenic foci on brain sonography occurs in the congenital infections, particularly CMV, rubella and HIV but may be seen in a myriad of other disorders such as asphyxia, chromosomal anomalies, fetal alcohol syndrome, and non-immune hydrops. Rubella is associated with vascular lesions and chronic meningoencephalitis, and HSV with necrotic foci and hemorrhage. Rubella and herpes are the infections most likely to have extensive cerebral cortical calcifications, while rubella and CMV lead to micrencephaly. Subependymal cysts occur in CMV and rubella, but also in Zellweger syndrome, following germinal matrix hemorrhage, and D-2-hydroxyglutaric aciduria. Hydrocephalus is common in toxoplasmosis, syphilis and enterovirus. Congenital myxoviruses, including mumps and parainfluenza, also have a predilection for ependymal cells, leading to congenital hydrocephalus[14,31,52,75,79].

Neuroimaging features of selected congenital infections (STORCH)

SYPHILIS

Syphilis infections follow transplacental transmission of treponema usually during or after the 4th month of pregnancy, although infection may be transmitted at any time during pregnancy. Infection of the placenta may lead to stillbirth and premature abortion. The most severely infected fetal survivors are infected relatively late, after week 24 of pregnancy, and there is a high perinatal mortality. The overwhelming majority of infected infants are clinically asymptomatic at birth necessitating careful review of maternal serology and follow-up to avoid long-term CNS complications. Fetal hydrops and hepatomegaly are common. Neonates may demonstrate exanthema, rhinitis and hepatosplenomegaly. 'Pseudoparalysis' of the limbs as a result of osteochondritis is a well-known clinical feature in the neonate. Additionally, necrotizing enterocolitis as a result of aortic vascular disease has been reported. There are both meningovascular and parenchymatous forms of neonatal neurosyphilis. Parenchymal disease leads to diffuse cerebral and cerebellar degeneration with microglial proliferation and inflammatory infiltrates. The meningovascular form is associated with perivascular inflammatory exudates, intimal proliferation and leptomeningeal spirochete masses, although parenchymal damage is usually slight. Hydrocephalus may result from syphilitic meningitis. There are occasional superficial cortical infiltrates and necrosis. Latent connatal syphilis (lues tarda) is associated with hearing loss, deformed incisors, saddle nose and tibial deformities. Tabes dorsalis is rare[1,34,64] (Fig. 10.10).

TOXOPLASMA

Toxoplasma is a protozoan parasite causing transplacental infection (toxoplasmosis) of the human fetus during or after the 3rd fetal month, and is the third most common fetal brain infection after CMV and HIV. Cats are the terminal host with oocysts excreted in feline feces. Maternal risk factors include exposure to cat excreta during pregnancy, or eating raw, pre-

viously unfrozen meat. Contaminated water supply has been linked to one outbreak. The maternal infection is usually asymptomatic, although involvement of the CNS occurs in approximately half of infected fetuses. The rate of infection increases with each trimester, while the actual severity of the infection decreases. Hydrops fetalis, ascites, pleural and pericardial effusions and hydrocephalus may be seen on fetal sonography. While neonates may be symptomatic at birth with clinical features similar to congenital CMV, they are usually asymptomatic. An important differentiating feature would be the head size, as neonates with congenital CMV are commonly microcephalic, while those with congenital toxoplasmosis are more likely to have hydrocephalus. Release of *Toxoplasma* from cysts leads to an intense inflammatory reaction and granulomatous necrosis. Progressive hydrocephalus occurs in association with turbid, proteinaceous CSF, ependymitis and subsequent aqueductal obstruction. Marked expansion of the atria of the lateral ventricles is common in patients with *Toxoplasma*-related hydrocephalus. Neuronal migration anomalies are not commonly seen, although delayed myelin maturation is seen on imaging. Basal ganglia and periventricular calcifications are common, may be seen even in asymptomatic children, and may even disappear over time without treatment. Chorioretinitis is extremely common, and may lead to progressive visual loss in otherwise asymptomatic children. Treatment *in utero* is available and improves outcome; treatment during the first year of life also improves neurological outcome[8,13,33,34,36,67] (Fig. 10.11).

RUBELLA

Rubella, a single-stranded RNA Togaviridae family virus, causes German measles, a usually self-limited and benign disease in children. Sequelae of congenital rubella, however, particularly acquired during the early part of the first trimester, are severe. The actual incidence of congenital rubella following maternal infection is reported to be low, although during the critical first 12 weeks of pregnancy the fetal infection rate can be as high as 80%. Congenital heart disease is reported in more than half, deafness due to damage to the organ of Corti in approximately half, and visual changes such as cataracts in approximately 40%. Additionally, 40% of survivors have developmental delay. Neurological symptoms are related to viral invasion and replication in brain tissue. Rubella appears to have an antimitotic effect on brain cell multiplication with micrencephaly a common outcome of fetal infection. The main brain tissue cell types infected with *in utero* rubella virus are the astrocyte and occasionally the neuron. The oligodendrocyte is relatively resistant, leading to a lack of significant demyelination, although delayed myelin maturation occurs.

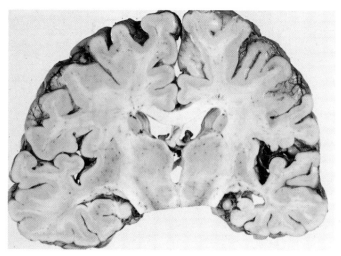

Fig. 10.10 Congenital syphilis. Coronal view of the brain in an adult survivor of congenital syphilis shows focal left cerebral atrophy with deepening of the sulci, superimposed on diffuse brain substance volume loss.

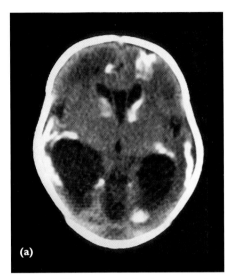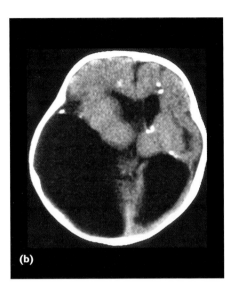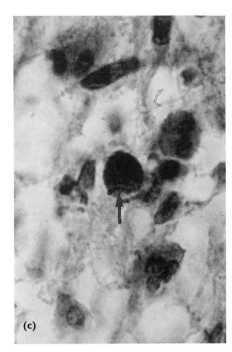

Fig. 10.11 Disappearing calcification in congenital toxoplasmosis. Unenhanced axial images of the brain in a 12-month-old infant shows ventricular enlargement **(a)**. CT at 4 years of age show that brain calcification is lessening over time **(b)**. HE stain, high-power view **(c)** shows a *Toxoplasma* cyst (*arrow*), characteristic of established infection surrounded by inflammatory cells. Cysts may be found around the periphery of necrotic lesions and may survive for years. (CTs of this case are used with permission of Dr Kling Chong of Hospital for Sick Children at Great Ormond Street.)

Rubella virus has a particular tendency to involve placental and fetal vascular endothelia. Abnormalities of the cerebral vascular system are present on pathologic specimens in more than half of cases. Focal destruction of the vascular walls, with thickening and proliferation results in luminal narrowing. Mineralizing microangiopathy with arterial occlusion and stroke occur. Outcomes include hydranencephaly, micrencephaly, particular cerebellar atrophy, and calcified brain. 'Branched candlestick' appearance of the vessels is seen on brain sonography of neonates. End vessels within the deep white matter and basal ganglia are the most frequently affected in pathologic studies of infants who died of congenital rubella syndrome. This ischemic pattern of involvement is felt to be responsible for the MR changes seen in adult survivors. Psychiatric disturbance in adult survivors has been reported in up to 50% of survivors of symptomatic congenital rubella. Congenital rubella has also been implicated as a significant cause of autism. Linear hyperintense foci in the deep white matter of the frontal and parietal lobes are common, seen in over half of adult survivors with schizophrenia-like symptoms, and in children normal except for deafness. Pediatric survivors may also demonstrate delay in myelin maturation and subcortical and periventricular white matter lesions. In another study of adults with congenital rubella and schizophrenia-like symptoms, small intracranial brain volumes and ventricular enlargement with sparing of the sulci were present[4,8,16,34,35,37,46,53,60,61,74,79,80,87] (Fig. 10.12).

Progressive brain damage with leukoencephalopathy, gliosis and atrophy occurs in a subgroup of infants who develop postnatal progressive rubella panencephalitis. Onset of symptoms, dementia, ataxia and seizures, in this slow virus infection, is between the ages of 8 and 21 years in males with clinical signs of congenital rubella syndrome[59]. Placental vascular and CNS vascular features in congenital infections with Venezuelan equine encephalitis virus infection are similar to those seen in rubella. Massive cerebral necrosis has been described[39].

CYTOMEGALOVIRUS (CMV)

CMV will infect most of us during our lifetimes. CNS complications are uncommon in the otherwise healthy child and adult. CMV poses its greatest risks to the fetus, the premature infant and the immunocompromised infant. The usual route of fetal infection is transplacental occurring during a primary infection of the mother. Thirty to 40% of cases of maternal primary infection will lead to fetal infection. Gestational age at time of infection has little correlation with rate of transmission, or severity of disease expression. Maternal antibodies, which protect the fetus in rubella and toxoplasmosis, do not prevent fetal transmission of the CMV virus, but do lessen the severity of the disease in CMV. Approximately 1% of neonates are born infected with CMV, but the majority will have silent infections following recurrent rather than primary maternal

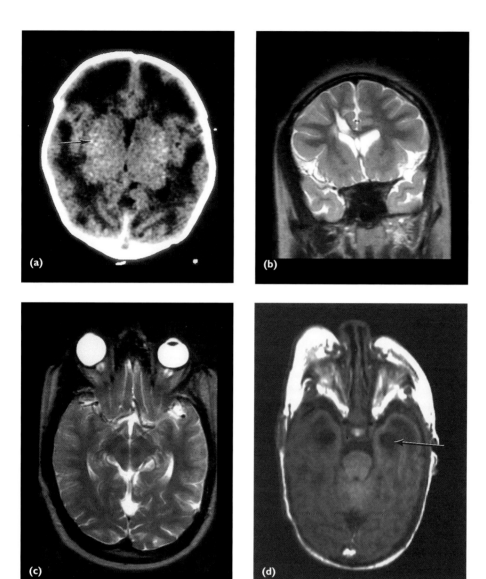

Fig. 10.12 Rubella. Unenhanced axial CT **(a)** in a 3-day-old with congenital rubella demonstrates punctate calcifications of the basal ganglia (*arrow*) and low attenuation of the white matter. Ultrasound (*not shown*) confirmed mineralizing vasculopathy. Axial and coronal MR **(b,c)** in a teenaged survivor of rubella who is deaf, blind and developmentally delayed demonstrates right frontal white matter and corpus callosum infarct and an abnormal right globe following cataract removal. T1W (860/20) axial image **(d)** in a term born infant imaged at 5 days. She presented with growth retardation, a petechial rash and thrombocytopenia. Congenital rubella infection was proven on serology. MR imaging showed widespread low SI within the WM and large focal cystic lesions in the temporal lobes (*arrow*). (With permission of Dr Mary Rutherford, Hammersmith Hospital.)

infection. CMV is thought to be the leading infectious cause of sensorineural hearing loss in the postrubella vaccination era, affecting approximately 10% of infected neonates. Mondini malformation with lack of interscalar septum, short and wide internal auditory canal and enlarged vestibular aqueduct are particularly common CT features of CMV survivors with hearing loss[7,35,50,77].

A small per cent of infants who have been infected *in utero* will be symptomatic with jaundice, hepatosplenomegaly, petechiae, microcephaly or chorioretinitis. Half to three-quarters of these infants will have abnormal neuroimaging. Prenatal documentation of atrophy, ventricular enlargement and prominent CSF spaces have been reported. Periventricular calcification and subependymal cysts have been documented on *in utero* and postnatal cranial imaging. 'Ring-like' areas of periventricular lucency have been shown

to precede the development of subependymal calcification and are felt to represent foci of subependymal degeneration and inflammation. Subsequent glial scarring and dystrophic calcification occurs. Increased echogenicity of the thalamo-striate arteries has been described on cranial sonography in the presence of congenital CMV, although this feature is not specific for CMV. The presence of an abnormal CT imaging during the neonatal period, with calcification the most common finding, has been shown to correlate well with an adverse neurodevelopmental outcome. Periventricular, and less frequently, basal ganglia, calcifications are reported on CT in 33–43%. This number is lower than that reported during the plain film era, likely due to the increasing identification of less severely affected patients. Periventricular foci of signal abnormality are common on MR, although it is difficult to differentiate calcification from punctate

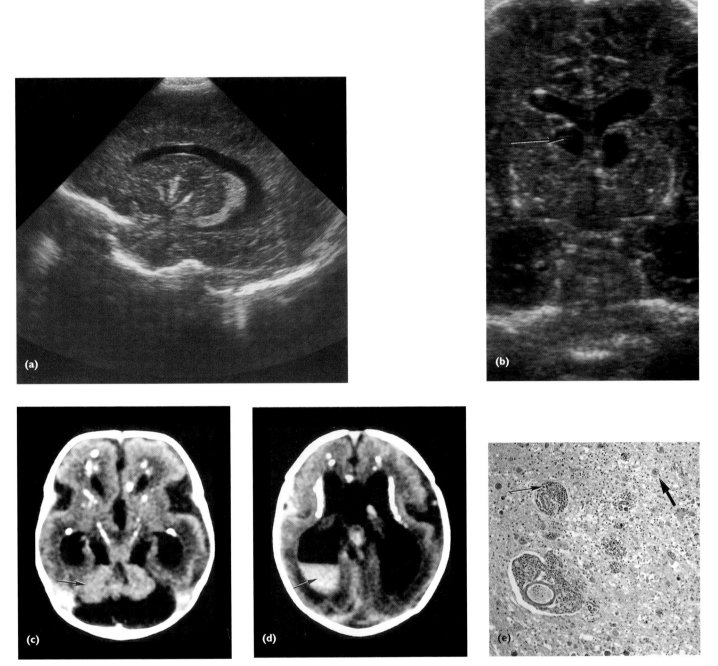

Fig. 10.13 Mineralizing microangiopathy and periventricular cysts in CMV. Sonography **(a)** in a neonate with documented CMV infection demonstrates the 'candelabra' configuration of mineralizing microangiopathy. Subependymal cysts (*arrow*) **(b)** are seen in a second neonate. Unenhanced CT **(c)** demonstrates typical calcifications as well as cerebellar hypoplasia (*arrow*), a common feature. Adjacent cut **(d)** from the same patient shows additional intraventricular hemorrhage (*arrow*). HE stain, low-power view **(e)** in pathologic specimen of CMV infection demonstrates intraparenchymal and perivascular (*thin arrow*) inflammatory infiltrates, as well as several cytomegalic cells (*thick arrow*) with intranuclear inclusions.

hemorrhage, as calcifications are less well appreciated on MR than on CT (Figs 10.13–10.15). Imaging features such as microcephaly and diffuse brain calcifications are shared with Aicardi–Gouthier syndrome, a familial disorder with CSF lymphocytosis[4,12,24,76,79].

Additionally, several different patterns of damage subsequent to congenital CMV infection have been described on MRI and reflect features well described on pathologic specimens. Lissencephaly with a thinned cerebral cortex, enlarged lateral ventricles, diminished white matter volume, delay in

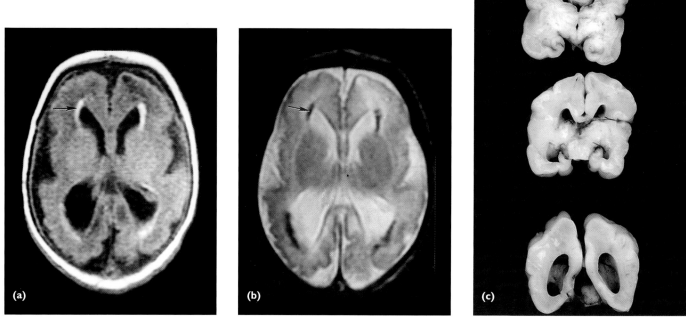

Fig. 10.14 Chronic CMV infection in term neonate. T1 (450/12) **(a)** and T2 (3000/80) **(b)** weighted images reveal arrested brain development with primitive Sylvian fissures and a smooth cortical surface in a full-term infant with microcephaly and documented congenital CMV infection. Note the periventricular calcifications (*arrows*). Coronal pathologic sections of brain **(c)** in another patient reveal periventricular and white matter calcifications (chalky white areas) in a case of congenital CMV infection and arrested brain development.

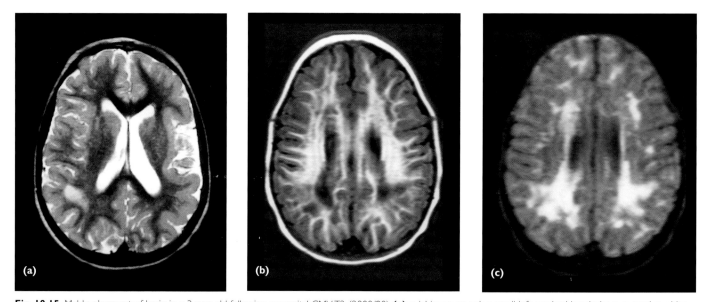

Fig. 10.15 Maldevelopment of brain in a 3-year-old following congenital CMV. T2 (2800/90) **(a)** axial image reveals a small left cerebral hemisphere, extensive white matter demyelination and destruction, and frontal lobes carpeted with polygyria in a 3-year-old with a known intrauterine infection occurring during the 8th fetal month. Abnormal white matter in CMV. T1 (860/20) **(b)** and T2 (2700/120) **(c)** weighted images in a 2-year-old infant with congenital CMV with maternal flu-like illness in the first trimester. There is widespread abnormal signal intensity within the white matter, this is most marked in the T2 weighted image. Her development at 7 years is within normal limits. (With permission of Dr Mary Rutherford, Hammersmith Hospital.)

myelination and small cerebellum support an insult to the germinal zone and therefore infection prior to 16–18 weeks of gestation. Localized dysplastic cortex (polymicrogyria) with thickened irregular cortices and diminished white matter is felt to indicate infection late in the migrational phase or in the organizational phase between 18 and 24 weeks. Focal polygyria in patients in this population is most commonly identified within the frontal lobes, and to a lesser degree within the temporal lobes. A normal gyral pattern with abnormal white matter signal supports infection in the third trimester, but it is not always possible to predict the pattern of brain abnormality from the reported timing of maternal infection[4,6,47] (Fig. 10.15).

CONGENITAL HIV

Congenital HIV is now the second most frequent viral infection of the newborn[43]. Usual transmission is *in utero*, although mother-to-child transmission may also occur post-partum via breast milk. Invasion of the CNS by HIV occurs at the time of the initial infection, prior to the period of symptomatic AIDS. Initially specific immune responses of neutralizing antibodies and cytotoxic T-lymphocytes inhibit viral replication. The virus, however, incites a subacute encephalitis with inflammatory T-cell reaction with perivascular mononuclear inflammatory cell infiltrates, leptomeningitis, and immune activation of brain tissue with increasing microglial cells and cytokine production. There is damage to the oligodendrocytes by cytokines and myelin pallor. Late neuronal loss occurs. Gliosis and brain atrophy are early features of adult infections, while impaired brain growth is characteristic of congenital infections. Multinucleated giant cell encephalitis and vacuolar myelopathy are less common in

pediatric AIDS than in adults, although corticospinal tract degeneration does occur[41,43].

Early clinical signs of HIV-related illness in the very young infant include failure to thrive, hepatosplenomegaly, pulmonary lymphoid hyperplasia, chronic diarrhea, thrush and recurrent bacterial infections. The most common sign of early HIV-related CNS encephalopathy is delay in acquisition of psychomotor milestones. Later on there may be loss of milestones, acquired microcephaly, and bilateral corticospinal tract involvement. Frequently, however, CNS symptomatology is minor in the first decade, with CNS disease ranging from 8% in asymptomatic children to 60% in children with advanced disease. CNS symptoms include a static–stable encephalopathy or a subacute, slowly progressive course. Progressive mineralizing vasculopathy of the basal ganglia, frequently present at birth, is the most common abnormal finding on neuropathology and imaging (Fig. 10.16). This calcification is shown on pathologic specimens to be in areas of intimal proliferation. Vascular striations are seen on brain sonography, and diffuse hazy increased density of the basal ganglia is often seen on CT. While cerebrovascular disease has been documented in one study to be present at autopsy in 24% of children with HIV, stroke occurs in 1–2%, less commonly in the older child than the infected adult and least commonly in the infant. Aneurysmal dilatation of the vessels of the circle of Willis occurs and has been reported as early as 6 months of age[11,71].

Routine MRI in congenital HIV is initially normal and despite the identification of HIV within fetal brain tissue as early as 15 weeks' gestation, there are no associated brain malformations. Delay in myelin maturation is common in the infected young infant. Atrophy, HIV white matter disease particularly involving the cortical white matter, and

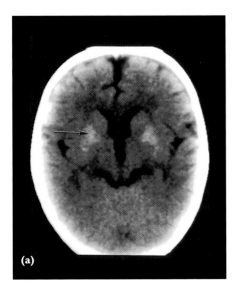

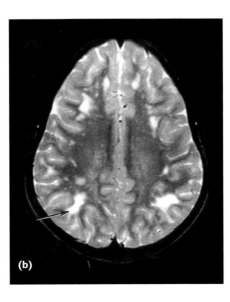

Fig. 10.16 Mineralizing microangiopathy and white matter lesions in congenital HIV. Axial CT **(a)** in a 2-month-old infant with known vertical transmission of HIV demonstrates hazy mineralizing microangiopathy of the basal ganglia and thalami (*arrow*). Axial T2W MR (2800/90) **(b)** in a 6-year-old child with vertically acquired HIV and failure to thrive shows focally abnormal signal within the subcortical white matter (*arrow*). This child subsequently succumbed to the sequelae of massive aneurysmal dilatation of the vessels of the circle of Willis.

progressive multifocal leukoencephalopathy (PML) are late findings in the child with vertically acquired disease, as is symptomatic brain involvement by opportunistic infections such as toxoplasmosis and CMV. MR spectroscopy may be useful even when the routine MRI is normal. Proton MR spectroscopy of the brain is abnormal in neonates exposed to HIV *in utero*, although this does not differentiate infected children from uninfected children. A non-specific amino acid peak in the 2.1–2.6 ppm area overlapping the N-acetyl-aspartic acid peak, high N-acetyl aspartate (NAA)-to-creatine and high choline-to-creatine ratios were felt to possibly result from the indirect effects of HIV, such as intrauterine growth retardation. Elevated choline is postulated to result from either myelin breakdown or from microglial and astrocytic hypertrophy. The decrease in the NAA-to-creatine ratio seen in older children and adults with symptomatic, progressive HIV encephalopathy was not seen in the HIV-exposed neonates. Loss of NAA in progressive HIV encephalopathy is likely secondary to loss of cortical neurons, as well as to loss of NAA within the axonal processes. Lactate has also been described, possible secondary to the glycolytic flux of the perivascular macrophages known to be present in symptomatic patients. The decreased NAA-to-creatine ratio and the lactate peak demonstrated in children with progressive HIV encephalopathy have been shown to improve following antiretroviral therapy[5,9,19,62,68].

HERPES SIMPLES VIRUS (HSV)

HSV, most commonly transmitted during birth, may cause significant damage to the developing brain whether acquired *in utero* or perinatally. HSV-2 infections account for 80–90%

of all neonatal and almost all of the congenital herpes virus cases. Endothelial cell infection with swelling and small vessel necrosis leads to early fetal brain destruction and fetal loss. Twenty per cent of infants with neonatal HSV present with isolated CNS involvement, typically during the second or third week of life. These infants may have non-specific clinical signs such as irritability, high-pitched cry, fever or poor feeding. Mortality is high if the CNS is involved in disseminated neonatal HSV. A smaller group, infected *in utero*, will present with microcephaly, cataracts and intrauterine growth retardation. Herpetic skin rashes are not universally seen and the maternal infection may be unsuspected, as primary infections, which are the highest risk to the fetus, are characteristically asymptomatic.

Brain involvement in neonatal encephalitis is diffuse, bilateral and typically does not spare the white matter. Predisposition for the temporal lobes does not occur. Sequential imaging typically demonstrates progressive brain edema with subsequent encephalomalacia and occasional cyst formation although unenhanced imaging early in the disease may be normal. Necrosis of brain substance may be severe and there is a predilection to involve the cerebellum, basal ganglia and brain stem. Increased cortical attenuation has been described in neonatal cases, possibly due to cortical vasodilatation rather than petechial hemorrhage or microcalcification. Hemorrhage or calcific densities are present in the thalamus, basal ganglia, peri-insular cortex, periventricular white matter and at the gray–white junction in infants. Progressive, diffuse brain calcification may rival only rubella in the degree of calcification. Mineralized depositions confined to the mitochondria have been reported in disintegrated cells which contain herpes simplex virions. Relapse or persistence of infection is

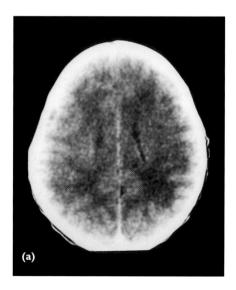
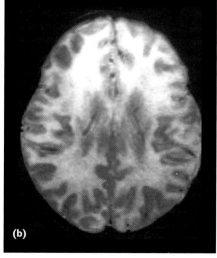
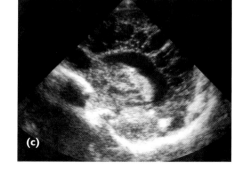

Fig. 10.17 *(Herpes simplex, see overleaf)*

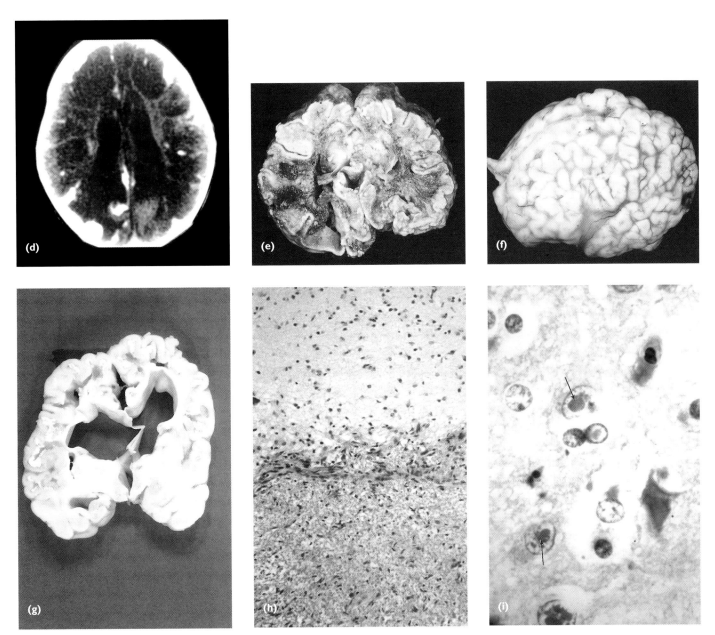

Fig. 10.17 Herpes simplex. Unenhanced axial CT in a 2-month-old infant **(a)** shows mild brain edema in a child presenting with fever, seizures and encephalopathy. T2W MR **(b)** shows more pronounced edema with high signal intensity most marked in the frontal white matter. Subacute sonogram demonstrates multifocal cystic lesions **(c)**, while follow-up unenhanced CT **(d)** shows severe multicystic encephalomalacia with extensive cortical calcifications. Extensive cerebral necrosis and encephalomalacia **(e)** is present in a case of HSV-2 encephalitis. Autopsy specimen in an infant with HSV-1 encephalitis **(f)**, shows evident cerebral atrophy with deep sulci, while the cut surface of the brain **(g)** demonstrates extensive calcification (chalky white material) and ventriculomegaly. H&E stain, medium-power view **(h)** demonstrates area of necrosis surrounded by reactive gliosis. H&E: high-power view **(i)** demonstrates intranuclear viral inclusions (*arrows*) in a different infant with HSV-1 encephalitis.

known despite appropriate antiviral therapy, particularly in association with frequent cutaneous relapses.

The pattern of destruction in infants, different from that in older children and adults, is likely due not only to the response of the developing brain to herpes encephalitis, but to the difference in acquisition of the infectious agent. HSV-1, typically, although not exclusively an infection of the older child and adult, usually enters the intracranial compartment via the olfactory nerve leading to specific involvement of the inferior and middle temporal gyri in older patients. Intrauterine acquired HSV-1 infection may also be associated with severe and progressive atrophy and calcification. Neuronal migration disorders have been reported in association with fetally acquired HSV-1[4,8,10,17,18,26,34,42,49,55,58,65,77] (Fig. 10.17).

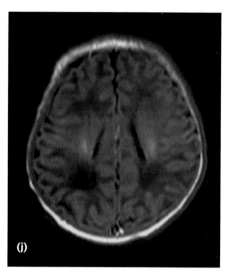
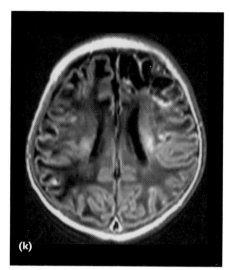
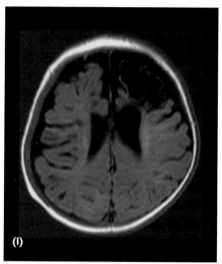

Fig. 10.17 Neonatal herpes simplex encephalitis. T1W MR (860/20) at 5 days **(j)**, 12 days **(k)** and 3 months **(l)** in an infant with seizures on day 3 of life. The initial images show minimal low signal intensity within the white matter normal in appearance but 1 week later there is extensive hemorrhagic infarction of WM and cortex **(k)** leading to atrophy **(l)**.

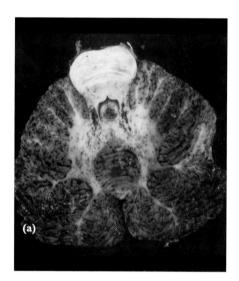
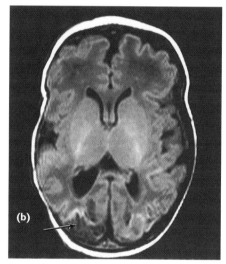

Fig. 10.18 Varicella. Fulminant varicella infection in an autopsy specimen of a 6-month-old infant with disseminated intravascular coagulation and extensive petechiae. **(a)** Term born infant with a maternal history of chickenpox at 15 weeks' gestation. He presented with scoliosis, cryptorchidism, micropthalmia and hypotonia. T1W (860/20) image at 8 days of age. **(b)** There is extensive cortical and WM infarction (*arrow*) in an appropriately mature brain. There were no congenital malformations within the brain. (With permission of Dr Mary Rutherford, Hammersmith Hospital.)

CONGENITAL VARICELLA ZOSTER

Congenital varicella zoster virus infections are less common than the other congenital infections. Maternal immunity is high, and infectivity of the fetus is apparently low. The congenital varicella syndrome typically follows 2–4% of maternal infection occurring prior to 20 weeks' gestation. A specific feature is cicatrix (lightning-flash skin lesions) in a dermatomal distribution. Limb hypoplasia and weakness follow intrauterine damage to the cervical or lumbosacral plexi; segmental spinal cord necrosis, intrauterine growth restriction (IUGR), cataracts, chorioretinitis and microphthalmia occur. Intracranial findings are the sequelae of necrotizing encephalitis and include hydrocephalus, porencephaly, hydra-nencephaly, calcifications, and malformations associated with intracranial vascular compromise, such as polymicrogyria or focal lissencephaly. Severe microcephaly may be an isolated feature and cerebellar hypoplasia is reported. Zoster may be the clinical presentation in infants infected after 20 weeks' gestation. Congenital varicella acquired during peripartum maternal infection leads to a presentation which resembles varicella in the immunocompromised host with pneumonia, progressive hepatic failure with clotting abnormalities and hemorrhage, and a high mortality rate (Fig. 10.18). Other infectious causes of disseminated intra-vascular coagulopathy in the neonate include enterovirus family, herpes simplex and, occasionally, toxoplasmosis[4,23,44,66,72].

Summary

- Neonatal brain infections may be acquired *in utero*, intrapartum or postnatally.

- Sequelae depend upon the stage of brain maturation at the time of infection, the status of the developing immune system, and the infectivity, dose and actual target cell of the infecting agent.

- Standard imaging protocols with contrast enhancement should be used with suspected infections.

- Computed tomography may be necessary to confirm the presence and the extent of calcification.

- Different patterns of pathologic damage in the developing brain lead to imaging appearances different from those in the fully formed brain; early infections affect organogenesis and later infections often lead to brain destruction.

- Despite the variability in patterns of damage, imaging differentiation amongst the infectious agents may be possible.

References

1. Aicardi J (1992) *Diseases of the Nervous System in Childhood*. Oxford, MacKeith Press.
2. Alliet P, Van Lierde S, Bruylants B *et al.* (1992) [Neonatal listeriosis]. *Tijdschr Kindergeneeskd* **60(1)**, 18–21.
3. Arvin B, Neville LF, Barone FC *et al.* (1996) The role of inflammation and cytokines in brain injury. *Neurosci Biobehav Rev* **20(3)**, 445–452.
4. Bale JF and Murph JR (1997) Infections of the central nervous system in the newborn. *Clinics in Perinatology* **24(4)**, 787–806.
5. Barker PB, Lee RR and McArthur JC (1995) AIDS dementia complex: evaluation with proton MR spectroscopic imaging. *Radiology* **195**, 58–64.
6. Barkovich AJ and Lindan CE (1994) Congenital cytomegalovirus infection of the brain: imaging analysis and embryologic considerations. *AJNR* **15(4)**, 703–715.
7. Bauman NM, Kirby-Keyser LJ, Dolan KD *et al.* (1994) Mondini dysplasia and congenital cytomegalovirus infection. *J Pediatr* **124(1)**, 71–78.
8. Becker LE (1992) Infections of the developing brain. *AJNR* **13**, 537–549.
9. Belman AL (1990) Aids and pediatric neurology. *Neurologic Clinics* **8(3)**, 571–603.
10. Benator RM, Magill HL, Gerald B *et al.* (1985) Herpes simplex encephalitis: CT findings in the neonate and young infant. *AJNR* **6(4)**, 539–543.
11. Bode H and Rudin C (1995) Calcifying arteriopathy in the basal ganglia in human immunodeficiency virus infection. *Pediatr Radiol* **25**, 72–73.
12. Boppana SB, Fowler KB, Vaid Y *et al.* (1997) Neuroradiographic findings in the newborn period and long-term outcome in children with symptomatic congenital cytomegalovirus infection. *Pediatrics* **99(3)**, 409–414.
13. Bowie WR, King AS, Werker DH *et al.* (1997) Outbreak of toxoplasmosis associated with municipal drinking water. *Lancet* **350**, 173–177.
14. Chang YC, Huang CC and Liu CC (1996) Frequency of linear hyperechogenicity over the basal ganglia in young infants with congenital rubella syndrome. *Clin Infect Dis* **22(3)**, 569–571.
15. Chang YC, Huang CC, Wang ST *et al.* (1997) Risk factor of complications requiring neurosurgical intervention in infants with bacterial meningitis. *Pediatr Neurol* **17(2)**, 144–149.
16. Chantler JK, Smyrnis L and Tai G (1995) Selective infection of astrocytes in human glial cell cultures by rubella virus. *Lab Invest* **72(3)**, 334–340.
17. Cleveland RH, Herman TE, Oot RF *et al.* (1987) The evolution of neonatal herpes encephalitis as demonstrated by cranial ultrasound with CT correlation. *Am J Perinatol* **4(3)**, 215–219.
18. Corey L, Whitley RJ, Stone EF *et al.* (1988) Difference between herpes simplex virus type 1 and type 2 neonatal encephalitis in neurological outcome. *Lancet* **1(8575–6)**, 1–4.
19. Cortey A, Jarvik JG, Lenkinski RE *et al.* (1994) Proton MR spectroscopy of brain abnormalities in neonates born to HIV-positive mothers. *AJNR* **15**, 1853–1859.
20. Dambska M and Laure-Kamionowska M (1998) The morphological picture of developing meningo-encephalitis in central nervous system. *Folia Neuropathol* **36(4)**, 205–210.
21. Dammann O and Leviton A (1998) Infection remote from the brain, neonatal white matter damage, and cerebral palsy in the preterm infant. *Semin Pediatr Neurol* **5(3)**, 190–201.
22. Daneman A, Lobo E and Mosskin M (1998) Periventricular band of increased echogenicity: edema or calcification? *Pediatr Radiol* **28**, 83–85.
23. Deasy NP, Jarosz JM, Cox TC *et al.* (1999) Congenital varicella syndrome: cranial MRI in a long-term survivor. *Neuroradiology* **41**, 205–207.
24. Dias JMJ, van Rijckevorsel GH, Landriue P *et al.* (1984) Prenatal cytolomegavirus infection and cerebral microgyria: evidence for perfusion failure, not disturbance of histogenesis, as the major cause of fetal cytomegalovirus encephalopathy. *Neuropediatrics* **15**, 18–24.
25. Egelhof JC (1997) Infections of the central nervous system. In: Ball WS (Ed.) *Pediatric Neuroradiology*. Philadelphia, Lippincott-Raven, pp. 273–318.
26. Enzmann D, Chang Y and Augustyn G (1990) MR findings in neonatal herpes simplex encephalitis type 2. *J Comput Assist Tomogr* **14(3)**, 453–457.
27. Eppes SC, Woods CR, Mayer AS *et al.* (1993) Recurring ventriculitis due to *Citrobacter diversus*: clinical and bacteriologic analysis. *Clin Infect Dis* **17(3)**, 437–440.
28. Epps RE, Pittelkow MR and Su WP (1995) TORCH syndrome. *Semin Dermatol* **14(2)**, 179–186.
29. Ersahin Y, Mutluer S and Guzelbag E (1994) Brain abscess in infants and children. *Childs Nerv Syst* **10(3)**, 185–189.
30. Felderhoff-Mueser U, Rutherford M, Squier W *et al.* (1999) Relation between magnetic resonance images and histopathological findings of the brain in extremely sick preterm infants. *Am J Neuroradiol* **20**, 1349–1357.
31. Ford-Jones EL (1999) An approach to the diagnosis of congenital infections. *Paediatr Child Health* **4(2)**, 109–112.

32. Ford-Jones EL and Ryan G (1999) Implications for the fetus of maternal infections in pregnancy. In: Armstrong A and Cohen J (Eds) *Infectious Diseases*. London, Mosby, pp. 55.1–55.14.

33. Foulon W, Villena I, Stray-Pedersen B *et al.* (1999) Treatment of toxoplasmosis during pregnancy: a multicenter study of impact on fetal transmission and children's sequelae at age 1 year. *Am J Obstet Gynecol* **180(2)**, 410–415.

34. Friede RL (1989) *Developmental Neuropathology*, 2nd edn. Berlin, Springer.

35. Friedman S and Ford-Jones EL (1999) Congenital cytomegalovirus infection – an update. *Paediatr Child Health* **4(1)**, 35–38.

36. Friedman S, Ford-Jones LE, Toi A *et al.* Congenital toxoplasmosis: prenatal diagnosis, treatment and postnatal outcome. *Prenat Diagn* **19**, 330–333.

37. Frey TK (1997) Neurological aspects of rubella virus infection. *Intervirology* **40(2–3)**, 167–175.

38. Gallagher PG and Ball WS (1991) Cerebral infarctions due to CNS infection with *Enterobacter sakazakii*. *Pediatr Radiol* **21(2)**, 135–136.

39. Garcia-Tamayo J (1992) Teratogenic effect of the Venezuelan equine encephalitis virus: a review of the problem. *Invest Clin* **33(2)**, 81–86.

40. Givner LB and Kaplan SL (1993) Meningitis due to *Staphylococcus aureus* in children. *Clin Infect Dis* **16(6)**, 766–771.

41. Gray F, Scaravilli F, Everall I *et al.* (1996) Neuropathology of early HIV-1 infection. *Brain Pathol* **6(1)**, 1–15.

42. Gray PH, Tudehope DI and Masel J (1992) Cystic encephalomalacia and intrauterine herpes simplex virus infection. *Pediatr Radiol* **22(7)**, 529–532.

43. Griffith BP and Booss J (1994) Neurologic infections of the fetus and newborn. *Neurol Clin* **12(3)**, 541–564.

44. Grose C (1994) Congenital infections caused by varicella zoster virus and herpes simplex virus. *Semin Pediatr Neurol* **1(1)**, 43–49.

45. Haimes AB, Zimmerman RD, Morgello S *et al.* (1989) MR imaging of brain abscesses. *AJR* **152**, 1073–1085.

46. Harwood-Nash DC, Reilly BJ and Turnbull I (1970) Massive calcification of the brain in a newborn infant. *AJR* **58(3)**, 528–532.

47. Hayward JC, Titelbaum DS, Clancy RR *et al.* (1991) Lissencephaly–pachygyria associated with congenital cytomegalovirus infection. *J Child Neurol* **6(2)**, 109–114.

48. Hazebroek FW, Tibboel D, Leendertse-Verloop K *et al.* (1991) Evaluation of mortality in surgical neonates over a 10-year period: nonpreventable, permissible, and preventable death. *J Pediatr Surg* **26(9)**, 1058–1063.

49. Herman TE, Cleveland RH, Kushner DC *et al.* (1985) CT of neonatal herpes encephalitis. *AJNR* **6(5)**, 773–775.

50. Hicks T, Fowler K, Richardson M *et al.* (1993) Congenital cytomegalovirus infection and neonatal auditory screening. *J Pediatr* **123(5)**, 779–782.

51. Huang CC, Chen CY, Yang HB *et al.* (1998) CNS candidiasis in very low-birth-weight premature neonates and infants: US characteristics and histopathologic and MR imaging correlates in 5 patients. *Radiology* **209**, 49–56.

52. Hughes P, Weinberger E and Shaw DW (1991) Linear areas of echogenicity in the thalami and basal ganglia of neonates: an expanded association. *Radiology* **179(1)**, 103–105.

53. Hwa HL, Shyu MK, Lee CN *et al.* (1994) Prenatal diagnosis of congenital rubella infection from maternal rubella in Taiwan. *Obstet Gynecol* **84(3)**, 415–419.

54. Incesu L, Akan H and Arslan A (1994) Neonatal cerebral candidiasis: CT findings and clinical correlation. *J Belge Radiol* **77(6)**, 278–279.

55. Jay V, Becker LE, Blaser S *et al.* (1995) Pathology of chronic herpes infection associated with seizure disorder: a report of two cases with tissue detection of herpes simplex virus 1 by the polymerase chain reaction. *Pediatr Pathol Lab Med* **15**, 131–146.

56. Kang GH and Chi JH (1990) Congenital tuberculosis – Report of an autopsy case. *J Korean Med Sci* **5(1)**, 59–64.

57. Kaufman D, Kilpatrick L, Hudson RG *et al.* (1999) Decreased superoxide production, degranulation, tumor necrosis factor, alpha secretion and CD11b/CD18 receptor expression by adherent monocytes from preterm infants. *Clin Diagn Lab Immunol* **6(4)**, 525–529.

58. Kubota T, Kusaka H, Hirano A *et al.* (1985) Ultrastructural study of early stage of calcification in herpes simplex encephalitis. *Acta Neuropathol* **68(1)**, 77–79.

59. Kuroda Y and Matsui M (1997) [Progressive rubella panencephalitis]. *Nippon Rinsho* **55(4)**, 922–925.

60. Lane B, Sullivan EV, Lim KO *et al.* (1996) White matter MR hyperintensities in adult patients with congenital rubella. *AJNR* **17**, 99–103.

61. Lim KO, Beal DM, Harvey RL *et al.* (1995) Brain dysmorphology in adults with congenital rubella plus schizophrenia like symptoms. *Biol Psychiatry* **37(11)**, 764–776.

62. Lu D, Pavlakis SG, Frank Y *et al.* (1996) Proton MR spectroscopy of the basal ganglia in healthy children and children with AIDS. *Radiology* **199**, 423–428.

63. Mathews VP, Kuharik MA, Edwards MK *et al.* (1989) Gd-DTPA-enhanced MR imaging of experimental bacterial meningitis: evaluation and comparison with CT. *AJR* **152**, 131–136.

64. Nathan L, Twickler DM, Peters MT *et al.* (1993) Fetal syphilis: correlation of sonographic findings and rabbit infectivity testing of amniotic fluid. *J Ultrasound Med* **12(2)**, 97–101.

65. Noorbehesht B, Enzmann DR, Sullender *et al.* (1987) Neonatal herpes simplex encephalitis: correlation of clinical and CT findings. *Radiology* **162(3)**, 813–819.

66. Ong CL and Daniel ML (1998) Antenatal diagnosis of a porencephalic cyst in congenital varicella-zoster virus infection. *Pediatr Radiol* **28**, 94.

67. Patel DV, Holfels EM, Vogel NP *et al.* (1996) Resolution of intracranial calcifications in infants with treated congenital toxoplasmosis. *Radiology* **199(2)**, 433–440.

68. Pavlakis SG, Lu D, Frank Y *et al.* (1998) Brain lactate and N-acetylaspartate in pediatric AIDS encephalopathy. *AJNR* **19**, 383–385.

69. Puvabanditsin S, Wojdylo E, Garrow E *et al.* Group B streptococcal meningitis: a case of transverse myelitis with spinal cord and posterior fossa cysts. *Pediatr Radiol* **27**, 317–318.

70. Sage MR and Wilson AJ (1994) The blood–brain barrier: an important concept in neuroimaging. *AJNR* **15**, 601–622.

71. Shah SS, Zimmerman RA, Rorke LB *et al.* (1996) Cerebrovascular complications of HIV in children. *AJNR* **17**, 1913–1917.

72. Sheffer IE, Baraitser M and Brett EM (1991) Severe microcephaly associated with congenital varicella infection. *Dev Med Child Neurol* **33(1)**, 916–920.

73. Stamos JK and Rowley AH (1994) Timely diagnosis of congenital infections. *Pediatr Clin North Am* **41(5)**, 1017–1033.

74. Sugita K, Ando M, Makino M *et al.* (1991) Magnetic resonance imaging of the brain in congenital rubella virus and cytomegalovirus infections. *Neuroradiology* **33(3)**, 239–242.

75. Takano T (1994) [Pathogenesis of congenital hydrocephalus: role of transplacental myxovirus infection]. *No To Hattatsu* **26(3)**, 206–210.

76. Tassin GB, Maklad NF, Stewart RR *et al.* (1991) Cytomegalic inclusion disease: intrauterine sonographic diagnosis using findings involving the brain. *AJNR* **12**, 117–122.

77. Tien RD, Felsberg GJ and Osumi AK (1993) Herpesvirus infections of the CNS: MR findings. *AJR* **161**, 167–176.

78. Tollofsrud PA, Kvittingen EA, Granum PE *et al.* (1998) [Botulism in newborn infants]. *Tidsskr Nor Laegeforen* **20**, 118(28), 4355–4356.

79. Toma P, Magnano GM, Mezzano P *et al.* (1989) Cerebral ultrasound images in prenatal cytomegalovirus infection. *Neuroradiology* **31**, 278–279.

80. Trottier G, Srivastava L and Walker CD (1999) Etiology of infantile autism: a review of recent advances in genetic and neurobiological research. *J Psychiatry Neurosci* **24(2)**, 103–115.

81. Tse G, Silver M, Whyte H *et al.* (1997) Neonatal meningitis and multiple brain abscesses due to *Citrobacter diversus. Pediatr Pathol Lab Med* **17(6)**, 977–982.

82. Weingarten K, Zimmerman RD, Becker LE *et al.* (1989) Subdural and epidural empyemas: MR imaging. *AJR* **152**, 615–621.

83. Weller RO, Engelhardt B and Phillips MJ (1996) Lymphocyte targeting of the central nervous system: a review of afferent and efferent CNS-immune pathways. *Brain Pathol* **6(3)**, 275–288.

84. Wong TT, Lee LS, Wang HS *et al.* (1989) Brain abscesses in children – a cooperative study of 83 cases. *Child's Nerv Syst* **5**, 19–24.

85. Woods CR, Mason EO and Kaplan SL (1992) Interaction of *Citrobacter diversus* strains with HEP-2 epithelial and human umbilical vein endothelial cells. *J Infect Dis* **166**, 1035–1044.

86. Yamaguchi K and Goto N (1993) An autopsy case of brain candidiasis in premature infant: morphology and intraparenchymal distribution of *Candida* foci. *No To Hattatsu* **25(4)**, 369–373.

87. Yoshimura M, Tohyama J, Maegaki Y *et al.* (1996) [Computed tomography and magnetic resonance imaging of the brain in congenital rubella syndrome]. *No To Hattatsu* **28(5)**, 385–390.

Congenital malformations in the neonate

11

Paolo Tortori-Donati and Andrea Rossi

Introduction and embryology

The first rudiment of the future central nervous system appears on the 15th day of gestation, when the primitive streak is formed on the surface of the bilaminar embryo; proliferating cells at its cranial end form the Hensen's node and subsequently migrate in the ectoderm–endoderm interface to form the intervening mesoderm, in a process called gastrulation. Specialized paired columns of migrating cells integrate along the mid-line to form the notochord, that induces the formation of the overlying neuroectoderm of the neural plate. The progressive thickening and infolding of the neural plate forms the neural groove, whose lips will fuse along the mid-line to form the neural tube. This process is called primary neurulation, and is traditionally conceived as beginning at about 20 days at level of somite 4 (future craniocervical junction) and proceeding bidirectionally in a zipper-like fashion, with the cranial end (anterior neuropore) closing at 25 days and the caudal end (posterior neuropore) at 26–28 days[15]. The cavity of the neural tube at the anterior neuropore progressively dilates into three primitive brain vesicles: prosencephalon, mesencephalon and rhombencephalon. Subsequently, the prosencephalon divides into the telencephalon (future cerebral hemispheres, caudate nuclei and putamina) and diencephalon (future thalami, hypothalamus and globi pallidi), and the rhombencephalon into the metencephalon (future pons and cerebellum) and myelencephalon (future medulla oblongata); the mesencephalon (future cerebral peduncles and quadrigeminal plate) remains undivided. Causes of brain malformations belong to four main categories: chromosomal aberrations, single gene mutations, extrinsic teratogens, and unknown. The latter category is the largest, accounting for as many as 75% of all malformations at term[15].

Neural tube closure defects

EMBRYOLOGY AND CLASSIFICATION

The process of infolding of the neural plate to form the neural tube (primary neurulation) characterizes the 4th gestational week. As previously stated, primary neurulation is traditionally believed to occur in a zipper-like fashion starting from the region of somite 4 and proceeding bidirectionally. However, recent evidence suggests that the neural tube starts closing simultaneously at five separate closure sites[21]. This concept is intriguing as (i) it points to the segmental nature of early embryonic development, and (ii) it explains why neural tube closure defects occur preferentially in certain sites, such as lumbosacral myelomeningoceles or occipito-cervical, occipital, frontal, and skull base cephaloceles. Probably, the interface between two adjacent closure sites is a sort of 'watershed'; that is, an intrinsically weaker area where closure defects are more likely to occur. As a consequence, cephaloceles and open spinal dysraphisms (prevailingly myelomeningoceles) may be schematically conceived as a single developmental disorder, with the main difference being the segmental location of the defect along the longitudinal embryonic axis. However, due to the need for uniform terminology, the separation between cephaloceles and the intracranial counterpart of myelomeningoceles (i.e. the Chiari II malformation) is preserved in this chapter. The intermediate form between these two entities (i.e. the Chiari III malformation) is also discussed separately.

CEPHALOCELES

Cephaloceles are characterized by a protrusion of cerebral and/or meningeal tissue through a congenital defect of the skull and dura, usually located at or near the mid-line. In Western populations, most cephaloceles are occipital in location. Although the diagnosis is usually made antenatally by means of ultrasound, magnetic resonance (MR) is used to assess the contents of the herniated sac; on this basis, five groups may be identified (Table 11.1)[14,17,18,20]. The skin and dura overlying the malformation may be incompletely formed, so that in some cases the arachnoid layer is directly exposed and may become infected and ulcerated.

MR (Fig. 11.1) provides a reliable depiction of the malformation, suggests its categorization according to the location (Table 11.2), and recognizes associated findings such as hydrocephalus, commissural anomalies and the Chiari II malformation; the association of the latter with an

occipito-cervical cephalocele is termed Chiari III malformation (Fig. 11.2)[17,18,20]. MR angiography detects blood vessels such as dural sinuses within the herniated sac, which may be responsible for major bleeding during surgery.

CHIARI II MALFORMATION

There is always a 1:1 association between an open spinal dysraphism (usually a lumbosacral myelomeningocele) (Fig. 11.3) and the Chiari II malformation, a complex congenital anomaly of the hindbrain characterized by caudal

Table 11.1 Cephaloceles: pathological classification

Name	Contents
Meningocele	CSF, lined by meninges
Gliocele	CSF, lined by glial tissue
Meningoencephalocele	CSF and brain
Meningoencephalocystocele	CSF, brain and ventricles
Atretic cephalocele	Small nodule of fibrous-fatty tissue

Table 11.2 Cephaloceles: anatomic classification

Cephaloceles of the vault	Cephaloceles of the base
Occipito-cervical	Frontoethmoidal
Inferior occipital	Sphenoorbitary
Superior occipital	Sphenomaxillary
Sagittal (interparietal)	Nasopharyngeal
Lateral	Temporal
Frontal	
Bregmatic	

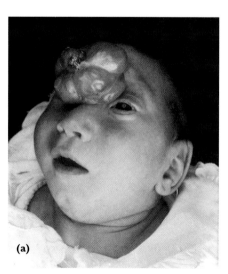
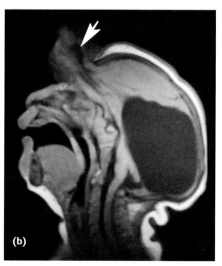
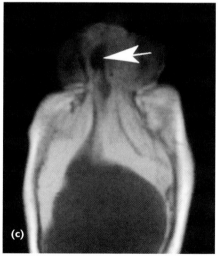

Fig. 11.1 Nasofrontal (glabellar) meningoencephalocystocele, 3-month-old baby. **(a)** Photograph of the patient; **(b,c)** MR at 0.5 T; **(b)** sagittal spin echo (SE) T1 weighted image, 500/20/2, repetition time/echo time/acquisitions; **(c)** axial MR T1 weighted image, 500/20/2. In this particular case, the cephalocele is associated with alobar holoprosencephaly. Notice the partially trapped right frontal horn within the cephalocele (*arrow*, **(b,c)**. There is concurrent cystic malformation in the posterior fossa whose precise attribution is difficult due to extreme distortion of the anatomical structures.

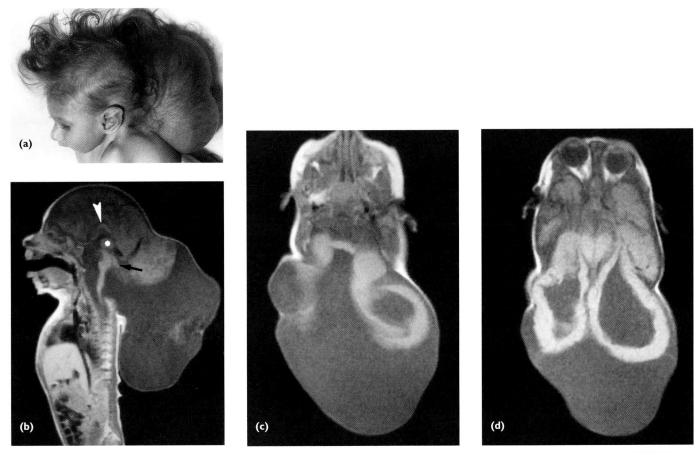

Fig. 11.2 Chiari III malformation, 3-day-old newborn. **(a)** Photograph of the patient at 8 months; **(b–d)** MR at 0.5 T; **(b)** sagittal SE T1 weighted image, 500/20/2; **(c,d)** axial SE T1 weighted images, 500/20/2. The herniated sac protrudes through a wide occipito-cervico-thoracic schisis, and contains the cerebellum, occipital lobes and ventricular trigones **(b–d)**. Associated Chiari II signs are present, i.e. low-lying brain stem, thickened interthalamic mass (*asterisk*, **b**), and tectal beak (*arrow*, **b**). Associated abnormalities in this particular case comprise callosal dysgenesis (*arrowhead*, **b**) and Dandy–Walker malformation.

displacement of the vermis, brain stem and fourth ventricle. It should be noted that such association is consistently present; that is, all neonates with myelomeningocele also harbor a Chiari II malformation. However, the severity of the hindbrain malformation may be variable, so that patients with a nearly normal-sized posterior fossa may sometimes be found; subtle, minimal features of Chiari II malformation should therefore be actively sought in all newborns with open spinal dysraphisms.

The original defect occurs in the phase of primary neurulation, and probably involves the interface between two adjacent neural tube closure sites, more frequently between sites 1 and 5 in the lumbosacral spine; at this level, the neuroectoderm is 'frozen' at a neural plate stage (placode). CSF leaks through the defect into the amniotic sac, resulting in chronic CSF hypotension within the developing neural tube, insufficient dilatation of the rhombencephalic vesicle (future fourth ventricle), and lack of induction of the perineural mesenchyma of the posterior cranial fossa[11]. Therefore, both

cerebellum and brain stem are eventually forced to develop within a smaller than normal posterior fossa, and consequently herniate through both the tentorial groove and the foramen magnum. CSF hypotension in the supratentorial brain may also impair neuronal migration and bony development, producing various associated malformations of the nervous tissue and osteomeningeal covering.

All infratentorial anomalies detected by MR (Fig. 11.3)[12,17,18,20] are generated by the lack of vital space for the cerebellum and brain stem into a smaller than normal posterior fossa. The inferior vermis herniates into the foramen magnum and wraps around the posterior surface of the cord (cerebellar peg). The medulla is stretched downwards into the foramen magnum while the cervical cord is anchored by the dentate ligaments, resulting in the cervicomedullary kink, best seen on sagittal views. The cerebellar hemispheres tend to engulf the brain stem, occupying the pontocerebellar angles. The cerebellum may also herniate upwards through the tentorial hiatus (towering cerebellum). The

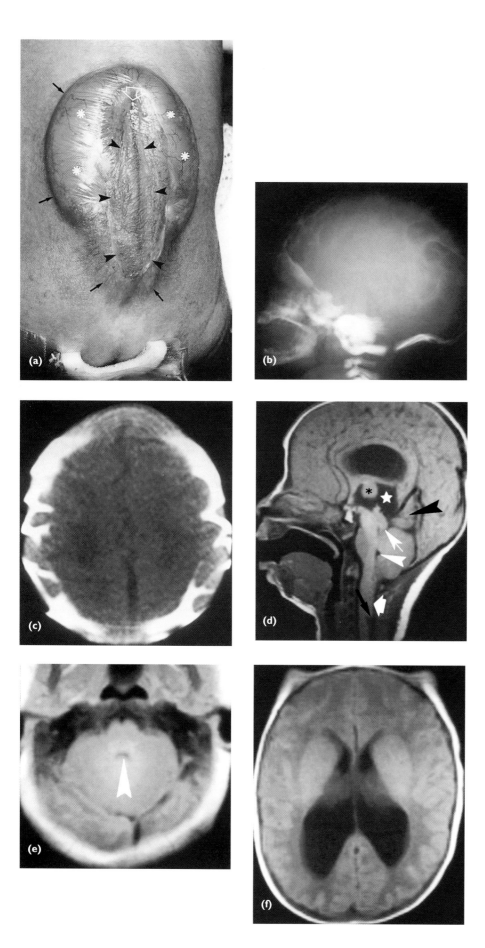

Fig. 11.3 Chiari II malformation. **(a–c)** 12-h-old newborn with thoracolumbar myelomeningocele; **(d–f)** 8-h-old newborn with sacral myelomeningocele. **(a)** Photograph of the patient; **(b)** plain X-ray radiograph, lateral view; **(c)** axial CT scan; **(d–f)** MR at 0.5 T; **(d)** sagittal SE T1 weighted image, 500/20/2; **(e,f)** axial SE T1 weighted images, 500/20/2. **(a)** This newborn has a large thoracolumbar myelomeningocele. The wide placode (*arrowheads*, **a**) is exposed to air and surrounded by a partially epithelized area (*asterisks*, **a**) and, more laterally, by intact skin (*arrows*, **a**). Dilatation of the underlying subarachnoid spaces produces the swollen appearance of the malformation. CSF leaks from the spinal canal at the cranial end of the placode (*empty arrow*, **a**). Skull X-rays **(b)** show multiple focal areas of radiolucency, consistent with lacunar skull. Notice the typical conformation of the skull in a Chiari II patient, with a shallow posterior fossa. On CT **(c)**, these lacunae are more clearly visible. In a different patient, the mid-sagittal MR image clearly shows the cerebellar peg (*thick white arrow*, **d**) and the cervicomedullary kink (*black arrow*, **d**), forming the typical cascade of herniations. The fourth ventricle is small (*white arrowhead*, **d**). The inferior quadrigeminal tubercles are thickened, although a typical tectal beak is not clearly visible in this particular case (*thin white arrow*, **d**). The apparently independent ('accessory') lobe visible right above the vermis (*black arrowhead*, **d**) is in fact the stretched medial surface of the temporal lobe. The suprapineal recess of the third ventricle is widened (*starlet*, **d**) and the interthalamic mass is thickened (*asterisk*, **d**). Axial views show a smaller than normal posterior fossa with a small fourth ventricle (*arrowhead*, **e**) and hydrocephalus **(f)**.

fourth ventricle is usually small or even completely effaced[17,18,20]. The inferior colliculi may be hypertrophied or fused, and point posteriorly to form the tectal beak. Hydrocephalus is a consistent finding in newborns within 48–72 h of repair of the spinal dysraphism, and is usually the first occasion for the neuroradiologist to see these patients, as MR is only rarely performed before surgery. The supra-pineal recess of the third ventricle and the interthalamic mass are especially prominent. Crowding of histologically normal cerebral convolutions in the parieto-occipital regions is known as stenogyria. Commissural (callosal) anomalies are commonly associated. Disorganization of the collagenous outer meninges from which the membranous calvarium forms produces irregularity of the surfaces of the inner and outer table of the skull; this feature, known as lacunar skull or *luckenschädel* (Fig. 11.3), was of diagnostic importance in the pre-MR era.

Chiari III malformation

It is characterized by the association of an occipito-cervical cephalocele with a number of typical features of the Chiari II malformation such as tectal beak, low-lying brain stem and thickened interthalamic mass (Fig. 11.2). The cephalocele must herniate through an occipito-cervical defect in order to meet the criteria for the Chiari III malformation [17,18,20].

Malformations of the lamina terminalis

ANOMALIES OF THE TELENCEPHALIC COMMISSURES

Mid-line telencephalic commissures are represented by the corpus callosum, hippocampal commissure and anterior commissure. The corpus callosum is the largest commissure in the brain, and is anatomically divided in four portions from anterior to posterior: the rostrum, genu, body and splenium. The hippocampal commissure or psalterium Davidi connects the posterior pillars of the fornix and lies along the inferior aspect of the posterior callosal body and splenium, so that the term 'calloso-hippocampal commissure' has been introduced to illustrate such continuity[16]. The anterior commissure cross-es the mid-line at the superior end of the lamina terminalis. Embryologically, the telencephalic commissures derive from the lamina reuniens, a dorsal thickening of the embryonic lamina terminalis. The recent concept that callosal development starts from the posterior portion of the genu and proceeds bidirectionally towards the splenium and rostrum has been questioned by Raybaud and Girard[16], who introduced a new classification of the abnormalities traditionally known as 'agen-

Table 11.3 Simplified new classification of agenesis of the telencephalic commissures

Callosal agenesis
Complete commissural agenesis
Calloso-hippocampal agenesis
Isolated callosal agenesis
Callosal hypoplasia
Partial posterior commissural agenesis
Diffuse commissural hypoplasia
Segmental callosal hypoplasia
Callosal agenesis with interhemispheric cyst
With diencephalic pseudocyst
With interhemispheric cyst

esis and hypoplasia of the corpus callosum', a simplified version of which is presented here (Table 11.3).

Callosal agenesis

Former callosal (now commissural) agenesis may be categorized into three subsets: complete commissural agenesis, calloso-hippocampal agenesis, and isolated callosal agenesis.

The most frequent among the three is calloso-hippocampal agenesis, in which the anterior commissure is preserved, and is sometimes hypertrophied; this variety represents the classical, widely described callosal agenesis. Calloso-hippocampal agenesis is characterized by a host of MR features, first and foremost the absent visualization of the corpus callosum and fornix in mid-sagittal scans (Fig. 11.4)[17,18,20]. Developing axons fail to cross the mid-line and remain in their native hemisphere, forming the so-called longitudinal callosal bundles of Probst. These run along the medial walls of the lateral ventricles, characteristically resulting in crescentic-shaped frontal horns in coronal sections. Because the cingulus (forming the white matter core of the cingulate gyrus) is consistently absent, the cingulate gyrus does not fold[16], the calloso-marginal sulcus does not form and the mesial cortical sulci show a radial arrangement; the evaluation of the calloso-marginal sulcus is especially useful in the neonate to assess callosal morphology indirectly, as absent or incomplete myelination results in physiologic isointensity of the corpus callosum with brain in the newborn. Moreover, absence of the cingulus produces thinning of the parahippocampal convolutions, leading to dilatation of the temporal horns and rudimentary hippocampal infolding[16]. Hypoplasia of occipital associative bundles allows dilatation of trigones of the lateral ventricles (colpocephaly)[16].

The rarer complete commissural agenesis and isolated callosal agenesis differ only in that the anterior commissure is hypoplastic and the psalterium is visible in mid-sagittal scans, respectively. Other than being frequently associated with other congenital brain abnormalities, calloso-hippocampal

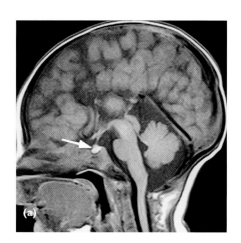
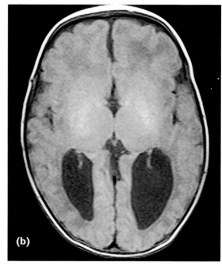
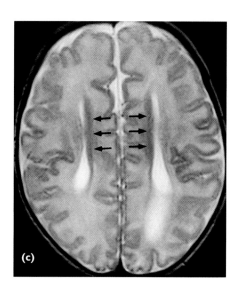
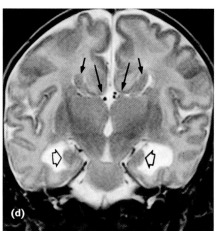

Fig. 11.4 Calloso-hippocampal agenesis, 23-day-old patient. MR at 1.5 T. **(a)**. Sagittal SE T1 weighted image, 600/20/2; **(b)** axial SE T1 weighted image, 614/20/2; **(c)** axial FSE T2 weighted image, 5000/112/4; **(d)** coronal FSE T2 weighted image, 5000/112/4. The corpus callosum and fornix are completely absent, resulting in the typical spokewheel-like arrangement of the mesial cortical sulci **(a)**. Notice physiologically hyperintense pituitary gland in this newborn (*arrow*, **a**). Dilatation of the posterior portions of the lateral ventricle is called colpocephaly **(b)**. On axial views, the longitudinal callosal bundles of Probst are visible along the medial walls of the lateral ventricles (*arrows*, **c**); the latter course parallel to the falx cerebri and the interhemispheric fissure. On coronal views, the frontal horns are crescentic due to the presence of the bundles of Probst along their medial walls (*short arrows*, **d**). Notice everted cyngulate gyri (*long arrows*, **d**) without formation of the callosomarginal sulci. Both hippocampi are rudimentary (*empty arrows*, **d**).

agenesis is consistently present in Aicardi syndrome. This entity has dominant X-linked transmission and is characterized by cortical dysplasia, chorioretinic lacunae, coloboma, cerebellar malformations, choroid plexus papillomas and holoprosencephaly.

Callosal hypoplasia

According to the new classification, callosal hypoplasia may in fact be divided into three categories: partial posterior commissural agenesis, diffuse commissural hypoplasia and segmental callosal hypoplasia. Partial posterior commissural agenesis is characterized by partial agenesis of the posterior portion of the corpus callosum; the extent of the agenetic portion may be variable, with only part of the genu (corresponding to the portion of the corpus callosum which forms first) present in the most severe cases, and is predictable based on the traditional theory of bidirectional development of the corpus callosum. Diffuse commissural hypoplasia, characterized by diffuse thinning of the three commissures, could be related to errors occurring later during commissur-

al plate development resulting in a lesser amount of fibers crossing the commissures. There is no widespread consensus as to whether segmental callosal hypoplasia, in which an intermediate portion of the corpus callosum is thinned, exists as a developmental abnormality, most cases being represented by secondary callosal destruction or resulting from white matter atrophy.

Former callosal hypoplasia/agenesis with interhemispheric cyst

CSF-filled cavities associated with commissural abnormalities belong to two main categories: diencephalic pseudocysts, representing superior bulging of the tela choroidea of the third ventricle, and interhemispheric cysts, which are independent from the ventricles and may in turn be intraparenchymal, subarachnoid, arachnoid, or even intradural. True interhemispheric cysts suggest that commissural development may influence, and in turn be influenced by, development of the meninx primitiva; this may also explain the high incidence of interhemispheric (so-called 'callosal') lipomas with commissural abnormalities (see below).

HOLOPROSENCEPHALY

This term refers to a complex developmental anomaly of the brain and skull, characterized by hypoplasia of the most rostral portions of the neural tube, resulting in fused cerebral hemispheres and absence of mid-line structures such as the rhinencephalon, corpus callosum and septum pellucidum. Both genetic factors (either chromosomal aberrations or single-gene mutations) and extrinsic teratogens may be involved in the pathogenesis[15]. The frequent association with neural tube closure defects suggests a common cellular disorder, possibly related to defective embryonic axial patterning and segmentation.

Holoprosencephaly is classically divided into alobar, semilobar and lobar types according to the severity of the malformation. However, a precise boundary among the three groups does not exist and intermediate cases may be identified[17,18,20].

Alobar holoprosencephaly (Fig. 11.5)

Mid-line structures such as the falx cerebri, superior sagittal sinus, interhemispheric fissure, septum pellucidum, corpus callosum, third ventricle, pituitary gland and olfactory bulbs are absent. The thalami are fused and abut a rudimentary ventricle freely communicating with a large cyst, the dorsal sac, extending upwards to the calvarium. Posterior fossa malformations and neuronal migration anomalies may be associated. The diagnosis is usually made antenatally by ultrasounds. Neonates are usually stillborn and are therefore rarely imaged by MR.

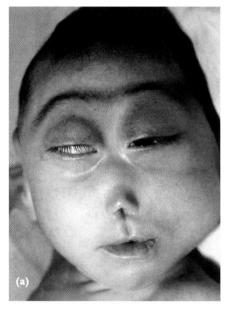 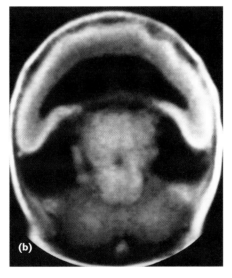 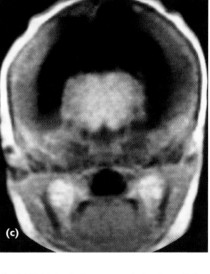 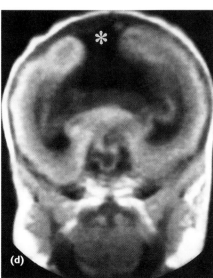 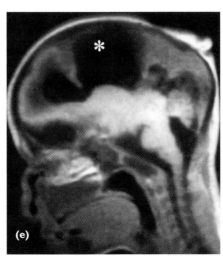

Fig. 11.5 Alobar holoprosencephaly, cebocephalic stillborn. (a) Photograph of the stillborn. (b–e) MR at 0.5 T; (b) axial SE T1 weighted image, 500/20/2; (c,d) coronal SE T1 weighted images, 500/20/2; (e) sagittal SE T1 weighted image, 500/20/2. The thalami are fused in the mid-line (b,c) and there is a crescentic holoventricle which communicates with a large dorsal sac (asterisk, d,e). There is associated Dandy–Walker variant (e).

Semilobar holoprosencephaly (Fig. 11.6)

The brain is less dysmorphic; rudimentary lateral ventricles are present and the cortex is more developed. The thalami may be partially separated and a rudimentary third ventricle may be seen. The interhemispheric fissure and the falx cerebri are partially developed posteriorly, whereas the frontal lobes are fused. The corpus callosum is absent in the fused regions, whereas a pseudosplenium is visible where the two cerebral hemispheres are separated[17,18,20]. The differentiation from the most severe alobar variant is usually easy by MR, and is based on the detection of the posterior part of the falx and interhemispheric fissure.

Lobar holoprosencephaly (Fig. 11.7)

This is the mildest form, usually found in asymptomatic or mildly retarded individuals. The lateral ventricles are formed; the frontal lobes may be partially fused in some cases and separated in others, but the septum pellucidum is constantly absent. The mildest forms show only the absence of the septum pellucidum, and therefore require differentiation from septo-optic dysplasia, in which, however, optic nerves are constantly hypoplastic. The differentiation from the semilobar variant is sometimes difficult by MR due to the large number of intermediate forms; the degree of anterior extension of the corpus callosum in midsagittal planes may be used as an indicator of the severity of the malformation.

SEPTO-OPTIC DYSPLASIA

It is characterized by the association of hypoplastic optic nerves and absent septum pellucidum. The clinical presentation is related to the association with either schizencephaly (presenting with seizures) or hypothalamic and pituitary hypoplasia (presenting with pituitary insufficiency).

The diagnosis of septo-optic dysplasia is based on ophthalmoscopy, showing hypoplastic optic discs, and an MR picture of small optic nerves and chiasm and absent septum

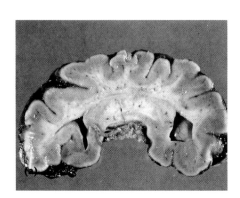
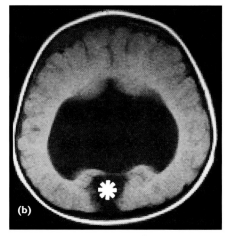
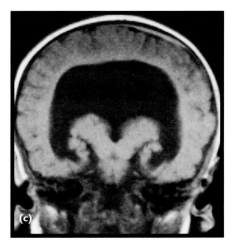
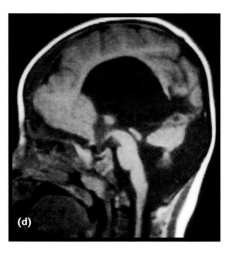

Fig. 11.6 Semilobar holoprosencephaly. **(a)** Anatomic specimen, coronal plane. There is complete fusion of the two hemispheres with absence of the interhemispheric fissure and corpus callosum. Temporal and occipital horns of the lateral ventricles are rudimentary. **(b–d)** MR at 0.5 T; **(b)** axial SE T1 weighted image, 500/20/2; **(c)** coronal SE T1 weighted image, 500/20/2; **(d)** sagittal SE T1 weighted image, 500/20/2. There is a single ventricular cavity with rudimentary trigones and temporal horns **(b,c)**. There is a concurrent small dorsal sac in this particular case (*asterisk*, **b**). There is absence of an interhemispheric fissure anteriorly with fusion of the two cerebral hemispheres. A rudimentary third ventricle separates the thalami. There is associated Dandy–Walker variant **(d)**.

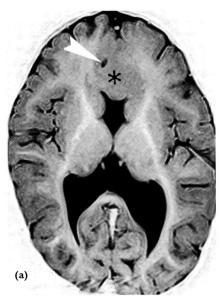
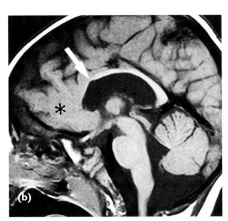
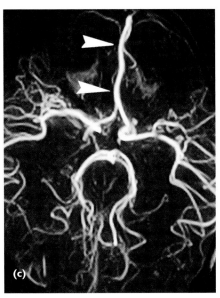

Fig. 11.7 Lobar holoprosencephaly, 14-month-old infant. MR at 1.5 T. **(a)** Axial MR FSE inversion recovery (IR) image, 8024/80/2 with 150 ms inversion time (TI); **(b)** sagittal SE T1 weighted image, 500/16/2; **(c)** 3D TOF MR angiography, 39/7.3/1 with 20° flip angle, axial reconstruction. There is fusion of the basal portions of the frontal lobes across the mid-line (*asterisk*, **a,b**). The septum pellucidum is absent and the shape of the lateral ventricles is rudimentary. In a mid-sagittal plane, the anterior edge of the corpus callosum (*arrow*, **b**) is an indicator of the degree of separation of the two cerebral hemispheres, and can be used to grade the severity of the abnormality. There is an azygous anterior cerebral artery (*arrowhead*, **a**), better demonstrated by MR angiography (*arrowheads*, **c**).

pellucidum (Fig. 11.8). The association with schizencephaly must be accurately scrutinized. The anterior recess of the third ventricle and the suprasellar cistern may be widened due to hypoplasia of the optic chiasm, infundibulum, and pituitary gland, whereas the frontal horns show a square-like shape due to the absence of the septum pellucidum, a feature in common with lobar holoprosencephaly[17,18,20].

Malformations of the cerebellum

EMBRYOLOGY

At the 28th–37th gestational day, the thin roof of the rhombencephalon is formed by an ependymal membrane coated by pia mater. The plica choroidea, a precursor of the

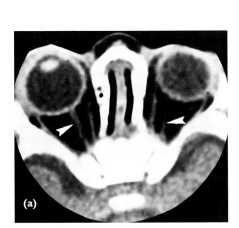
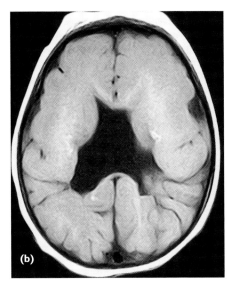
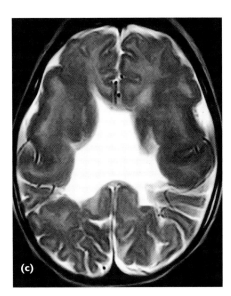

Fig. 11.8 Septo-optic dysplasia, 7-month-old patient. **(a)** Axial CT scan; **(b–f)** MR at 1.5 T; **(b)** axial SE T1 weighted image, 600/16/2; **(c)** axial FSE T2 weighted image, 4500/112/2; **(d)** coronal SE T1 weighted image, 600/16/2; **e)** coronal FSE T2 weighted image, 4500/112/2; **(f)** sagittal SE T1 weighted image, 500/16/2. Both optic nerves are markedly thin (*arrowheads*, **a**). The septum pellucidum is absent **(b–e)**. Several schizencephalic clefts are recognizable in both cerebral hemispheres.

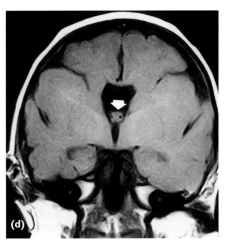 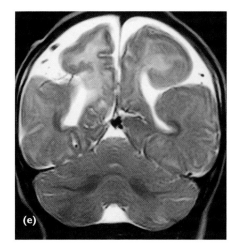 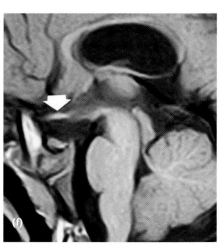

Fig 11.8 *continued* Scattered calcified foci in the white matter are depicted as hyperintense spots in T1 weighted images **(b)**. In coronal views, the frontal horns are square-shaped due to the absence of the septum pellucidum; the anterior pillars of the fornix are fused in this particular case (*arrow*, **d**). More posteriorly **(e)**, two open-lipped schizencephalic clefts bordered by dysplastic cortex are detected. In a mid-sagittal view, the optic chiasm is hypoplastic (*arrow*, **f**), whereas the pituitary stalk is not visualized.

future choroid plexus, divides the rhombencephalic roof in two portions: the anterior membranous area (AMA) lying cephalad, and the posterior membranous area (PMA) lying caudad. The edges of AMA thicken progressively by cellular proliferation, forming the rhombic lips. These paired structures approach each other until they eventually fuse in the mid-line to form the vermis; the intervening AMA progressively involutes until its remnants are incorporated in the choroid plexus. Meanwhile, the PMA shows a transient posterior finger-like expansion, the Blake's pouch, which will then disappear as the foramen of Magendie opens[18].

Cerebellar malformations derive from an inbalance between the formation of the rhombic lips and of the choroid plexuses at one side, and the involution of the AMA and PMA at the other[18]. A further categorization distinguishes cystic malformations, in which a CSF collection of variable nature is found within the posterior cranial fossa, and non-cystic malformations, which are usually dominated by vermian dysgenesis[18]. The most important group of cystic malformations is the Dandy–Walker complex[1], whose main differential diagnosis is with infratentorial arachnoid cysts (Table 11.4).

DANDY–WALKER COMPLEX

This term was introduced by Barkovich to designate a group of cystic malformations of the cerebellum resulting from a defective development of the structures originating

Table 11.4 Differential diagnosis of cystic cerebellar malformations

Diagnosis	Hydrocephalus	Vermis	Cerebellar hemispheres	Fourth ventricle	Posterior fossa	Torcular Herophili	Cisterns
Dandy–Walker malformation	80% of cases	Rotated, partial or total agenesis	Hypoplastic	Dilated, cystic	Widened	High-lying	Virtual
Dandy–Walker variant	Uncommon	Rotated, partial or total agenesis	Hypoplastic	Normal	Normal	Normal	Variable
Mega cisterna magna	Absent	Usually normal	Usually normal	Normal	Normal or widened	High-lying in 12% cases	Dilated
Persisting Blake's pouch	Tetraventricular	Usually normal	Deformed	Dilated	Normal or widened	Normal	Virtual
Arachnoid cyst	Triventricular	Normal or deformed	Normal or deformed	Compressed	Normal	Normal	Compressed

from the rhombencephalic roof that represent an embryological continuum[1]. A further categorization is possible based on the prevailing involvement of the AMA or PMA (Table 11.5)[17,18,20]. Because the AMA is the initiator of cerebellar development, anomalies of the AMA will be dominated by major vermian hypoplasia, whereas in anomalies of the PMA the cerebellum is grossly normal. In fact, persistence of part of the AMA in between the cerebellar hemispheres implies that the corresponding portion of the vermis does not form, while the AMA itself balloons into a cyst that is in fact a dilated fourth ventricle.

Dandy–Walker malformation (DWM)

The definition of DWM classically includes partial or complete vermian agenesis associated with hypoplastic cerebellar hemispheres, cystic dilatation of the fourth ventricle, and expansion of the posterior fossa associated with high insertion of the tentorium, torcular Herophili and transverse sinuses (Fig. 11.9)[1,17,18,20]. Vermian hypogenesis may be more or less severe; however, the hypoplastic superior vermis is constantly rotated in a counter-clockwise fashion, and often lies posterior to the quadrigeminal plate. Cerebellar hemispheres are also hypoplastic and abut the petrous ridges. As previously stated, the posterior fossa is occupied by a large cyst corresponding to a dilated fourth ventricle, while the cisterna magna, albeit present, is effaced. Hydrocephalus develops in up to 80% of untreated cases. The diagnosis of DWM is important for treatment and prognostic implications. In fact, shunting of the fourth ventricle allows re-expansion and growth of the cerebellar hemispheres in about 80% of cases, while hydrocephalus invariably disappears[18].

Dandy–Walker variant (DWV)

In some cases, some key features of DWM, such as a rotated, hypoplastic vermis and a cystic dilatation of the fourth ventricle, may be found in patients with an essentially normal posterior fossa (Figs 11.5, 11.6 and 11.10). The incidence of DWV is actually higher than that of the full-blown DWM,

Table 11.5 The Dandy–Walker complex

Anomalies of anterior membranous area	Anomalies of posterior membranous area
Dandy–Walker malformation	Mega cisterna magna
Dandy–Walker variant	Persisting Blake's pouch

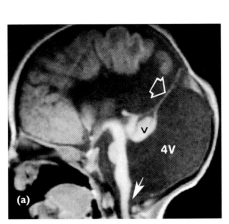
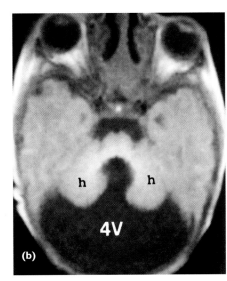
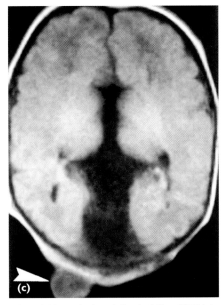

Fig. 11.9 Dandy–Walker malformation. A 3-day-old newborn with craniofacial dysmorphia, hypertelorism, palatoschisis and right parietal cephalocele. MR at 0.5 T. **(a)** Sagittal SE T1 weighted image, 500/20/2; **(b,c)** axial SE T1 weighted images, 600/20/2. The posterior fossa is larger than normal due to the presence of a cyst-like fourth ventricle (4V) **(a,b)**, whose inferior tip protrudes into the foramen magnum (*white arrow*, **a**). The vermis (v) is hypoplastic and rotated in a counterclockwise fashion **(a)**. The tentorium is elevated (*empty arrow*, **a**) so that the torcular comes to lie cranial to the lambda (so-called torcular-lambdoid inversion). Notice the scalloped profile of the occipital squama in the sagittal section **(a)**. In the axial plane, the hypoplastic cerebellar hemispheres (h) are winged outward **(b)**. The pons is hypoplastic **(a)**. The third ventricle appears to communicate with a dilated interhemispheric fissure **(c)**. Associated malformations in this particular case include agenesis of the corpus callosum with the classical spokewheel-like arrangement of the mesial cortical sulci **(a)** and a right parietal cephalocele (*arrowhead*, **c**).

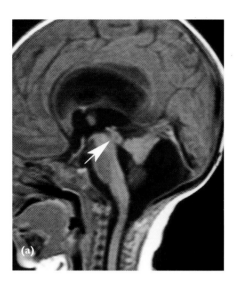

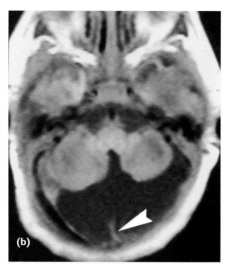

Fig. 11.10 Dandy–Walker variant, 26-day-old newborn. MR at 0.5 T. **(a)** Sagittal SE T1 weighted image, 544/16/3; **(b)** axial SE T1 weighted image, 573/16/3. The fourth ventricle is dilated and the vermis is hypoplastic and rotated in a counterclockwise fashion; however, the global size of the posterior fossa is normal, different to what is found in the full-blown Dandy–Walker malformation. The cerebellar hemispheres are winged outward and displaced against the petrous ridges. The falx cerebelli is present (*arrowhead*, **b**). Supratentorial hydrocephalus is caused by concurrent aqueductal stenosis (*arrow*, **a**).

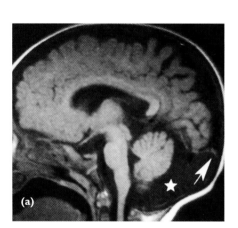

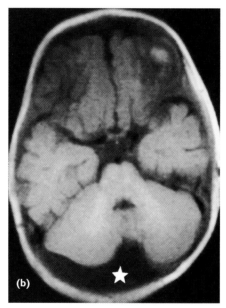

Fig. 11.11 Mega cisterna magna. MR at 0.5 T. **(a)** Sagittal SE T1 weighted image, 500/20/4; **(b)** axial SE T1 weighted image, 500/20/4. There is dilatation of the cisterna magna (*starlet*, **a,b**). The vermis is normal, whereas the right cerebellar hemisphere is mildly hypoplastic (**b**). The CSF collection protrudes through a partially split tentorium (*arrow*, **a**). The fourth ventricle has a normal shape and there is no hydrocephalus.

representing at least one-third of all cerebellar malformations[1,17,18,20]. Probably, DWM and DWV represent two ends of the spectrum of AMA anomalies, with the main difference being in the degree of dilatation of the fourth ventricle and, therefore, of the posterior fossa.

Mega cisterna magna

It is a common posterior fossa anomaly, secondary to evagination of the tela choroidea of the fourth ventricle and characterized by a sometimes marked dilatation of the cisterna magna which is, however, freely communicating with both the fourth ventricle and the adjacent subarachnoid spaces. The vermis and cerebellar hemispheres are normal or only mildly hypoplastic, and the fourth ventricle has

normal shape and size (Fig. 11.11)[19]. Hydrocephalus is never associated and the anomaly is constantly clinically silent, being usually encountered during MRI for other indications.

Persisting Blake's pouch

If the Blake's pouch fails to regress, it may persist throughout childhood. This anomaly is characterized by a retrocerebellar CSF collection communicating with a dilated and deformed fourth ventricle (Fig. 11.12). Because the foramen of Magendie never opens, CSF obstruction with tetraventricular hydrocephalus results. Shunting of the retrocerebellar pouch restores normal CSF outflow, so that both hydrocephalus and the pouch itself disappear[19].

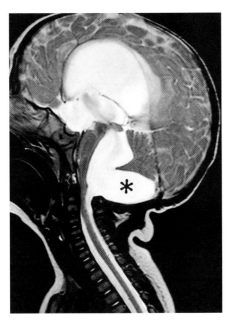

Fig. 11.12 Persisting Blake's pouch, 5-month-old infant. MR at 1.5 T. Sagittal FSE T2 weighted image, 4070/96/5. The Blake's pouch (*asterisk*) widely communicates with a dilated fourth ventricle. There is marked tetraventricular hydrocephalus. Turbulent CSF flow generates artifacts in the third ventricle, aqueduct, and fourth ventricle, seen as relative signal decay. The inferior vermis is compressed.

NON-CYSTIC CEREBELLAR MALFORMATIONS

A wide group of syndromes, some with a genetic background, fall into this heterogeneous group. Pathologically, they are mainly characterized by vermian dysgenesis. Only the main entities are discussed here.

Rhombencephalosynapsis

This rare abnormality is characterized by vermian agenesis, fused cerebellar hemispheres and peduncles, and apposed or fused dentate nuclei. MR detects the absence of the vermis and the mid-line fusion of the cerebellar hemispheres (Fig. 11.13)[18]. In axial MR images, the folia and sulci are continuous throughout the mid-line; in sagittal MR images, the structure lying in the mid-sagittal plane is not the vermis but a monolobated cerebellum. The posterior fossa is small and the fourth ventricle has a characteristic keyhole shape. Associated supratentorial abnormalities may be found.

Tectocerebellar dysraphism

This rare abnormality is characterized by vermian hypo-aplasia, occipital cephalocele, and marked deformation of the quadrigeminal plate and brain stem. The colliculi are fused to form a 'beak' pointing towards the site of the cephalocele. On MR (Fig. 11.14)[18], vermian hypo-aplasia is well depicted, and the tectal beak is visible both in the sagittal and axial planes. The cerebellar hemispheres usually tend to engulf the brain stem. Associated supratentorial anomalies and hydrocephalus are common findings. This anomaly should probably be classified as a particular form of neural tube closure defect associated with vermian agenesis.

Joubert syndrome

This entity typically presents clinically in the neonatal age with hyperpneic–apneic spells, ataxia, nystagmus and

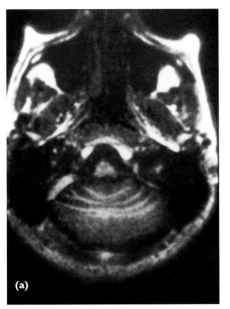
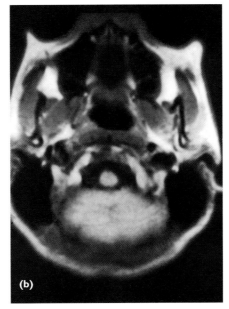
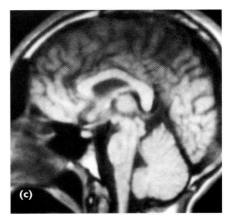

Fig. 11.13 Rhombencephalosynapsis, 9-year-old patient with truncal ataxia and psychomotor delay. MR at 0.5 T. **(a)** Axial SE IR image, 2000/20/1 with TI 150 ms; **(b)** axial SE T1 weighted image, 500/20/2; **(c)** sagittal SE T1 weighted image, 500/20/2; **(d)** coronal SE T1 weighted image, 500/20/2. The posterior fossa is small.

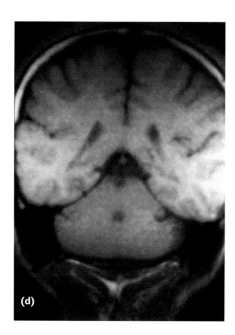

Fig. 11.13 *continued* Cerebellar convolutions are orientated transversely and the white matter is continuous across the mid-line **(a,b)**. The tonsils and the vallecula are not visible **(b,d)**. On a mid-sagittal section **(c)**, the 'vermis' is actually a mid-line cut through the monolobated cerebellum, whose fissures are clearly visible **(c)**.

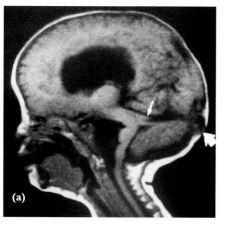

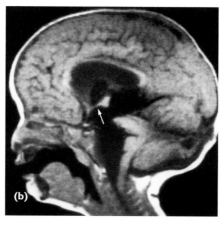

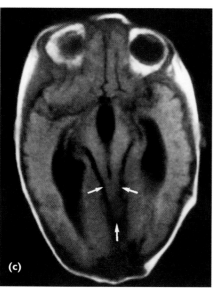

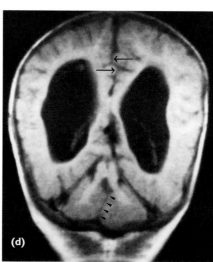

Fig. 11.14 Tectocerebellar dysraphism. Patient operated for small occipital cephalocele containing cerebellar tissue. MR at 0.5 T. **(a,b)** Sagittal SE T1 weighted images, 500/20/2; **(c)** axial SE T1 weighted image, 600/20/2; **(d)** coronal SE T1 weighted image, 500/20/2. The brain stem is markedly distorted and stretched towards the cephalocele site (*thick arrow,* **a**); the corpus callosum is thin, and the mammillary bodies are hypoplastic (*arrow,* **b**). The mesial cortex is diffusely arranged into multiple small gyri (stenogyria) **(a)**. There is extreme beaking of the quadrigeminal plate (*thin arrows,* **a,c**). The vermis is agenetic, and the two cerebellar hemispheres face one another at the mid-line (*arrowheads,* **d**). The falx cerebri is fenestrated, resulting in interdigitation of gyri across the interhemispheric fissure (*arrows,* **d**).

developmental delay. The inheritance is autosomal recessive. Pathologically, vermian dysgenesis is the key feature. Absence of the pyramidal decussation and medullary olivary nuclei is often associated. On MR (Fig. 11.15)[18], the vermis is completely or partially absent with only the anterior lobules visible. The fourth ventricle is high-riding and has an umbrella shape in axial images, whereas its roof is convex superiorly in sagittal images. The superior cerebellar peduncles are elongated, thin, and project straight back, running parallel with each other. An occipital cephalocele is present in 30% of cases.

Malformations of the cerebral cortex

EMBRYOLOGY AND CLASSIFICATION

The complex events leading to the formation of the cerebral cortex may be simplified in three main steps: proliferation, migration and organization[15]. Proliferation begins during the 7th gestational week, when cells in the subependymal layer of the walls of the lateral ventricles form the germinal matrix. During the following weeks, neurons generated by intense mitotic activity in the germinal matrix begin to migrate radially towards the surface of the brain; such migration follows a track laid by specialized radial glial fibers. There is a 1:1 correspondence between the site of cell proliferation within the germinal matrix and its eventual location within the cortical plate. It is not clear at what time migration in the cortex of the human fetus stops. However, distal processes of the radial glia disappear by 20–28 weeks' gestation, suggest-

ing no or little migration on glial guides at this stage[15]. Organization of the cortex to the eventual six-layer configuration occurs next, and is completed by the 7th lunar month[15].

The current classification[6] categorizes cortical malformations in defects of proliferation, migration, and organization (Table 11.6). However, the terminology used to describe these anomalies is still not uniform, and there is a tendency to employ different terms to describe malformations which are in fact identical in clinical, histological and neuroradiological terms.

HEMIMEGALENCEPHALY

According to the current classification[6], this anomaly results from a disorder in neuronal and glial proliferation in the germinal matrix. It may be isolated or occur in patients with neurocutaneous syndromes such as the Klippel–Trenaunay–Weber syndrome, linear nevus sebaceous syndrome, hypomelanosis of Ito, neurofibromatosis type 1, and Proteus syndrome[20]. MR shows enlargement of a whole hemisphere (Fig. 11.16). The cortex is affected by diffuse migration anomalies, while the white matter is gliotic and dysmyelinated. The ipsilateral ventricle is frequently dilated and the frontal horn is stretched. The homolateral cerebellar hemisphere is usually enlarged as well. Affected newborns suffer from untreatable epilepsy, so that hemispherectomy is often necessary. However, because hemispherectomy is contraindicated if the contralateral hemisphere has cortical malformations, assessment of the contralateral hemisphere is crucial.

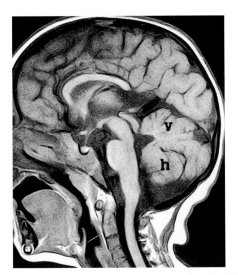
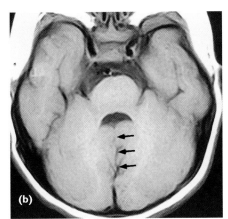
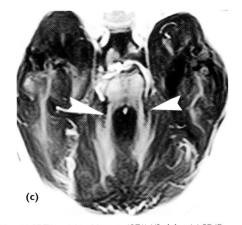

Fig. 11.15 Joubert syndrome, 23-month-old infant. MR at 1.5 T. **(a)** Sagittal SE T1 weighted image, 500/14/2; **(b)** axial SE T1 weighted image, 437/16/2; **(c)** axial SE IR image, 2500/30/1 with T1 150 ms. The vermis (v) is partially agenetic, and the cerebellar hemispheres (h) are seen as they abut one another at the mid-line **(a)**. There is concurrent callosal dysgenesis with absence of the splenium and genu. Axial sections show the cleft between the two adjoining cerebellar hemispheres (*arrows*, **b**) and the resulting umbrella-like fourth ventricle. On a slightly higher section, the two hypoplastic superior cerebellar peduncles project straight back, running parallel to each other (*arrowheads*, **c**).

Table 11.6 Simplified classification of cortical malformations

Disorders of proliferation	Focal transmantle dysplasia (Taylor's type focal cortical dysplasia with balloon cells)
	Hemimegalencephaly
Disorders of migration	Type I (classical) lissencephaly (agyria–pachygyria complex)
	Miller–Dieker syndrome (chromosome 17)
	X-linked lissencephaly
	Band heterotopia (X-linked)
	Type II (cobblestone) lissencephaly
	Fukuyama congenital muscular dystrophy
	Walker–Warburg syndrome
	Muscle-eye-brain disease
	Heterotopia
	Subependymal
	Subcortical
	Marginal glioneuronal heterotopia
Disorders of organization	Focal cortical dysplasia without balloon cells
	Polymicrogyria
	Schizencephaly

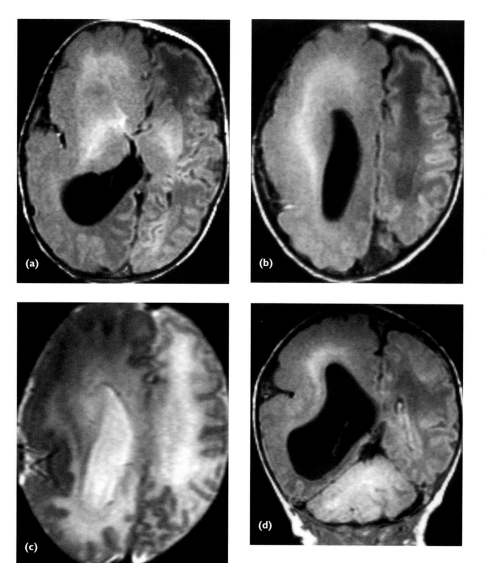

Fig. 11.16 Hemimegalencephaly, 20-day-old newborn with Proteus-like syndrome. **(a,b)** Axial SE T1 weighted images, 820/20/2; **(c)** axial SE T2 weighted image, 2700/120/2; **(d)** coronal SE T1 weighted image, 820/20/2. There is asymmetric macrocrania due to abnormal enlargement of the right cerebral hemisphere as compared to the left. In the posterior parietal region, the cortex is relatively normal. However, the remainder of the hemisphere shows a lissencephalic appearance with marked cortical thickening **(a–c)**. The Sylvian fissure is rudimentary, and the ipsilateral lateral ventricle is enlarged. There is high signal in T1 and low signal in T2 in the white matter of the affected hemisphere resulting from arrested neurons and glial cells as well as, probably, by hypermyelination. The right cerebellar hemisphere is enlarged as well **(d)**. (Case courtesy Dr Mary Rutherford, London, UK.)

LISSENCEPHALY (AGYRIA–PACHYGYRIA)

The term lissencephaly refers to a complete lack of sulcation of the cortical plate and should therefore be considered synonymous with agyria, whereas pachygyria indicates few, broad gyri with shallow sulci[5]. However, there is a wide spectrum of intermediate features in which variably combined areas of agyria and pachygyria co-exist; this may validate the use of the term agyria–pachygyria complex[6]. Embryologically, the anomaly results from diffusely abnormal neuronal migration.

Type 1 (classical) lissencephaly

Type 1 (classical) lissencephaly is usually found in children with Miller–Dieker syndrome (caused by partial deletion of chromosome 17), but some patients have X-linked lissencephaly; histologically, there is a four-layered cortex with a thick sparse cell layer interposed between the external and internal cellular layers. On MR (Fig. 11.17)[17,18,20], the cortical surface is flat and the Sylvian cisterns are broad and vertically oriented; therefore, the brain has a figure-of-eight shape in axial sections. The cortex is thickened and the hyperintense sparse cell layer is usually visualized.

Band heterotopia

Band heterotopia is presently categorized as a particular subset within the type 1 X-linked lissencephaly group[6]; in this entity, the majority of radial glial fibers are damaged, manifesting with bilateral, thick layers of arrested neurons located approximately half-way between the ventricles and the cortical plate, resembling a doubling of the cortex (Fig. 11.18)[17,18,20].

Type 2 (cobblestone) lissencephaly

Type 2 (cobblestone) lissencephaly is usually found in children with Fukuyama congenital muscular dystrophy, Walker–Warburg syndrome, and muscle–eye–brain disease. There is a more anarchic disorganization of the cortex, with

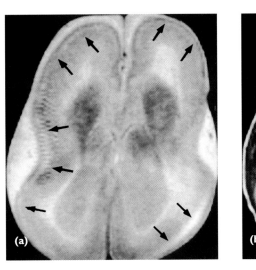
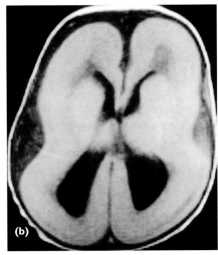
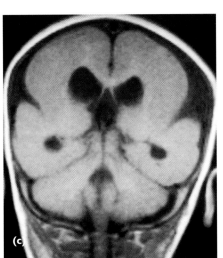
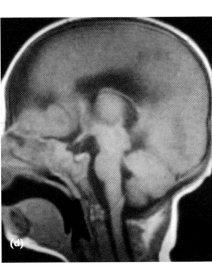

Fig. 11.17 Type 1 (classical) lissencephaly. A 13-day-old newborn with Miller–Dieker syndrome. MR at 0.5 T. **(a)** Axial SE T2 weighted image, 2000/90/1; **(b)** axial SE T1 weighted image, 600/20/2; **(c)** coronal SE T1 weighted image, 600/20/2; **(d)** sagittal SE T1 weighted image, 500/20/2. The brain has a figure-of-eight shape in the axial plane **(a,b)** and a 'chicken brain' shape in the coronal plane **(c)**. The surface of the brain is flat due to the lack of sulcation, and the Sylvian fissures are shallow and vertically oriented. The cortex is markedly thickened, and a hyperintense band corresponding to the sparse cell layer is clearly visible in T2 weighted images (*arrows*, **a**). There is also marked callosal hypoplasia **(d)**.

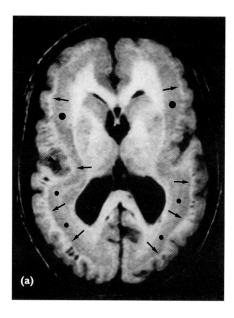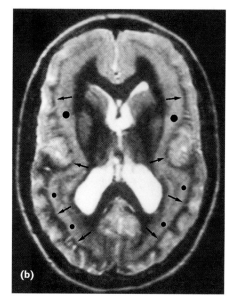

Fig. 11.18 Band heterotopia, 25-month-old infant. MR at 0.5 T. **(a)** Axial T1 weighted image, 600/20/2; **(b)** axial FSE T2 weighted image, 3000/96/2. A large band of isointense tissue (*dots*, **a,b**) is interposed between the ventricles and the cortex. Between the band heterotopia and the cortex is a thin layer of myelinated white matter (*arrows*, **a,b**). There is poor, irregular sulcation of the cerebral cortex. (Case courtesy Dr Claudio Fonda, Florence, Italy.)

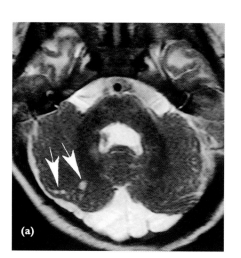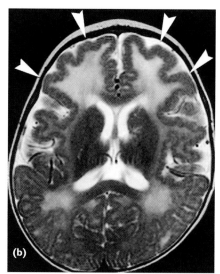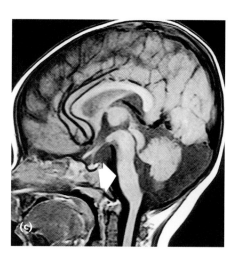

Fig. 11.19 Type 2 (cobblestone) lissencephaly, 6-month-old female with muscle–eye–brain disease. MR at 1.5 T. **(a,b)** Axial FSE T2 weighted image, 4500/108/4; **(c)** sagittal T1 weighted image, 500/12.5/2. There is cortical thickening with abnormal gyri and shallow sulci in the frontal lobes (*arrowheads*, **b**); the cortex shows a bumpy surface and is less markedly thickened than in type I lissencephaly. The underlying white matter is abnormally hyperintense due to abnormal myelination; also the paratrigonal white matter shows the same features. In the posterior fossa cerebellar cortical dysgenesis is revealed by the bumpy surface of both hemispheres and multiple subcortical cysts (*arrows*, **a**) There is also hypoplasia of the pons (*arrow*, **c**) and inferior vermis with concurrent cisterna magna.

zones of typical lissencephaly interspersed among areas of polymicrogyria. Cortical lamination is absent and subcortical heterotopia may be found. On MR (Fig. 11.19), the cortex is thinner than in type 1, and there may be concurrent hypomyelination of the white matter[5].

HETEROTOPIA

Damage of radial glial fibers may arrest neuronal migration at anomalous sites, where neurons conglomerate in a disor-ganized fashion. Patients almost always present with a seizure disorder. Gray matter heterotopia may be subependymal, subcortical or meningeal, whereas band het-erotopia is presently classified among the lissencephalies (see above). In all cases, heterotopia is isointense with normal gray matter in all MR sequences. Subependymal heterotopia is more common, and may in turn be focal or diffuse; focal nodules are found as sporadic cases (Fig. 11.20), whereas diffuse heterotopia bordering the walls of the lateral

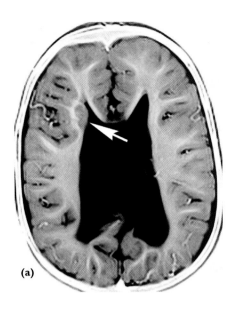 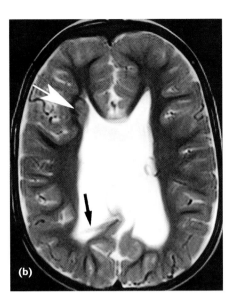

Fig. 11.20 Subependymal heterotopia, 28-month-old child with Chiari II malformation. MR at 1.5 T. **(a)** Axial SE T1 weighted image, 500/16/2; **(b)** axial FSE T2 weighted image, 4000/96/2. There is a subependymal heterotopic nodule in the lateral wall of right frontal horn (*white arrow*, **a,b**). The nodule is isointense with gray matter both in T1 and T2 weighted images. Notice abnormal configuration of the lateral ventricles in this Chiari II patient and the presence of a shunt catheter (*black arrow*, **b**).

ventricles are more likely to be X-linked[3]. Subcortical heterotopia is less frequent (Fig. 11.19). In other cases, radial glial fibers may develop excessively, resulting in neuronal overmigration; eventually, neurons come to lie within the meninges (marginal glio-neuronal heterotopia)[18].

FOCAL CORTICAL DYSPLASIA

The term *cortical dysplasia* has been widely used in the neuroradiological literature to refer to diffuse, focal, and monobilateral cortical anomalies whose ultimate categorization as polymicrogyria or agyria–pachyigyria was difficult by means of MR alone. With the advent of more refined MR technology and the tumultuous development in the understanding of normal and abnormal cortical development, it has become apparent that focal cortical dysplasias (FCD) exist as autonomous malformations and that their differentiation from both polymicrogyria and agyria–pachygyria is feasible

by MR. However, not every problem has been solved, and a certain degree of confusion probably still exists; this is mainly due to the fact that different types of FCD have been identified histologically and that these different varieties result from abnormalities occurring in different steps of neuronal development[9]. The main entities that are discussed here are Taylor type FCD (FCD with balloon cells) and FCD without balloon cells.

FCD with balloon cells (Taylor type FCD) is presently classified among proliferation disorders. According to Barkovich[2], this abnormality is coincidental with focal transmantle cortical dysplasia; however, we have seen cases in which the abnormality did not involve the whole cerebral mantle thickness, and we therefore believe that there is a spectrum of abnormality ranging from restricted cortical involvement to transmantle abnormalities, in which abnormal cells extend along the full thickness of a hemisphere (from the subependymal layer to the brain surface).

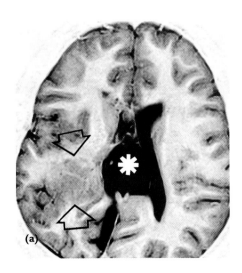 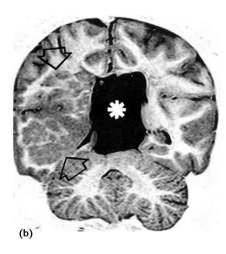

Fig. 11.21 Focal cortical dysplasia with balloon cells (focal transmantle cortical dysplasia), 24-month-old patient with status epilepticus. MR at 1.5 T. **(a)** Axial FSE IR image, 8024/80/2 with TI 150 ms; **(b)** coronal FSE IR image, 8024/80/2 with TI 150 ms. There is a giant conglomerate of heterotopic nodules with interspersed white matter in the right cerebral hemisphere extending from the ependymal to the brain surfaces (*empty arrows*, **a,b**). There also is concurrent interhemispheric cyst (*asterisks*, **a,b**).

Histologically, both atypical neurons and glial are found, and balloon cells (large cells with abundant eosinophilic cytoplasm, showing intermediate features between neuronal and glial elements) are consistently present.

On MR (Fig. 11.21), there is an abnormal gyral pattern in the involved region. The abnormal tissue may extend radially inwards to the ventricular surface, and typically shows mixed signal intensity, with areas that are isointense to gray matter and other areas isointense to white matter. The underlying white matter is hyperintense in T2 weighted images[9]. The gray–white matter interface is blurred.

FCD without balloon cells or microdysgenesis is characterized histologically by abnormal cortical lamination without the presence of balloon cells. It is presently categorized among disorders of cortical organization. Affected children almost always present with complex partial seizures. MR scans may be deceptively normal; however, focal atrophy in the affected areas has been described in the majority of cases[9].

POLYMICROGYRIA

Polymicrogyria is the most frequent cause of partial epilepsy in the pediatric age[5]. Strictly speaking, polymicrogyria is a histological diagnosis. In polymicrogyria, the causal insult produces selective laminar necrosis of layer 5, resulting in excessive infolding of the cortex with thin, numerous microconvolutions separated by narrow and often obliterated sulci. The insult occurs after the end of neuronal migration, that is in the phase of cortical organization.

Polymicrogyria may be unilateral or bilateral (congenital bilateral perisylvian syndrome); in the latter case, both Sylvian fissures are maldeveloped and lined by dysplastic cortex, frequently extending to the perirolandic regions. Clinically, this anomaly presents with congenital Foix–Chavany–Marie syndrome (facio-pharyngo-glosso-masticatory diplegia or diparesis)[7]. Bilateral polymicrogyria may also involve the frontal, occipital and temporal lobes. Because genetic as well as acquired (cytomegalovirus infection, *in utero* ischemia) causes may result in polymicrogyria, this abnormality represents a sort of watershed between true malformations and destructive events.

On MR (Fig. 11.22), polymicrogyria appears as an area of increased cortical thickness and may therefore mimic pachygyria when thick sections are acquired; thin cuts reveal that the abnormality is composed of multiple, small gyri. The gray–white matter junction is generally irregular, whereas the cortical surface may be flat or extend inward, producing a cortical infolding around an abnormally oriented sulcus. The abnormal cortex itself is isointense to normal gray matter, whereas the underlying white matter may show T2 prolongation; in these cases, the differentiation from Taylor's type focal cortical dysplasia is possible only by means of histology. Anomalous venous drainage is common in dysplastic cortical areas, and large veins may often be seen within the abnormal sulci.

SCHIZENCEPHALY

Schizencephaly is characterized by a cleft extending through the whole hemisphere, from the ependymal lining of the lateral ventricle to the pia covering the brain. The cleft may be uni- or bilateral and is constantly lined by polymicrogyric cor-

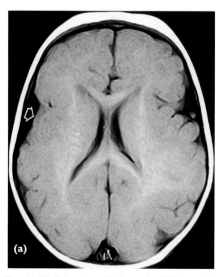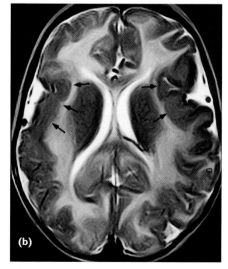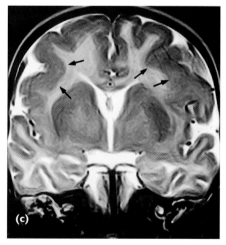

Fig. 11.22 Polymicrogyria, 8-month-old infant with connatal cytomegalovirus infection. MR at 1.5 T. **(a)** Axial SE T1 weighted image, 700/16/2; **(b)** axial FSE T2 weighted image, 4500/112/2; **(c)** coronal FSE T2 weighted image, 4500/112/2. A shallow Sylvian fissure is visible in T1 weighted images (*empty arrow*, **a**). T2 weighted images are better suited to depict the cortical anomaly by detecting bilateral thickening of the brain cortex (*arrows*, **b,c**). A few broad, shallow sulci are visible in the anomalous area.

tex; as a consequence, schizencephaly may be viewed as an extreme of the spectrum of polymicrogyria, in which the cortical infolding reaches the lateral ventricle. The genetic nature of schizencephaly has been proved recently[8], and the traditional clastic theory has been dismissed.

The walls of the cleft may be widely separated (open lips); in this case, the cleft is occupied by CSF and the anomaly is easily detected by MR (Fig. 11.23). When the walls abut one another (fused lips), the cleft may not be easily visible; however, a dimple may be seen in the wall of the lateral ventricle where the cleft communicates (Fig. 11.24). In all cases, the detection of the dysplastic cortex lining the cleft is essential in order to distinguish schizencephaly from a porencephalic cavity[4,17,18,20].

Chiari I malformation

Contrary to what the term might suggest, this anomaly is not related with Chiari II or III malformations except for the name of Dr H. Chiari, who first described these entities in 1891[18]. The Chiari I malformation is characterized by bilateral or, less frequently, unilateral ectopia of the cerebellar tonsils into the foramen magnum (Fig. 11.25). The posterior fossa is generally normal, and the vermis is normally shaped and located. Associated hydrocephalus and hydromyelia are frequent, and may be secondary to restricted CSF flow at the level of the crowded foramen magnum[18]. In rare cases, the medulla oblongata is dysmorphic, thickened in the sagittal plane, and shows a prominent obex. This associated feature depicts a myelencephalic variant of Chiari

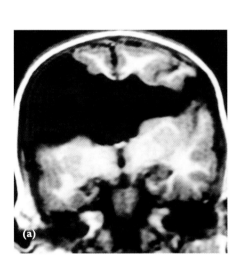
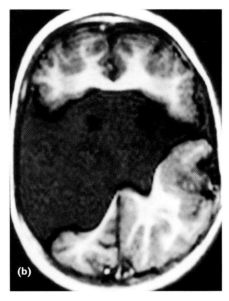

Fig. 11.23 Open lips schizencephaly, 26-month-old child. MR at 0.5 T. **(a)** Coronal SE T1 weighted image, 500/16/2; **(b)** axial SE T1 weighted image, 500/16/2. The cleft is bilateral and involves the full thickness of the brain. The margins of the cleft are composed of polymicrogyric cortex. There is no septum pellucidum. (Case courtesy Dr M. Gallucci, L'Aquila, Italy.)

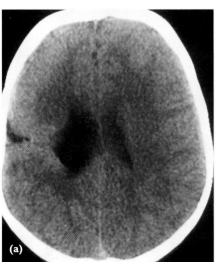
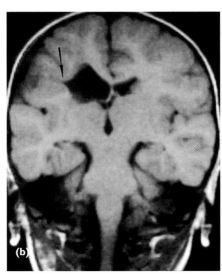

Fig. 11.24 Fused lips schizencephaly, 3-year-old patient. **(a)** Axial CT scan; **(b)** MR at 0.5 T, coronal SE T1 weighted image, 500/20/2. Both CT and MR adequately depict the presence of cortex bordering the cleft. A dimple along the lateral wall of the right lateral ventricle is visible in the coronal section (*arrow*, **b**), and correspondes to the opening of the schizencephalic cleft. The opening on the brain surface is best seen in the CT image in this particular case **(a)**.

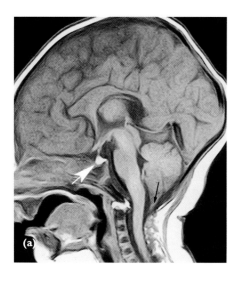

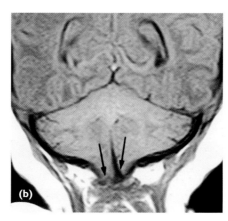

Fig. 11.25 Chiari I malformation, 18-day-old newborn. MR at 1.5 T. **(a)** Sagittal SE T1 weighted image, 600/16/2; **(b)** Coronal SE T1 weighted image, 591/16/2. The ectopic tonsils (*thin black arrows*, **a,b**) lie posterior to the medulla–cord junction. The brain stem is normal. Notice diffusely hyperintense pituitary gland (*large black arrow*, **a**), a typical finding in the neonate.

I as opposed to the classical form, in which the medulla, albeit stretched caudally, is otherwise normal[17,18,20].

Patients with Chiari I malformation may be asymptomatic or present with headache, torticollis, cervical pain and cranial nerves palsies. When suspecting a Chiari I malformation, other causes of cerebellar tonsils herniation (especially acute intracranial hypertension) must be ruled out. In addition, all patients with Chiari I should undergo spinal MR in order to detect hydromyelia. The reverse is also true in that all cases of unexplained hydromyelia should be scrutinized for an associated Chiari I.

Malformations of the meninx primitiva

LIPOMAS

Their commonest location is in the deep interhemispheric fissure (so called lipomas of the corpus callosum), where they are almost consistently associated with commissural plate abnormalities, but they may also be located in the quadrigeminal plate, suprasellar, interpeduncular, cerebellopontine angle and Sylvian cisterns[18]. Lipomas are not tumors, but true malformations of the meninx primitiva, abnormally differentiating into fatty tissue. They are almost always midline in location and lie in the subarachnoid spaces.

MR depicts lipomas as hyperintense masses on T1 weighted images, becoming hypointense on T2 weighted images as TE increases, except for FSE-T2 weighted images, where they remain hyperintense (Fig. 11.26). Signal intensity in both T1 and T2 weighted images is nulled when fat saturation pulses are applied. Large lipomas will show the chemical shift artifact. Pericallosal lipomas are subdivided according to morphology into curvilinear and tubulonodular varieties[10]: the former is thinner, has a more or less linear morphology, and lies usually along the callosal body and splenium (Fig. 11.26), whereas the latter is found along the anterior corpus callosum, is bulkier, and has a higher incidence of calcifications.

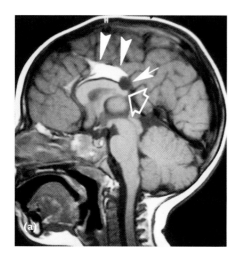

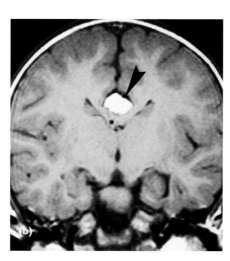

Fig. 11.26 Lipoma of the interhemispheric fissure, 17-month-old child. MR at 1.5 T. **(a)** Sagittal SE T1 weighted image, 600/16/3; **(b)** coronal SE T1 weighted image, 600/14/3. This curvilinear lipoma lies along the superior aspect of the corpus callosum (so-called 'callosal lipoma') (*arrowheads*, **a,b**). There is concurrent partial posterior commissural agenesis (*empty arrow*, **a**) as well as a small interhemispheric cyst (*arrow*, **a**). (Case courtesy Dr F. Triulzi, Milan, Italy.)

ARACHNOID CYSTS

Arachnoid cysts are CSF-filled cavities coated by a membrane made of arachnoid–neurothelial tissue which may secrete fluid, as do normal arachnoid villi. Although the pathogenesis of these malformations is still incompletely understood, they could result from anomalous differentiation of the leptomeninges, a process occurring between the 6th and 8th gestational weeks. Arachnoid cysts are more frequently supratentorial (about 75% of cases) (Fig. 11.27), particularly at the temporal poles[13]. Other relatively common locations include the posterior fossa (Fig. 11.28) and the suprasellar and quadrigeminal cisterns (Table 11.7). MR (Figs. 11.27 and 11.28) depicts arachnoid cysts as round to oval masses with signal intensity paralleling that of CSF, although increased protein content in excluded cysts may shorten T1

and increase T2. CSF pulsation tends to slowly but progressively enlarge the cyst, producing a certain degree of mass effect and even a deformation of the skull in some cases. Although the diagnosis is usually relatively straightforward, arachnoid cysts in the posterior fossa require careful differentiation with other cystic malformation belonging to the Dandy–Walker complex (Table 11.4).

Table 11.7 Anatomic location of arachnoid cysts

Supratentorial (77.5%)	Infratentorial (22.5%)
Temporal	Retrocerebellar
Suprasellar	Hemispheric
Convexity	Mid-line
Quadrigeminal	Clival
Interhemispheric	Pontocerebellar angle

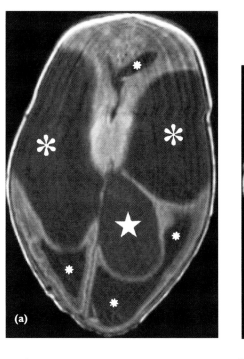
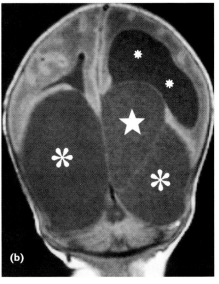
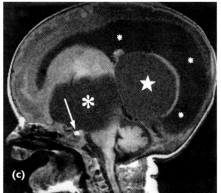
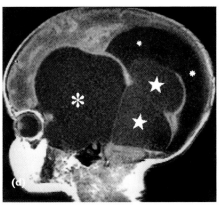

Fig. 11.27 Multiple supratentorial arachnoid cysts, 3-day-old newborn with macrocrania. MR at 0.5 T. **(a)** Axial SE T1 weighted image, 600/16/2; **(b)** coronal SE T1 weighted image, 600/16/2; **(c,d)** sagittal SE T1 weighted images, 600/16/2. Two large temporal cysts (*large asterisks*, **a–d**) and a bilobate left interhemispheric cyst (*starlets*, **a–d**) are detected. The latter is slightly higher intensity, probably due to higher protein content. The ventricular system is in part dilated (*small asterisks*, **a–d**). Notice the uniformly hyperintense pituitary gland (*arrow*, **c**), a typical finding in the newborn.

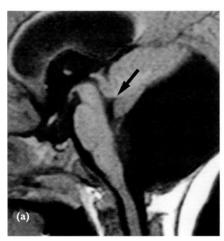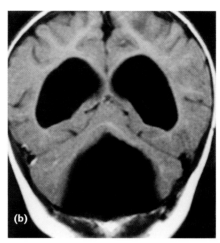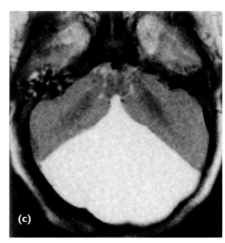

Fig. 11.28 Retrocerebellar arachnoid cyst, 21-month-old infant. MR at 0.5 T. **(a)** Sagittal SE T1 weighted image, 600/20/2; **(b)** coronal SE T1 weighted image, 600/20/2; **(c)** axial FSE T2 weighted image, 3500/90/2. This huge cyst splays the cerebellar hemispheres and displaces the vermis superiorly. On axial sections this arachnoid cyst could be mistaken for a Dandy–Walker malformation, but the mid-sagittal section clearly shows a normally developed, albeit compressed, fourth ventricle (*arrow*, **a**). There is marked triventricular hydrocephalus.

Summary

- MRI provides detailed multiplanar imaging which is essential for identifying congenital malformations.

- A knowledge of normal brain development is essential for correctly identifying abnormalities.

- The classification of congenital malformations is continually changing with new insights into brain development.

- As the genetics of congenital malformations becomes more complex MRI can provide important information on specific brain phenotypes.

References

1. Altman NR, Naidich TP and Braffman BH (1992) Posterior fossa malformations. *Am J Neuroradiol* **13**, 691–724.
2. Barkovich AJ (2000) *Pediatric Neuroimaging*, 3rd edn. Philadelphia, Lippincott Williams & Wilkins, pp. 281–318.
3. Barkovich AJ and Kjos BO (1992) Gray matter heterotopias: MR characteristics and correlation with developmental and neurological manifestations. *Radiology* **182**, 483–489.
4. Barkovich AJ and Kjos BO (1992) Schizencephaly: correlation of clinical findings with MR characteristics. *Am J Neuroradiol* **13**, 85–94.
5. Barkovich AJ, Gressens P and Evrard P (1992) Formation, maturation, and disorders of brain neocortex. *Am J Neuroradiol* **13**, 423–446.
6. Barkovich AJ, Kuzniecky RI, Dobyns WB *et al.* (1996) A classification scheme for malformations of cortical development. *Neuropediatrics* **27**, 59–63.
7. Cama A, Tortori-Donati P, Piatelli GL *et al.* (1995) Chiari complex in children. Neuroradiological diagnosis, neurosurgical treatment and proposal of a new classification (312 cases). *Eur J Pediatr Surg* **5** (Suppl 1), 35–38.
8. Capra V, De Marco P, Moroni A *et al.* (1996) Schizencephaly: surgical features and new molecular genetic results. *Eur J Pediatr Surg* **6** (Suppl 1), 27–29.
9. Colombo N, Tassi L, Galli C *et al.* (1998) Malformations of cortical development. Clinical-neuroradiologic correlations in 38 patients. *Bull Lega It Epil* **102/103**, 17–28.

10. Kash F, Brown G, Smirniotopoulos JA *et al.* (1996) Intracranial lipomas. Pathology and imaging spectrum. *Int J Neuroradiol* **2**, 109–116.
11. McLone DG and Knepper PA (1989) The cause of Chiari II malformation: a unified theory. *Pediatr Neurosci* **15**, 1–12.
12. Naidich TP, McLone DG and Fulling KH (1983) The Chiari II malformation. Part IV. The hindbrain deformity. *Neuroradiology* **25**, 179–197.
13. Naidich TP, McLone DG and Radkowski MA (1986) Intracranial arachnoid cysts. *Pediatr Neurosci* **12**, 112–122.
14. Naidich TP, Altman NR, Braffman BH *et al.* (1992) Cephaloceles and related malformations. *Am J Neuroradiol* **13**, 655–690.
15. Norman MG, McGillivray BC, Kalousek DK *et al.* (1995) *Congenital Malformations of the Brain. Pathological, Embryological, Clinical, Radiological and Genetic Aspects.* New York, Oxford University Press.
16. Raybaud C and Girard N (1998) Étude anatomique par IRM des agénésies et dysplasies commissurales télencéphaliques (agénésies du corps calleux et anomalies apparentées). Corrélations cliniques et interprétation morphogénétique. *Neurochirurgie* **44 (Suppl 1)**, 38–60.
17. Tortori-Donati P (http://medic-online.net/mr/tortori-donati/) (1996–1998) MRI – Congenital brain malformations. In: Passariello R *et al.* (Eds) (http://medic-online.net/mr/) *Magnetic Resonance in Medicine Multimedia Virtual Textbook.* Luxembourg S:A.

18. Tortori-Donati P, Taccone A and Longo M (Eds) (1996) *Malformazioni Cranio-encefaliche. Neuroradiologia*. Torino, Minerva Medica.

19. Tortori-Donati P, Fondelli MP, Rossi A *et al.* (1996) Posterior fossa malformations originating from a defect of the posterior membranous area. Mega cisterna magna and persisting Blake's pouch: two separate entities. *Child's Nerv Syst* **12**, 303–308.

20. Tortori-Donati P, Fondelli MP and Rossi A (1998) Anomalie congenite. In: Simonetti G, Del Maschio A, Bartolozzi C *et al.* (Eds) *Trattato Italiano di Risonanza Magnetica*, Vol. 1. Naples, Gnocchi-Idelson, pp. 155–203.

21. Van Allen MI, Kalousek DK, Chernoff GF *et al.* (1993) Evidence for multisite closure of the neural tube in humans. *Am J Med Genet* **47**, 723–743.

Vascular malformations of the neonatal brain

12

Pierre Lasjaunias, Georges Rodesch and Hortensia Alvarez

Contents

Introduction

Vascular 'malformations' include anatomical, pathophysiological and clinical entities as diverse as cerebral arteriovenous shunts, dural meningeal arteriovenous shunts, and arterial aneurysms. The differences between these disorders is now well recognized, but there are additional differences within each group: within the group of cerebral arteriovenous shunts, for instance, age of onset of initial signs. This is best illustrated by comparing aneurysmal malformations of the vein of Galen with true cerebral (or pial) malformations (see below). The distinction is both anatomical and clinical and suggests that the underlying mechanisms may differ[2]. A similar difference occurs within the group of dural lesions. Although they have been well defined in adults because of their prevalence, little is known about them in children because of their rarity. Venous sinuses of the cranial cavity are formed within the dura during the fetal and postnatal periods, at which times malformations may occur. Venous sinus malformations are found in infants but are never found in adults who present with dural lesions. Aneurysms are also a heterogeneous group. They are difficult to manage in children, because they are so seldom encountered, and because the etiology is different from aneurysms found in adults.

The concept conveyed by the word 'congenital' is that an individual with a vascular malformation was born with the lesion, which has remained basically unchanged. Consequently the clinical goals that we have set are early diagnosis and early treatment, whether it be preventive or curative, in an effort to prevent or cure the disorder's natural history which, we suppose, begins at birth[2,3].

However, there is much evidence to show that it is not that simple. In Rendu–Osler's disease (regardless of the presence of cerebral arteriovenous lesions), polycystic kidney disease (with arterial aneurysms), fibromuscular dysplasia, or type 1 neurofibromatosis, no morphological lesions can be detected in children belonging to affected families. The first signs do not usually appear until early adulthood. The best-known example of this is polycystic kidney disease, in which the first aneurysms are not diagnosed until approximately 30 years of age, 'only' 10 years earlier than in unaffected families. This suggests that familial and genetic predisposition are not enough in themselves to cause aneurysms, but that other intrinsic or extrinsic phenomena (mutation, traumatic triggering factor such as a virus) must occur to morphologically reveal the disease. Likewise, what we consider to be acquired lesions may actually be malformations that are systematically revealed in the same conditions by a factor that has been identified but that does not truly cause the disorder.

Hence the concept of malformation shifts from a morphological to a biological entity. Congenital vascular malformations date from the first stages of development, irrespective of when they are detected (Table 12.1).

The brain's specific vulnerability during the perinatal period is such that most arteriovenous malformations diagnosed in children are associated with structural alterations. During his or her first years, a child is not a miniature adult, nor are his or her pathologies those of an adult's. Conversely there is little chance that lesions discovered in adults were present during infancy or childhood without having left any detectable marks[2].

Every structural and hemodynamic change occurring in the cardiovascular system acts as a shear stress on blood vessels. This stress influences the modeling and remodeling of vessels. A persisting active arteriovenous communication may also cause hypertrophy of the right ventricle and atrium (Fig. 12.3). It may also, depending on its severity, result in respiratory, renal or hepatic failure, and peripheral arterial diastolic steal. Note, however, that adult carriers of cerebral arteriovenous shunts never have a history of perinatal heart failure, regardless of the flow rate within the lesion.

In infants, cerebrospinal fluid is reabsorbed via the cortical and deep cerebral veins, as the Pacchioni granulations in the sagittal sinus are still immature. This explains why venous

hypertension (induced by arteriovenous shunts) prevents CSF reabsorption and causes macrocrania, because of excess fluid in the brain (Figs 12.4 and 12.5). When this pressure imbalance is marked, hydrocephalus occurs, as a way of alleviating the stress induced by the abnormal venous hemodynamics. Once again, note that adult carriers of arteriovenous shunts rarely have macrocrania.

The venous hemodynamic balance required for synaptogenesis, myelogenesis and the maturation of granulations is essential for normal brain growth. Arteriovenous shunts that are active from birth are associated with rapid brain atrophy, most likely due to apoptosis, and cause the brain to 'melt' (Figs. 12.2 and 12.6). The disorder is bilateral and

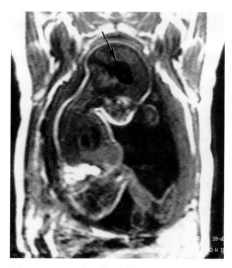

Fig. 12.1 Typical appearance of a vein of Galen aneurysmal malformation on fetal MRI. T1 weighted images. The lesion is seen as low signal intensity (*arrow*).

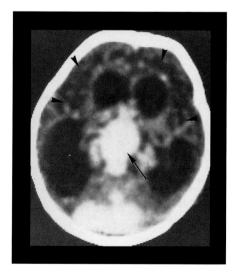

Fig. 12.2 A 1-day-old baby with severe cardiac failure. Infant with a vein of Galen aneurysmal malformation. CT scan shows the lesion as a rounded mid-line lesion with increased attenuation (*arrow*). There is, however, diffuse bilateral severe brain damage (*arrowheads*), which represents a contraindication to treatment.

Table 12.1 So-called congenital or malformative intracranial vascular lesions

Familial (seldom symptomatic at pediatric age)

Arterial aneurysm (polycystic kidney disease, Chr 16, Chr 6)

Pial arteriovenous shunts (Rendu–Osler–Weber, Chr 12, Chr 9) (the cerebral phenotype is not transmitted: in children lesions are usually high-flow multifocal AV fistulae)

Cavernomas (Chr 7); often multiple located in the brain and even the cord

Sporadic or primitive

Vein of Galen aneurysmal malformations (30% diagnosed *in utero*)

Pial arteriovenous shunts (cerebral), isolated, multiple, systematized (Bonnet Dechaume et Blanc or Wyburn–Mason syndromes)

Dural sinus malformation: torcular, transverse sinus, sagittal sinus, sigmoid sinus (50% diagnosed *in utero*)

Single cavernoma

Sturge–Weber syndrome

Acquired or secondary

Dural arteriovenous shunt (juvenile and adult types, sigmoid and transverse sinus, cavernous plexus)

Vascular anomalies

Developmental venous anomaly

Sinus pericranii

Embryonic vessel persistence

Chr = chromosome

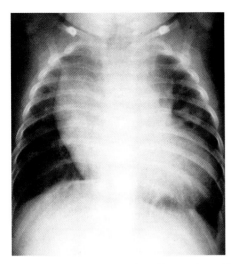

Fig. 12.3 Chest X-ray of a neonate presenting with acute heart failure due to a high-flow arteriovenous brain malformation. Cardiac enlargement due to cardiac overload is apparent, with predominantly right-sided enlargement of the cardiac silhouette.

Table 12.2 Clinical presentation

In utero
  Congestive cardiac failure (heart rate >200/min, ventricular extrasystoles, tricuspid insufficiency); macrocrania, ventriculomegaly
Neonate
  Systemic disorders: congestive cardiac failure, multiorgan failure, consumption coagulopathies
  Intracranial hemorrhage (hematoma, venous infarct, subarachnoid hemorrhage, convulsions)
Infant
  Hydrovenous disorders: macrocrania, hydrocephalus, convulsions
  Intracranial hemorrhage, (hematoma, venous infarct, subarachnoid hemorrhage)
Child
  Intracranial hemorrhage (hematoma, venous infarct, subarachnoid hemorrhage), convulsions
  Progressive neurological deficits
  Headaches

symmetrical when venous drainage is located on either side of the deep venous or dural sagittal system; it is focal when drainage is lateral, in the cortical veins of a single hemisphere. Once again, this phenomenon is specific to the pediatric population: focal cerebral atrophy is never detected in adult carriers of arteriovenous shunts. Finally, the deleterious effect of arteriovenous shunts on both myelination and synaptogenesis is associated with neurocognitive impairment in children, while adult carriers of this type of lesion are not usually intellectually impaired.

Thus, we can define congenital vascular lesions as the structural translation of a genetic defect, whether inherited or not, in the arterial or venous system. It can be expressed at any stage of life, when the vascular system is being either modeled or remodeled. It is induced by a secondary event (Table 12.2).

Prenatally diagnosed lesions

As a result, we cannot expect to offer prenatal diagnosis for every type of vascular lesion that belongs to the category entitled 'malformation', since a number of them are not expressed until adulthood, while others may even be caused

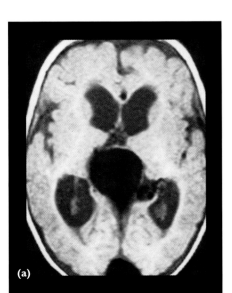

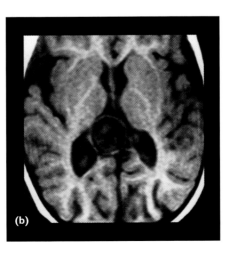

Fig. 12.4 Example of hydrodynamic disorders at the supratentorial level in an infant with a vein of Galen aneurysmal malformation. Note the ventriculomegaly **(a)** that resolves after partial embolization of the lesion **(b)**.

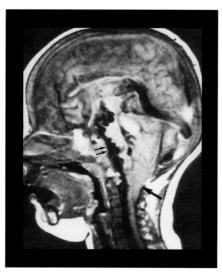

Fig. 12.5 Example of hydrodynamic disorders at the infratentorial level in an infant with a vein of Galen aneurysmal malformation. Note the tonsilar prolapse giving rise to a pseudo-Chiari appearance (*large arrow*). The brain stem is surrounded by tortuous veins (*double small arrows*), that represent the diversion of blood flow because of bilateral sigmoid thrombosis.

Table 12.3 Vascular lesions per age group in order of frequency

In utero
1. Aneurysmal malformations of the vein of Galen
2. Dural sinus malformation

Neonates
1. Aneurysmal malformation of the vein of Galen
2. Dural sinus malformation
3. Pial arteriovenous shunt
4. Cavernoma
5. Arterial aneurysm

Infants
1. Aneurysmal malformation of the vein of Galen
2. Dural sinus malformation
3. Pial arteriovenous shunt
4. Cavernoma
5. Arterial aneurysm

Children
1. Pial arteriovenous malformation
2. Cavernoma
3. Arterial aneurysm
4. Dural arteriovenous shunt (juvenile type)

by a postnatal event (Table 12.3). From a practical point of view, two types of malformations are detected before birth: aneurysmal malformations of the vein of Galen and defective dural sinuses.

Aneurysmal malformations of vein of Galen[1,4] can be diagnosed as early as the 28th week of pregnancy by ultrasonography or MRI (Fig. 12.1). They appear as a rounded intracranial mass behind the third ventricle in which flow compatible with an arteriovenous shunt can be detected. Associated signs may include heart failure with tachycardia,

ventricular extrasystoles, and tricuspid regurgitation. Vein of Galen malformations are rare congenital connections occurring between intracranial vessels. They occur within the first months of development and there is a strong association with persistent venous anomalies such as an absent straight sinus and persistent falcine and occipital sinuses. This does not imply that intrauterine straight sinus thrombosis with subsequent recanalization is responsible for the malformation but represents a time marker for an event that occurred prior to the straight sinus development. Despite their early origins

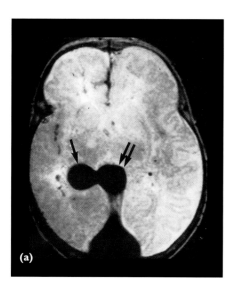

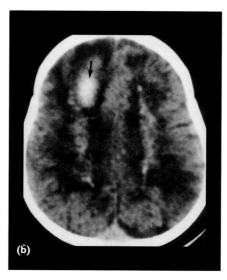

Fig. 12.6 Three-week old neonate presenting with seizures and progressive macrocrania. On T2 weighted MRI (**a**), although the vein of Galen is dilated (*double arrow*), the bilobed aspect of the venous ectasia is not consistent with a classical aneurysmal malformation of the vein of Galen. The lesion was diagnosed as a pial arteriovenous fistula draining into the deep venous system (*arrow*) ending in the vein of Galen that dilated because of the high flow. Urgent embolization to reduce the hydrovenous effects of the shunt was recommended, but refused by the parents. One month later a control CT scan was performed (**b**) which showed massive brain destruction ('melting brain syndrome').

only about half the aneurysmal malformations of vein of Galen are diagnosed antenatally even with good quality ultrasonographic investigations. *In utero* macrocrania is infrequent and does not imply a poor prognosis. It is usually linked to the volume of the aneurysmal sac rather than to accumulated fluid within the cranial cavity. The natural progression of the disorder is now well established, as are treatment and intervention techniques, which are discussed below.

Malformations of the dural sinuses originate during the fetal period, when sagittal and transverse sinuses differentiate after a normal phase of substantial enlargement around the torcular[2]. The size of the sinuses spontaneously decreases before birth as they open into a venous system within the dura mater along the edge of the foramen magnum. Malformations that develop at this stage will cause giant venous 'lakes' extending on either side of the mid-line. Because of the immaturity of the sinuses, they thrombose spontaneously and cause venous brain infarction and hemorrhage as the process spreads throughout the cerebral venous system. Only a third of dural sinus malformations are diagnosed before birth. The development of the jugular bulbs ends several weeks after birth. Postnatal malformations are due to defective maturation of the jugular bulb, which is due to regression of the embryonic sinus around the occiput. The malformations only affect sigmoid sinuses with secondary arteriovenous communications, are usually easy to treat, and have a good prognosis.

Vein of Galen aneurysmal malformations and malformations of the dural sinuses are the only two true intracranial malformations that we have diagnosed antenatally on ultrasound. Failure to detect pial arteriovenous malformations (AVMs) before birth suggests that they only appear secondarily, after age 2 years, when the brain is more mature and the vulnerable period has finished or that they may be dormant and only manifest clinically later in life. Very rarely pial AVM are diagnosed neonatally but they represent less than 1% of all AVMs seen in our center at Bicêtre, and 5% of those brain AVMs seen in children below 15 years.

Familial lesions

There are no familial disorders that cause AVMs. Although one of the phenotypes of Rendu–Osler disease, which preferentially affects the head, neck, and sometimes the lungs, is associated with cerebral vascular lesions, these lesions are not inherited and seem to follow an independent distribution among families. The AVMs found in children carrying the Rendu–Osler disease all conform to a specific architecture: focal or multifocal fistulae with high flow rates and large venous ectasia. Signs appear later on in life with

mental deficiency or more seldom hemorrhage. They are well tolerated for many years. There is no aneurysmal malformation of the vein of Galen in either child or adult carriers of the Rendu–Osler disease. Their flow rate and the lack of cardiac effects suggest that the AVMs do not become active until early childhood, once again after the age of 2 years. Murmurs can be heard on skull auscultation, but children fail to complain about them because they are a part of their primary acoustic environment. Diagnosis is made after having established the family history, with epistaxis in parents and other relatives. Mucocutaneous telangiectasia, although characteristic of the disease in adults, is not present at this age.

Cavernomas[1,4,5] are focal or multifocal venous malformations that may be familial but that rarely occur in children. They are usually small, well-delineated, intraparenchymal lesions that spontaneously appear as dense lesions, which enhance well with contrast, but are angiographically occult. Nevertheless, their diagnosis must be considered when facing relatively well-tolerated intracerebral hemorrhage (or more rarely intraventricular hemorrhage) in infants presenting with convulsions (Fig. 9.20). In familial forms, multiple cavernomas can appear *de novo* over the course of time. This is a further example of a dormant genetic disorder that requires either a second mutation or an unknown triggering factor to become active.

Familial forms of aneurysm are rare, and mainly found in dominant renal polycystic disease. Recessive forms can nevertheless be found in children. Subarachnoid hemorrhage is usually the initial presenting sign. When these malformations do exist in the pediatric population, they occur mainly in children aged 5 years or more and infants are rarely affected. Familial forms of aneurysm with no known genetic disorder have been reported. However, the ratio of children presenting with intracranial hemorrhage is no higher among these families than in the general population. Consequently, it is difficult to recommend systematic screening of the members of a family; in addition, it is difficult to provide guidelines on the frequency of follow-up examinations. Thus, the mere fact of belonging to a family in which several relatives are affected with aneurysms does not necessarily imply that a child will develop aneurysms during his or her early years, much less during the neonatal period.

Sporadic lesions

Sporadic lesions can be linked to congenital diseases as defined above, with an initial defect that is deciphered secondarily. The structural lesion may be detected or cause clinical signs at any stage of life.

Clinical presentation and management of intracranial arteriovenous shunts

ANEURYSMAL MALFORMATIONS OF THE VEIN OF GALEN

The natural history of aneurysmal malformations of the vein of Galen is now thoroughly understood and appropriate management of these disorders yields satisfactory results[2]. While about half the aneurysmal malformations of the vein of Galen are diagnosed before birth, the first clinical signs (systemic disorders) appear after birth and vary in their severity. Conditions range from heart failure with acute multi-organ failure and cerebromalacia that began *in utero*, to the accidental discovery of an enlarged cardiac silhouette with neither respiratory signs nor consequences on feeding. Clinical management depends on the severity of the clinical manifestations. Diagnosis is often easily made by auscultation of the skull, cranial ultrasound, CT scan or MRI. Angiography is not indicated for diagnostic purposes, as it will be performed with the first treatment. Lesions that are identified early on usually have a good prognosis: most infants who have aneurysmal malformations of the vein of Galen thrive until the age of 5 or 6 months, at which time endovascular treatment should begin regardless of the symptoms. Infants with heart failure require medical treatment (digitalis and diuretics or diuretics alone) until they can be embolized, which will also stabilize their hemodynamic status. More severe forms with intractable cardiac failure may require earlier or even immediate embolization of the main shunts. These infants may be identified using a neonatal score that we have developed over the last 10 years. The object of urgent intervention is to disconnect at least 30% of the initial malformation so as to bring the infant to a clinically stable condition. A more complete treatment can be performed later with more technical ease and with less risk for subsequent neurocognitive impairment. Contraindications to treatment are a poor initial neurological score and evidence of brain damage on imaging, both a reflection on the severity of multiple organ failure (Fig. 12.2). Embolization, when it is well performed, produces satisfactory results in this type of disorder.

Aneurysmal malformations of vein of Galen cause venous hemodynamic disorders that induce macrocrania or ventriculomegaly (Figs 12.4 and 12.5). The ventricular enlargement is not caused by compression of the aqueduct but by venous sinus congestion; later it may be secondary to atrophy of the brain. Although surgical ventricular drainage may temporarily solve the clinical problems due to intracranial hypertension it does not treat the venous hypertension. Transarterial endovascular treatment is the treatment of choice for it deals with venous hypertension, the basic cause of the lesion. Embolization must be performed before the symptoms become irreversible. Only by anticipating each stage in the natural history of the disease can severe consequences such as neurocognitive retardation, epileptic seizures and hemorrhage (secondary to occlusion of the jugular bulb and retrograde pial venous flow) be avoided. Embolization has its own complications. Stroke may occur from inadvertent embolization of arteries supplying functional tissue or iatrogenic compromise of the venous outlets.

MALFORMATIONS OF THE DURAL SINUS

Approximately one-third of dural sinus malformations are diagnosed *in utero*. They appear as a large sac that may already be thrombosed. This can rapidly cause diffuse bilateral cerebral venous ischemia as a result of venous hypertension. A consumption coagulopathy may also develop secondary to the large volume of coagulated blood within the sac. Moderate cardiac hypertrophy may develop later in infancy. Even when arteriovenous communications in the walls of the malformed sinuses do exist (Fig. 12.11), the prognosis depends on the alternative drainage for cerebral venous blood. An infant's vascular system has not yet acquired the capacity to drain cerebral venous blood into the cavernous sinus, and consequently cortical veins are affected by thrombosis within the malformation. Thrombosis usually develops 2–3 months after birth, later if the sinus lesion is lateral. The use of anticoagulants is generally resorted to at this point, for it is more efficient than endovascular or surgical reconstruction of the sinuses and stabilizes the situation while allowing maturation, however late it may be, of the sinus. These malformations have a severe prognosis. Diagnosis is often made in the presence of macrocrania due to the size of the lesion. Cranial murmurs may not be heard on auscultation. Formal diagnosis is made with cranial ultrasound performed through the fontanel, and confirmed by the MRI and the CT scan.

CEREBRAL (PIAL) VASCULAR MALFORMATIONS (FIG. 12.10)

These are very rare in neonates and infants. They tend to present with clinical convulsions as a result of irritation or from ischemia of the cerebral veins on the cortex (Fig. 12.7). In infants, they are usually identified following a hemorrhage (Fig. 12.8), more often than by the presence of neurodevelopmental delay. Hemorrhage combined with

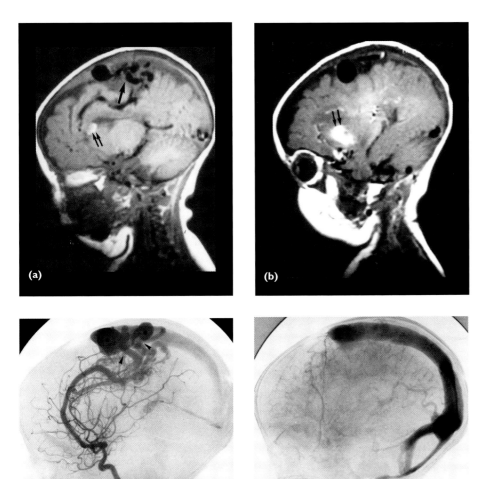

Fig. 12.7 Three-month-old baby presenting with seizures. T1 weighted MRI in sagittal views **(a, b)** shows an AVM (*arrow*, **a**) in the posterior part of the frontal lobe. Diffuse hemorrhagic infarcts (*double arrows*, **a, b**) are noted remote from the shunt. Angiography **(c, d)** demonstrated an AVM of fistulous type (*arrowheads*, **c**) draining into venous ectasias (*asterisks*, **c**). Poor hemispheric venous drainage was apparent because of the venous congestion in the pathological venous system and in the superior sagittal sinus **(d)**.

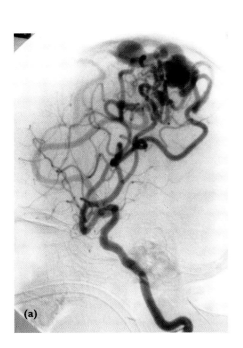
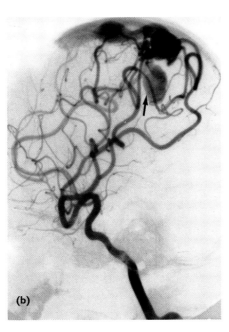

Fig. 12.8 A 3-day-old neonate presenting with seizures. A brain AVM was diagnosed at MRI (not shown) and confirmed at angiography **(a)**. Embolization was planned but could not be performed because of intracranial hemorrhage. Analysis of the angio-architecture of the lesion after this hemorrhagic stroke **(b)** revealed an annexed venous false aneurysm (*arrow*) pointing to the exact rupture point of the AVM.

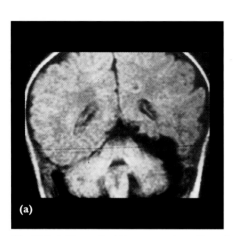
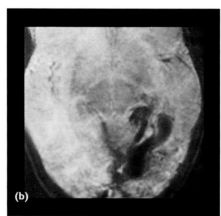
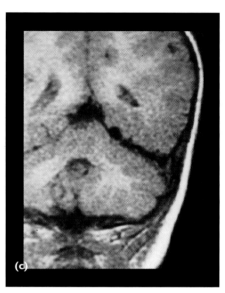

Fig. 12.9 A 20-month-old boy presenting with cardiac failure treated by digitalis and diuretics. Ultrasound of the brain detected a probable temporal AVM, confirmed by T1 weighted MRI in coronal **(a)** and axial **(b)** planes. Embolization was performed in order to counterbalance the effects of this high-flow AVM on the maturing brain. A repeat MRI **(c)** confirmed the subtotal occlusion of the AVM and the normal aspect of the brain parenchyma. Total occlusion of the lesion was obtained with a later procedure.

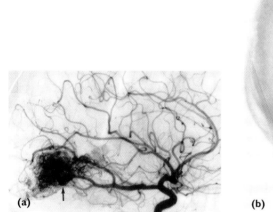
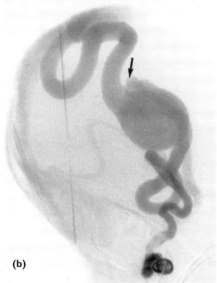
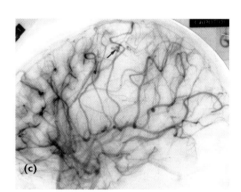

Fig. 12.10 Different architectural types of brain AVMs that can be encountered in the pediatric population: nidus type **(a)** with interposition of a pathological vascular network (*arrow*) between feeding arteries and draining veins; fistula type **(b)** with direct communication (*arrow*) between an enlarged artery and an ectatic vein; micro-AVM type (*arrow*, **c**) with normal-sized artery draining into a normal-sized vein.

suggestive findings on a CT scan and especially the MRI should lead to emergency endovascular treatment, even in neonates, to prevent focal brain 'melting'. We maintain that although symptoms caused by aneurysmal malformation of vein of Galen often do not require immediate attention, rapid intervention is mandatory in confirmed true cerebral malformations (Fig. 12.6).

The growth and maturation of both the vascular system and brain at this age influence the management of vascular lesions. Indeed, whereas aneurysms and AVMs are relatively stable in adults, in children they are continually changing. Potential spontaneous remodeling, the extreme case being spontaneous thrombosis, or florid angiogenesis may not necessarily lead to rapid and total exclusion of the lesions. The

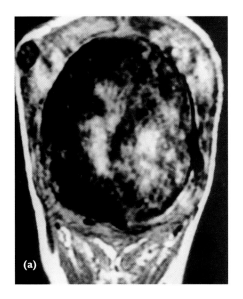

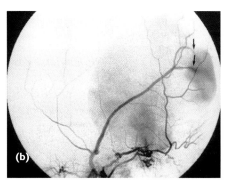

Fig. 12.11 Dural sinus malformation diagnosed in an infant. T1 weighted MRI shows the giant venous lake corresponding to the malformed sinus **(a)**, confirmed at angiography **(b)**. Arteriovenous shunts into the malformation, fed by the middle meningeal artery (*arrows*) are demonstrated.

current therapeutic objective is the minimum procedure that will ensure normal growth and maturation of the nervous system whilst preventing hemorrhage (Fig. 12.9). Experience shows that transarterial endovascular treatment is more flexible than surgery or radiotherapy and is associated with a low morbidity. Several procedures can be performed over a period of time and adjusted to the maturational stage of the brain.

ANEURYSMS

Very few aneurysms can be called 'congenital' apart from those that occur in fetal life due to inabilities to remodel the vascular system. This is illustrated by the small number of aneurysms diagnosed during infancy[1,2,4,5]. Aneurysms are mainly classified according to their site.

'Spontaneous' aneurysms (non-traumatic) are divided into giant and non-giant aneurysms. An appearance of pseudodissection is often seen. A further category includes postinfectious and mycotic aneurysms, very rare occurrences in comparison with the prevalence of infection in the pediatric population. These aneurysms are often multiple. The type of infection that causes mycotic cerebral vascular lesions (meningitis, encephalitis or septicemia) is still unclear. Some multiple forms of aneurysm are linked to immune deficiencies transmitted *in utero* or acquired later in infancy, for example familial candidiasis, HIV infection.

When aneurysms are not found incidentally, the main presenting sign is intracranial hemorrhage and sometimes compression. The latter will cause a variety of symptoms depending on the site and size of the aneurysm. Focal neurological signs may be secondary to the volume of the lesion, but may also occur secondary to thrombosis or due to distal emboli sent out by the aneurysmal sac.

Conclusions

The technical management of congenital vascular disorders has been greatly modified over the past few years. The complete obliteration of lesions for 'cosmetic' purposes used to be the main objective. At times, its clinical toll was too high. Today, care and management of patients with vascular disorders is clearly multidisciplinary and involves neuropediatricians, interventional neuroradiologists and neurosurgeons who may, if need be, complete the endovascular treatment. Clinical follow-up examinations in a neuropediatric clinic are mandatory to assess the team's previous decisions and measure results over the course of time. Although vascular lesions were thought to be rare several years back, they form an important part of Bicêtre's activity (Table 12.4).

Techniques have become more precise because of the development of the finer, more supple and more hydrophilic

Table 12.4 Breakdown of vascular diseases managed per age group (458 cases <16 years) Bicêtre 1985–1998

Vein of Galen aneurysmal malformation (n = 213)	Neonates 95	Infants 83	Children 35
Dural sinus malformation and arteriovenous shunts (n = 29)	Neonates 8	Infants 14	Children 7
Pial arteriovenous shunts (n = 197)	Neonates 7	Infants 25	Children 165
Arterial aneurysms (n = 19)	–	Infants 4	Children 15

microcatheters. Our objectives and the time required to reach them have been modified by a better understanding of the natural history and of the etiology of the disorders. Our therapeutic goal is to allow the child's normal neurological development and normal brain maturation whilst minimizing the risk of complications from the lesion, for example hemorrhage.

Summary

- 'Congenital vascular malformation' is a biological concept rather than a structural one. Malformations can be present and detected *in utero*, but in most instances they appear to be 'triggered' and revealed postnatally.

- Two lesions may be diagnosed *in utero*: the vein of Galen aneurysmal malformation and dural sinus malformation.

- Cerebral arteriovenous malformations and arterial aneurysms are diagnosed much later during life.

- During the first 2 years of life there is significant cardiovascular maturation, as well as cerebral venous and dural sinus maturation. The brain is very vulnerable to ischemic injury during this period. Management of any malformation must allow for satisfactory brain maturation.

- Brain damage from vascular malformations during this period usually arises from ischemia secondary to venous congestion or thrombosis.

- Ventriculomegaly is primarily caused by venous congestion, but it may occur later as a result of cerebral atrophy. In some cases an active hydrocephalus may develop.

- Treatment of these lesions is optimally by a transarterial endovascular approach at all stages of the diseases.

- Familial vascular diseases are rarely diagnosed in the perinatal period. In particular, familial diseases giving aneurysms lead to arterial problems in adulthood, which most likely require a secondary mutation to reveal the underlying genetic defect.

References

1. Edwards M and Hoffman H (1989) *Cerebral Vascular Disease in Children and Adolescents*. Baltimore, Williams & Wilkins.
2. Lasjaunias P (1997) *Vascular Disease in Neonates, Infants and Children. Interventional Neuroradiology Management*. Berlin, Springer.
3. Levene M, Lilford R, Bennett M *et al.* (1995) *Fetal and Neonatal Neurology and Neurosurgery*. Edinburgh, Churchill Livingstone.
4. Raimondi A, Choux M and di Rocco C (1991) *Cerebrovascular Diseases in Children*. New York, Springer.
5. Roach ES and Riela AR (1995) *Pediatric Cerebrovascular Disorders*. New York, Futura.

Non-accidental head injury in the young infant

Maeve McPhillips

Contents

Head injury is a leading cause of morbidity and mortality in children. In the absence of a history of significant accidental trauma, up to 95% of serious head injury in children less than 1 year is caused by abuse[3].

Mechanism of injury

Caffey described the effects of shaking on infants, and its association with bilateral retinal hemorrhage and the typical metaphyseal corner fracture[7]. His theory of whiplash-shaking was supported by the finding of bilateral subdural hemorrhage, and the frequent absence of evidence of impact injury. It is true that while it is unusual to slap or spank an infant, the significance of shaking or jerking has only been realized in recent times. Shaking produces repeated acceleration–deceleration forces, so-called whiplash, mainly in an antero-posterior direction, but the brain will also rotate within the calvarium, as a secondary motion. These movements can cause tearing of the delicate bridging veins, which course from the cerebral cortex, through the subarachnoid space and the potential subdural space, to drain into the venous sinuses. This results in hemorrhage into the subarachnoid or subdural spaces (Fig. 13.3b,e) or both. The infant brain is more at risk from a shaking injury due to its greater relative weight, the lack of tone in the supporting muscles of the neck, and the poor myelination associated with a higher water content. The relative degree of myelination contributes to the development of shearing injuries, most com-

monly at the gray–white interface, with a subcortical or callosal location. This may be a reflection of the different densities of gray and white matter.

There is often controversy as to the precise mechanism of injury, whether it be a pure shaking-whiplash injury, or whether there is an additional impact injury. The forces generated with an impact are of an order of magnitude greater than with shaking[9]. Impact against a soft surface, such as a mattress or sofa, does not significantly reduce the effect of the impact, but it does dissipate the trauma. Therefore the resulting signs of external injury are few, and there is no evidence of a focal impact type cerebral injury. However, it is accepted that the forces generated during a vigorous shaking alone are sufficient to cause devastating cerebral damage[5]. The American Academy of Pediatrics Committee on Child Abuse describes such an act as 'so violent that competent individuals observing would recognize it as dangerous'[1].

Primary injury

Primary injury is that which is caused by the trauma itself. The most subtle finding is that of subarachnoid blood. This is well described on computed tomography (CT), and has a typical location in the interhemispheric fissure posteriorly. It is recognizable as subarachnoid in location as the blood can be seen in the parasagittal sulci of the cerebral hemispheres. Recognizable blood in the basal cisterns and around the brain stem is unusual in abuse, and is more suggestive of a

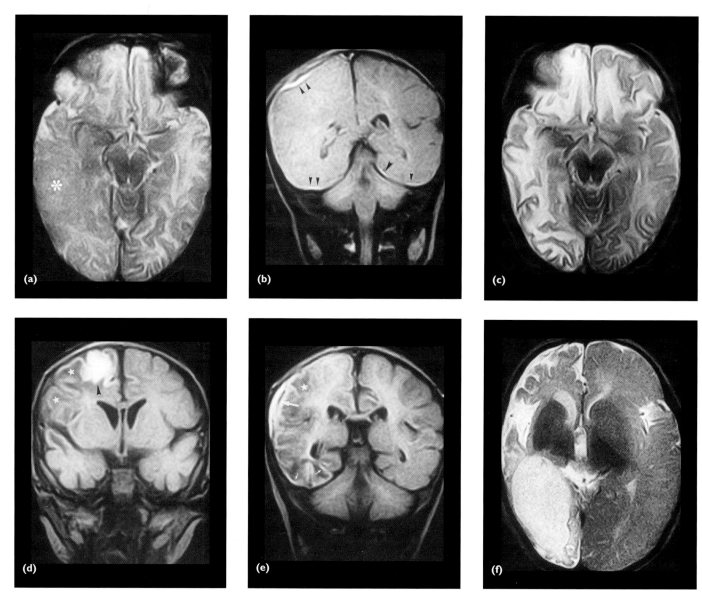

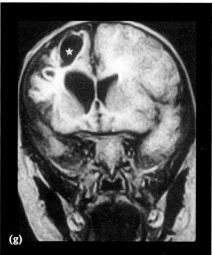

Fig. 13.1 37-day-old infant presenting with a tense fontanel and fits. All examinations performed on Picker Outlook 0.23 system. **(a)** T2 weighted (FSE 5100/80; FA 90°) sequence, transverse plane. Presentation scan. There is loss of the normal gray–white matter differentiation on the right (*asterisk*), sparing the frontal lobe and the occipital lobes. The left hemisphere is normal. **(b)** FLAIR (IRSE 3564(1600)/120 FA 90°) sequence, coronal plane. Loss of gray–white matter differentiation involving the right hemisphere, with some compression of the right lateral ventricle. High signal is seen over the convexity on the right and in the subtemporal region bilaterally (*arrowheads*), representing subdural hemorrhage. **(c)** T2 weighted (FSE 5100/80 FA 90°) sequence, transverse plane. Scan 10 days after presentation. There is increased intensity of the white matter of the right cerebral hemisphere, and of the frontal lobe on the left. Sulci are prominent, due to early loss of cerebral substance. **(d)** FLAIR (IRSE 3564 (1600)/120 FA 90°) sequence, coronal plane. There is reduced intensity of the parietal white matter on the right (*stars*), but the deep gray matter has been spared. There is a high intensity lesion in the right para-sagittal region (*arrowhead*) which appears to extend to the cortex. This is consistent with a white matter tear. **(e)** FLAIR (IRSE 3564 (1600)/120 FA90°) sequence, coronal plane. A more posterior image from the same examination shows a high intensity subdural hemorrhage over the right lateral parietal convexity (*thick arrow*). There is also increased intensity of the gyri on the right (*thin arrows*), and poor gray–white matter differentiation (*star*) compared to the normal left hemisphere. **(f)** T2 weighted (FSE 5100/80 FA 90°) sequence, transverse plane. Scan 9 months after presentation. The left cerebral hemisphere remains normal at this level. There is extensive atrophy on the right, sparing only the basal ganglia. There is white matter loss and prominence of the sulci. There is marked dilatation of the occipital horn of the right lateral ventricle. **(g)** FLAIR (IRSE 3564(1600)/120 FA90°) sequence, coronal plane. The previously noted white matter tear is now seen as a low intensity cystic area (*star*) surrounded by high signal gliosis. Again the white matter loss and atrophy of the right cerebral hemisphere is visible. The lateral ventricle is dilated. The hemicranium on the right is also smaller.

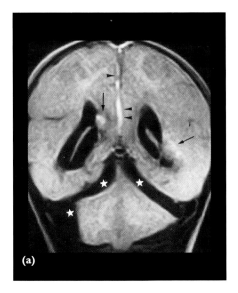
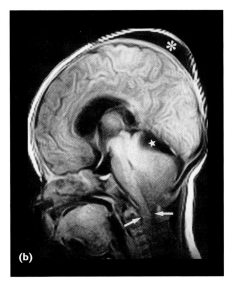
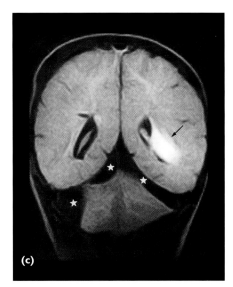
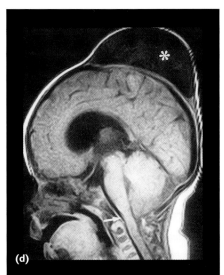

Fig. 13.2 A 26-day infant presenting with a high-pitched cry. She had an increasing head circumference and her eyes showed 'sunsetting'. There was occipital and facial swelling. Skeletal survey showed rib fractures and a periosteal reaction along the left humerus. **(a)** FLAIR (IRSE 3567(1600)/120 FA 90°) sequence, coronal plane, 24 h after presentation. There is high intensity in the interhemispheric fissure on this posterior image (*arrowheads*), indicating subdural hemorrhage. Bilateral infratentorial low-intensity collections are also visible (*stars*). There was herniation of the cranio-cervical junction on the sagittal images. There is ill-defined high intensity in the subependymal regions of both lateral ventricles (*arrows*) suggesting hemorrhage from shearing injury. **(b)** T1 weighted (FE 3D 35/13 FA 40°) sequence, sagittal plane. Examination obtained 10 days after presentation. There is a low intensity posterior fossa subdural collection (*star*) with herniation of the cranio-cervical junction (*arrows*), which was seen on the presentation images also. There is a subgaleal collection over the vertex (*asterisk*). **(c)** FLAIR (IRSE 3567(1600)/120 FA 90°) sequence, coronal plane. Bilateral low-intensity collections in the posterior fossa (*stars*). The left sided subependymal high intensity has developed into obvious hemorrhage (*arrow*). **(d)** T1 weighted (FE 3D 35/13 FA 40°) sequence, sagittal plane. Follow-up examination obtained 10 weeks after presentation. There is a large persisting subgaleal collection (*asterisk*). The position of the cranio-cervical junction has returned to normal (*arrow*). The posterior fossa collections have resolved.

ruptured aneurysm. The previous relative insensitivity of magnetic resonance (MR) scanning to the presence of subarachnoid blood is one of the major reasons why CT scanning is still regarded as the most appropriate modality in the imaging of the acute phase of suspected non-accidental injury. However, with the advent of fluid-attenuated inversion recovery (FLAIR) sequences, which suppress the normal high signal from fluid in an otherwise T2 weighted sequence, small amounts of subarachnoid blood have become visible on MR[16].

SUBDURAL HEMORRHAGE

Subdural hemorrhage is a hallmark of non-accidental shaking head injury. The blood is usually bilateral, and is described as being visible typically in the interhemispheric fissure (Fig. 13.2a). Since MR, with its multiplanar capabilities and lack of bony artifact, has become more widely used in the assessment of non-accidental injury, it is recognized that the subdural blood is usually a continuous collection and so is visible over the convexity, and in the subtemporal and subfrontal regions (Figs 13.1b and 13.3b). Hemorrhage may be seen on either side of the tentorium, as well as along the falx. Posterior fossa subdurals may be found, although uncommonly (Fig. 13.2a,b,c).

Subdural collections may show loculation, septation or fluid–fluid levels. This is often thought to imply repeated injury or hemorrhage. The evolution of a subdural hemorrhage which was uniform in intensity at initial imaging may, however, show apparent loculation with varying intensities,

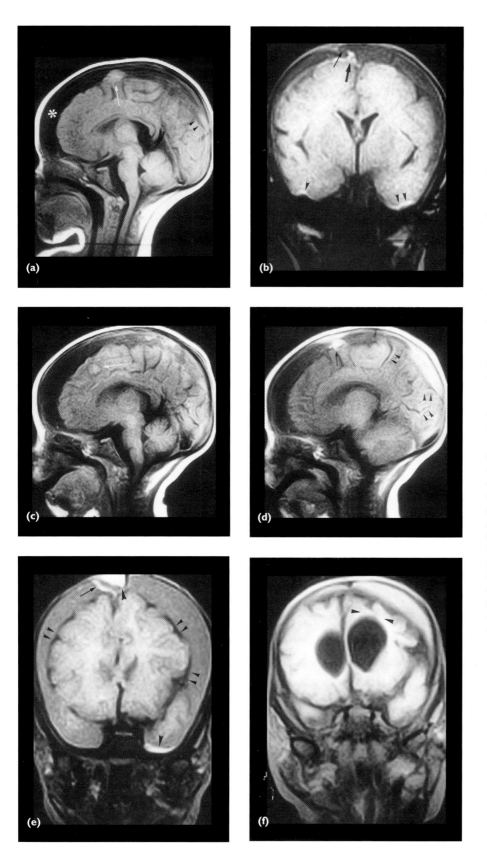

Fig. 13.3 A 6-week-old infant presenting with convulsions. Skeletal survey showed a spiral fracture of the tibia. **(a)** T1 weighted (FE 3D 75/28 FA 110°) sequence, sagittal plane. Presentation scan. There is widening of the pericerebral space (*asterisk*), with increasing intensity posteriorly (*arrowheads*), in keeping with layering of a subdural hemorrhage. In addition there is a focal area of high intensity over the fronto-parietal convexity (*arrow*), suggesting focal clot formation. **(b)** FLAIR (IRSE 3564(1600)/ 120 FA 90°) sequence, coronal plane. The increased intensity of subdural hemorrhage is seen in the subtemporal region bilaterally (*arrowheads*). In the right fronto-parietal region there is focal high signal (*arrow*), in keeping with clot, and the suggestion of a visible bridging vein (*thin arrow*). **(c)** T1 weighted (SE 3D 75/21 FA 110°) sequence, sagittal plane. Six days after presentation. This left para-sagittal image shows irregular increase in intensity posteriorly. In the fronto-parietal subcortical white matter there is ill-defined increase in intensity (*arrow*) representing a white matter tear. **(d)** T1 weighted (SE 3D 75/21 FA 110°) sequence, sagittal plane. This slightly more lateral image shows the variable intensity of the subdural hemorrhage, and the constant focal high signal over the fronto-parietal surface (*arrow*). There is also high signal from the occipital and parietal gyri (*arrowheads*). **(e)** FLAIR (IRSE 3564(1600)/120 FA 90°) sequence, coronal plane. Clear CSF is seen as low intensity in the enlarged subarachnoid space (*small arrowheads*). It is seen separately from the subdural space due to the different intensity of their contents. The subdural space is of medium intensity due to the presence of blood products, with focal areas of high intensity persisting in the left subtemporal and right para-falcine locations (*large arrowheads*). Again the suspected bridging vein is seen (*thin arrow*). **(f)** FLAIR (IRSE 3567(1600)/120 FA 90°) sequence, coronal plane. Two months after presentation. There is generalized atrophy with dilatation of the lateral ventricles and prominence of the sulci. There is focal atrophy on the left in the region of the previous white matter tear (*arrowheads*). There is residual high signal in the subdural space, more so on the left.

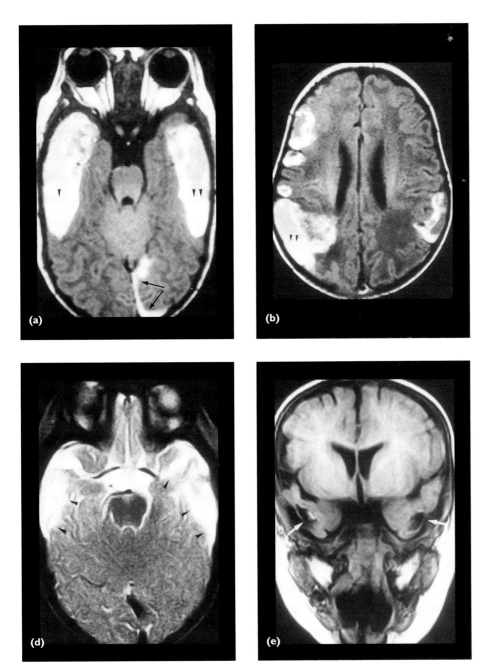

(a) **(b)** **(c)**

(d) **(e)**

interhemispheric subdural hemorrhage seen as a high intensity stripe (*arrows*). There are bilateral temporal hemorrhagic contusions, with layering of blood products faintly visible within (*arrowheads*). **(b)** T1 weighted (SE 600/15) sequence, transverse plane. A more cranial image shows further areas of contusion in the parieto-occipital region bilaterally, worse on the right, where layering of blood products is visible (*arrowheads*). **(c)** T1 weighted (SE 600/15) sequence, transverse plane. Two weeks after initial scan. High signal intensity around the periphery of the bitemporal hemorrhagic contusions (*arrowheads*), with clearing of the central area seen as low intensity (*asterisks*). There is reduced signal seen in the adjacent uninvolved white matter (*star*) in keeping with changes of encephalomalacia. **(d)** T2 weighted (FSE 5100/80 FA 90°) sequence, transverse plane. Follow-up scan 7 months after presentation. There is high signal in the temporal lobes bilaterally, in keeping with cystic encephalomalacia (*arrowheads*), but the remainder of the brain appears remarkably normal. **(e)** FLAIR (IRSE 3567(1600)/120 FA 90°) sequence, coronal plane. The temporal lobes are small and atrophied (*arrows*) with some dark areas of cystic change.

Fig. 13.4 A 6-week-old infant referred because of facial bruising. Fitting on admission. **(a)** T1 weighted (SE 600/15) sequence, transverse plane. Scan obtained 2 days after presentation. There is a left-sided posterior

and the intensity may vary from anterior to posterior, or, indeed, from one side to the other (Fig. 13.3d,e)[15]. This is particularly seen in large collections. It is therefore important for future reference and for estimating the age of the hematoma, to obtain an early scan. Ideally, this should be done before any invasive procedure such as insertion of an access device or diagnostic or therapeutic aspiration.

Much work has been done on the temporal evolution of the intensity of intracerebral hemorrhage[4] (see Chapter 9).

Hyperacute subdural hemorrhage may be of high, low or iso-intensity on T1 weighted images. It will be high intensity on T2 weighted images, but thin collections may not be readily visible with this sequence (Fig. 13.1a). The FLAIR sequence which suppresses the high signal of normal CSF has been of particular use in very recent hemorrhage (Fig. 13.1b). The typical acute (1–3 days) subdural hemorrhage is low intensity on both T1 and T2 or FLAIR images, evolving to high intensity on these sequences in the late subacute (1–2 weeks) phase.

Unfortunately due to several possible reasons, blood in the extra-axial spaces does not always appear to behave in a totally predictable fashion (see chapter 9). High intensity may persist longer than expected (Fig. 13.2a and 13.4a). This may be because of the higher oxygen concentration in the sub-arachnoid space, because of layering within large collections, or because of a dilutional effect of CSF[15]. It may also reflect repeated bleeds, perhaps associated with therapeutic subdural aspirations. As there is rarely a precise history of the timing of the inflicted trauma in these cases, it is difficult to study the temporal evolution of the intensity of extra-axial hemorrhage.

INTRACEREBRAL INJURY

Primary injury to the cerebrum itself occurs by a contusion as a result of a focal impact, by shearing of white matter due to acceleration during shaking or deceleration on impact, or rarely by compression.

Direct impact can cause cortical contusion without evidence of fracture, with an injury at the site of impact, and a contre-coup injury on the opposing aspect of the brain. The most common sites for cortical contusions are the antero-lateral and inferior surfaces of the frontal and temporal lobes. Rarely the infant's head may be compressed, with symmetrical contusions (Fig. 13.4). Hemorrhage associated with the contusion may show layering into different intensities, visible as a fluid–fluid level (Fig. 13.4a,b). A hyperintense margin on T1 imaging is likely to be due to the presence of met-hemoglobin in the wall of the hemorrhage. The long-term outcome following contusion can vary, from marked atrophy and encephalomalacia to a surprising degree of recovery from an apparently devastating hemorrhage (Fig. 13.4d).

Diffuse axonal injury (DAI) is caused by shearing of the white matter, typically at the gray–white matter junction. It can also be seen in the corpus collosum, the basal ganglia, the subependymal region and in the brain stem (Fig. 13.2a). Hemorrhagic contusion is best seen as hyperintense petechial hemorrhage on T1 images, or hypointensities on T2 images. In the absence of hemorrhage, FLAIR images show DAI as hyperintensities. Resolution is with focal or diffuse atrophy with gliosis and encephalomalacia.

White matter tears are well recognized, and well seen on ultrasound[12]. These are seen in the anterior parietal or frontal lobes (Figs 13.1d and 13.3c), and, again, may be hemorrhagic or non-hemorrhagic[18]. They probably represent a more marked shearing injury. Located in the subcortical white matter they may, rarely, extend to the cortex. Hemorrhagic tears may show fluid–fluid level formation. Healing is by cyst formation (Fig. 13.1g) or total collapse of the damaged area (Fig. 13.3f), which at autopsy may look like artifactual cleft formation.

Secondary injury

Secondary injury occurs as an indirect result of trauma. It is associated with raised intracranial pressure and may be seen as cerebral edema, diffuse brain swelling due to hyperemia, or the spectrum of hypoxia–ischemia.

EDEMA

The mechanisms by which cerebral edema occurs are not well understood. Edema is seen as a consequence of direct injury such as contusion or shearing. It has been postulated that there may be an element of strangulation or suffocation associated with the inflicted injury, but this cannot be substantiated. Vascular occlusion, arterial or venous, may occur due to entrapment of vessels by herniation.

Diffuse brain swelling is associated with rapid neurological deterioration to a Glasgow Coma Score (GCS) of 3–5. Despite being labelled as diffuse it is frequently confined to one hemisphere. It does not seem to be due to edema, or increase in water volume, as it has been shown on CT not to be associated with a decrease in density[6]. The swelling is therefore due to an increase in blood volume due to increased blood flow, or hyperemia. Bruce demonstrated increased cerebral blood flow in six patients with diffuse cerebral swelling, which reverted to normal when the swelling was no longer visible. How this comes about is unclear. It is possible that it is a reactive hyperemia in response to an episode of reduced perfusion or prolonged fitting. Trauma to the brain stem may produce chemical mediators which cause changes in capillary permeability. Defective autoregulation is unlikely to be responsible, as there would be accompanying raised systemic blood pressure in the presence of the raised intracranial pressure in these infants. If the injured infant survives the initial stage of diffuse brain swelling, a second stage of edema is seen some 3 days later. This then progresses to loss of cerebral bulk, with enlarged extra-axial fluid spaces and apparent atrophy. In up to 43% there is possible recovery of brain substance, perhaps as denatured myelin is reconstituted and brain protein is replenished[6].

HYPOXIA–ISCHEMIA

The mechanism of the development of cerebral hypoxia–ischemia in the abused infant is not clear. It is postulated that the crying infant may be shaken into silence, which in fact is a period of apnea. Other factors may include deliberate strangulation or suffocation, or prolonged squeezing of the chest. The presence of rib fractures would be evidence for the latter. Gray matter and areas of active metabolism, such as active myelination, seem to be particularly at risk from hypoxia–ischemia.

MR findings of swelling, edema or hypoxic–ischemic change may be immediately visible or may be delayed. Diffuse cerebral swelling, which may be unilateral or bilateral, is seen as reduction in size of CSF spaces, with compression of the lateral ventricles being most obvious. Depending on the stage of evolution, gray–white matter differentiation may be lost (Fig. 13.1a,b). In the presence of edema and hypoxia–ischemia, gray matter will be hypointense on T1 weighted images, and hyperintense on T2 and FLAIR images, in keeping with an increased water content.

As early as 1 week after the initial insult, some infants with hypoxia–ischemia develop a pattern of subcortical hyperintensity on T1 weighted images, which is hypointense on T2 weighted images. The changes may persist for months, or may disappear within weeks. These findings have also been described on CT where the density may suggest calcification[19], but hemorrhagic change with hemosiderin formation could also account for the appearance[8,13].

In the longer term, cerebral atrophy becomes evident. There is great variability in the timing of its appearance, with earlier loss of brain substance associated with greater severity of the initial insult (Fig 13.1d, 13.3f, and 13.4e). There is widening of the extra-axial spaces, with increased prominence of the sulci, widening of the subarachnoid space and dilatation of the ventricles (Fig. 13.3e,f). Areas of previous hypoxic–ischemic change may be hyperintense on T2 weighted images, but hypointense on T1 and FLAIR images, in keeping with the changes of cystic encephalomalacia. Focal areas of porencephaly may also be seen where localized damage has resulted in cyst formation which may become confluent with the lateral ventricle.

Associated findings

Retinal hemorrhage is found in over 70% of non-accidental head injuries in infants. Typically bilateral in location, hemorrhage may be retinal, subretinal, preretinal, along the optic nerves or into the vitreous. Other retinal injuries such as folds, lacerations or detachments may be seen. The hemorrhages are thought to be due to a sudden rise in intravascular pressure associated with an increase in intrathoracic pressure during an episode of shaking or shaking-impact. They are not, however, pathognomonic of non-accidental injury as they may rarely be seen in severe decelerating head trauma such as deceleration injuries in road traffic accidents[14]. Cardiopulmonary resuscitation is recognized as a cause of retinal hemorrhage, though the incidence is disputed[11,14], through the same postulated mechanism of raised intrathoracic pressure.

Intracerebral injury can occur in the absence of obvious focal head trauma. The presence of facial or cranial bruising is, however, evidence of injury. Swelling may be from impact or from hair-pulling, and result in subgaleal collections (Fig. 13.2b,d). Skull fractures in non-accidental injury may be simple or complex. A simple fracture is linear, confined to one bone, well defined and usually less than 3 mm in width. A complex fracture may be branching or stellate, it can cross suture lines to involve more than one bone, or the fracture line may be diastased with separation of the edges.

Rib fractures in non-accidental injury usually occur from squeezing of the chest, commonly by adult hands. Less often they can occur by direct compression, such as kneeling on the chest. The rib may break at any point in the arc, but posterior rib fractures are perhaps the most common. They occur at the head of the rib where it articulates with the vertebral body or at the tubercle which articulates with the transverse process. Lateral and anterior rib fractures are more easily seen, while fractures of the costo-chondral junction may be difficult to see, even on oblique views[15]. Rib fractures which are not readily evident on a skeletal survey at the time of presentation, may be seen on a follow-up survey at 10–14 days, when callus renders them more obvious. Ultrasound has been suggested as a method of identifying rib fractures which are not obvious on radiographs[22].

Apart from the finding of long bone fractures which do not fit with the history provided, the classical fracture of non-accidental injury is the metaphyseal injury. This is a subtle fracture involving the metaphysis. Depending on the radiographic projection, it may appear as a corner fracture or a bucket-handle fracture. This pattern of fracture is due to flailing and twisting of the limbs during shaking, to pulling by an extremity or direct twisting of the limb. Again, a skeletal survey is needed to detect fractures, and in selected cases follow-up radiographs of suspected sites are useful to assess healing, and to aid in dating of injuries.

Differential diagnosis

Retinal hemorrhages are not pathognomonic of non-accidental injury. Goetting reports hemorrhages in 20–50% of newborns after vaginal delivery, but almost exclusively following a cephalad delivery, not breech[11]. He also reports an incidence of less than 1% after cesarian section. Baum found an incidence of 31% in newborns examined in the first 12 h of life, but the incidence dropped markedly in those whose eyes were first examined after 12 h of age, with an incidence of 15.5% in the first week[2]. It is generally accepted that retinal hemorrhages will have cleared within a month after delivery. Smith examined with MR a small group of full-term, vaginally delivered neonates who had documented retinal hemorrhage. None showed any evidence of intracranial injury[20].

Intracranial injury may be seen following a difficult or instrumental delivery. Subarachnoid and subdural hemorrhage is recognized in both normal breech and vacuum deliveries, typically in the posterior fossa[17]. Intraventricular hemorrhage may also be identified. In infants who are subsequently delivered normally, maternal injury in the prenatal period may cause intracranial injury in the fetus *in utero*[21].

Premature infants with subsequent intraventricular hemorrhage may develop communicating hydrocephalus with dilated ventricles and widening of the extra-axial spaces. It would seem likely that tearing of bridging veins would occur more readily in these circumstances, but this has not been proven scientifically[15]. In any case, the degree of force needed to cause intracranial hemorrhage would still be in excess of that used in normal care of infants.

Meningoencephalitis may initially present with an obtunded infant, where the possibility of non-accidental injury cannot be discounted. Widened extra-axial spaces may be identified, which on MR will show slightly increased intensity on T1 and FLAIR sequences, reflecting an increase in protein content, or the presence of inflammatory cells. Biochemical or cytological examination of the CSF may be able to distinguish meningoencephalitis from hemorrhage.

The presence of a coagulopathy may contribute to the development of subarachnoid or subdural hemorrhage, in the absence of a history of significant trauma. Again, laboratory testing should clarify the diagnosis.

Falls and accidental injuries do occur, but, in the absence of a history of severe trauma, are rarely associated with significant intracerebral injury. Subdural hemorrhage is seen following motor vehicle accidents, but is rare following falls or crush injury[10]. Extensive intracranial injury, when not accompanied by an appropriate history of severe trauma, should lead to the search for other corroborative evidence of inflicted injury.

Clinicians, and in particular radiologists, must not only be aware of the possibility of non-accidental injury, but search for it and alert colleagues to the possibility. It is also of utmost importance to be aware of the conditions to be considered in the possible differential diagnosis, and positively exclude them. Only in this way will children be protected both from abuse and from over-zealous protection.

Summary

- Magnetic resonance imaging of the brain is an essential part of the investigation of any infant with suspected non-accidental head injury.

- FLAIR images are recommended for the detection of acute subdural hemorrhage.

- The known patterns of abuse produce well-recognized intracranial pathology.

- Lesions in the brain may be primary or secondary.

- Evidence for pathology elsewhere in the body must always be sought to corroborate the diagnosis of non-accidental injury.

References

1. American Academy of Pediatrics (1993) Shaken baby syndrome: inflicted cerebral trauma. *Pediatrics* **92**, 872–875.
2. Baum JD and Bulpitt CJ (1970) Retinal and conjunctival hemorrhage in the newborn. *Arch Dis Child* **45**, 344–349.
3. Billmire ME and Myers PA (1985) Serious head injury in infants: accident or abuse? *Pediatrics* **75**, 340–342.
4. Bradley WG (1993) MR appearance of hemorrhage in the brain. *Radiology* **189**, 15–26.
5. Brown JK and Minns RA (1993) Non-accidental head injury, with particular reference to whiplash shaking injury and medico-legal aspects. *Dev Med Child Neurol* **35**, 849–869.
6. Bruce DA, Alavi A, Bilaniuk L *et al.* (1981) Diffuse cerebral swelling following head injuries in children: the syndrome of 'malignant brain edema'. *J Neurosurg* **54**, 170–178.
7. Caffey J (1972) On the theory and practice of shaking infants. *Amer J Dis Child* **124**, 161–169.
8. Close PJ and Carty HM (1991) Transient gyriform brightness on non-contrast enhanced computed tomography (CT) brain scan of seven infants. *Pediatr Radiol* **21**, 189–192.
9. Duhaime AC, Gennarelli TA, Thibault LE *et al.* (1987) The shaken baby syndrome. *J Neurosurg* **66**, 409–415.
10. Ewing-Cobbs L, Kramer L, Prasad M *et al.* (1998) Neuroimaging, physical and developmental findings after inflicted and noninflicted traumatic brain injury in young children. *Pediatrics* **102**, 300–307.
11. Goetting MG and Sowa B (1990) Retinal hemorrhage after cardiopulmonary resuscitation in children: an etiological reevaluation. *Pediatrics* **85**, 585–588.
12. Jaspan T, Narborough G, Punt JAG *et al.* (1992) Cerebral contusional tears as a marker of child abuse – detection by cranial sonography. *Pediatr Radiol* **22**, 237–245.
13. Jaspan T and Stevens KJ (1999) Radiological imaging of craniocerebral non-accidental injury in infancy. *RAD Magazine* **25(288)**, 66–69.
14. Kanter KK (1986) Retinal hemorrhage after cardiopulmonary resuscitation or child abuse. *J Pediatr* **108**, 430–432.
15. Kleinman PK and Barnes PD (1998) Head trauma. In: Kleinman PK

(Ed.) *Diagnostic Imaging of Child Abuse*, 2nd edn. St Louis: Mosby, pp. 296–325.

16. Noguchi K *et al.* (1995) Acute subarachnoid hemorrhage: MR imaging with fluid-attenuated inversion recovery pulse sequences. *Radiology* **196**, 773–777.

17. Odita JC and Hebi S (1996) CT and MRI characteristics of intracranial hemorrhage complicating breech and vacuum delivery. *Pediatr Radiol* **26**, 782–785.

18. Sato Y, Yuh WT, Smith WL *et al.* (1989) Head injury in child abuse; evaluation with MR imaging. *Radiology* **173**, 653–657.

19. Sener RN (1993) Gyral calcifications detected on the 45th day after cerebral infarction. *Pediatr Radiol* **23**, 570–571.

20. Smith WL, Alexander RC, Judisch GF *et al.* (1992) Magnetic resonance imaging evaluation of neonates with retinal hemorrhages. *Pediatrics* **89**, 332–333.

21. Stephens RP, Richardson AC and Lewin JS (1997) Bilateral subdural hematomas in a newborn infant. *Pediatrics* **99**, 619–621.

22. Wischhofer E, Fenkl R and Blum R (1995) Ultrasound detection of rib fractures for verifying fracture diagnosis. A pilot project. *Unfallchirug* **98(5)**, 296–300.

The neonate with a neuromuscular disorder

Eugenio Mercuri and Francesco Muntoni

Contents

Introduction

Neuromuscular disorders may present with hypotonia, weakness and/or contractures in the newborn period[10]. However, these may also be the presenting signs in infants with abnormalities of the central nervous system. With the easier access to brain MRI in the neonatal period, it is possible to identify those infants whose hypotonia is related to congenital or acquired brain lesions and those infants in whom there is both central and peripheral nervous system involvement. In many cases it is possible to differentiate infants with a primary neuromuscular disorder from those with involvement of the CNS by detailing the obstetric history, by careful observation and by performing a careful physical examination[10,12]. In this manner, only selected infants will need further investigation with imaging techniques.

Obstetric history and clinical assessment

Reduced fetal movements, breech presentation and polyhydramnios are frequently observed in children with weakness with onset *in utero*. Contractures, skin dimpling and poor dermatoglyphic patterns are all indicators of poor fetal movements and can provide information on the severity and timing of onset of the immobility. These signs are highly suggestive of a 'peripheral' lesion and with the exception of a few conditions are rarely associated with CNS involvement. The exceptions include those conditions that affect the fetus in the first months of pregnancy, such as neuronal migration disorders (e.g. bilateral opercular syndrome), or antenatal basal ganglia injury from a severe hypoxic–ischemic insult (e.g. attempted maternal suicide)[22].

The presence or absence of antigravity movements is also important. These have to be observed when the infant is at the peak of the activity, such as when crying or when in discomfort. While infants with neuromuscular disorders will show little change in their movement pattern in response to pain or when crying, children with CNS, metabolic or syndromic disorders may have a severely floppy posture which is interrupted by occasional antigravity movements. The distribution of wasting, weakness and hypotonia is also important, but might differ in individual conditions and only rarely can provide a diagnostic clue.

Reflexes are also an important part of the examination. Normal reflexes in a floppy infant almost exclude a severe peripheral neuropathy or motor neuron disorder and make a severe myopathy unlikely.

Other signs, such as an abnormal pattern of respiratory muscle involvement, major bulbar weakness with inability to suck and to clear secretions are frequently observed in children with some of the congenital myopathies, but can also be a feature of 'central' involvement, as observed in the infants with basal ganglia or brain stem lesions (see Chapter 6).

In this chapter we focus on the involvement of the central nervous system in infants with conditions that affect primarily the skeletal muscle or the motoneuron, or in diseases in which both central and peripheral nervous system are involved as part of more general multisystemic involvement.

Congenital muscular dystrophies

The term 'congenital muscular dystrophies' includes a group of disorders which share several clinical and pathological features such as contractures, weakness and hypotonia at birth or in the following few months and a dystrophic pattern on muscle biopsy. The spectrum of clinical signs in the neonatal period is variable, and in some of the congenital muscular dystrophy syndromes involvement of the CNS can dominate the clinical picture.

Three well-defined syndromes, Fukuyama congenital muscular dystrophy, Walker–Warburg syndrome, muscle–eye–brain disease, which are all associated with structural brain changes, were separated from a 'pure', or classical form of congenital muscular dystrophy, not associated with

structural brain changes by an International Consortium in 1993[11,13]. Imaging studies, however, have demonstrated that a proportion of children with 'pure' congenital muscular dystrophy showed white matter changes, and these changes were consistently related to the deficiency of the laminin α2 chain of merosin, an extracellular matrix protein. In contrast, children with normal expression of merosin were initially described as having a normal MRI[30]. More recently, however, there have been a few descriptions of other brain changes, such as cortical dysplasia and cerebellar hypoplasia, not only in the merosin-deficient group but also in the children with normal merosin, suggesting that the involvement of the brain in congenital muscular dystrophy is more complex than initially assumed[47]. Table 14.1 illustrates the current but ever growing classification of congenital muscular dystrophy based on clinical and MRI findings, and when known, on protein and molecular data.

FUKUYAMA CONGENITAL MUSCULAR DYSTROPHY

This form of muscular dystrophy was first described by Fukuyama *et al.* in 1960 and is almost exclusively confined to Japan[18]. The inheritance is autosomal recessive and the

Table 14.1 Classification of the congenital muscular dystrophies

Form	MRI findings	Protein	Molecular data
Fukuyama CMD	Mycropolymicrogyria, pachygyria, cerebellar involvement, abnormal signal in white matter	Fukutin	9q31
Walker–Warburg syndrome	Type II lyssencephaly, hydrocephalus, brainstem and cerebellar hypoplasia		
Muscle–eye–brain disease	Pachgyria and polymicrogiria		1p
	Brain stem and cerebellar hypoplasia, periventricular white matter frequent but not constantly observed		
CMD with primary merosin-deficiency			
Typical form	Diffuse white matter changes		
With cortical dysplasia	WM changes and cortical dysplasia	Laminin α2 (merosin)	6q2
With cerebellar hypoplasia	WM changes and cerebellar hypoplasia		
CMD with secondary merosin-deficiency			
With muscle hypertrophy, rigidity of the spine	Normal		1q-42
With severe phenotype and normal brain MRI	Normal		
With microcephaly and mental retardation	Normal		
With microcephaly, and cerebellar hypoplasia	Cerebellar hypoplasia		
With mental retardation and cerebellar cysts	Cerebellar cysts		
Merosin positive CMD			
Typical form	Normal or non-specific changes		
+ Mental retardation	Normal or non-specific changes		
+ Cerebellar hypoplasia	Cerebellar hypoplasia		

CMD, congenital muscular dystrophy; WM, white matter.

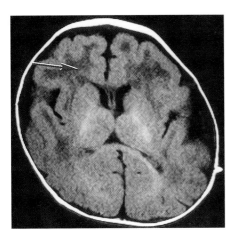

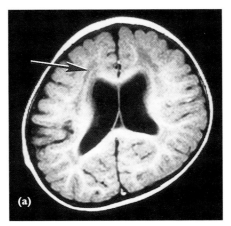

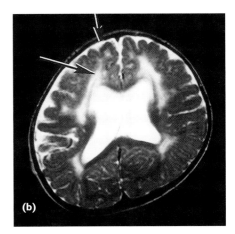

Fig. 14.1 Fukuyama muscular dystrophy (severe). Infant aged 7 months with the severe form of Fukuyama muscular dystrophy. The severe type makes up approximately 10% of all cases. The MRI appearances are more marked with more prominent white matter changes (*arrow*) that are clearly seen on the T1 weighted (SE 450/15) sequence. This infant also had a right-sided micro-ophthalmia and retinal detachment (*not shown*). (With permission, Professor Yukio Fukuyama.)

Fig. 14.2 Fukuyama muscular dystrophy. Infant aged 9 months of age. T1 weighted spin echo (SE 450/15) **(a)** and T2 weighted fast spin echo (FSE 4000/100) **(b)** sequences. There is abnormal signal intensity within the white matter. This is most marked in the frontal lobes (*long arrow*) and is more clearly seen on the T2 weighted images. The appearance of the frontal cortex is consistent with polymicrogyria (*short arrow*). This is also most clearly seen on the T2 weighted images. (With permission, Professor Yukio Fukuyama.)

locus has been assigned to chromosome 9. Recently, the gene responsible for this form has been identified and the protein product named fukutin. The clinical features of the Fukuyama congenital muscular dystrophy are early onset with mild to moderate hypotonia at birth and a progressive course with more increasing weakness, joint contractures, marked elevation of creatine kinase, moderate to severe mental retardation and frequent association with epilepsy. Ocular abnormalities, such as myopia and optic nerve atrophy occur in approximately 70% of these children but are rarely severe.

A severe form has been demonstrated in approximately 10% of cases (Fig. 14.1).

Brain MRI

MRI shows structural changes consisting of pachygyria and polymicrogyria and abnormal signal intensity within the white matter (Fig. 14.2). Sequential MRI studies have demonstrated that the abnormal white matter appearance is associated with delayed myelination rather than with dysmyelination or demyelination as the abnormal signal intensity improves with age. In fact, in these children myelination, though very delayed, still occurs, following the patterns normally observed at earlier ages in normal children. The frontal lobes are the last areas in which the abnormal signal persists. Ventricular dilatation has also been frequently recorded. Cerebellar hypoplasia may be seen but is not frequent[28].

Pathology

The abnormal cortex shows localized areas of pachygyria and polymicrogyria with markedly irregular arrangements of neurons. Areas of normal cortex can be observed. Recent studies in fetuses have suggested that a defect of the basement membrane might play a role in the genesis of the brain lesions[38].

WALKER–WARBURG SYNDROME

This is an autosomal recessive disorder characterized by the combination of muscular, brain and ocular involvement. The clinical picture can be very variable and signs of CNS involvement predominate[7-9]. Although milder phenotypes have been described, these infants generally show severe hypotonia, poor visual attention and decreased alertness. Muscle weakness in the first year of life can be mild. Serum creatine kinase can also be normal in the initial phases of the disorder or only mildly elevated, but tends to increase with age.

Muscle pathological studies show a dystrophic pattern but the changes may, however, be less severe with only minimal variation in fiber size in the first months of life.

Ocular abnormalities consist of retinal dysgenesis in all cases but other abnormalities such as microphthalmia, cataracts, optic nerve hypoplasia and anterior chamber malformations have also been described.

Brain MRI

Brain MRI shows a type II lissencephaly with the typical micropolygyric cobblestone cortex. Cerebellar hypoplasia, mainly affecting the vermis, is also a constant feature. White matter is also severely abnormal showing dysmyelination or cystic changes. Other features, such as brain stem hypoplasia, Dandy–Walker syndrome or encephaloceles have been described, in various combinations.

Pathology

The cobblestone cortex consists of cortical and leptomeningeal abnormalities. These abnormalities are more severe than the ones observed in Fukuyama and muscle–eye–brain disease. Some children have widespread agyria, whereas other show a combination of pachygyria and polymicrogyria with only small areas of agyria. The whole brain can be covered by glial tissue and the cortex completely disorganized with no horizontal layers.

CASE 14.1 WALKER–WARBURG SYNDROME

Perinatal history

This Indian male infant was born at 34 weeks' gestation by cesarian section. Early antenatal ultrasound scan detected cerebral ventricular dilatation. At birth the infant showed some dysmorphic features, such as torricephaly, small jaw and low set ears. He had poor visual alertness and did not feed well.

Clinical course

At 2 weeks a ventriculoperitoneal shunt was inserted because of an increasing head circumference. At 5 weeks he still showed generalized hypotonia and muscle weakness, more severe in the proximal distribution associated with mild anti-gravity strength in the limbs. The pattern of movements was very poor. There was some visual fixation but no tracking. Sucking movements were present but there was poor stripping.

Serum creatine kinase were markedly elevated (5620 IU).

At 3 months he showed a variable tone and better anti-gravity power in the limbs despite the persistent proximal weakness. Visual alertness was still very reduced but sucking had improved. Ophthalmology review demonstrated lamellar cataracts but no retinal abnormalities.

A muscle biopsy showed some variability in fiber size.

MRI

Brain MRI at 5 weeks (Fig. 14.3) demonstrated marked ventricular dilatation with a thickened featureless cortex, consis-

tent with type II lissencephaly. There was also hypoplasia of the brain stem and cerebellar hemispheres. The basal ganglia were rudimentary, the lateral and third ventricle were grossly enlarged.

MUSCLE–EYE–BRAIN DISEASE

Muscle–eye–brain disease is an autosomal recessive form of congenital muscular dystrophy originally described by Santavuori in 1977. It is relatively frequent in Finland and has been recently mapped to chromosome 1p.

Clinical signs are usually present at birth or in the first months of life. Late presentation is less common. Ocular abnormalities consist of myopia, retinal defects and abnormal electroretinogram. Some of the ocular symptoms can become evident only after the first years of life. These children show severe mental retardation and, often, epilepsy[35].

Brain MRI

Brain MRI shows extensive abnormalities of neuronal migration, such as pachygyria and polymicrogyria. Brain stem and cerebellar hypoplasia are also frequent but not constantly observed. The white matter can show areas of abnormal signal but these are not very prominent and, when present, are localized in the periventricular areas.

Pathology

Neuropathological studies have shown coarse gyri with a nodular appearance of the surface and agyric areas. Microscopically, the cortex appeared disorganized without horizontal lamination. The cerebellar cortex is also disorganized.

MEROSIN-NEGATIVE CONGENITAL MUSCULAR DYSTROPHY

In 1994 Tome first reported that a proportion of children with pure congenital muscular dystrophy showed a deficiency of the laminin α2 chain (merosin), an extracellular membrane protein normally present in skeletal muscle[44]. The laminin α2 chain gene has been mapped to chromosome 6q22–23[47]. Children with merosin deficiency have, in general, a more severe clinical course than the children with congenital muscular dystrophy but normal merosin. They are usually symptomatic at birth or in the first few weeks of life with hypotonia and muscle weakness, a weak cry and, in 10–30% of cases, with contractures. Motor nerve conduction velocity is generally reduced[36].

White matter changes on MRI are a constant feature in these children. The changes diffusely involve the hemispheres,

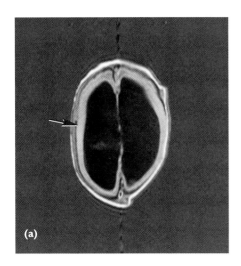

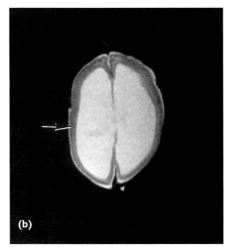

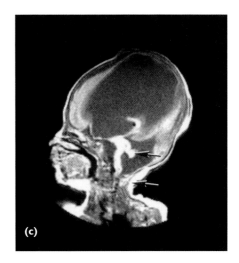

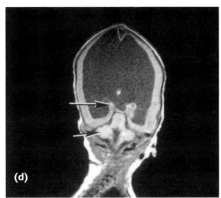

Fig. 14.3   Walker–Warburg syndrome: case 14.1. Imaged at 5 weeks of age. Inversion recovery (IR 3800/30/950) sequence **(a)** and T2 weighted spin echo (SE 2700/120) sequence **(b)**. Transverse plane. There is gross ventricular dilation with a smooth thick cortical rim (*arrow*). T1 weighted spin echo (TE 860/20) in sagittal **(c)** and coronal **(d)** planes. There is cerebellar hypoplasia (*short arrow*) and rudimentary basal ganglia (*long arrow*).

sparing the corpus callosum and the brain stem. The degree of involvement can be variable between individuals but is consistent within siblings[29,30]. The changes may be difficult to identify within the first months of life (Figs 14.4 and 14.7) when it can be difficult to differentiate between unmyelinated white matter and abnormal myelination but become more evident around 6 months and, by the age of 12 months the pattern is similar to that observed in older children[24,25] Fig. 14.7. Despite their dramatic appearance on imaging, these changes do not result in significant functional impairment in these children and cognitive abilities are usually within normal limits. Visual and somatosensory evoked potentials, in con-

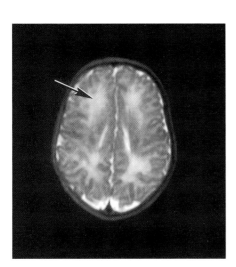

Fig. 14.4   Merosin-negative congenital muscular dystrophy. Male infant born at term with marked hypotonia and weakness. He had mild contractures. His creatine kinase was markedly elevated. Imaged at 5 days of age. T2 weighted fast spin echo (FSE 300/120) sequence. There is abnormal high signal intensity within the periventricular white matter (*arrow*).

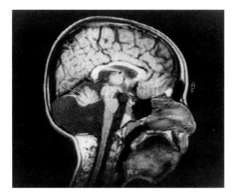

Fig. 14.5 Merosin-negative congenital muscular dystrophy. Male child aged 9 years. T1 weighted spin echo (SE 860/20) sequence in the sagittal plane. There is marked hypoplasia of the cerebellar vermis (*arrow*) and the cerebellar hemispheres (not shown).

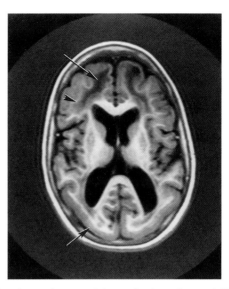

Fig. 14.6 Merosin-negative congenital muscular dystrophy: case 14.2. Male child aged 11 years. Inversion recovery (IR 3400/30/800) sequence. There is abnormal low signal intensity within the white matter (*long arrow*). There is preservation of the normal signal form myelin within the U fibers (*arrowhead*). The cortex of the occipital and temporal lobes is lissencephalic (*short arrow*).

trast, are generally delayed or absent[23]. The only other sign of the involvement of the central nervous system is epilepsy, which has been observed in 10–30% of children[47].

The significance of the white matter changes is not clear as laminin α2 expression appears to be limited to the blood–brain barrier[45]. A pathological study has suggested that the changes observed on MRI might be the result of an increase in water content in the brain[15]. This would explain why the changes seem so striking on imaging yet do not give a significant functional impairment.

Recent studies have demonstrated, however, that besides the diffuse white matter changes, which have been observed in all the patients with merosin-deficient congenital muscular dystrophy, other patterns of brain lesions may also be observed. The association of white matter changes and cerebellar hypoplasia has now been described by several authors. The hypoplasia generally involves the vermis and is not associated with severe mental retardation (Fig. 14.5)[25,42,47]. In contrast, the association of white matter changes and cortical dysplasia is normally associated with severe mental retardation and epilepsy (Fig. 14.6)[25,32,37,47] although children with normal mental function have been reported[4].

CASE 14.3: MEROSIN-NEGATIVE CONGENITAL MUSCULAR DYSTROPHY

Perinatal

This caucasian female infant was born at 42 weeks' gestation by forceps for failure to progress. Birth weight was 3.410 kg. She was noted to be floppy soon after birth and transferred to the neonatal unit on day 1 because of hypoglycemia, slow feeding and difficulty in maintaining body temperature.

At 3 weeks she still showed generalized hypotonia with marked head lag, no effort against gravity in ventral suspension and mild equino-varus talipes deformities. Some antigravity movements were present in both arms and legs but the pattern of spontaneous movements was very poor.

Investigations

Creatine kinase was grossly elevated at 4000 IU/l (normal = <200 IU/l). Electromyography of the quadriceps was interpreted as normal. A needle muscle biopsy of the quadriceps at 5 weeks of age showed dystrophic changes. On immunocytochemistry, the laminin α2 chain of merosin was deficient but not entirely absent, confirming a diagnosis of merosin-deficient congenital muscular dystrophy.

Clinical development

The child is now 3 years old. She has remained floppy and her motor milestones were all delayed. At 3 years she is able to sit without support and to stand with support. Intellectual development is appropriate for her age. Her head circumference is above the 90th centile.

Magnetic resonance imaging

MRI was done at 3 weeks and 6, 12 and 17 months (Fig. 14.7).

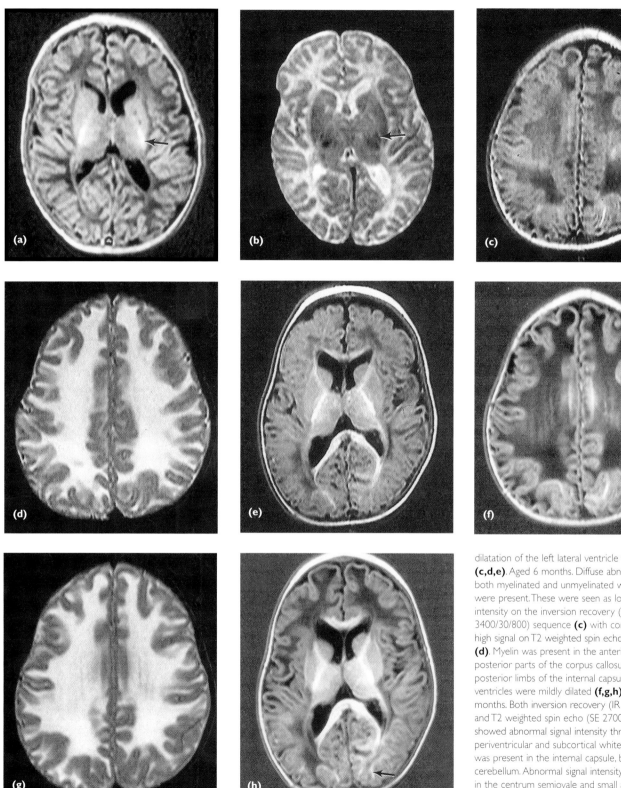

Fig. 14.7 Merosin-negative congenital muscular dystrophy: case 14.3. Female child aged 3 weeks. Inversion recovery (IR 3800/30/950) **(a)** and T2 weighted spin echo (SE 2700/120) **(b)** sequences showed the appropriate pattern for her age. Myelin was present in the posterior limb (*arrow*) of the internal capsule, brain stem, pons and cerebellum. Areas of unmyelinated white matter had abnormal low signal intensity on IR but were unremarkable on T2 weighted images. There were small cysts in the left lentiform nucleus and mild dilatation of the left lateral ventricle were seen **(c,d,e)**. Aged 6 months. Diffuse abnormalities of both myelinated and unmyelinated white matter were present. These were seen as low signal intensity on the inversion recovery (IR 3400/30/800) sequence **(c)** with corresponding high signal on T2 weighted spin echo (SE 2700/120) **(d)**. Myelin was present in the anterior and posterior parts of the corpus callosum, anterior and posterior limbs of the internal capsule **(e)**. The ventricles were mildly dilated **(f,g,h)**. Aged 12 months. Both inversion recovery (IR 3400/30/800) and T2 weighted spin echo (SE 2700/120) images showed abnormal signal intensity throughout the periventricular and subcortical white matter. Myelin was present in the internal capsule, brain stem and cerebellum. Abnormal signal intensity was also seen in the centrum semiovale and small amounts of myelinated white matter were present in the occipital lobes. At 17 months, there was no discernible change from the scan performed at 12 months.

Congenital muscular dystrophy with secondary merosin-deficiency

In the last few years there have been several description of other forms of congenital muscular dystrophy with secondary merosin-deficiency which do not link to the LAMA 2 gene. Brain MRI plays an important role in the differential diagnosis of these forms. Although this is a heterogeneous group, none of these cases reported so far has shown the typical white matter changes invariably observed in patients with primary deficiency of merosin. Brain MRI is also helpful in the characterisation of the phenotype in the different forms which have recently been reported.

Congenital muscular dystrophy with secondary merosin deficiency, muscle hypetrophy and rigidity of the spine linked to chromosome 1q42

This form, characterized by proximal girdle weakness, generalized muscle hypertrophy, rigidity of the spine and contractrures of the tendo Achilles, was originally described in a consanguineous family from the United Arab Emirates and has recently been assigned to chromosome 1q42. Brain MRI is normal[5].

Other forms of secondary merosin deficiency have been described in which all the known loci of CMD were executed by linkage analysis. The variability in clinical phenotype suggest genetic heterogeneity.

Congenital muscular dystrophy with secondary merosin deficiency and normal brain MRI

We have recently described a form of CMD in which the clinical phenotype strongly resembles that observed in the 6q-merosin deficient form with the exception of the brain MRI which is completely normal[26].

Congenital muscular dystrophy with secondary merosin deficiency, microcephaly and normal structural brain

Another form of CMD with secondary merosin deficiency and normal brain MRI has been reported in 2 siblings by Topaloglu et al[41]. At variance with the previous cases however, these siblings have microcephaly and mental retardation.

Congenital muscular dystrophy with secondary merosin deficiency, microcephaly-muscle hypertrophy-cerebellar hypoplasia

Villanova et al have recently reported 5 patients from 4 Italian families with a severe phenotype characterised by severed hypotonia, weakness and joint contractures since birth, muscle hypertrophy and severe mental retardation[46]. Brain MRI showed an abnormal posterior cranial fossa with enlargement of the cisterna magna, variable hypoplasia of the vermis of cerebellum and periventricular white matter changes.

Congenital muscular dystrophy with secondary merosin deficiency and cerebellar cysts

A consanguineous Turkish family with this phenotype was recently reported[39]. Characteristic features were early-onset hypotonia, generalized muscle wasting, weakness, join contractures and moderate mental retardation. Brain MRI revealed multiple small cysts in the cerebellum, without cerebral cortical dysplasia or white matter changes.

MEROSIN-POSITIVE CONGENITAL MUSCULAR DYSTROPHY

The diagnosis of merosin-positive congenital muscular dystrophy is usually made after having excluded all the remaining congenital muscular dystrophy syndromes. The clinical picture of children with merosin-positive congenital muscular dystrophy is very heterogeneous. Classically, this form has been described as having normal MRI, but recent studies have shown that a small proportion of these children show some brain changes, ranging from non-specific localized white matter changes, possibly secondary to antenatal or perinatal insults, to the presence of structural abnormalities, such as cerebellar hypoplasia[17,31,43].

Recently, the locus for a form of merosin-positive congenital muscular dystrophy characterized by marked rigidity of the spine and respiratory failure in the first or second decade of life has been assigned to chromosome 1p.

CASE 14.4: MEROSIN-POSITIVE CONGENITAL MUSCULAR DYSTROPHY

Perinatal

This Asian female infant was born at 26 weeks' gestation by emergency cesarian section for fetal distress. Her birth weight was 3.240 kg. She required ventilation and was transferred to the neonatal unit. On examination she presented dysmorphic features, was floppy and showed a limited range of movements, slow feeding and reduced visual alertness. She also had contractures of her knees, elbows and neck.

Investigations

Creatine kinase was grossly elevated at 4000 IU/l (normal = <200 IU/l). Electromyography of the quadriceps was suggestive of a myopathic process. A needle muscle biopsy of the quadriceps at 5 days of age showed dystrophic changes.

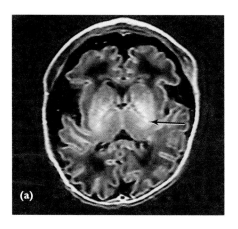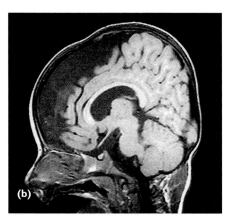

Fig. 14.8 Merosin-positive congenital muscular dystrophy: case 14.4. Inversion recovery (IR 3800/30/950) sequence **(a)**. Infant born at 36 weeks' gestation and imaged at 2 days of age. There is a widened extracerebral space frontally. The cortical folding of the frontal lobes is slightly immature. There is a small amount of high SI consistent with early myelination in the posterior limb of the internal capsule (*arrow*) **(a)** T1 weighted spin echo (SE 860/20) aged 16 months. The frontal space is still markedly widened **(b)**. Myelination has progressed appropriately.

On immunocytochemistry, the laminin α2 chain of merosin was present, confirming a diagnosis of merosin-positive congenital muscular dystrophy.

Clinical development

The child showed a progressive improvement. She was weaned off the ventilator after the neonatal period and feeding was established soon after. Her tone and her weakness have also improved. She is now 4 years old and she is able to walk and almost to run.

Magnetic resonance imaging

MRI of the brain was performed at 2 days and repeated at 16 months (Fig. 14.8).

Congenital myotonic dystrophy

The main presenting features of congenital myotonic dystrophy in the newborn are generalized hypotonia, contractures and marked difficulty in sucking and swallowing, usually requiring tube feeding. Respiratory difficulties are also frequent and often responsible for neonatal death[34]. These infants show a striking facial diplegia with a triangular-shaped open mouth and are unable to close their eyes completely. Skeletal deformities, such as talipes, are very common. Unlike the adult form, in the neonatal period there is no evidence of myotonia and the EMG is usually normal. The typical myotonic discharges only appear later on in life. The muscle pathology may be confusing as this can show either minimal non-specific changes or features suggestive of myotubular myopathy.

A good clinical and antenatal history and a careful examination of the mother provide the diagnostic clue. A history of reduced fetal movements in pregnancy and polyhydramnios can be elicited in most instances. The demonstration of grip or percussion myotonia and facial weakness in the mother establishes the diagnosis of myotonic dystrophy.

The severe neonatal weakness involving the respiratory and swallowing muscles shows a gradual improvement tending to resolve after the first months of life. Very severely affected neonates can, however, require ventilator support for weeks and some may never be weaned off the ventilator. Although the brain is structurally normal in these children, non-specific abnormalities are often observed (Fig. 14.9). The incidence of ventricular dilatation in these infants has been reported to be between 70 and 80%. Other abnormalities, such as intraventricular hemorrhage and periventricular leukomalacia have also been reported[19,40].

Hashimoto *et al.* have reviewed the MRI in seven cases with congenital myotonic dystrophy showing ventricular dilatation in all, associated with periventricular or deep white matter changes (6/7), cortical atrophy (3/7), small corpus callosum (4/7) and small brain stem (2/7)[19].

Congenital myopathies

Involvement of the CNS may also be observed in some of the congenital myopathies, such as the severe variant of nemaline myopathy and X-linked myotubular myopathy.

NEMALINE MYOPATHY

This myopathy is characterized by the presence of rods on muscle biopsy. The classical congenital form, observed in early infancy, is characterized by mild floppiness and swallowing problems, and is not usually associated with CNS involvement. In contrast, the more severe and usually fatal congenital form characterized by arthrogryposis and ventilator dependency at birth, is more frequently associated with brain involvement, such as mild dilatation of the ventricles or

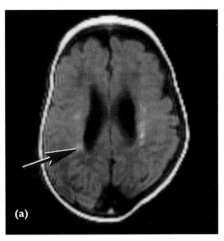 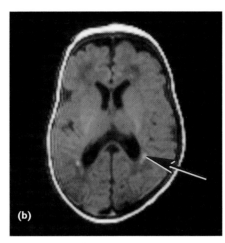 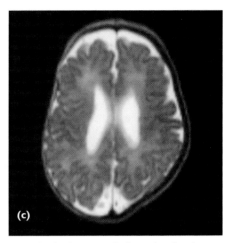

Fig. 14.9 Congenital myotonic dystrophy: case 14.5. Female infant born at 36 weeks' gestation. Her mother was diagnosed as having myotonic dystrophy after the birth of a previously affected child. This pregnancy was complicated by polyhydramnios. The infant was born by emergency cesarian section with Apgar scores of only 3 at 1 min. She was intubated for lack of respiratory effort and remained ventilator dependent for 41 days. She was imaged at 6 weeks of age. T1 weighted (SE 860/20) **(a,b)** and T2 weighted (SE 2700/120) **(c)** spin echo sequences. There is mild ventricular dilation. There are additional small probably hemorrhagic lesions seen as high signal intensity on T1 weighted images (*long arrow*). These are not easily visible on the T2 weighted images **(c)**. Myelination within the posterior limb of the internal capsule is appropriate for age **(a,b)**.

cortical atrophy. Structural brain abnormalities are, however, not observed in this form.

CASE 14.6: NEMALINE MYOPATHY

Perinatal

This African male infant was born at 34 weeks' gestation by emergency cesarian section for breech presentation. His birth weight was 2.360 kg. He was intubated soon after birth showing very poor respiratory movements. On examination he showed severe hypotonia, with absence of spontaneous movements, mild contractures in the wrist, reduced visual alertness and poor sucking.

Investigations

His creatine kinase was normal (123 U/l). A needle muscle biopsy of the quadriceps at 5 days of age showed the classical features of nemaline myopathy. Cranial ultrasound showed marked posterior echo densities and diffuse echo densities over the cerebellum. He died at 4 months of age.

Magnetic resonance imaging

Brain MRI was performed at 10 days of age (Fig. 14.10).

X-LINKED MYOTUBULAR MYOPATHY

Children affected with X-linked myotubular myopathy have a very similar clinical picture to the severe congenital form of

myotonic dystrophy, with the additional involvement of the extraocular muscles, giving rise to ophthalmoplegia. The long-term survival in this form is extremely poor because of the severity of the respiratory and bulbar muscle involvement.

CASE 14.7: X-LINKED MYOTUBULAR MYOPATHY

Perinatal

This African male infant was born at 35 weeks' gestation by cesarian section for fetal distress. Early antenatal ultrasound scan detected polyhydramnios. The mother also felt reduced fetal movements. At birth the infant showed no respiratory effort and was intubated. On examination he showed ophthalmoplegia, facial weakness, severe hypotonia, no antigravity movements, and no visual alertness. Sucking and rooting were also absent.

Investigations

Creatine kinase was grossly elevated at 4000 IU/l (normal = <200 IU/l). Electromyography of the quadriceps was suggestive of a myopathic process. A needle muscle biopsy of the quadriceps at 5 days of age showed dystrophic changes. Cranial ultrasound was normal.

Magnetic resonance imaging

Brain MRI showed diffuse abnormal signal intensity in white matter with small petecchial foci consistent with hemorrhage. There was a widened extracerebral space (Fig. 14.11).

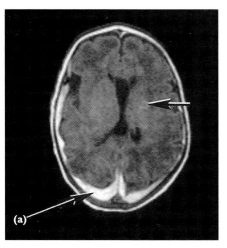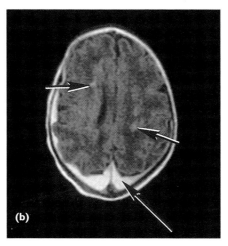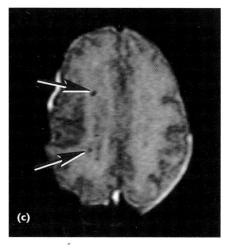

Fig. 14.10 Nemaline myopathy: case 14.6. T1 weighted (SE 860/20) **(a,b)** and T2 weighted (SE 2700/120). There is a large subdural hemorrhage (*long arrow*). Multiple small areas (*short arrows*) of high signal intensity on T1 weighted images **(a,b)** and low signal intensity on T2 weighted images **(c)** are consistent with hemorrhagic lesions.

Clinical development

At 5 months the infant is still oxygen dependent, is still very floppy and has shown only a minimal improvement with onset of some antigravity movements. His alertness is also very poor with no auditory orientation and only occasional opening of the eyes.

Motoneuron disorders

Spinal muscular atrophy (SMA) type 1 (Werdnig–Hoffman disease) is the most common disease of the motoneuron in the newborn. The condition characteristically involves the proximal limb and the intercostal respiratory muscles more severely, while it spares the facial muscles and the diaphragm; clinically evident bulbar involvement is frequent but relatively mild. Infants affected by this form usually die within the first year, or before 18 months of age. The recent discovery of the gene defect for SMA (deletion of the telomeric copy of the SMN (survival motor neuron) provides a very useful and rapid diagnostic tool as a deletion of this gene can be found in more than 98% of children with SMA 1. Although in Werdnig–Hoffman disease there is usually no associated central nervous system involvement, non-specific changes such as cerebral atrophy or other ischemic changes have been observed in some of these children, mainly associated with prematurity or birth asphyxia[33].

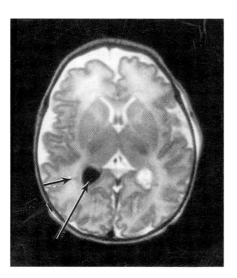

Fig. 14.11 X-linked myotubular myopathy: case 14.7. T1 weighted spin echo (SE 860/20) sequences. Infant aged 10 days. There is an intraventricular hemorrhage (*long arrow*) and small parenchymal hemorrhagic lesions in the white matter (*short arrow*). The parenchymal hemorrhagic lesions are easier to see using a T1 weighted sequence.

PONTOCEREBELLAR HYPOPLASIA TYPE I

Unlike Werdnig–Hoffman disease, clinical and radiological evidence of CNS involvement is a major feature of the form of spinal muscular atrophy associated with pontocerebellar hypoplasia type I[3]. Studies have shown that this form is not allelic to SMA[14] and the gene responsible for this form has not yet been identified.

Affected infants show a combination of clinical signs related to both motoneuron disorder and central nervous system involvement. The clinical course is progressive and respiratory and feeding difficulties, already present at birth or in early infancy, become more severe.

The MRI shows hypoplasia of the cerebellar vermis and, often also of the cerebellar hemispheres, associated with a thin brain stem and pons (Fig. 14.12). Pathological studies have shown normal brain weight with extreme hypoplasia of pons and cerebellum. Cerebellar folia were poorly developed while vermal folia were relatively well preserved with general loss of granular cells and atrophy of dentate and inferior olivary nuclei. A near total loss of nuclei was also observed in the pons with reactive gliosis[3].

The differential diagnosis is with other forms, which show cerebellar and brain stem hypoplasia and peripheral nerve involvement, such as the carbohydrate-deficient glycoconjugate syndromes.

CASE 14.8: PONTOCEREBELLAR HYPOPLASIA TYPE I

Perinatal

This female infant was the first child born to healthy non-consanguineous parents of Asian origin. At 28 weeks' gestation polyhydramnios was noted and at 32 weeks there was poor fetal growth and movement. End diastolic flow velocities were absent. The mother was given dexamethasone and the baby was delivered by cesarian section. The infant had poor respiratory effort requiring immediate intubation and ventilation; her birth weight was on the third centile. She had widespread contractures involving large and small joints. Her posture was characterized by hypotonia, internal rotation of arms and ulna deviation of fingers with adducted thumbs in clenched fists. There was virtually no spontaneous movement, even after painful stimuli. The baby was unable to swallow.

Clinical development

She never opened her eyes spontaneously and remained ventilator dependent. At 1 month of age she became progressively more difficult to ventilate, with sepsis and increasing acidosis. Intensive care was withdrawn and the child died soon afterwards.

Magnetic resonance imaging

Brain MRI revealed a large subcerebellar space with symmetrical cerebellar and mesencephalon hypoplasia. The midbrain also appeared small and the ventricular system was dilated (Fig. 14.12).

Only a limited postmortem examination was allowed and this revealed generalized muscle atrophy, affecting the distal muscles more severely. The brain was small and immature with a hypoplastic cerebellum and moderate dilatation of the lateral ventricles. The spinal cord was grossly normal.

PERIPHERAL NERVE DISORDERS ASSOCIATED WITH CNS INVOLVEMENT

Several metabolic diseases can affect both the peripheral nerves and brain but in the majority of them the onset occurs after the neonatal period. A possible underlying metabolic

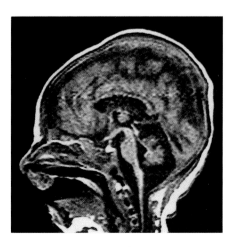

Fig. 14.12 Pontocerebellar hypoplasia type I: case 14.8. Female infant born at 32 weeks' gestation and imaged at 3 weeks of age. T1 weighted spin echo (SE 860/20) sequence. There is hypoplasia of the cerebellum, medulla and mid-brain.

disorder, however, must always be considered when investigating a severely ill and floppy newborn. These infants often present with respiratory or cardiac problems and an abnormal neurological examination with reduced tone and a reduced level of alertness or seizures. A clinical examination can provide some useful additional information such as the presence of dysmorphic features or visceromegaly which can aid the differential diagnosis.

The carbohydrate-deficient glycoconjugate syndromes deserve a particular mention, because of structural changes observed in the cerebellum and in the brain stem. These syndromes include a group of genetic disorders characterized by a deficiency of the carbohydrate moiety of glycoconjugates[20,21]. Type I is the most common and has been related to a deficit in phosphomannomutase. Infants present with dysmorphic features, hypotonia, and hyporeflexia, abnormal eye movements and poor feeding. The clinical presentation, however, can be variable, even within siblings and other signs in the neonatal period are skeletal abnormalities, hepatomegaly, proteinuria and cardiomyopathy. Retinitis pigmentosa, joint contractures, epilepsy and stroke-like episodes are frequent but usually occur at a later stage. The involvement of the peripheral nerves is shown by abnormal motor and sensory nerve conduction velocity.

Serial MRI is useful in differential diagnosis, showing brain stem and cerebellar hypoplasia[20,21].

The diagnosis is made by isoelectrofocusing and immunofixation of serum transferrin and can be confirmed by finding decreased phosphomannomutase in fibroblasts or leukocytes.

Other conditions, such as Refsum's disease and some peroxisomal disorders can show similar signs, with dysmorphic features, slow nerve conduction and global delay. In some of these such as neonatal adrenoleukodystrophy (Fig. 14.13) or Refsum's, the involvement of the brain may not be easily detectable in the neonatal period when it is difficult to differentiate between the unmyelinated white matter and signs of dysmyelination.

Mitochondrial encephalomyopathies

Mitochondrial disorders are described separately from the other metabolic disorders because of the possible association of brain changes with peripheral nerve and skeletal and cardiac muscle involvement. Only a few of the mitochondrial disorders affecting children and adults have neonatal onset (see chapter 17). Lactic acidosis is the landmark of most of these forms which, in the neonatal period, are mainly related to defects of the respiratory chain and, in particular to deficiency of complex I and III and, more commonly, of complex IV. There have been several descriptions of a fatal infantile form with cardiac and renal involvment, seizures, hypotonia and respiratory distress. In these cases CT and MRI generally show cortical and subcortical atrophy and dysmyelination[1] (Fig. 14.14). The muscle can be normal, or reveal lipid–glycogen storage.

A neonatal onset has also been described for the Leigh syndrome or subacute necrotizing encephalopathy[6]. The underlying enzyme defect can only be detected in 20–25% of the cases and is often related to complex IV or I deficiency and, in some cases to pyruvate dehydrogenase deficiency. The clinical manifestations of Leigh syndrome are very variable and often the overt symptoms appear, even in the infantile form, after a relatively symptom-free period. Clinical signs consist of hypotonia and developmental regression with onset of movement disorders and seizures. In the

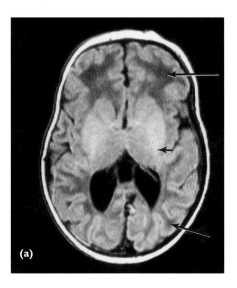

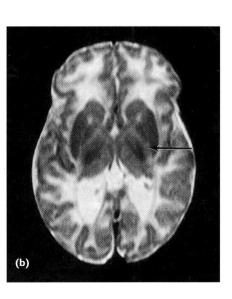

Fig. 14.13 Neonatal adrenoleukodystrophy. Female infant born at 38 weeks' gestation with dysmorphic features, hypotonia and contractures at the knee. She developed neonatal seizures. Imaging was performed at 5 weeks of age. T1 weighted spin echo (SE 860/20) sequence **(a)**. There is minimal high signal intensity from myelin within the internal capsule (*short arrow*). The level of myelination is at least 1 month behind. The white matter has a very low signal intensity (*long arrows*). T2 weighted spin echo (SE 2700/120) sequence **(b)**. The white matter has a very high signal intensity. There is no obvious signal from myelin within the posterior limb of the internal capsule (*arrow*).

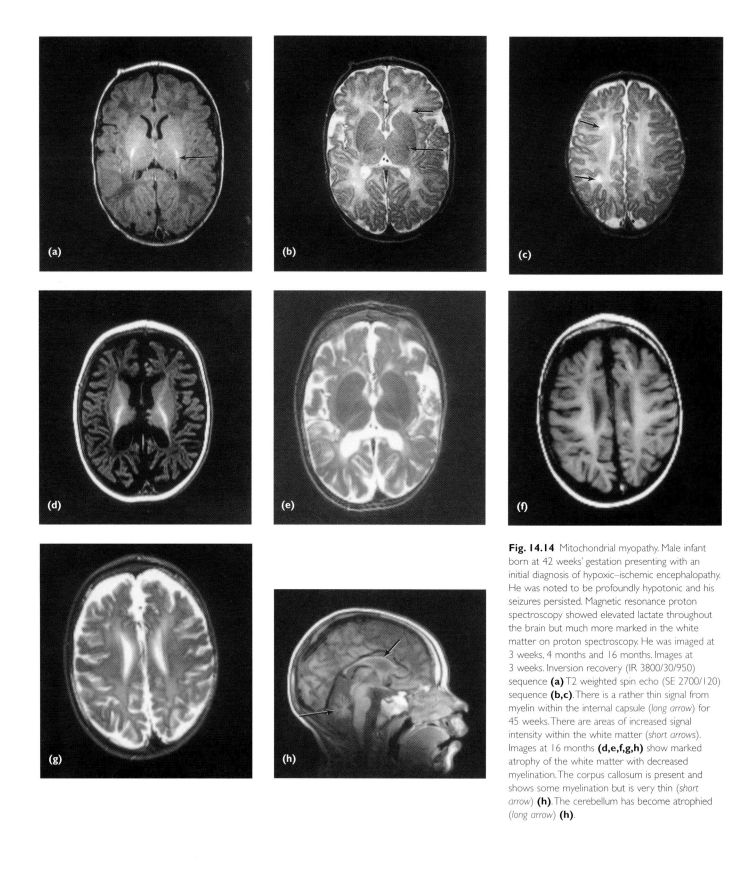

Fig. 14.14 Mitochondrial myopathy. Male infant born at 42 weeks' gestation presenting with an initial diagnosis of hypoxic–ischemic encephalopathy. He was noted to be profoundly hypotonic and his seizures persisted. Magnetic resonance proton spectroscopy showed elevated lactate throughout the brain but much more marked in the white matter on proton spectroscopy. He was imaged at 3 weeks, 4 months and 16 months. Images at 3 weeks. Inversion recovery (IR 3800/30/950) sequence **(a)** T2 weighted spin echo (SE 2700/120) sequence **(b,c)**. There is a rather thin signal from myelin within the internal capsule (*long arrow*) for 45 weeks. There are areas of increased signal intensity within the white matter (*short arrows*). Images at 16 months **(d,e,f,g,h)** show marked atrophy of the white matter with decreased myelination. The corpus callosum is present and shows some myelination but is very thin (*short arrow*) **(h)**. The cerebellum has become atrophied (*long arrow*) **(h)**.

neonatal forms the symptoms are evident soon after birth with absence of poor acquisition of new milestones.

The MRI in Leigh syndrome shows a typical pattern with abnormal signal in the bilateral lenticular nuclei and in the caudate with subsequent cavitation. Cerebellar hypoplasia is also frequent. MRI spectroscopy shows high levels of lactate in the basal ganglia, even in the absence of increased serum lactate. Muscle biopsy may be morphologically normal or show only non-specific changes but show biochemical abnormalities. Nerve conduction velocity (NCV) can be abnormal.

Summary

■ MR brain imaging will help in correctly diagnosing infants with signs of neuromuscular disease.

■ MRI is identifying an increasing range of associated brain abnormalities within the congenital muscular dystrophies.

■ Follow-up imaging in infants with neuromuscular disorders may show progressive changes within the white matter.

■ MR spectroscopy may be useful for differentiating metabolic disease from primary neuromuscular disorders.

Acknowledgments

We thank Mary Rutherford for preparing all the images and legends.

References

1. Aicardi J (1998) *Diseases of the Nervous System in Childhood*. London, MacKeith Press.
2. Akaboshi S, Ohno K and Takeshita K (1995) Neuroradiological findings in the carbohydrate-deficient glycoprotein syndrome. *Neuroradiology* **37**, 491–495.
3. Barth PG (1993) Pontocerebellar hypoplasia. An overview of a group of inherited neurodegenerative disorders with fetal onset. *Brain Dev* **15**, 411–422.
4. Brett FM, Costigan D, Farrell MA *et al.* (1998) Merosin-deficient congenital muscular dystrophy and cortical dysplasia. *Eur J Paed Neurol* **2**, 77–82.
5. Brockington M, Sewry CA, Herrmann R, *et al.* (2000). Assignment of a form of congenital muscular dystrophy with secondary merosin deficiency to chromosome 1q42. *A J Hum Gen*, 66, 428–435.
6. Cocker SB and Thomas C (1995) Connatal Leigh disease. *Clin Pediatr* **34**, 349–352.
7. Dobyns WB and Truwitt CL (1995) Lissencephaly and other malformations of cortical development: 1995 update. *Neuropediatrics* **26**, 132–147.
8. Dobyns WB, Kirkpatrick JB, Hittner HM *et al.* (1985) Syndromes with lyssencephaly II. Walker–Warburg and cerebro-oculo-muscular syndromes and a new syndrome with type II lyssencephaly. *Am J Med Genet* **22**, 157–195.
9. Dobyns WB, Pagon RA, Armstrong D *et al.* (1989) Diagnostic criteria for Walker–Warburg syndrome. *Am J Med Genet* **32**, 195–210.
10. Dubowitz V (1969) The floppy infant. *Clinics in Developmental Medicine* **31**, London, Spastics International/Heinemann.
11. Dubowitz V (1994) Workshop report on 22nd ENMC-sponsored meeting on congenital muscular dystrophy held in Baarn, The Netherlands, May 14–16 1993. *Neuromusc Disord* **4**, 75–81.
12. Dubowitz V (1995) *Muscle Disorders in Childhood*, 2nd edn. London, Saunders.
13. Dubowitz V, Fardeau M (1995) Workshop report on 27th ENMC-sponsored meeting on congenital muscular dystrophy held in Baarn, The Netherlands, April 22–24 1994. *Neuromusc Disord* **4**, 253–258.
14. Dubowitz V, Daniels RJ and Davies KE (1995) Olivopontocerebellar hypoplasia with anterior horn cell involvement (SMA) does not localize to chromosome 5q. *Neuromusc Disord* **5**, 25–29.
15. Echenne B, Pages M and Marty Double C (1984) Congenital muscular dystrophy with cerebral white matter spongiosis. *Brain Dev* **6**, 491–495.
16. Echenne B, Rivier F, Jellali AJ *et al.* (1997a) Merosin positive congenital muscular dystrophy with mental deficiency, epilepsy and MRI changes in the cerebral white matter. *Neuromusc Disord* **7**, 187–190.
17. Echenne B, Rivier F, Tardieu M *et al.* (1997b) Congenital muscular dystrophy and cerebellar atrophy. *Neurology* (1998) **50**, 1477–80.
18. Fukuyama Y, Kawazura M and Haruna H (1960) A peculiar form of congenital muscular dystrophy. *Paediatr Univ Tokyo* **4**, 5–8.
19. Hashimoto T, Tayama M, Myazaki M *et al.* (1995) Neuroimaging study of myotonic dystrophy I. Magnetic resonance imaging of the brain. *Brain Dev* **17**, 24–27.
20. Jaeken J and Casaer P (1997) Carbohydrate-deficient glyconjugate (CDG) syndromes: a new chapter of neuropaediatrics. *Eur J Paed Neurol* **2/3**, 61–66.
21. Jaeken J, Stibler H and Hagberg B (1991) The carbohydrate-deficient glycoprotein syndrome: a new inherited multisystemic disease with severe nervous system involvement. *Acta Paediatr Scand Suppl* **375**, (monograph).
22. Maalouf E, Battin M, Counsell S *et al.* (1997) Arthrogryposis multiplex congenita and bilateral mid-brain infarction following maternal overdose. *Eur J Paed Neurol* **5/6**, 183–186.
23. Mercuri E, Muntoni F, Berardinelli A *et al.* (1995) Somatosensory and visual evoked potentials in congenital muscular dystrophy: correlation with MRI changes and muscle merosin status. *Neuropediatrics* **26**, 3–7.
24. Mercuri E, Pennock J, Goodwin F *et al.* (1996) Sequential study of central and peripheral nervous system involvement in an infant with merosin-deficient CMD. *Neuromusc Disord* **6**, 425–429.

25. Mercuri E, Gruter-Andrew J, Philpot J *et al.* (1999) Cognitive abilities in children with congenital muscular dystrophy: correlation with brain MRI and merosin status. *Neuromusc Disord* **9**, 383–387.

26. Mercuri E, Sewry CA, Brown SC, *et al.* (2000). Congenital muscular dystrophy with secondary merosin deficiency and normal brain MRI: a novel entity? *Neuropediatrics* 31:186–189.

27. Mercuri E, Rutherford M, De Vile C, *et al.* (2001) Early white matter changes on brain magnetic resonance imaging in a newborn affected by merosin-deficiency congenital muscular dystrophy. *Neuromusc Disord*, 11:297-9.

28. Osawa M, Sumida S, Suzuki N *et al.* (1997) Fukuyama type congenital progressive muscular dystrophy. In: Fukyama Y, Osawa M and Saito K (Eds) *Congenital Muscular Dystrophies.* Amsterdam, Elsevier Science.

29. Philpot J, Sewry C, Pennock J *et al.* (1995) Clinical phenotype in congenital muscular dystrophy: correlation with expression of merosin in skeletal muscle. *Neuromusc Disord* **5**, 301–305.

30. Philpot J, Topaloglu H, Pennock J *et al.* (1995) Familial concordance of brain magnetic resonance imaging changes in congenital muscular dystrophy. *Neuromusc Disord* **5**, 227–231.

31. Philpot J, Pennock J, Cowan F, *et al.* (2000) Brain magnetic resonance imaging abnormalities in merosin-positive congenital muscular dystrophy. *Europ J Paediatr Neurol* 4:109–14.

32. Pini A, Merlini L, Tome FMS *et al.* (1996) Merosin negative congenital muscular dystrophy, occipital epilepsy with periodic spasms and focal cortical dysplasia. Report from three Italian cases in two families. *Brain Dev* **18**, 316–322.

33. Rudnick-Schoneborn, Forkert R, Hahnen E *et al.* (1996) Clinical spectrum and diagnostic criteria of infantile spinal muscular atrophy: further delineation on the basis of SMN deletion findings. *Neuropediatrics* **27**, 8–15.

34. Rutherford MA, Heckmatt JZ and Dubowitz V (1989) Congenital myotonic dystrophy: respiratory function at birth determines survival. *Arch Dis Child* **64**, 191–195.

35. Santavuori P, Somer H, Saino K *et al.* (1989) Muscle–eye–brain disease (MEB). *Brain Dev* **11**, 147–153.

36. Shorer Z, Philpot J, Muntoni F *et al.* (1995) Demyelinating peripheral neuropathy in merosin-deficient congenital muscular dystrophy. *J Child Neurol* **10**, 472–475.

37. Sunada Y, Edgar TS, Lotz BP *et al.* (1995) Merosin-negative congenital muscular dystrophy associated with extensive brain abnormalities. *Neurology* **45**, 2084–2089.

38. Takashima S and Mizuguchi M (1997) Cytoarchitectonic alterations of the cerebral cortex in Fukuyama type congenital muscular dystrophy and other cortical dysplasia syndrome. In: Fukuyama Y, Osawa M, and Saito K (Eds) *Congenital Muscular Dystrophies.* Amsterdam, Elsevier Science, pp. 125–142.

39. Talim B, Ferreiro A, Cormand B, *et al.* (2000). Merosin-deficient congenital muscular dystrophy with mental retardation and cerebellar cysts unlinked to the LAMA2, FCMD and MEB loci. *Neuromusc Disord* **10**, 548–52.

40. Tanabe Y, Iai M, Tamai K *et al.* (1992) Neuroradiological findings in children with congenital myotonic dystrophy. *Acta Paediatr* **81**, 613–617.

41. Topaloglu H, Talim B, Vignier N, *et al.* (1998) Merosin-deficient congenital muscular dystrophy with severe mental retardation and normal cranial MRI: a report of two siblings. *Neuromusc Disord* **8**, 169–174.

42. Trevisan CP, Martinello F, Ferruzza E *et al.* (1996) Brain alteration in the classical form of congenital muscular dystrophy. Clinical and neuroimaging follow up of 12 cases and correlation with the expression of merosin in muscle. *Child Nerv Syst* **12**, 604–610.

43. Trevisan CP, Martinello F, Armani M *et al.* (1997) Brain involvement in a series of cases with merosin-positive congenital muscular dystrophy. *Neuromusc Disord* **7**, 433.

44. Tome FM, Evangelista T, Leclerc A *et al.* (1994) Congenital muscular dystrophy with merosin deficiency. *CR Acad Sci III* **317(4)**, 351–357.

45. Villanova M, Malandrini A, Toti P *et al.* (1996) Localization of merosin in the normal human brain: implications for congenital muscular dystrophy with merosin deficiency. *J Submicrosc Cytol Pathol* **28(1)**, 1–4.

46. Villanova M, Mercuri E, Bertini E, *et al.* (2001). Congenital muscular dystrophy associated with calf hypertrophy, microcephaly and severe mental retardation: A new CMD syndrome. *Neuromusc Disord* **10**: 541–547.

47. Voit T (1998) Congenital muscular dystrophies: 1997 update. *Brain Dev*, **20** 65–74.

48. Vuolteenalho R, Nissinen M, Sainio K, *et al.* (1994). Human laminin M chain (merosin): complete primary structure, chromosomal assignment, and expression of the M and A chain human fetal tissues. *J Cell Biol*, 124:381–394.

Magnetic resonance imaging of the fetal brain

15

Annick Sévely and Claude Manelfe

Contents

Introduction

Fetal magnetic resonance imaging (MRI) is still in its infancy but as MR systems have become more widely available it is now the technique of choice when ultrasonography (US) detects abnormalities of the fetal brain and further elucidation is required. MRI is more sensitive than US because of its higher spatial resolution, contrast abilities and multiplanar acquisition. The first description of MRI during pregnancy was published by Smith *et al.* in 1983[25]. At that time the potential of MR was limited by the long acquisition time, fetal motion and maternal respiratory artifact[3,21,22,28]. The development of ultrafast imaging sequences such as fast spin echo (FSE), half-Fourier single-shot FSE, one side image reconstruction techniques, and echoplanar imaging now allow a clinically useful MR study of the fetus without the use of sedation[15,17]. T1 weighted sequences are less satisfactory than half-Fourier FSE techniques because of degradation from motion artifact, although they may be useful for confirming the presence of hemorrhage or fat.

Safety issues

Although there are no documented ill-effects to the fetus[23,27], current guidelines recommend that, as dividing cells in the embryo are more susceptible to many forms of injury, the use of MR in the first trimester of pregnancy should be avoided in normal volunteers[17,27]. In addition, at the present time the quality of images below about 17 weeks' gestation is limited by fetal size. Gadolinium-based contrast material has been used without ill-effect during pregnancy[18]. Gadolinium crosses the placenta and passes to the fetus. It is excreted from the fetal bladder into the amniotic fluid and is then swallowed. This potential reabsorbtion by the fetus means that the half-life of gadolinium-based contrast agents may persist for extended times. Gadolinium has been safely used in preterm infants *ex utero*. It is usually not necessary to monitor the fetal heart during scanning. Imaging times are also very short. However, with the development of techniques that could be used to monitor and investigate the stressed fetus or the fetus during labor, monitoring may become necessary. This could be achieved with modifications to standard Doppler ultrasound[24].

Developments

Most fetal imaging is performed in the routine adult body coil. The use of arrays of surface coils should improve image quality. Vaginal ultrasound now allows good quality images of the fetus at very early stages of development and it may be mimicked in the future by the construction of internal coils for per vaginal MRI of the fetus. There has been little development of either sequences or coils that are specific for fetal imaging and there are likely to be many advances that improve signal to noise and hence the quality of images over the next decade.

MR sequences

The images used to illustrate this chapter were all acquired on a 1.5 T (Magnetom Vision, Siemens, Erlangen, Germany) with a phased-array surface coil using a HASTE sequence (half-Fourier single shot turbo spin echo)[14,16,29]. This sequence uses a 90° excitation pulse, followed by an echo train of up to 128 refocusing pulses. The half-Fourier reconstruction algorithm is used to generate a spin echo image with a matrix of 240 × 256 in 2 s. A strongly T2 weighted image is obtained with TR = 10.9 ms and TE = 87 ms.

Five images are acquired in 10 s in the axial, sagittal and coronal planes using a field of view of 400 × 400 mm and a slice thickness of 5 mm. For T1W imaging we use a FLASH 2D sequence, TR = 158 ms, TE = 4.8 ms with a matrix of 256 x 107, one acquisition and 5 slices of 5 mm. Total acquisition time is 17 s. In the event of motion artifact the sequences may be repeated. Total examination time is usually about 5 min.

Patients are usually referred because of concern over fetal brain development on antenatal ultrasound. This usually takes the form of ventricular dilation or possible agenesis of the corpus callosum.

Normal development

Maturation of the normal fetal brain may be compared to the anatomic atlas of Fees-Higgins and Larroche[5] (Fig. 15.1). MRI can be used to study brain maturation[9], fetal brain cellular migration[7] and cortical development which is often delayed in fetuses with CNS abnormalities[13]. The images produced are comparable with those taken *ex utero* in very preterm infants (see Chapter 3). Studies of formalin-fixed embryos and fetuses give some indication of the development of different brain structures which may be used as a guide for *in vivo* imaging of the very immature brain[20]. The task for radiologists involved in MR imaging of the fetus is to know which appearances are within the normal range. This can only be ascertained by serial imaging with long-term follow-up of the infants following delivery. Several groups have noted that some ventricular asymmetry is frequently seen in both fetuses and preterm infants. The left posterior horn is slightly bigger than the right in the majority of cases. In addition, it is clear that fetuses and preterm infants up to approximately 32 weeks' gestation have a large posterior extracerebral space which decreases with increasing gestation[8]. This appears to be a normal developmental feature rather than an external hydrocephalus. The evolution of cortical folding may be shown antenatally and postnatally. The maturation of the

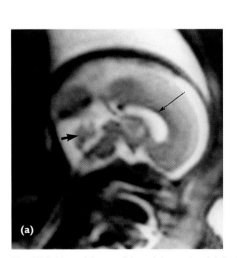 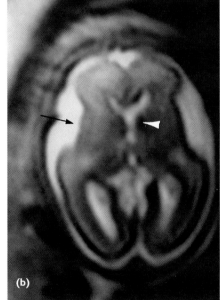 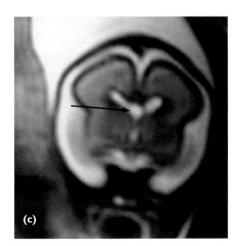

Fig. 15.1 Normal fetus at 26 weeks' gestation. **(a)** Sagittal T2 weighted image (HASTE) shows a low signal intensity corpus callosum (*long arrow*) and small vermis (*short arrow*). **(b)** Axial T2 weighted image (HASTE) shows large ventricles, open Sylvian fissures (*long arrow*), a low signal intensity cortical ribbon and normal germinal matrix over the caudate head (*white arrowhead*). **(c)** Coronal T2 weighted image (HASTE) shows normal smooth cerebral surface and a septum pellucidum cyst (*arrow*).

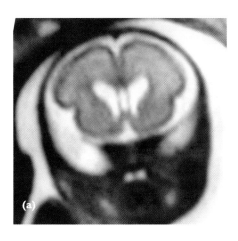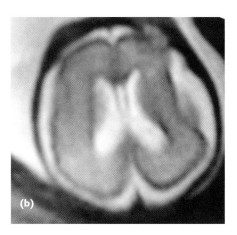

Fig. 15.2 Ventricular dilatation at 27 weeks' gestation. **(a)** Coronal T2 weighted image (HASTE) shows ventricular dilatation with a cavum septum pellucidum but no other abnormalities. **(b)** Axial T2 weighted image (HASTE) shows the asymmetrical ventricular dilatation.

cortex may be influenced by factors such as sex, intrauterine growth retardation and multiple pregnancy. Postnatal studies suggest that there may be a 2-week individual variation between infants (see Chapter 3). Visual analysis is sufficient to identify major abnormalities of cortical development but is insufficient for identifying small differences in folding. A comparison of *in utero* and *ex utero* brain development using computer quantification (see Chapter 3) would enable us to address important issues on the role of extrinsic (*ex utero*) factors on brain development in the infant born prematurely.

Fetal cerebral abnormalities

VENTRICULAR DILATION

The most frequent indication for fetal MRI is ventriculomegaly detected by ultrasound. MRI may be used to identify any underlying abnormalities in the brain associated with the dilated ventricles. Abnormal size and shape to the ventricles may arise as a congenital malformation (see Chapter 11),

as a result of obstruction to the flow or absorption of cerebrospinal fluid, or as a result of brain atrophy. It is important to differentiate 'normal' ventricular asymmetry from unilateral dilatation associated with a porencephalic cyst. The increased resolution of MR may be useful to ascertain the presence of a normal regular ventricular outline and the presence of old hemorrhage. Intraventricular hemorrhage is also easily depicted by MRI because of the sensitivity of MR to the presence of blood (Fig. 15.8) (see Chapter 9). Antenatal fetal hemorrhage may be secondary to fetal clotting abnormalities, the presence of which would alter the management of the pregnancy and delivery.

In many cases, MRI is able to confirm the presence of an otherwise normal structure to the brain in the presence of ventricular dilatation (Fig. 15.2).

AGENESIS OF CORPUS CALLOSUM

Ventricular dilation may occur with or without visualization of the corpus callosum (Figs. 15.2 and 15.3). Corpus callosal agenesis may be associated with agenesis of other commis-

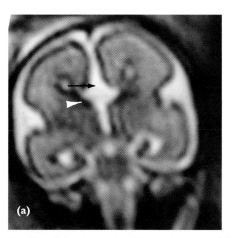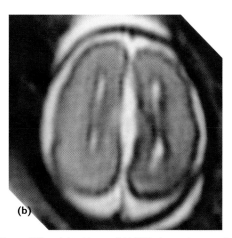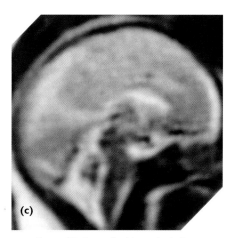

Fig. 15.3 Callosal agenesis at 25 weeks' gestation. **(a)** Coronal T2 weighted image (HASTE) shows absence of corpus callosum (*black arrow*) with continuity between the inter hemispheric fissure and ventricular system. The normal germinal matrix can be visualized as low signal intensity (*white arrow*). **(b)** Axial T2 weighted image (HASTE) shows dilated posterior portion of one lateral ventricle. **(c)** Sagittal T2 weighted image (HASTE): confirms the absence of corpus callosum.

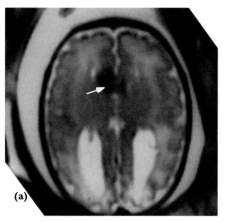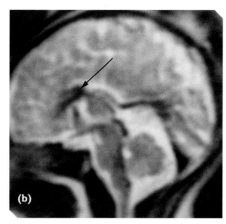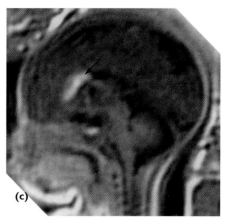

Fig. 15.4 Callosal agenesis with lipoma at 34 weeks' gestation. **(a)** Axial T2 weighted image (HASTE) shows splaying of the frontal horns, posterior ventricular dilatation and median low signal intensity between the frontal horns (*white arrow*). **(b)** Sagittal T2 weighted image (HASTE): there is absence of the corpus callosum and low signal intensity at the level of the genu (*arrow*). **(c)** Sagittal T1 weighted image shows the lipoma as a high signal intensity (*arrow*).

sures and with other brain malformations. These may be more easily depicted using MRI when compared with ultrasound[4]. An associated lipoma may be easily visualized (Fig. 15.4). The acquisition of both T1 and T2 weighted sequences will allow good differentiation of lipomatous lesions. The diagnosis of agenesis of the corpus callosum is not possible before 22 weeks' gestation[2].

ARACHNOID CYST

MRI contributes in the diagnosis (Fig. 15.5) and therapeutic management of arachnoid cysts as some of these need surgical treatment after birth (Fig. 15.6). MRI is helpful in clarifying US findings in cystic malformations of the posterior fossa: Dandy–Walker malformation (Fig. 15.7),

Dandy–Walker variant, vermian agenesis or arachnoid cyst or a cisterna magna (see Chapter 11, Table 11.4).

MYELOMENINGOCELE

MRI is useful for evaluating neural tube defects, particularly caudal abnormalities that may be difficult to detect with ultrasound. MR has been used to identify hindbrain herniation as a complication of myelomeningocele and then to monitor its evolution following antenatal closure of the neural tube defect[26].

PARENCHYMAL LESIONS

Sometimes antenatal ultrasound (US) only shows ventricular enlargement and is not able to detect the associated

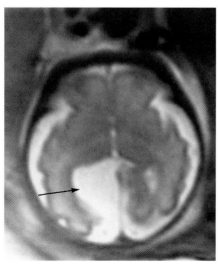

Fig. 15.5 Arachnoid cyst at 29 weeks' gestation. Axial T2 weighted image (HASTE) shows a right well circumscribed interhemispheric cyst (*arrow*).

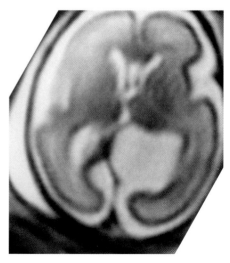

Fig. 15.6 Arachnoid cyst at 27 weeks' gestation. Axial T2 weighted image (HASTE) shows a water signal intensity extra axial cystic formation displacing the cortex. Surgical treatment was required after birth.

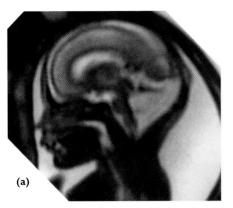 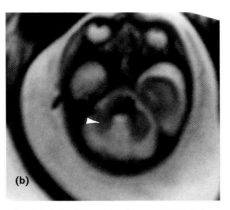 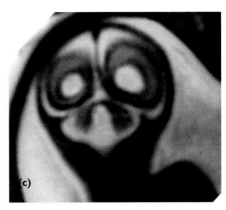

Fig. 15.7 Dandy–Walker malformation at 24 weeks' gestation. **(a)** Sagittal T2 weighted image (HASTE) shows an increase in CSF signal intensity in the posterior fossa with vermian agenesis. **(b)** Axial T2 weighted image (HASTE) shows hypoplasic cerebellar hemispheres (*arrow*). **(c)** Coronal T2 weighted image (HASTE) shows associated ventricular dilatation.

parenchymal lesions. MRI can depict those periventricular lesions (Fig. 15.8) which have a bad prognosis and modify family counselling. Definition of white matter structures may not at present be sufficient to identify more subtle abnormalities. It is hoped that future sequence development will allow MRI to detect more subtle WM injury in the fetal brain.

TUBEROUS SCLEROSIS

The diagnosis of tuberous sclerosis is difficult with antenatal US which only shows cardiac rhabdomyoma and may not detect cerebral anomalies. MRI may improve the detection of subependymal nodules and tubers[19].

The present

US evaluation remains the screening modality of choice to depict fetal CNS abnormalities. However, many series now report the potential of MRI to improve US diagnosis of cerebral anomalies, which may modify both the counselling of the family and the management of the pregnancy.

In our experience of all patients referred for fetal MR examinations, 25% of fetal images were normal. MRI confirmed the US findings in 50% of cases and provided additional diagnostic information in 50% of cases, which in some cases changed the management of the pregnancy.

The future

Fast MRI sequences allow an excellent study of the fetal brain without the need for sedation and already has the ability to supply valuable information about the fetus prior to delivery. This assessment could include the position of the umbilical cord, subtle abnormalities in fetal lie, and evidence of cephalo-pelvic disproportion. The future development of sequences could substantially improve the image quality, particularly for T1 weighted sequences. The additional use of contrast agents may help improve detection of lesions in certain pathological states. Perfusion/diffusion techniques could provide a unique tool for identifying areas of ischemia and for monitoring the development of white matter tracts. The acquisition of non-motion artifacted volume images will

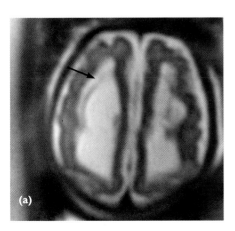 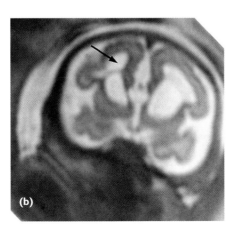

Fig. 15.8 Severe periventricular leukomalacia at 35 weeks, gestation. **(a)** Axial T2 weighted image (HASTE) shows ventricular enlargement with periventricular high signal intensity (*arrow*). There is marked atrophy of the white matter and secondary abnormal cortical folding. **(b)** Coronal T2 weighted image (HASTE) shows the cavities in the frontal parenchyma (*arrow*).

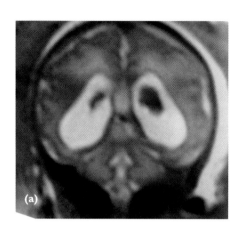
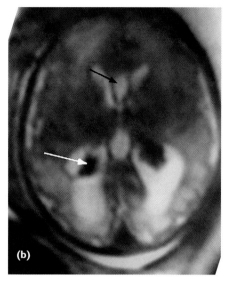

Fig. 15.9 Intraventricular hemorrhage and ventricular dilatation at 34 weeks' gestation. **(a)** Coronal T2 weighted image (HASTE) shows ventricular dilatation with a low signal intensity consistent with hemorrhage within the choroid plexuses (*arrow*). **(b)** Axial T2 weighted image (HASTE) shows the dilatation of occipital horns, the hypointense choroid plexuses (*white arrow*) and a cavum septum pellucidum (*black arrow*).

allow measurements of fetal brain structures providing normal ranges for brain development[1]. Subtle or new appearances on fetal brain imaging still need to be compared with the long-term clinical outcome of the child, with postnatal imaging and with histopathological study where relevant. Placental studies have been used to assess the normal and abnormal placenta[6,10] and to identify abnormal insertion of the placenta[17] and MR spectroscopy may also help assess placental function in health and disease[12]. MR offers an exciting new tool for assessing the function of the maternal–placental–fetal unit. Functional MRI in response to auditory stimulus has been reported[11]. As with all functional imaging studies, the interpretation of small imaging changes in the face of motion artifact remains a problem, though not an insoluble one.

Summary

- US evaluation remains the screening modality of choice to depict fetal CNS abnormalities.

- The use of fast MRI sequences, however, does allow an excellent study of the fetal brain without the need for sedation.

- The use of MR in the first trimester of pregnancy should be avoided.

- The maturation of the normal fetal brain can be compared to the anatomic atlas of Fees-Higgins and Larroche[5] and to published data on imaging in the preterm infant.

- The most frequent clinical indication for fetal MRI is ventriculomegaly detected with US with or without visualization of the corpus callosum.

- MRI contributes in the diagnosis and therapeutic management of arachnoid cysts and is helpful in clarifying US findings in cystic malformations of the posterior fossa.

- MRI can depict periventricular lesions more easily than fetal US.

- Fetal MRI is in its infancy. Coil and sequence development over the next few years should result in significant improvements in image quality.

References

1. Baker PN, Johnson IR, Gowland PA *et al.* (1995) Measurement of fetal liver, brain and placental volumes with echo-planar magnetic resonance imaging. *Br J Obstet Gynaecol* **102(1)**, 35–39.
2. Bennet GL, Bromley B and Benacerraf BR (1996) Agenesis of the corpus callosum: prenatal detection usually is not possible before 22 weeks of gestation. *Radiology* **199**, 447–450.
3. D'Ercole C, Girard N, Boubli L *et al.* (1993) Prenatal diagnosis of fetal cerebral abnormalities by ultrasonography and magnetic resonance imaging. *Eur J Obstet Gynecol Reprod Biol* **50(3)**, 177–184.
4. D'Ercole C, Girard N, Cravello L *et al.* (1998) Prenatal diagnosis of fetal corpus callosum agenesis by ultrasonography and magnetic resonance imaging. *Prenat Diagn* **18**, 247–253.
5. Fees-Higgins A and Larroche J-C (1987) *Le Développement du Cerveau Foetal Humain, Atlas Anatomique.* INSERM CNRS Masson Paris.
6. Francis ST, Duncan KR, Moore RJ *et al.* (1998) Non-invasive mapping of placental perfusion. *Lancet* **351**, 1397–1399.
7. Girard NJ and Raybaud C (1992) *In vivo* MRI of foetal brain cellular migration. *J Comput-Assist Tomogr* **16(2)**, 265–267.
8. Girard N and Raybaud C (2000) Can benign hydrocephalus be recognised *in utero*? *Child's Nerv Syst* **16**, 70.

9. Girard N, Raybaud C and Poncet M (1995) *In vivo* MR study of brain maturation in normal fetuses. *Am J Neuroradiol* **16 (2)**, 407–413.

10. Gowland PA, Freeman A, Issa B *et al.* (1998) *In vivo* relaxation time measurements in the human placenta using echoplanar imaging at 0.5 T. *Magn Reson Imaging* **16**, 241–247.

11. Hykin J, Moore R, Duncan K *et al.* (1999) Fetal brain activity demonstrated by functional magnetic resonance imaging. *Lancet* **354(9179)**, 645–646.

12. Kay HH, Hawkins SR, Gordon JD *et al.* (1992) Comparative analysis of normal and growth-retarded placentas with phosphorus nuclear magnetic resonance spectroscopy. *Am J Obstet Gynecol* **167**, 548–553.

13. Levine D and Barnes PD (1999) Cortical maturation in normal and abnormal fetuses as assessed with prenatal MR imaging. *Radiology* **210**, 751–758.

14. Levine D, Keedy G, Hatabu H *et al.* (1996) Obstetrical magnetic resonance imaging with HASTE. *Proceeding SIRMS* 159.

15. Levine D, Keedy J, Hatabu H *et al.* (1996) Obstetrical magnetic resonance imaging with HASTE (abstr). *Proceedings of the Fourth Meeting of the International Society for Magnetic Resonance in Medicine.* Berkeley, CA, International Society for Magnetic Resonance in Medicine, **1**, p. 159.

16. Levine D, Barnes P, Sher S *et al.* (1998) Fetal fast MR imaging: reproducibility, technical quality and conspicuity of anatomy. *Radiology* **206**, 549–554.

17. Levine D, Barnes PD and Edelman RR (1999) Obstetric MR imaging. *Radiology* **211**, 609–617.

18. Marcos HB, Semelka RC and Worawattanakul S (1997) Normal placenta: gadolinium-enhanced dynamic MR imaging. *Radiology* **205(2)**, 493–496.

19. Mirlesse V, Wener H, Jacquemard F *et al.* (1992) Magnetic resonance imaging in antenatal diagnosis of tuberous sclerosis. *Lancet* **340(7)**, 1163.

20. Nakayama T and Yamada R (1999) MR imaging of the posterior fossa structures of human embryos and fetuses. *Radiat Med* **17(2)**, 105–114.

21. Powel MC, Worthington BS, Buckley JM *et al.* (1988) Magnetic resonance imaging (MRI) in obstetrics. II. Fetal Anatomy. *Br J Obstet Gynecol* **95**, 38–46.

22. Revell M-P, Morell M-P, Bessis R *et al.* (1994) IRM du foetus *in utero*: une étude de 40 cas réalisés sans curarisation. *Rev Im Med* **6**, 91–100.

23. Schwartz J and Crooks L (1982) NMR imaging produces no observable mutations or cytotoxicity in mammalian cells. *AJR* **139**, 583–585.

24. Shakespeare SA, Moore RJ, Crowe *et al.* (1999) A method for foetal heart rate monitoring during magnetic resonance imaging using Doppler ultrasound. *Physiol Meas* **20**, 363–368.

25. Smith FW, Adam AH and Philips WDP (1983) NMR imaging in pregnancy. *Lancet* **1**, 61–62.

26. Sutton LN, Adzick NS, Bilaniuk LT *et al.* (1999) Improvement in hindbrain herniation demonstrated by serial fetal magnetic resonance imaging following fetal surgery for myelomeningocele. *JAMA* **17**, 1826–1831.

27. US Food and Drug Administration (1988) *Guidance for content and review of a magnetic resonance diagnosis device 510 (k) application.* Washington DC, US Food and Drug Administration, August 2.

28. Weinreb JC, Lowe TW, Santos-Ramos R *et al.* (1985) Magnetic resonance imaging in obstetric diagnosis. *Radiology* **154**, 157–167.

29. Yamashita Y, Namimoto T, Abe Y et al. (1997) MR imaging of the fetus by a HASTE sequence. *AJR* **168**, 513–519.

Magnetic resonance spectroscopy of the neonatal brain

Nicola J Robertson and I Jane Cox

Contents

Technical aspects

INTRODUCTION

Nuclear magnetic resonance (NMR) spectroscopy is one of the most important tools for quantitative analysis of chemical composition and structure; in the last two decades this technique has been applied *in vivo* to study biochemical processes in the preterm and term infant brain. Interpretation of a clinical MR spectrum can provide information about cellular energetics, membrane turnover, neuronal function, selected neurotransmitter activity, the fate of anesthetic agents and of certain drugs.

The first set of 1.5–2.0 Tesla (T) horizontal magnets in the early 1980s had a bore of approximately 20 cm, so it was feasible to study cerebral metabolism only in newborn infants[15]. It is now possible to obtain clinical MR spectra using whole-body 1.5–2.0 T MR systems[24], either as an adjunct to an MRI examination or as a separate study. The availability of routine clinical MRI systems with localized spectroscopy capabilities has considerably widened the applicability of clinical magnetic resonance spectroscopy (MRS). On some systems, generally those in a research setting, there is scope for obtaining spectra from a number of different nuclei, which allow different aspects of *in vivo* biochemistry to be studied.

OBTAINING MULTINUCLEAR SPECTRA

The NMR phenomenon underlies both MRI and clinical MRS[34]. While MRI demonstrates anatomy and highlights structural abnormalities, MRS may be used to obtain non-invasive metabolic information in health and disease. Certain atomic nuclei, such as hydrogen-1 (proton, ^1H), phosphorus-31 (^{31}P), carbon-13 (^{13}C), fluorine-19 (^{19}F) and nitrogen-15 (^{15}N), can be induced to produce radiofrequency signals in the presence of a strong magnetic field. In a static magnetic field (B_0) these nuclei become weakly magnetized along the direction of the field and can be imagined to be acting like tiny bar magnets. An MR signal is generated by applying a second time-dependent magnetic field (B_1), which changes the direction of magnetization. The induced magnetization then relaxes back to the original direction after the B_1 pulse has been removed, producing the MR signal which is known as the free induction decay (FID). The resonance frequency of a nucleus is primarily influenced by its magnetogyric ratio as well as B_0. For MRS applications, the FID can be resolved into a frequency spectrum by the mathematical function of Fourier transformation. The local magnetic environment of a nucleus and therefore the resonance frequency is subtly influenced by its immediate chemical environment. The relative frequency position can be described by a parameter known as chemical shift, a dimensionless unit accounting for the strength of the static magnetic field and measured in parts per million (ppm). In principle, the intensity of the metabolite signal is directly related to its concentration, but in practice absolute quantitation is difficult to achieve *in vivo*[14]. Many *in vivo* MRS studies, therefore, report results in terms of metabolite ratios. Since the technique is relatively insensitive only compounds present in millimolar concentrations are detectable using clinical *in vivo* MRS.

The phosphorus nucleus has proved to be particularly valuable in clinical *in vivo* MRS since it is technically straightforward to collect a spectrum and because the resonances observable are from phosphate groups in metabolites of central importance in energy metabolism.

The proton is the most common nucleus in biological systems and has the highest absolute NMR sensitivity. *In vivo* ^{1}H MRS studies are a technical challenge for a number of reasons: (i) the water signal is 10 000 times larger than signals from metabolites of interest; (ii) the chemical shift encountered covers a narrow range, so peak overlap is a problem. Furthermore there are stringent demands on magnetic field homogeneity; interaction between nearby protons within a molecule (spin–spin coupling) complicates the spectral pattern; and (iii) the scalp lipid signal is 100 times larger than the metabolite signals and produces broad features which can overlap and partially obscure the sharper resonances from smaller, more mobile species.

HARDWARE REQUIREMENTS

A clinical MR system comprises a magnet, shim coils, gradient coils, a radiofrequency transmitter/receiver system and a computer to perform the function of equipment control, acquisition, processing and data storage. For MRS applications, a multinuclear radiofrequency capability is required if nuclei other than protons are to be studied.

The static magnetic field needs to be at least 1 T to achieve adequate sensitivity within a clinical examination time, and also to achieve adequate dispersion of signals from different moieties.

A critical step prior to the acquisition of spectroscopy data is the process known as shimming, by which the magnetic field is made as uniform as possible within the selected volume of interest.

SEQUENCES

An important prerequisite for the detailed interpretation of a clinical MR spectrum is some knowledge of the region from which the spectrum is obtained. Combining an MRS study with an MRI examination allows definition and visualization of the region of interest. Spatial localization in MRS has generally been achieved by one or more of the following four techniques: image selected *in vivo* spectroscopy (ISIS), point-resolved spectroscopy (PRESS), stimulated echo acquisition mode (STEAM) and phase encoding (also known as chemical shift imaging, [CSI]). The first three are generally single volume techniques: the ISIS method is often used for ^{31}P MRS and the STEAM and PRESS methods are used for ^{1}H MRS in conjunction with water suppression techniques. Spectroscopic information can be obtained simultaneously from a number of voxels in the whole slice or volume using CSI methods.

As mentioned previously, the appearance of a spectrum is influenced by interactions between neighboring nuclei, which causes line splitting of the NMR signal. This interaction, known as spin–spin coupling, is generally stronger the closer the nuclei. Some nuclei are adjacent to nuclei with a zero magnetic moment and therefore the resonance is a single peak, for example the N-$(CH_3)_3$ peak in choline-containing compounds. The coupling pattern however can become very complex as is the case for the $-CH_2$-protons in glutamate and glutamine. If there is a time delay between excitation and the start of sampling of the FID (time to echo (TE)), for example if localization sequences are required, the phase of the coupled peaks is modulated and the resultant pattern will depend on both the delay before data acquisition and the coupling pattern. A good example of this is lactate; the methyl group in lactate is a doublet which will be inverted when the delay before data acquisition is 135 ms and upright when the delay is 270 ms.

Various sequences have been developed for minimizing the water signal in proton MRS, for example using chemical shift excitation pulses (CHESS) preceding the localization pulses, the excited transverse magnetization of the water is nulled by dephasing with spoiler gradients prior to the spatial localization sequence. Another approach is to use frequency selective excitation pulses, which have a null in the region of the water resonance and maximum excitation in the region of the metabolite signals, for example the 1331 binomial pulses. The water signal has a shorter T2 than the signal from metabolites so using a T2 weighted sequence will additionally suppress the water signal.

Suppression of scalp lipid signals may become necessary when the volume of interest is near to the brain surface, or when phase encoding techniques are used and voxels containing lipid are included in the matrix. The lipid signal can be separated from the lactate doublet by exploiting differences in relaxation properties and phase modulation characteristics; a long delay before data acquisition will preferentially reduce signals from lipids.

QUANTITATION

The NMR measurement of absolute *in vivo* metabolite concentrations will provide a more detailed insight into basic neurochemistry and mechanisms of damage than can be achieved using measurement of peak area ratios. However, in order for the measurement of metabolite concentrations to be more useful than peak area ratios a longer examination time is needed to collect all the required data. This is particularly a problem for neonatal studies when the study time is dictated by the length of time the neonate will remain sufficiently still. Therefore a decision often has to be made between the range of data collected (e.g. MRI, ¹H MRS and ³¹P MRS) and the extent to which specific spectral peak areas can be interpreted as metabolite concentrations.

Many MRS quantification techniques have been proposed and applied during the last 10 years[10,21,27,28,30,31,50,53,54,66,82,100]. In general, a reference MR signal is required from a standard of known or assumed concentration and a knowledge of the relaxation parameters of the metabolites of interest are required to interpret the MR parameters from a specific spectrum as metabolite concentrations. A number of studies have been undertaken reporting the T1 and T2 values in neonates[17,18,53,100].

The routine applicability of three reference methods has been compared in a recent multicenter trial[50]. The three methods used were: (i) an internal water standard[21], (ii) a phantom replacement method[12,30]; and (iii) a combined external standard/compartmental analysis method[31,54]. Using the internal standard the reference signal was collected from water, one of the compounds naturally existing in the region of interest. Using the phantom replacement method, the position of the volume of interest was constant, the patient being replaced by an external standard. Using the external phantom method, a sample was placed next to the patient in the receiver coil, so the reference signal was obtained during the patient examination but using different regions of interest. Variations arising from differing proportions of cerebral spinal fluid (CSF), gray and white matter could be accounted for by using compartmental analysis. Only the internal water standard technique could be readily implemented at all participating sites and provided acceptable precision and interlaboratory reproducibility[50].

The advantage of the internal water standard technique is that it is not necessary to compensate for any effects related to coil loading and to inhomogeneities in the pulse profile. There are no requirements for a phantom to be positioned, which can be practically difficult when the patient size varies considerably (e.g. comparing a preterm infant with a 1-month old healthy neonate). However, the internal water standard method requires knowledge of the MR-visible water concentration, that is not only what the water concentration is but how MR visible it is. For example, water bound to myelin is generally considered invisible since the T2 is 10–20 ms[61]. Corrections are required for the proportion of CSF, gray and white matter within the region of interest and also the NMR visible water content of gray and white matter fractions. In practice, fully relaxed *in vivo* water signals need to be acquired from the same region of interest as the metabolite signals at a range of TE values. If it is assumed that the water signal consists of contributions from CSF (with a long T2) and water within the brain (with a short T2), then a biexponential fit to the full set of water echoes will allow calculation of the brain tissue water signal and the CSF water signal. A consideration for applying this method to clinical studies of the neonate is that both the brain water concentration and the MR visible fraction may change with age, particularly prematurity[29], and also with pathology.

COMPARTMENTATION

Several types of cells are anatomically, biochemically and physiologically integrated to make up normally functioning brain tissue. The neuron is the communicating cell whose function is strongly shaped and sustained by the neuroglial cells. In a typical neuron, three major parts can be defined: i) the cell body or perikaryon which contains the nucleus and major cytoplasmic organelles ii) a variable number of dendrites which emanate from the perikaryon and ramify over a certain volume of gray matter and iii) a single axon which extends further from the perikaryon than the dendritic arbor. During development axons become surrounded by a myelin sheath which facilitates rapid impulse conduction. In addition to the ependyma lining the ventricles and central canal, there are three types of neuroglia or supporting cells in the brain: oligodendrocytes, astrocytes and microglia.

Cellular localization of function is referred to as compartmentation which may be either intercellular or intracellular. Due to the intrinsically low sensitivity of MR methods it is generally not possible *in vivo* to obtain spectra of single cells. Instead the spectrum is the sum of the signal from millions of cells and multiple cell types. In a few situations metabolic pathways and metabolites are localized to specific cell types and this can be seen using MRS. An example of this is the glutamate/glutamine neurotransmitter cycle in which glutamate released by neurons during neurotransmission is transported out of the synaptic cleft by surrounding glial cell membranes and converted to glutamine. This cycle is critical for normal brain function and protection against excitotoxicity. MRS measurements of isotopic labeling of metabolites involved allows information to be obtained about neuronal and glial metabolism and their interplay. This is discussed further in the section on glutamine and glutamate.

Normal brain development in infants and children

Major maturational processes such as neuronal organization, proliferation, differentiation of glial cells and myelination occur before and after birth. These processes are reflected by changes occurring in brain metabolites detected by ^{31}P and ^{1}H MRS. Metabolite concentrations also vary in different parts of the brain, for example the white matter and basal ganglia. An understanding of age-dependent and regional changes in metabolite ratios and absolute concentrations of ^{31}P and ^{1}H metabolites is important to enable accurate identification and recognition of metabolite abnormalities in pathological states.

In the following section, peaks detected by *in vivo* ^{31}P and ^{1}H MRS are assigned followed by a discussion of the role of the individual metabolites.

PHOSPHORUS-31 (^{31}P) MRS

The first ^{31}P MR spectrum was obtained in 1982 in a preterm infant[15]. [31]P MR spectra are generally taken from the whole brain because of the relatively low concentration.

Seven main peaks can be assigned in a cerebral phosphorus spectrum: phosphomonoesters (PME), inorganic phosphate (Pi), phosphocreatine (PCr), phosphodiesters (PDE) and the three phosphate groups (α, β, γ) in nucleotide triphosphate (NTP) (Fig. 16.1). Notably absent from the spectrum are signals from membrane phospholipids such as phosphatidylcholine. The phosphorus nuclei in such large molecules have reduced mobility and the signals are NMR invisible. Similarly the signal from adenosine diphosphate (ADP) bound to proteins is not detectable using NMR methods, and therefore the small ADP signal observed only represents free ADP. The dominant contribution to the NTP peaks is from adenosine triphosphate (ATP), but 10–20% of the peak area may be due to guanosine triphosphate (GTP) and uridine triphosphate (UTP). An unresolved peak from nicotinamide adenine dinucleotide (NAD[+]/NADH) may be observed as a right-hand shoulder on the αATP resonance[36]. In clinical studies this shoulder is often difficult to distinguish from αATP.

^{31}P MRS can also measure intracellular pH (pH_i), a measurement which is difficult to obtain by other means *in vivo*.

Phosphomonoesters (PME) and phosphodiesters (PDE)

The peak assigned to PME is multicomponent, and may contain contributions from phosphoethanolamine (PE) and phosphocholine (PC), metabolites on the pathway of membrane synthesis, as well as intermediates of carbohydrate metabolism such as glucose-6-phosphate. The PDE signal predominantly contains contributions from glycerophosphoethanolamine (GPE) and glycerophosphocholine (GPC), which represent phospholipid breakdown products.

Spectra from a newborn infant are characterized by a high peak from PME relative to the lower concentrations of PCr, Pi and PDE (Fig. 16.1). PME decreases and PDE increases during the first 2–3 years after birth[8,103]. The high PME peak at birth is attributed to the abundance of compounds destined for the production of membrane phospholipids and myelin whereas the PDE peak mainly represents phospholipid breakdown products. The change in the ratio of PME/PDE with maturation is therefore related to the process of myelination and proliferation and growth of glial cells. Quantification studies confirm this decrease in PME and increase in PDE with maturation; in addition there is a change in the chemical shift and width of the PME peak, indicating that the relative proportions of contributing metabolites, PE and PC, alter[13] (Table 16.1).

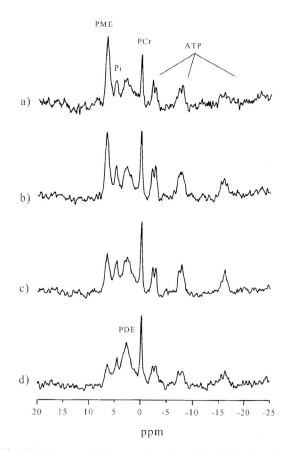

Fig. 16.1 ^{31}P MR spectra of **(a)** a normal preterm infant (GA 29[+3] weeks (age at scan 35[+1] weeks)), **(b)** a normal term infant, **(c)** an infant aged 6 months with normal neurodevelopmental outcome and **(d)** an adult control. These spectra illustrate the relative decrease in PME/ATP and increase in PDE/ATP with maturation.

Table 16.1 Concentrations of ³¹P metabolites in healthy brains of human neonates, infants and adults. (Reproduced with permission of the International Pediatric Research Foundation, Inc. from Buchli et al.[13])

		Mean concentration ±SD (mmol/l = mmol/dm³)					
	n	PME	Pi	PDE	PCr	ATP	³¹P total
Neonates	16	4.5 ± 0.7*	0.6 ± 0.1†	3.2 ± 0.8†	1.4 ± 0.2†	1.6 ± 0.2†	14.9 ± 2.3†
Infants	17	3.6 ± 0.9	0.6 ± 0.1	4.2 ± 0.7	1.7 ± 0.3	1.8 ± 0.3	16.1 ± 2.5
Adults	28	3.5 ± 0.6*	1.0 ± 0.2†	11.7 ± 2.2†	3.4 ± 0.5†	2.9 ± 0.4†	29.3 ± 3.1†

* Significant difference p <0.01.

† Significant difference p <0.001.

Phosphocreatine/inorganic phosphate (PCr/Pi)

When ATP generation is impaired, energy flux is maintained by the creatine kinase equilibrium with the breakdown of PCr and increase in Pi, so that a decline in the ratio of PCr/Pi is a valuable indicator of impaired energy metabolism even in the presence of normal or near normal ATP. PCr/Pi therefore gives a non-invasive measure of the adequacy of cerebral oxidative metabolism.

There is a significant increase with postnatal age in PCr/Pi in infants from 26 to 42 postconceptional weeks. As seen from the metabolite concentrations in Table 16.1, this reflects a more pronounced increase in PCr compared with Pi[13].

Adenosine triphosphate (ATP)

ATP is the energy currency of the cell and is produced more efficiently by oxidative phosphorylation (36 moles of ATP per mole of glucose) than anaerobic glycolysis (2 moles of ATP per mole of glucose). ATP concentrations have been presumed to be constant in the brain during maturation and have in the past been used as a stable reference to compare other metabolite changes[103]. This presumption was based on observations made in the biochemical analysis of the developing rat brain in which the cerebral [ATP] in both neonatal and adult rats were independent of age[62,67]. However, caution may be necessary since in one *in vivo* study using a calibration phantom as a concentration standard, [ATP] was almost double in adult brain compared to a healthy neonate[13].

Intracellular pH (pH$_i$)

In 1973, Moon and Richards demonstrated that ³¹P MRS could be used to measure pH$_i$ – a key variable controlling cell metabolism and function[69]. The theory underlying this is that Pi is an acid which titrates in the physiological pH range. The acidic form of Pi resonates at 3.29 ppm and the basic form at 5.68 ppm; however, because the protonation – deprotonation reaction is extremely fast, usually a single peak is seen, the position of which depends on the relative concentrations of acid or base. The pH$_i$ is calculated from the chemical shift difference between Pi relative to PCr using the Henderson–Hasselbalch equation and a suitable titration curve, for example:

$$pH_i = 6.77 + \log \frac{(Pi\ shift - 3.29)}{(5.68 - Pi\ shift)}$$

where Pi shift = chemical shift difference between PCr and Pi (Fig. 16.2)[81]

Estimation of pH$_i$ is accurate to about 0.1 pH units, and it is generally accepted that changes in pH can be measured to within 0.5 pH units or better[34]. Factors likely to affect the titration curve include temperature, ionic strength, presence of protein and the concentrations of sodium, potassium, phosphate, calcium and especially magnesium[81].

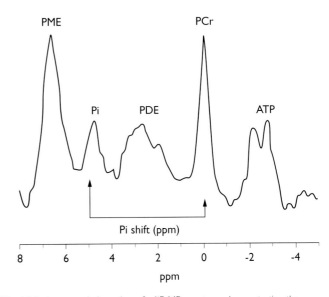

Fig. 16.2 An expanded portion of a ³¹P MR spectrum demonstrating the chemical shift difference between Pi and PCr which is the basis of pH$_i$ measurement. The unit of measure of Pi shift is ppm (parts per million); ppm = 10⁶ × (sample Hz – ref Hz)/ref Hz. The Pi chemical shift is independent of magnetic field strength allowing comparison of data from different spectrometers.

Table 16.2 pH$_i$ in healthy brains of human neonates, infants and adults. (Reproduced with permission of the International Pediatric Research Foundation, Inc. from Buchli et al.[13])

	n	Chemical shift difference shift (Pi-PCr) ppm	pH$_i$*
Neonates	16	4.93 ± 0.07	7.11 ± 0.06†
Infants	17	4.9 ± 0.08	7.09 ± 0.07
Adults	28	4.82 ± 0.08	7.02 ± 0.07†

$$* \; pH_i = 6.73 + \log \frac{Pi\ shift - 3.28}{5.69 - Pi\ shift}$$

† Significant difference: $p < 0.01$.

The chemical shift of the PME peak is also pH-sensitive and can be used to measure the intracellular pH$_i$ *in vivo*, although at physiological pH$_i$ values (from pH$_i$ range 6.9 to 7.2) this is less sensitive than the Pi shift[23].

The normal adult pH$_i$ has been reported to be 7.02 (+/−0.07) and this is thought to reflect the intracellular cytoplasmic pH. In our studies, normal infants born at term had a pH$_i$ of 7.05 +/− 0.06; in other studies however, the pH$_i$ was more alkaline at birth (7.11 +/− 0.06) with a subsequent decrease during postnatal maturation (Table 16.2)[3,13,71].

At high field strengths and under certain physiological conditions such as hypothermia, the Pi peak can be resolved into extra- and intracellular[83] and perhaps also mitochondrial[35,39] compartments, implying the presence of compartments of different pH. Our group has recently visualized a doublet Pi peak in some infants although it is presently unclear whether this doublet reflects extracellular and intracellular compartments[83], neuronal/glial compartmentation[98] or different intracellular compartments[35].

Regional variation

Owing to the low sensitivity of the phosphorus nucleus and the large voxel size required, most neonatal ^{31}P spectra are taken from the entire brain and cannot differentiate between gray and white matter. Regional differences in gray and white matter have been demonstrated in the adult and are likely to apply to the infant. Gray matter was found to have significantly higher ratios of PCr to γ-ATP whereas the PCr/Pi ratio and pH$_i$ were not significantly different[64].

PROTON (^{1}H) MRS

The first ^{1}H MR spectrum from the neonatal brain was obtained in the early 1990s – almost a decade after the first neonatal ^{31}P MR spectrum. The information obtained in a ^{1}H MR spectrum is complementary to that obtained in a ^{31}P

MR spectrum. Because of the greater sensitivity of the ^{1}H nucleus, data can be obtained from smaller regions of the brain. In addition, different TEs can be used to obtain more metabolite information. At short TEs, *myo*-inositol, Glx, lipids and macromolecules are more easily seen. Long TEs are usually used to obtain information about lactate as there will be less contamination from lipids and macromolecules.

Three singlet peaks can be readily assigned in the proton spectrum to N-acetylaspartate (NAA), choline-containing compounds (Cho) and creatine plus phosphocreatine (Cr). In addition more complex peaks can be identified from protons in a range of metabolites, if present, including lactate, inositols (specifically *myo*-inositol (mI)), alanine, glutamine (Gln) and glutamate (Glu).

Physiological changes in the ^{1}H MR spectrum occur during the first 2–3 years of postnatal life with the most important changes occurring in the first year. Age-specific, reproducible, regional studies with absolute quantitation of ^{1}H MR metabolites are difficult to obtain[73]. Adult norms are more established and are achieved by 3 years of age, reflecting the successful completion of most myelination and organization events.

N-acetylaspartate (NAA)

All studies have documented an increase in NAA after birth, with it becoming the dominant peak by 6 months of age[51,53,103] (Fig. 16.3). Quantification studies have confirmed an almost doubling of NAA from birth levels of 4.82 mM to adult levels of 8.89 mM[53].

NAA is an amino acid found exclusively in the nervous system and is synthesized in brain mitochondria from acetyl-CoA and aspartate by the enzyme L-aspartate N-acetyl transferase. NAA has been used as a neuronal marker, as apart from oligodendrocyte type 2 astrocyte precursors, NAA is present primarily in neurons[102]. More recently, studies have demonstrated that mature oligodendrocytes can express NAA *in vitro* when trophic factors are used[6]; this observation challenges the concept that NAA changes observed *in vivo* ^{1}H MRS reflect neuronal function alone. The exact functions and roles of this amino acid are unclear although it is thought to have a role in myelination in the developing brain, metabolism of specific brain fatty acids, ion balance and neuromodulation. NAA can be detected in the cerebral cortex and white matter of fetuses as early as 16 weeks' gestation and shows an age-dependent increase in synthetic rate which is reflected in total brain levels of NAA[49].

Using *in vivo* ^{1}H MRS and high performance liquid chromatography, a marked regional variation in NAA concentrations was demonstrated in healthy preterm (gestational age (GA) 27–34 weeks studied at postconceptional age (PCA) 31–37 weeks) and term infants with higher concentrations in

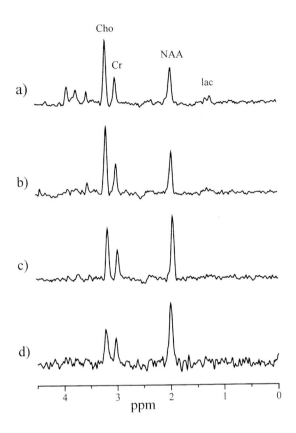

Fig. 16.3 ¹H MR spectra (TE 270 ms) from an 8 cm³ voxel within the basal ganglia of **(a)** a normal preterm infant (GA 29⁺³ weeks (age at scan 35⁺¹ weeks)), **(b)** a normal preterm infant, **(c)** an infant aged 6 months with normal neurodevelopmental outcome, and **(d)** an adult control. This series demonstrates that by 6 months NAA has become the dominant peak in the spectrum, the Cho/Cr ratio decreases with maturation and that lactate is only easily visible in the preterm infant.

the thalamus and basal ganglia than the frontal lobe and pre-central gyrus[47]. Of note, the NAA concentrations of these healthy preterm infants at 40 weeks PCA were no different to NAA concentrations of term newborns studied shortly after birth.

Choline-containing compounds (Cho)

The Cho peak includes free choline, phosphocholine and glycerophosphocholine. These compounds are intermediates in phospholipid metabolism. The Cho/Cr ratio decreases with increasing postnatal age until about 3 years of age. Quantification studies confirm that the newborn brain contains higher concentrations of Cho than the adult brain[53]. The reduction in Cho/Cr mirrors the fall in PME with age and it has been suggested that the accelerated myelination during the first few months of life incorporates a proportion of these 'NMR-visible' choline residues into an 'invisible' macromolecule associated with myelin[53]. Cho/Cr is high in the acute state of demyelinating disease and some infants with neurologic abnormalities: this may represent the inverse process described above or an abnormality in phospholipid metabolism.

Creatine plus phosphocreatine (Cr)

The equilibrium enzyme creatine kinase converts Cr to PCr, which is the short-term energy storage form of the tissue. The total measured Cr (sum of PCr and Cr), therefore, may reflect the energy potential available. As seen from Table 16.3, the concentration of Cr increases rapidly before and around term[53].

TABLE 16.3 Absolute concentrations of different age groups in mmol/kg brain tissue (mean +/−1 SEM) and significance tests for the differences found. (Reproduced with permission of Wiley from Kreis et al.[53])

Group	n (ROIs)	GA (weeks)	pn age (weeks)	NAA	Cr	Cho	ml
<42 GA	11	38.7 ± 0.7	3.9 ± 1.6	4.82 ± 0.54ª	6.33 ± 0.32	2.41 ± 0.11	10.1 ± 1.1
42–60 GA	8	50.2 ± 1.8	9.3 ± 1.9	7.03 ± 0.41	7.28 ± 0.28	2.23 ± 0.06	8.52 ± 0.92
<2 pn	6	40.0 ± 1.0	0.8 ± 0.2	5.52 ± 0.64	6.74 ± 0.43	**2.53 ± 0.12**	**12.4 ± 1.4**
2–10 pn	7	41.9 ± 1.5	3.8 ± 0.9	5.89 ± 0.21	6.56 ± 0.44	2.16 ± 0.09	7.69 ± 0.62
Adult	10		1440 ± 68	**8.89 ± 0.17**	**7.49 ± 0.12**	**1.32 ± 0.07**	**6.56 ± 0.43**
p value: 42 GA versus adult				<0.0001	<0.0001	<0.0001	0.001
p value: 42 GA versus 42 to 60 GA				0.0007	0.02	0.07	0.10
p value: 42 to 60 GA versus adult				<0.0001	0.16	<0.0001	0.0003
p value: <2 pn versus adult				<0.0001	0.005	<0.0001	<0.0001
p value: <2 pn versus 2 to 10 pn				0.7	0.8	0.02	0.004
p value: 2–10 pn versus adult				<0.0001	0.001	<0.0001	0.007

ª Minima and maxima are highlighted in bold. ROI, region of interest; pn, postnatal; GA, gestational age; NAA, N-acetyl aspartate; Cr, creatine; Cho, choline; ml, *myo*-inositol.

Regional variation and differing rates of increase in Cr concentrations have been demonstrated in healthy preterm infants. At term, Cr is significantly higher in the thalamus and basal ganglia compared to the frontal lobe and precentral gyrus[47]. These findings are in concordance with positron emission tomography studies showing local cerebral metabolic rates for glucose to be highest in the thalamus and basal ganglia[22].

Several MRS studies of term infants after hypoxic injury (HI) have used Cr as a metabolite of reference because the Cr concentration has been reported to be relatively stable after such an insult[18].

Studies in neonatal rats have explored whether systemic injections of creatine are neuroprotective – in one study creatine injection 3 days prior to a hypoxic insult increased survival and suppressed seizures in the immature rat[45]. Further studies are needed.

Lactate

The doublet signal at 1.33 ppm is easily observed when cerebral lactate levels are increased, although good spatial localization is required to eliminate interfering resonances from extracranial lipids. Confirmation of the assignment of the lactate doublet resonance is readily established by varying the echo time (TE 135 ms doublet inverted, TE 270 ms doublet upright) (Fig 16.4).

Lactate and its redox partner pyruvate have a central position as the terminal metabolites of glycolysis within the cytosol and pyruvate as the initial substrate for the mitochondrial tricarboxylic acid (TCA) cycle. The lactate concentration must rise whenever the glycolytic rate in a volume of tissue exceeds the capacity to catabolize lactate or export it to the bloodstream. The prospect of measuring cerebral lactate was one of the driving forces for the development of localized *in vivo* ^{1}H MRS because of its importance as a marker of tissue ischemia and hypoxia. During normal aerobic conditions, lactate is present in the normal adult brain at concentrations of approximately 0.3 to 1 mM, which is close to the NMR detectable limit. In hypoxia and stroke brain lactate can increase to concentrations above 10 mM. Lactate can be detected in the brain of healthy preterm infants; indeed studies estimate brain lactate concentrations to be 0.9–2.4 mM in this patient group, the concentration increasing with decreasing gestational age and degree of growth restriction[57]. This may be a reflection of the immature stage of enzyme development in the preterm brain[9,85] and is explained by the increasing dependence on glycolysis compared with mitochondrial respiration with immaturity. This less efficient method of energy production may be sufficient for the

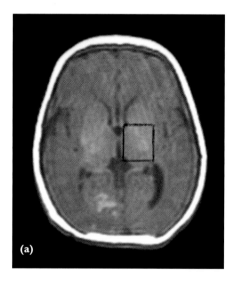
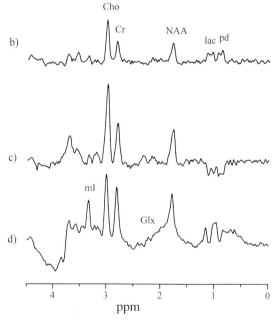

Fig. 16.4 Male term infant aged 5 days following neonatal encephalopathy due to birth asphyxia. **(a)** T1 weighted spin echo transverse image (SE 500/20) at the level of the basal ganglia. There is some abnormal signal intensity in the thalami and the posterior lentiform nucleus on the right. There is a diminished signal from myelin in the posterior limb of the internal capsule. **(b,c,d)** [1]H MR spectra (PRESS) from a 2 cm[3] voxel encompassing the left basal ganglia in the same infant with neonatal encephalopathy demonstrating modulation of lactate doublet at various echo times, **(b)** the lactate doublet is upright at TE 270 ms, **(c)** the lactate doublet is inverted at TE 135 ms, and **(d)** the lactate doublet is out of phase at TE 40 ms. This modulation pattern is determined by the 7 Hz coupling constant of the lactate doublet. Propan-1,2-diol, the carrier for phenobarbital and phenytoin, resonates at 1.1 ppm and also undergoes phase modulation at different echo times.

preterm brain as the energy requirement (measured by oxygen uptake) is low at 26 to 32 weeks for example, when it is around one sixth that of the adult brain and one half of the term brain[1]. Regional variation in lactate ratios have been demonstrated with higher concentrations seen in the occipitoparietal regions compared to the basal ganglia suggesting a relative immaturity and a reduction in oxidative phosphoylation in this particularly vulnerable area[79].

For some time it has been known that plasma lactate can be used as a fuel in the normal preweaning neonatal brain[104]; studies on monocarboxylate transporters have clarified this further. These transporters, present on the blood-brain barrier in early life, transport lactate from plasma to brain, however after weaning these transporters disappear and plasma lactate can no longer be used as a major fuel by the brain[76].

Although plasma lactate cannot substitute for glucose as a metabolic substrate in the post weaning brain because of its limited permeability across the blood brain barrier, it is now clear that in physiological states lactate formed *within* the brain parenchyma (for example through glutamate-activated glycolysis in astrocytes) can fulfill the energetic needs of neurons. Indeed *in vivo* ^{1}H MRS studies in humans demonstrate a *transient* lactate peak in the primary visual cortex during physiological stimulation; this is consistent with *neuronal activation-induced glycolysis*[84]. The following mechanism for glutamate-induced glycolysis in astrocytes during physiological activation has been proposed and confirmed by *in vitro* experimental evidence[77,78] (Fig. 16.5).

Glial cells make up approximately half of the brain volume and the astrocyte is one of the predominant glial cells. Astrocytes outnumber neurons by as much as 10:1 even in the healthy brain and are ideally suited to couple local changes in neuronal activity with adaptations in energy metabolism. Astrocytic perivascular endfeet surround brain capillaries; this therefore is a likely site for the predominant uptake of glucose. In addition astrocytes have processes which ensheathe synaptic contacts. Neuronal activity leads to release of glutamate, which depolarizes postsynaptic neurons. The action of glutamate is terminated by an efficient glutamate uptake system located in astrocytes. Glutamate is co-transported with Na[+], leading to an increase in the intra-astrocytic concentration of Na[+], which in turn leads to an activation of the astrocyte Na[+], K[+]-ATPase. Activation of the Na[+], K[+]-ATPase stimulates glycolysis (glucose utilization and lactate production). Lactate is then released into the extracellular space to be used by neurons.

myo-Inositol

myo-inositol is a naturally occurring sugar and is normally present at about 5 mM in the adult brain. It can be visualized by ^{1}H MRS at short echo times (keeping T_2 and *J*-coupling effects to a minimum). One resonance can be observed at approximately 3.56 ppm (Fig. 16.6) and a second distinct resonance of *myo*-inositol at 4.06 ppm, however this is too close to the partially suppressed water peak to be reliably quantified. Seventy per cent of the major *myo*-inositol resonance is *myo*-inositol itself, 15% *myo*-inositol-monophosphate, and 15% glycine[94].

myo-Inositol is one of the dominant peaks at short TEs in newborn proton spectra (Fig. 16.6). The intracerebral concentration of *myo*-inositol at birth is approximately 12 mM and it decreases rapidly after birth to reach adult levels at around 2 months. Although there is a trend toward a higher *myo*-inositol concentration the more premature the baby, the concentration of *myo*-inositol is mostly determined by postnatal age[51]. This agrees with reports of newborn CSF having 20 times the concentration of *myo*-inositol than adult CSF and being twice as high in umbilical artery blood than adult plasma. There is evidence to suggest that *myo*-inositol is associated with surfactant production – administration of *myo*-inositol to immature animals increased levels of pulmonary surfactant[2] and supplementation with *myo*-inositol in preterm infants reduced severity of respiratory distress syndrome, although exogenous natural surfactant had a more striking effect[40].

In 1984, Berridge discovered the activity for which inositols are now best known[5] – as an intermediate in the cerebral inositol polyphosphate (IPP) cascade, they are active in releasing Ca[2+] from endoplasmic reticulum and mitochon-

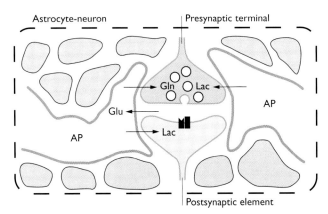

Fig. 16.5 The astrocyte-neuron metabolic unit. Glutaminergic terminals and the astrocytic processes that surround them can be viewed as a highly specialized metabolic unit in which the activation signal (glutamate) is manufactured by the neuron and presented to the astrocyte. Glutamate is then taken up by the astrocyte, thus removing glutamate from the extracellular space (ECS) and protecting surrounding cells from excitotoxicity from glutamate. Glutamate taken up by the astrocyte is converted to glutamine, then released into the ECS where it is taken up by neurons and converted back to glutamate for further signaling. In the astrocyte, meanwhile, glutamate stimulates glucose uptake and glycolysis to lactate. The lactate is then 'shuttled' to the neuron where it can be used as a fuel. (Reproduced with permission of the Academic Press from Zigmond et al[113].)

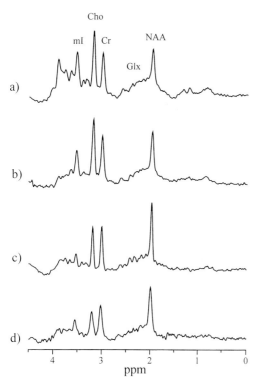

Fig. 16.6 ¹H MR spectra (TE 40 ms) from an 8 cm³ voxel within the basal ganglia of **(a)** a normal preterm infant (GA 29⁺³ weeks (age at scan 35⁺¹ weeks)), **(b)** a normal term infant, **(c)** an infant aged 6 months with normal neurodevelopmental outcome, and **(d)** an adult control. This series demonstrates the added metabolite information obtained at short TE time, particularly from *myo*-inositol and glutamine/glutamate. *Myo*-Inositol is prominent in the spectra from the preterm and newborn infants.

dria, thus linking hormone receptor binding with intracellular activity. The inositols therefore are second messengers for the hormone actions of vasopressin, thyrotrophin and angiotensin II for example. *myo*-Inositol also functions as a major non-nitrogenous osmoregulator in the CNS[94]. Clinical evidence for such a function is a reversible increase in brain *myo*-inositol detected with ¹H MRS in an infant with severe hypernatremia[56] and a decrease in *myo*-inositol in several patients with severe hyponatremia[105] (Fig. 16.7). Other roles proposed for *myo*-inositol are cell nutrition[46] and detoxification[52]. The *myo*-inositol peak visible by MR represents free *myo*-inositol acting as an intracellular osmolyte as *myo*-inositol involved in signal transduction is mostly bound and present in very small concentration.

There is no consensus on the metabolic significance of an increased or decreased concentration of brain *myo*-inositol. Increased ratios of cerebral mI have been described in Alzheimer's disease[68,86], Down's syndrome[97] (Fig. 16.8) and HIV dementia[20]. Decreased levels of *myo*-inositol have been described in hepatic encephalopathy[52]. Possible mechanisms for an increase in *myo*-inositol are: (i) loss of neurons and replacement by glia (gliosis) as this might result in a reciprocal loss of NAA and increase in *myo*-inositol/Cr. This presumption rests on the *in vitro* work by Brand *et al.* on embryonic nervous tissue in culture which identified *myo*-inositol as a marker for glia[11] although other more recent *in vitro* studies have documented high levels of *myo*-inositol in neuronal cultures[70]; and (ii) osmotic stress, which may upregulate the expression of the sodium/*myo*-inositol cotransporter (SMIT), thereby increasing intracellular *myo*-inositol levels. Evidence for this comes from *in vitro* work where the abundance of SMIT mRNA and the transcription rate of the SMIT gene were increased when brain glial cells were cultured in hypertonic medium[33]. Upregulation of SMIT has been demonstrated in cultured fibroblasts in Down's syndrome; this may explain the increased *myo*-inositol seen in these patients (Fig. 16.8).

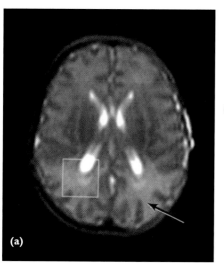

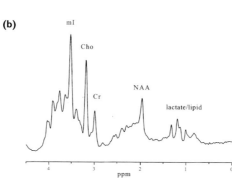

Fig. 16.7 This male infant was born at 23 weeks' gestation and scanned at 36 weeks. He had severe respiratory distress syndrome and was ventilator dependent for several weeks. One week prior to the scan he developed diarrhea and became dehydrated. His serum sodium increased to 179 mmol/l 2 days prior to the scan and was still elevated on the day of scan. **(a)** T2 weighted images show slightly high signal intensity (*arrow*) in the posterior white matter bilaterally. **(b)** ¹H MRS spectrum acquired from an 8 cm³ voxel in the posterior periventricular white matter demonstrating a raised *myo*-inositol/Cr of 3.63. This increase in *myo*-inositol is likely to be in response to the hypernatremia.

We have observed changes in *myo*-Inositol during the first week after birth in infants with severe neonatal encephalopathy. This will be discussed in the section below.

Glutamate, glutamine and γ amino butyric acid (GABA)

Glutamate is the major neurotransmitter for brain excitatory function and GABA is the major neurotransmitter for inhibitory function. Both of these neurotransmitters are taken up by the surrounding glial cells after release from the nerve terminal. Glutamate re-uptake and synthesis is required or else the nerve terminal precursor pool will become depleted. Glial cells are able to transport glutamate from the synaptic cleft so maintaining low concentrations of extracellular glutamate. Glutamate taken up by glia is converted to glutamine by glutamine synthetase, an enzyme exclusively in glia. Glutamine is released from the glia to the ECF where it is taken up by neurons and converted back to glutamate. The localization of glutamate and glutamine as well as the enzyme glutamine synthetase provides the basis for studying neuronal/glial interactions *in vivo* by MRS. Carbon-13 (^{13}C) MRS has been used to obtain information about glial and neuronal metabolism as well as metabolic flux, enzyme activities and metabolic regulation *in vivo* of the ^{13}C isotopic enrichment of specific carbon positions of glutamate and glutamine.

Cerebral pathology

In the following section ^{31}P and ^{1}H MRS findings are discussed with reference to term neonatal encephalopathy and preterm brain injury. Recently considerable doubt has been cast on the assumption that perinatal hypoxia-ischemia (HI) is the primary cause of neonatal encephalopathy and cerebral palsy. Important epidemiological studies have suggested a wide range of alternative causal pathways such as maternal fever during labor, chorioamnionitis, maternal thyroid disease and abnormalities of the haemostatic system. There appears, however, to be at least a subgroup of infants with neonatal encephalopathy who have cerebral metabolic changes entirely characteristic of acute cerebral hypoxia–ischemia in the perinatal period.

Damage to the preterm brain is an increasingly important problem as more extremely low birth weight infants are surviving. Less is known about the cerebral metabolic events associated with preterm brain injury; however, there is increasing evidence of a major role of infection or inflammatory processes while secondary energy failure is unlikely to have a central role.

TERM NEONATAL ENCEPHALOPATHY AND FOLLOW-UP

Secondary energy failure

ATP is the energy currency for the cell. In situations where oxidative phosphorylation is impaired, such as hypoxia–ischemia, [ATP] will fall; the fall is initially extremely small because of the buffering effect of the creatine kinase reaction. While this reaction maintains [ATP] close to normal, [PCr] falls and [Pi] increases, that is the PCr/Pi ratio decreases. This ratio is proportional to the phosphorylation potential of the tissue and is a measure of the energy reserve of the tissue. Only when [PCr] becomes depleted to 1 mM does the [ATP] fall.

^{31}P MRS has been important in demonstrating the biphasic pattern of energy failure during and after hypoxia–ischemia. Experimental studies in several species of mammal have confirmed this biphasic pattern of cerebral metabolic abnormality during and after cerebral hypoxia–ischemia. In the piglet during global hypoxia–ischemia[59,80] and during focal stroke in rat pups[7,108] there was 'primary' energy failure: intracerebral

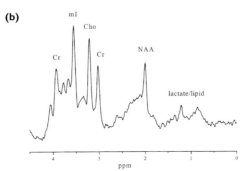

(b)

Fig. 16.8 Term-born infant with Down's syndrome. **(a)** T2 weighted images show some slightly high signal intensity (*arrow*) throughout the white matter only. The head is brachycephalic. **(b)** ^{1}H MRS spectrum (TE 40 ms) acquired from the same infant demonstrating a raised *myo*-inositol/Cr of 1.71.

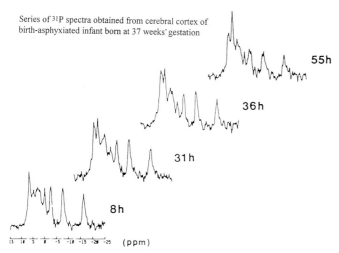

Series of ^{31}P spectra obtained from cerebral cortex of birth-asphyxiated infant born at 37 weeks' gestation

55h

36h

31h

8h

(ppm)

Fig. 16.9 ^{31}P spectra from a birth-asphyxiated infant born at 37 weeks' gestation: postnatal ages at the time of study are indicated. At 8 h PCr/Pi was 0.99, ATP/total P was 0.09, and pH$_i$ was 7.06: pH$_i$ rose to a maximum of 7.28 at 36 h. Minimum value for PCr/Pi was 0.32 at 55 h when ATP/total P was 0.04 and pH$_i$ 6.99. The infant died at 60 h. (Reproduced with permission of the International Pediatric Research Foundation, Inc., from Azzopardi et al.[3].)

PCr/Pi fell and the pH$_i$ became acidotic. Eventually [ATP] fell, but on resuscitation, metabolites returned to normal within 1–2 h. Some 6–12 hours later, the period of secondary energy failure began during which PCr/Pi again declined, lactate increased and the pH$_i$ became alkaline. There was a dose response between the severity of HI insult and the magnitude of the secondary changes in cerebral energy metabolism. The more severe the cerebral metabolic injuries, the worse the histological injury.

MRS of term infants with neonatal encephalopathy demonstrated identical abnormalities of cerebral energy metabolism. The primary event cannot be observed but newborn infants following HI were seen to have normal phosphorylation potential and pH$_i$ on the first day of life. 8 to 24 h after birth a delayed decline in PCr/Pi or 'secondary' energy failure occurred[4] (Fig. 16.9) accompanied by an alkalotic pH$_i$ and an increase in brain lactate[43]. The magnitude of PCr/Pi drop during secondary energy failure was seen to correlate with subsequent neurodevelopmental abnormality and reduced cranial growth 1 and 4 years later[95,96]. Elevated cerebral lactate within 18 h of birth asphyxia predicted adverse outcome at 1 year of age[43] (Figs 16.10 and 16.11). Recent data from our laboratory suggest that brain *myo*-inositol/Cr is increased during the period of secondary energy failure in those infants with neonatal encephalopathy associated with increased lactate/Cr, MRI changes of severe injury and a poor neurodevelopmental outcome at one year. A possible explanation for this acute change in *myo*-inositol/Cr may be the induction of the sodium/*myo*-inositol cotransporter (SMIT), one of the many gene expressions to be influenced by an acute insult[109,110].

Follow-up after neonatal encephalopathy

Lactate can persist in the brain for weeks or months in infants who develop neurodevelopmental impairment (Fig. 16.12). Lactate was detected in the brain using ^{1}H MRS after 4 weeks of age in seven out of eight infants with

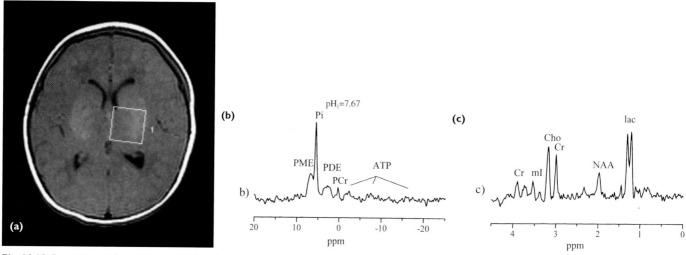

Fig. 16.10 Female term infant with severe birth asphyxia imaged at 2 days of age. MR data obtained on a Picker Eclipse system. **(a)** A T1 weighted spin echo sequence (SE 500/20) in the transverse plane at the level of the basal ganglia. The brain is normally formed although edematous. There is abnormal high signal intensity in the lentiform and thalami nuclei and an absence of signal from myelin in the posterior limb of the internal capsule. There is loss of gray/white matter differentiation **(b)** ^{31}P MR spectrum taken from a 125 cm^3 voxel encompassing the whole brain in the same baby demonstrating a depletion of ATP and PCr, a markedly raised Pi and an alkaline pH$_i$ consistent with an abnormal outcome with severe neurodevelopmental impairment. **(c)** ^{1}H MR spectrum from an 8 cm^3 voxel (left basal ganglia) in the same baby demonstrating a decreased NAA and markedly increased lactate levels. The MR findings are associated with an abnormal outcome with severe neurodevelopmental impairment and this baby died on day 5.

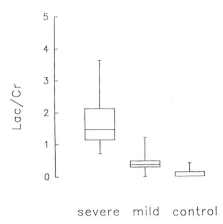

Fig. 16.11 Medians, interquartile ranges, 5th and 95th centiles of lactate/Cr measured by ^{1}H MRS during the first 18 h after birth in asphyxiated infants in whom later measurements found PCr/Pi <0.75 (severe) or PCr/Pi >0.75 (mild) and in controls (control). Values in the three groups are significantly different (Kruskall–Wallis). (Reproduced with permission of MacKeith Press from Hanrahan et al.[43].)

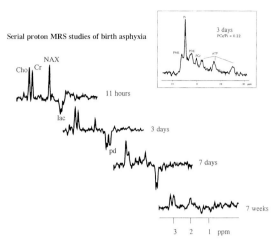

Fig. 16.12 Representative ^{1}H MR spectra from the basal ganglia of a term infant with severe birth asphyxia. The ^{1}H MR data were collected using chemical shift imaging techniques with TE 130 ms. A signal from lactate could be detected at all the time points studied. The inset ^{31}P MR spectrum at 2 days of age showed severe secondary energy failure, consistent with an abnormal outcome.

abnormal neurodevelopmental outcome at 1 year after perinatal asphyxia; none of the infants with normal outcome at 1 year showed evidence of persisting lactate[42]. A recent study of 43 babies following perinatal asphyxia demonstrated a significant relationship between persisting increased cerebral lactate levels and alkaline pH_i, that is a persisting lactic alkalosis (Fig. 16.13) and also decreased phosphorylation potential (increased Pi/PCr)[89]. Comparing those infants with normal or abnormal neurodevelopmental outcomes at 1 year of age, there were significant differences for lactate/Cr measured at most times, pH_i measured at all times, Pi/PCr measured in the first 2 weeks and NAA/Cr measured after the first 2 weeks. pH_i was the strongest predictor of outcome at all times up to 30 weeks postnatal age.

Possible causes for this persisting cerebral intracellular lactic alkalosis are: (i) an altered redox state caused by an inability to regenerate NAD[+]; (ii) infiltration of activated phagocytes which have an enhanced glycolytic rate thus increasing lactate production[58]; (iii) altered buffering mechanisms (e.g. Na[+]/H[+] antiporter) in the remaining cells[32] and/or (iv) stimulation of glycolysis in the astrocyte with production of lactate which can then be used as a fuel for neurons. Glutamate uptake is known to stimulate glycolysis, similarly an alkaline milieu inside the cell will stimulate glycolysis due to the pH dependency of the glycolytic enzyme phosphofructokinase. Further understanding of the mechanisms leading to these prolonged changes may lead to other modalities of intervention with the aim of improving neurodevelopmental outcome[88].

We found a significantly lower NAA/Cr in infants with an abnormal outcome at 1 year after neonatal encephalopathy after 2 weeks of age[89]. Other studies have shown a reduced NAA/Cr at 7 days[37], 14 days[75] and at 3 months[37] and this has been shown to be indicative of an abnormal outcome after

(a)

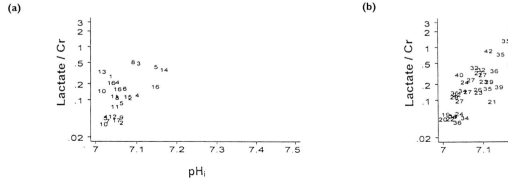

(b)

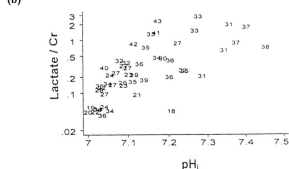

Fig. 16.13 Lactate/Cr plotted against pH_i for normal **(a)** and abnormal **(b)** outcome. Linear regression analysis showed a significant relationship between lactate/Cr and pH_i. The relationship was the same irrespective of outcome. (Reproduced with permission of the International Pediatric Research Foundation, Inc. from Robertson et al.[89].)

perinatal HI. A further study done in infants at an earlier stage after birth asphyxia (median of 1.3 days)[79] showed no convincing reduction with age-matched controls, however in some very severely damaged infants we have demonstrated a reduction in NAA/Cr at <24 h.

In summary, ^{1}H and ^{31}P MRS have been important in furthering our understanding of the metabolic response to injury of the brain in the term infant and have led us to suspect an on-going metabolic derangement following HI in those with abnormal neurodevelopmental outcome.

PRETERM BRAIN INJURY

The more subtle effects of prematurity in the absence of detectable brain injury are now well recognized and include minor neurocognitive impairments, behavioral difficulties and specific learning disorders. It is unknown whether prematurity itself affects brain development with data suggesting either delay, acceleration or no effect. A comparison of ex-preterm infants (mean GA 30.5 +/− 1.8 weeks) at a corrected age of term with term-born infants using ^{1}H MRS revealed no statistically significant differences in concentrations of NAA, Cho and *myo*-inositol between groups[48], although there were differences in imaging findings and in some behavior parameters.

It is well known that structural brain injury occurring in preterm infants, such as periventricular leukomalacia (PVL) and hemorrhagic parenchymal infarction (HPI), have an impact on later cognitive and neuromotor performance[106]. It is now generally accepted that white matter damage (WMD) in the premature infant is a better predictor of poor neurologic outcome than isolated intraventricular hemorrhage (IVH)[74] and that IVH with ventricular dilatation are powerful predictors of WMD occurrence[55]. In a 2-year cohort study of infants born at <30 weeks' gestation there was a high incidence of MRI abnormality in the white matter (WM)[60]. This was associated with high concentrations of pro-inflammatory cytokines and T-cell activation in umbilical cord blood, which accords well with other data suggesting that fetoplacental infection is a cause of both preterm birth and cerebral WM injury[25]. There are at present no MRS studies looking at the characteristics of this WM.

White Matter Damage (WMD)

We have recently assessed the biochemical characteristics of WMD (consisting of both PVL and HPI) using ^{1}H and ^{31}P MRS and compared this to preterm infants with no WMD at a corrected age of term. 30 infants (gestational age 27.9 ± 3.1 weeks, birth weight 1122 ± 4459) were studied at a postnatal age of 9.8 ± 4.1 weeks (corrected age 40.3 ± 3.9 weeks[92]). In the WMD group, mean lactate/Cr and *myo*-

inositol/Cr were higher than the normal WM group. There was no difference in the NAA/Cr, Cho/Cr or pH$_i$ between the two groups. We found the absence of an alkaline pH$_i$ in cases with a markedly elevated brain lactate interesting; the relationship between pH$_i$ and lactate/Cr appears to differ in preterm infants compared to term infants following neonatal encephalopathy. For a given lactate/Cr in a preterm infants the pH$_i$ was never as alkaline as it was in term infants after perinatal HI. Both the type of injury and response of the extremely preterm brain to an insult may differ from that in the term brain (Fig. 16.14).

Periventricular leukomalacia (PVL)

Few studies have looked at the preterm brain with PVL. Hyperechoic areas ('flares' or echo densities) on cerebral ultrasound are thought to reflect disturbances in the periventricular blood circulation, resulting in some cases, in local destruction of tissue and development of cysts in the periventricular white matter which are in turn demonstrable as hypoechoic areas (cysts), consistent with periventricular leukomalacia[26]. Many of the hyperechoic regions seen on ultrasound will disappear and leave no visible trace on ultrasound. ^{31}P MRS was used to study 27 preterm and term infants with increased echo densities on cranial ultrasound in the first few days of life and compared these findings to 18 normal infants. This showed that the PCr/Pi ratio was predictive of outcome[41].

Groenendaal *et al.*[38] used localized PRESS ^{1}H MRS to study preterm infants with PVL and term infants with subcortical leukomalacia. A low NAA/Cho predicted poor outcome although some infants developed unfavorably despite a normal NAA/Cho ratio. The absence or presence of lactate did not improve prediction of outcome. Failure of ^{1}H MRS to accurately predict outcome may be due to partial volume effects or difficulties with localization.

Intraventricular hemorrhage (IVH)

A small number of studies have been done in preterm infants with IVH. Two studies are discussed here. High energy phosphorus metabolites and pH$_i$ were measured in five babies with grade 3 to 4 IVH and compared to 15 preterm infants without IVH[112]. The group of babies with the IVH had significantly lower estimated gestational age (GA) (mean 26.8 versus 30.0 weeks), 5 min Apgar score and required a longer period of ventilation and had lower PCr/Pi and PCr/ATP ratios than those without an IVH.

^{1}H MRS was used to investigate the metabolic consequences of germinal matrix hemorrhage in the striatal region of 12 preterm infants of GA mean (SD) 29.3 +/− 2.5 weeks[101]. Both sides were studied twice and in most infants

the hemorrhage was unilateral or larger on one side: the side with the (larger) hemorrhage was compared to the less-affected side. The findings were that germinal matrix hemorrhage (GMH) was initially followed by lactate accumulation and a presumed delay in maturation as indicated by transiently low Cr and NAA indices. At a corrected age of 3 months, there was no difference in these metabolite indices; however, there was an increase in the Cho index suggesting a more persistent metabolic change after GMH.

Conclusions

This review has illustrated that a wide range of MR spectral changes are observed in neonatal pathologies. After HI, lactate/Cr and *myo*-inositol/Cr may be markedly elevated, PCr/Pi dramatically reduced and pH$_i$ alkaline. Changes in lactate/Cr and *myo*-inositol/Cr have been observed in prematurity. For all these studies, knowledge of age-related normative ranges are essential for spectral interpretation.

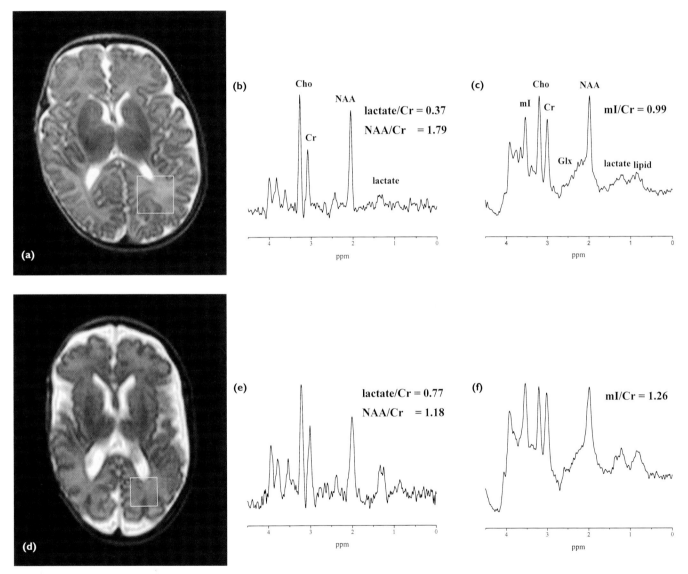

Fig. 16.14 (a) T2-weighted magnetic resonance (MR) image and the 8-cm³ voxel localized to the posterior periventricular white matter (WM) from where MRS data were obtained from an infant born at 24 weeks gestation and scanned at 46 weeks corrected age with normal WM on MRI. The MRS data acquired using **(b)** echo time (TE) of 270 milliseconds and **(c)** TE of 40 milliseconds from the posterior periventricular WM are shown. **(d)** T2-weighted MR image gestationa nd the 8-cm³ voxel localized to the posterior periventricular WM from where MRS data were obtained from an infant born at 26 weeks gestation and scanned at 36 weeks corrected age. The MRI demostrated multiple abnormal high signal intensity lesions in the white matter and widespread atrophy. The MRS data acquired using **(e)** TE of 270 milliseconds and **(f)** TE of 40 milliseconds from the posterior periventricular WM are shown. These spectra demonstrate an increased lactate/Cr and *myo*-inositol/Cr in the infant with WMD **(e** and **f)** compared with those from the infant with the normal MRI **(b** and **c)**; these differences were significant between groups even when age of scan was included in the analysis. Although the NAA/Cr in the infant with white matter damage **(e)** was less than the infant with normal WM **(b)**, this difference was not significant when all infants in each group were compared and age of scan was included in analysis. Cr, creatine plus prosphocreatine; Cho, choline-containing compounds; NAA, N-acetyl aspartate; Glx, glutamine/glutamate. (Reproduced with permission of Lipincott Williams and Wilkins, inc. from Robertson et al[92].)

However, data from normal subjects are difficult to obtain, not only because of a general reluctance to examine healthy infants but also because they do not keep still enough for long.

MRS has particularly contributed to the understanding of brain injury after HI, in illustrating the concept of delayed cerebral energy failure, in defining a possible 'therapeutic window' some hours after the insult when intervention may ameliorate brain injury, and also in contributing to the concept that there are persisting metabolic changes in the brain months after HI. Combined with laboratory and cell work, these findings may aid in the understanding of mechanisms leading to these biochemical changes.

Exploiting the non-invasive nature of multinuclear MRS, a major advantage of the technique is that longitudinal studies can be readily achieved enabling insights into how pathophysiological processes evolve *in vivo*. It may also be used to assess the effectiveness of treatment regimens.

One of the major challenges in clinical *in vivo* MRS is the necessity to quantify accurately metabolite concentrations within the timescale of a neonatal examination. It continues to be difficult to obtain enough measurements to interpret a spectral peak in terms of a metabolite concentration rather than a metabolite ratio. Improvements in technical methodologies are central to further developments in clinical MRS. For example, chemical MRS studies have benefited from the use of higher magnetic fields, and the same may be expected for clinical MRS studies. A whole-body MR system based on an 8 T magnet is available[93], and 3 T systems are becoming more widely available for clinical use. Better resolution from smaller voxel sizes and improved editing of artifacts can be expected in the future; for example, improved definition of spectral changes due to voluntary or involuntary movements[72].

Other recently developed ^{1}H MRS techniques take advantage of the interaction of the proton nucleus with other nuclei such as the ^{13}C and ^{15}N nuclei. Studies of glucose and amino acid metabolism in the human brain have been performed using ^{13}C-labeled glucose permitting measurements of Kreb's cycle, glutamine synthesis and glycolytic fluxes *in vivo*[63]. This technique is likely to be useful in understanding mechanisms of neurologic disorders in infants.

In summary, MRS studies can provide a non-invasive insight into *in vivo* brain biochemistry. Combined with newer MRI techniques such as diffusion weighted imaging enabling visualization of tracts, MRS can be expected to define brain injury in the neonate with more precision.

Summary

- Nuclear magnetic resonance spectroscopy is one of the most important tools for quantitative analysis of chemical composition and structure, and this technique is now being applied *in vivo* to study biochemical process in the term and preterm infant.

- Interpretation of a clinical MR spectrum can provide information about cellular energetics, membrane turnover, neuronal function, selected neurotransmitter activity and intracellular pH.

- Proton MR spectra can be acquired using a standard MRI system with appropriate sequences but the static magnetic field should be at least 1 Tesla to achieve adequate sensitivity. For other nuclei a multinuclear radiofrequency capability is required.

- An understanding of age-dependent and regional changes in metabolite ratios and absolute concentrations of ^{31}P and ^{1}H metabolites is important to enable accurate identification and recognition of metabolite abnormalities in pathological states.

- Seven main peaks can be assigned in a cerebral phosphorus spectrum to phosphomonoesters (PME), inorganic phosphate (Pi), phosphocreatine (PCr), phosphodiesters (PDE) and the three phosphate groups (α, β, γ) in nucleoside triphosphate (NTP).

- Three singlet peaks can be readily assigned in the proton spectrum to N-acetylaspartate (NAA), choline-containing compounds (Cho) and creatine plus phosphocreatine (Cr). In addition more complex peaks can be identified from protons in a range of metabolites, if present, including lactate, inositols (specifically *myo*-inositol), alanine, glutamine (Gln) and glutamate (Glu).

- Cerebral ^{1}H and ^{31}P MRS have been important in furthering our understanding of the response to injury of the brain following hypoxia–ischemia. Newborn infants with neonatal encephalopathy show a 'secondary' energy failure 8–24 h after birth. The magnitude of the spectral abnormalities during secondary energy failure are predictive of adverse outcome at 1 year of age. Increased lactate levels and an alkaline intracellular pH can persist for weeks or months in those infants who develop neurodevelopmental impairment.

- Cerebral ^{1}H and ^{31}P MRS findings are discussed in preterm brain injury, specifically white matter damage, periventricular leukomalacia and intraventricular hemorrhage.

References

1. Altman DI, Perlman JM, Volpe JJ (1993) Cerebral oxygen metabolism in newborns. *Pediatrics* 92: 99–104.
2. Anceschi MM, Petrelli A, Zaccardo G *et al.* (1988) Inositol and glucocorticoid in the development of lung stability in male and female rabbit fetuses. *Pediatr Res* 24, 617–621.
3. Azzopardi D, Wyatt JS, Hamilton PA *et al.* (1989) Phosphorus metabolites and intracellular pH in the brains of normal and small for gestational age infants investigated by magnetic resonance spectroscopy. *Pediatr Res* 25, 440–444.
4. Azzopardi D, Wyatt JS, Cady EB *et al.* (1989) Prognosis of newborn infants with hypoxic–ischemic brain injury assessed by phosphorus magnetic resonance spectroscopy. *Pediatr Res* 25, 445–451.
5. Berridge MJ (1993) Inositol triphosphate and calcium signalling. *Nature* 361, 315–325.
6. Bhakoo KK, Pearce D (2000) *In vitro* expression of N-acetyl aspartate by oligodedrocytes: implications for proton magnetic resonance spectroscopy signal *in vivo*. *J Neurochem* 74, 254–62.
7. Blumberg RM, Cady EB, Wigglesworth JS *et al.* Relation between delayed impairment of cerebral energy metabolism and infarction following transient focal hypoxia ischaemia in the developing brain. *Exp Brain Research* 113, 130–137.
8. Boesch C, Gruetter R, Martin E *et al.* (1989) Variations in the *in vivo* P-31 MR spectra of the developing human brain during postnatal life. Work in progress. *Radiology* 172(1), 197–199.
9. Booth REG, Patel TB and Clark JB (1980) The development of enzymes of energy metabolism in the brain of precocial (guinea pig) and non-precocial (rat) species. *J Neurochem* 34, 17–25.
10. Bovee W, Canese R, Decorps M *et al.* (1998) Absolute metabolite quantification by *in vivo* NMR spectroscopy: IV. Multicentre trial on MRSI localisation tests. *Magn Reson Imaging* 16(9), 1113–1125.
11. Brand A, Richter-Landsberg C and Leibfritz D (1993) Multinuclear NMR studies on the energy metabolism of glial and neuronal cells. *Dev Neurosci* 15, 289–298.
12. Buchli R and Boesiger P (1993) Comparison of methods for the determination of absolute concentrations in human muscles by ^{31}P MRS. *Magn Reson Med* 30, 552–628.
13. Buchli R, Martin E, Boesiger P *et al.* (1994) Developmental changes of phosphorus metabolite concentrations in the human brain: a ^{31}P magnetic resonance spectroscopy study *in vivo*. *Pediatr Res* 35(4), 431–435.
14. Cady EB (1995) Quantitative combined phosphorus and proton PRESS of the brains of newborn human infants. *Magn Reson Med* 33, 557–563.
15. Cady EB, Costello AM, Dawson JM *et al.* (1983) Non-invasive investigation of cerebral metabolism in newborn infants by phosphorus nuclear magnetic resonance spectroscopy. *Lancet* 8333, 1059–1062.
16. Cady EB, Lorek A, Penrice J *et al.* (1994) Detection of propan-1, 2-diol in neonatal brain by *in vivo* proton magnetic resonance spectroscopy. *Magn Res Med* 32, 764–776.
17. Cady EB, Penrice J, Amess PN *et al.* (1996) Lactate, N-acetylaspartate, choline and creatine concentrations, and spin–spin relaxation in thalamic and occipito-parietal regions of developing human brain. *Magn Reson Med* 36(6), 878–886.
18. Cady EB, Amess P, Penrice J *et al.* (1997) Early cerebral-metabolite quantification in perinatal hypoxic–ischaemic encephalopathy by proton and phosphorus magnetic resonance spectroscopy. *Magn Reson Imaging* 15(5), 605–611.
19. Chang L, Ernst T, Osborn D *et al.* (1998) Proton spectroscopy in myotonic dystrophy: correlations with CTG repeats. *Arch Neurol* 55, 305–311.

20. Chang L, Ernst T, Leonido-Yee M *et al.* (1999) Cerebral metabolite abnormalities correlate with clinical severity of HIV-1 cognitive motor complex. *Neurology* 52(1), 100–108.
21. Christiansen P, Toft PB, Gideon P *et al.* (1994) MR-visible water content in human brain: a proton MRS study. *Magn Reson Imaging* 12, 1237–1244.
22. Chugani HT, Phelps ME and Mazziotta JC (1987) Positron emission tomography study of human brain functional development. *Ann Neurol* 22, 487–497.
23. Corbett RJT, Laptook AR and Nunnally RL (1987) The use of the chemical shift of the phosphomonoester P-31, magnetic resonance peak for the determination of intracellular pH in the brains of neonates. *Neurology* 37, 1771–1779.
24. Cox IJ (1996) Development and applications of *in vivo* clinical magnetic resonance spectroscopy. *Prog Biophys Molec Biol* 65, 45–81.
25. Dammann O and Leviton A (1997) Maternal intrauterine infection, cytokines and brain damage in the preterm newborn. *Pediatr Res* 42, 1–8.
26. Dammann O and Leviton A (1997) Duration of transient hyperechoic images of white matter in very low birthweight infants; a proposed classification. *Dev Med Child Neurol* 39, 2–5.
27. de Beer R, Van den Boogaart A, Cody E *et al.* (1998) Absolute metabolite quantification by *in vivo* NMR spectroscopy: V. Multicentre quantitative data analysis on the overlapping background problem. *Magn Reson Imaging* 16(9), 1127–1137.
28. de Beer R, Barbiroli B, Gobbi G *et al.* (1998) Absolute metabolite quantification by *in vivo* NMR spectroscopy: III. Multicentre 1H MRS of the human brain addressed by one and the same data-analysis protocol. *Magn Reson Imaging*, 16(9), 1107–1111.
29. Dobbing J and Sands J (1973) Quantitative growth and development of the human brain. *Arch Dis Child* 48, 757–767.
30. Duc CO, Weber OM, Trabesinger AH *et al.* (1998) Quantitative ^{1}H MRS of the human brain *in vivo* based on the stimulation phantom calibration strategy. *Magn Reson Med* 39, 491–496.
31. Ernst T, Kreis R and Ross BD (1993) Absolute quantification of water and metabolites in the human brain. I. Compartments and water. *J Magn Reson* B102, 1–8.
32. Ferimer HN, Kutina KL and LaManna JC (1995) Methyl isobutyl amiloride delays normalization of brain intracellular pH after cardiac arrest in rats. *Crit Care Med* 23(6), 1106–1111.
33. Fruen BR and Lester BR (1990) Down's syndrome fibroblasts exhibit enhanced ml uptake. [Abstract] *Biochem J* 270, 119–123.
34. Gadian DG and Gadian DG (Eds) (1995) *NMR and its Applications to Living Systems*, 2nd edn. New York, Oxford University Press, pp. 139–170.
35. Garlick PB, Brown TR, Sullivan RH *et al.* (1993) Observation of a second phosphate pool in the perfused heart by ^{31}P NMR; is this the mitochondrial phosphate? *J Mol Cell Cardiol* 15, 855–858.
36. Glonek T, Kopp SJ, Kot E *et al.* (1982) P-31 nuclear magnetic resonance analysis of brain: the perchloric acid extract spectrum. *J Neurochem* 39, 1210–1219.
37. Groenendaal F, Veenhoven RH, van der Grond J *et al.* (1994) Cerebral lactate and N-acetyl-aspartate/choline ratios in asphyxiated full-term neonates demonstrated *in vivo* using proton magnetic resonance spectroscopy. *Pediatr Res* 35, 148–151.
38. Groenendaal F, van der Grond J, Eken P *et al.* (1997) Early cerebral proton MRS and neurodevelopmental outcome in infants with cystic leukomalacia. *Dev Med Child Neurol* 39(6), 373–379.
39. Gruwel MLH, Kuzio B, Deslauriers R *et al.* (1998) Observation of two inorganic phosphate NMR resonances in the perfused hypothermic rat heart. *Cryobiology* 37, 355–361.

40. Hallman M, Bry K, Hoppu K *et al.* (1992) Inositol supplementation in premature infants with respiratory distress syndrome. *N Eng J Med* **326**, 1233–1239.

41. Hamilton PA, Cady EB, Wyatt JS *et al.* (1986) Impaired energy metabolism in brains of newborn infants with increased cerebral echodensities. *Lancet* i, 1242–1246.

42. Hanrahan D, Cox IJ, Edwards AD *et al.* (1998) Persistent increases in cerebral lactate concentrations after birth asphyxia. *Pediatr Res* **44**, 304–311.

43. Hanrahan D, Cox IJ, Azzopardi D *et al.* (1999) Relation between proton magnetic resonance spectroscopy within 18 hours of birth asphyxia and neurodevelopmental outcome at one year of age. *Dev Med Child Neurol* **41**, 76–82.

44. Hashimoto T, Tayama M, Yoshimoto T *et al.* (1995) Proton magnetic resonance spectroscopy of brain in congenital myotonic dystrophy. *Pediatr Neurol* **12(4)**, 335–340.

45. Holtzman D, Togliatti A, Khait I *et al.* (1998) Creatine increases survival and suppresses seizures in the hypoxic immature rat. *Pediatr Res* **44(3)**, 410–414.

46. Holub BJ (1992) The nutritional importance of inositol and the phosphoinositides. *N Eng J Med* **326(19)**, 1285–1287.

47. Hüppi PS, Fusch C, Boesch C *et al.* (1995) Regional metabolic assessment of human brain during development by proton magnetic resonance spectroscopy *in vivo* and by high-performance liquid chromatography/gas chromatography in autopsy tissue. *Pediatr Res* **37**, 145–150.

48. Hüppi PS, Schuknecht B, Boesch C *et al.* (1996) Structural and neurobehavioural delay in postnatal brain development of preterm infants. *Pediatr Res* **39(5)**, 895–901.

49. Kato T, Nishina M, Matsushita K *et al.* (1997) Neuronal maturation and N-acetyl-L-aspartic acid development in human fetal and child brains. *Brain Dev* **19**, 131–133.

50. Keevil SF, Barbiroli B, Brooks JC *et al.* (1998) Absolute metabolite quantification by *in vivo* NMR spectroscopy: II. A multicentre trial of protocols for *in vivo* localised proton studies of human brain. *Magn Reson Imaging*, **16(9)**, 1093–1106.

51. Kimura H, Fujii Y, Itoh S *et al.* (1995) Metabolic alterations in the neonate and infant brain during development: evaluation with proton MR spectroscopy. *Radiology* **194(2)**, 483–489.

52. Kreis R, Ross BD, Farrow NA *et al.* (1992) Metabolic disorders of the brain in chronic hepatic encephalopathy detected with ¹H MRS. *Radiology* **182**, 19–27.

53. Kreis R, Ernst T and Ross BD (1993) Development of the human brain: *in vivo* quantification of metabolite and water content with proton magnetic resonance spectroscopy. *Magn Reson Med* **30(4)**, 424–437.

54. Kries R, Ernst T and Ross BD (1993) Absolute quantitation of water and metabolites in the human brain.II.Metabolite concentrations. *J Magn Reson* **B102**, 9–19.

55. Kuban K, Sanocka U, Leviton A *et al.* (1999) White matter disorders of prematurity: association with intraventricular haemorrhage and ventriculomegaly. *J Pediatr* **134**, 539–546.

56. Lee JH, Arcinue E and Ross BD (1994) Brief report: organic osmolytes in the brain of an infant with hypernatraemia. *N Eng J Med* **331(7)**, 439–442.

57. Leth H, Toft PB, Pryds O *et al.* (1995) Brain lactate in preterm and growth-retarded neonates. *Acta Pediatr* **84**, 495–499.

58. Lopez-Villegas D, Lenkinski RE, Wehrli SL *et al.* (1995) Lactate production by human monocyte/macrophages determined by proton MR spectroscopy. *Magn Reson Med* **34(1)**, 32–38.

59. Lorek A, Takei Y, Cady EB *et al.* (1994) Delayed ('secondary') cerebral energy failure following acute hypoxia–ischaemia in the newborn piglet: continuous 48-hour studies by 31P magnetic resonance spectroscopy. *Pediatr Res* **36**, 699–706.

60. Maalouf EF, Duggan PJ, Rutherford MA *et al.* (1999) Magnetic resonance imaging of the brain in extremely preterm infants: normal and abnormal findings from birth to term. *J Pediatr* **135**, 351–357.

61. MacKay A, Whittall K, Adler J *et al.* (1994) *In vivo* visualisation of myelin water in brain by magnetic resonance. *Magn Reson Med* **31**, 673–677.

62. Mandel P and Edel-Harth S (1966) Free nucleotides in the rat brain during postnatal development. *J Neurochem* **13**, 591–595.

63. Mason GF, Gruetter R, Rothman DL *et al.* (1995) Simultaneous determination of the rates of the TCA cycle, glucose utilization, α-ketoglutarate/glutamate exchange and glutamine synthesis in human brain by NMR. *J Cereb Blood Flow Metab* **15**, 12–25.

64. Mason GF, Chu WJ, Vaughan JT *et al.* (1998) Evaluation of ³¹P metabolite differences in human cerebral gray and white matter. *Magn Reson Med* **39**, 346–353.

65. Merboldt KD, Bruhn H, Hanicke W *et al.* (1992) Decrease of glucose in the human visual cortex during photic stimulation. *Magn Reson Med* **25(1)**, 187–194.

66. Michaelis T, Merboldt KD, Bruhn H *et al.* (1993) Absolute concentrations of metabolites in the adult human brain *in vivo*: quantification of localized proton MR spectra. *Neuroradiology* **187**, 219–227.

67. Miller AL and Shamban A (1977) A comparison of methods for stopping intermediary metabolism of developing brain. *J Neurochem* **28**, 1327–1334.

68. Miller BL, Moats RA, Shonk T *et al.* (1993) Alzheimer disease: depiction of increased cerebral *myo*-inositol with proton MR spectroscopy. *Radiology* **187**, 433–437.

69. Moon RB and Richards JH (1973) Determination of intracellular pH by ³¹P magnetic resonance. *J Biol Chem* **248**, 7276–7278.

70. Moore GJ, Koch S, Chen G *et al.* (1999) *myo*-Inositol is not exclusively glial in the human CNS. [Abstract] *Proc Intl Soc Mag Reson Med* 7, 33.

71. Nioka S, Chance B, Lockard SB *et al.* (1991) Quantitation of high energy phosphate compounds and metabolic significance in the developing dog brain. *Neurol Res* **13(1)**, 33–38.

72. Nguyen Q, Clemence M and Ordidge RJ (1998) The use of intelligent re-acquisition to reduce scan time in MRI degraded by motion. [Abstract] 6th Annual meeting of the International Society for Magnetic Resonance in Medicine, 134.

73. Novotny E, Ashwal S and Shevell M (1998) Proton magnetic resonance spectroscopy: an emerging technology in pediatric neurology research. *Pediatr Res* **44(1)**, 1–10.

74. Paneth N (1999) Classifying brain damage in preterm infants. *J Pediatr* **134(5)**, 527–529.

75. Peden CJ, Rutherford MA, Sargentoni J *et al.* (1993) Proton spectroscopy of the neonatal brain following hypoxic-ischaemic injury. *Dev Med Child Neurol* **35**, 502–510.

76. Pellerin L, Pellegri G, Martin JL, *et al.* (1998) Expression of monocarboxylate transporter RNAs in mouse brain: support for a district role of lactate as an energy substrate for the neonatal vs adult brain. *Proc Natl Acad Sci* USA 95: 3990–3995.

77. Pellerin L, Magistretti P 1994 Glutamate uptake into astrocytes stimulates aerobic glycolysis: a mechanism coupling neuronal activity to glycose utilization. *Proc Natl Acad Sci* 91(22): 10625–10629.

78. Pellerin L, Pellegri G, Biltar P *et al.*(1998) Evidence supporting the existance of an activity-dependent astrocyte-neuron lactate shuttle. *Dev Neurosci* 20(4–5): 291–299.

79. Penrice J, Cady E, Lorek A (1996) Proton magnetic resonance spectroscopy of the brain in normal preterm and term infants, and early changes after perinatal hypoxia–ischaemia. *Pediatr Res* **40**, 6–14.

80. Penrice J, Lorek A, Cady EB *et al.* (1997) Proton magnetic resonance spectroscopy of the brain during acute hypoxia-ischemia and delayed cerebral energy failure in the newborn piglet. *Pediatr Res* 41(6), 795–802.

81. Petroff OAC, Pritchard JW, Behar KL *et al.* (1985) Cerebral intracellular pH by ³¹P magnetic resonance spectroscopy. *Neurology* **35**, 781–788.

82. Podo F, Henriksen O and Bovee WM *et al.* (1998) Absolute metabolite quantification by *in vivo* NMR spectroscopy: I. Introduction, objectives and activities of a concerted action in biomedical research. *Magn Reson Imaging* **16(9)**, 1085–1092.

83. Portman MA and Ning X (1990) Developmental adaptations in cytosolic phosphate content and pH regulation in the sheep heart *in vivo*. *J Clin Invest* **86**, 1823–1828.

84. Pritchard J, Rothman D, Novotny E *et al.* (1991) Lactate rise detected by ¹H NMR in human visual cortex during physiologic stimulation. *Proc Natl Acad Sci* USA 88: 5829–5831.

85. Pysh JJ (1970) Mitochondrial changes in rat inferior colliculus during postnatal development: an electron microscopic study. *Brain Res* **18**, 325–342.

86. Rai GS, McConnell JR, Waldman A *et al.* (1999) Brain proton spectroscopy in dementia: an aid to clinical diagnosis. *Lancet* **353(9158)**, 1063–1064.

87. Robbins RC, Balahan RS and Swain JA (1990) Intermittent hypothermic asanguineous cerebral perfusion (cerebroplegia) protects the brain during prolonged circulatory arrest. A phosphorous 31 nuclear magnetic resonance study. *J Thoracic Cardiovasc Surg* **99**, 878–884.

88. Robertson NJ and Edwards AD (1998) Recent advances in developing neuroprotective strategies for perinatal asphyxia. *Curr Opin Pediatr* **10**, 575–580.

89. Robertson NJ, Cox IJ, Cowan FM *et al.* (1999) Cerebral intracellular lactic alkalosis persisting months after neonatal encephalopathy measured by magnetic resonance spectroscopy. *Pediatr Res* **46(3)**, 287–296.

90. Robertson NJ, Cox IJ, Cowan FM *et al.* (1999) Brain intracellular pH measured by phosphorus-31 MRS correlates with outcome after perinatal asphyxia. [Abstract] *Early Hum Dev* **54(1)**, 76–77.

91. Robertson NJ, Lewis RH, Cowan FM *at al.* (2001) Early increases in brain *myo*-inositol measured by proton magnetic resonance spectroscopy in term infants with neonatal encephalopathy. *Pediatr Res* (in press).

92. Robertson NJ, Kuint J, Counsell TJ *et al.* (2000) Characterisation of cerebral white matter damage in preterm infants using ¹H and ³¹P magnetic resonance spectroscopy. *J Cereb Blood Flow Metab* 20: 1446–1456.

93. Robitaille PM, Abduljalil AM, Kangarlu A *et al.* (1998) Human magnetic resonance imaging at 8 T. *NMR Biomed* **11**, 263–265.

94. Ross BD (1991) Biochemical considerations in ¹H spectroscopy. Glutamate and glutamine: myo-inositol and related metabolites. *NMR in Biomedicine* **4**, 59–63.

95. Roth SC, Edwards AD, Cady EB *et al.* (1992) Relation between cerebral oxidative metabolism following birth asphyxia and neurodevelopmental outcome and brain growth at one year. *Dev Med Child Neurol* **34**, 285–295.

96. Roth SC, Baudin J, Cady EB *et al.* (1997) Relation of deranged neonatal cerebral oxidative metabolism with neurodevelopmental outcome and head circumference at 4 years. *Dev Med Child Neurol* **39**, 718–725.

97. Shonk T and Ross BD (1995) Role of increased cerebral myo-inositol in the dementia of Down Syndrome. *Mag Reson Med* **33**, 858–861.

98. Sunagawa S, Buist RJ, Hruska FE *et al.* (1994) Hydrogen ion compartmentation during and following cerebral ischaemia evaluated by ³¹P NMR spectroscopy. *Brain Res* **641**, 328–332.

99. Thurston JH, Sherman WR, Hauhart RE *et al.* (1989) myo-Inositol: a newly identified nonnintrogenous osmoregulatory molecule in mammalian brain. *Pediatr Res* **26**, 482–485.

100. Toft PB, Christiansen P, Pryds O *et al.* (1994) T1, T2, and concentrations of brain metabolites in neonates and adolescents estimated with H-1 MR spectroscopy. *J Magn Reson Imaging* **4**, 1–5.

101. Toft PB, Leth H, Peitersen B *et al.* (1997) Metabolic changes in the striatum after germinal matrix haemorrhage in the preterm infant. *Pediatr Res* **41(3)**, 309–316.

102. Urenjak J, Williams SR, Gadian DG *et al.* (1992) Specific expression of N-acetylaspartate in neurons, oligodendrocyte-type 2 astrocyte progenitors and immature oligodendrocytes *in vitro*. *J Neurochem* **59**, 55–61.

103. van der Knapp MS, van der Grond J, van Rijen PC *et al.* (1990) Age-dependent changes in localised proton and phosphorus MR Spectroscopy of the brain. *Radiology* **176**, 509–513.

104. Vicario C, Arizmendi C, Malloch G, *et al.* (1991) Lactate utilization by isolated cells from early neonatal rat brain. *J Neurochem* 57: 1700–1707.

105. Videen JS, Michae IT, Pinto P *et al.* (1995) Human cerebral osmolytes during chronic hyponatraemia. A proton magnetic resonance spectroscopy study. *J Clin Invest* **95**, 788–793.

106. Volpe JJ (1998) Neurologic outcome of prematurity. *Arch Neurol* **55**, 297–300.

107. Volpe JJ and Volpe JJ (Eds) (1995) *Neurology of the Newborn*, 3rd edn. Philadelphia, Saunders, pp. 634–671.

108. Yager JY, Brucklacher RM and Vannucci RC (1992) Cerebral energy metabolism during hypoxia–ischemia and early recovery in immature rats. *Am J Physiol* **262**, H672–677.

109. Yamashita T, Kohmura E, Yamauchi A *et al.* (1996) Induction of SMT mRNA after focal cerebral ischaemia: evidence for extensive osmotic stress in remote areas. *J Cerebral Blood Flow Metab* **16**, 1203–1210.

110. Yamashita T, Shimada S, Yamauchi A *et al.* (1997) Induction of SMIT mRNA after rat cryogenic injury. *Mol Brain Res*, **46**, 236–242.

111. Yamashita T, Yamauchi A, Miyai A *et al.* (1999) Neuroprotective role of SMIT against veratidine cytotoxicity. *J Neurochem* **72**, 1864–1870.

112. Younkin D, Medoff-Cooper B, Guillet R *et al.* (1988) *In vivo* ³¹P nuclear magnetic resonance measurement of chronic changes in cerebral metabolites following neonatal intraventricular haemorrhage. *Pediatrics* **82(3)**, 331–336.

113. Zigmond MJ, Bloom FE, Story C et al. (1999) Fundamental Neuroscience. Academic Press; p. 409.

Metabolic disorders in the neonate

17

Zoltan Patay, Nicola J Robertson and I Jane Cox

Contents

Introduction

Metabolic diseases are classically divided into two groups: inborn errors of metabolism and acquired metabolic disorders. Inborn errors of metabolism present with systemic metabolic abnormalities (acidosis, ketosis, ketoacidosis, etc.) and/or clinical signs and symptoms related to the involvement of one or more of the organ systems. These include the central and the peripheral nervous system (spinal cord, brain stem, cerebellum, basal ganglia, cerebral white and gray matter or peripheral nerve lesions), the musculoskeletal system (myopathy, dysostosis), some of the visceral organs (cardiomyopathy, hepatosplenomegaly) and even the skin (alopecia, dermatitis, petechiae).

Inborn errors of metabolism that involve exclusively the nervous system are referred to as neurometabolic diseases. They include L-2-hydroxyglutaric aciduria, glutaric aciduria type 1, 4-hydroxybutyric aciduria, alpha-ketoglutaric aciduria, mevalonic aciduria and N-acetylaspartic aciduria (Canavan's

disease), none of which is encountered in neonates. Some of the metabolic disorders have no neurological manifestations at all (e.g. glycogen storage disorders).

Acquired metabolic disorders are relatively frequent in neonates receiving intensive care. They often present with disturbances of the central nervous system but there are few reports of associated brain imaging abnormalities. In acquired metabolic disorders, neurological complications may occur as a direct effect of the abnormality, from associated hypoxic–ischemic injury or may be secondary to the treatment. Benign forms of hyperbilirubinemia are often seen in neonates and typically resolve without sequelae; however, delayed or inappropriate treatment of more severe forms potentially leads to basal ganglia disease. Kernicterus is associated with abnormalities within the globus pallidum, subthalamic nuclei and hippocampus. Spectroscopy in this disorder may be unremarkable (Fig. 17.1). Hypoglycemia is a relatively common cause for admission on to a neonatal unit and is occasionally associated with severe white matter injury (see Chapter 6).

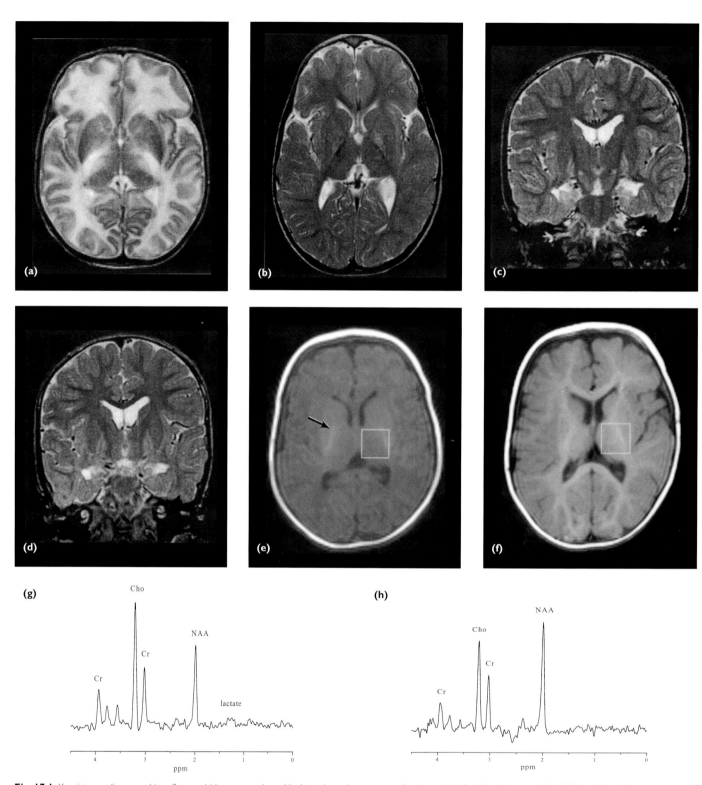

Fig. 17.1 Kernicterus discovered in a 3-year-old boy presenting with dystonia and movement disorders. Axial **(a–b)** and coronal **(c–d)** T2 weighted fast spin echo sequences. The lesions in the globus pallidum are well appreciated on both the axial and coronal images, but signal changes within the subthalamic nuclei are visible only on the coronal image **(c)**. T1 weighted images of a term-born infant with hyperbilirubinemia examined at 6 days **(e)** and at 7 months **(f)**. There is a normal appearance to the brain. Myelination is appropriate for age. There is a slightly widened appearance to the anterior portion of the posterior limb of the internal capsule (*arrow*). This increased signal intensity was seen more clearly and bilaterally on the lower slice and was consistent with abnormal signal intensity within the globus pallidum. **(g)** ^{1}H MRS spectrum (TE 270 ms) from a 2 cm × 2 cm voxel in the basal ganglia. The spectrum was acquired at 6 days of age and demonstrates a lactate/Cr of 0.23 and a NAA/Cr of 1.47. These values are within the normal range for a term infant. **(h)** ^{1}H MRS spectrum (TE 270 ms) from a 2 cm × 2 cm voxel in the basal ganglia. This spectrum was acquired at 7 months of age and demonstrates a lactate/Cr of 0.1 and a NAA/Cr of 1.74. These values are within the normal range for an infant at this age; the NAA/Cr has increased with maturation. The neurodevelopmental outcome was normal at one year of age.

Clinical and biochemical aspects of inborn errors of metabolism

Most of the inborn errors of metabolism of neonatal onset fall into the category of the devastating metabolic diseases, which refers to a fairly well-defined clinical syndrome, typically seen in neonates and infants. In the devastating metabolic diseases the underlying metabolic derangements result in global brain toxicity leading to diffuse brain edema and neurological manifestations that reflect the varying patterns and degrees of white or gray matter involvement. The clinical hallmarks of the condition are poor feeding, vomiting, seizures, stupor and lethargy rapidly leading to deep coma and subsequently to death or severe neurological impairment in the survivors.

AGE OF ONSET

The age of onset is often an important diagnostic and prognostic factor in metabolic diseases. Some diseases are exclusive to the neonatal age group; the onset of the underlying metabolic derangement may, however, be either pre- or postnatal. Neonatal or early infantile onset is usually related to a more profound metabolic derangement, whereas later onset often but not always reflects a less severe metabolic derangement with better prognosis.

In some of the diseases (primary lactic acidosis, type 2 glutaric aciduria, very long-chain acyl coenzyme A dehydrogenase, hydroxymethylglutaryl (HMG)-CoA lyase, ornithine transcarbamylase and carbamyl phosphatase synthetase deficiencies) the metabolic derangements manifest immediately at birth. In others clinical signs and symptoms develop a few days later (isovaleric acidemia, methylmalonic acidemia, propionic acidemia, non-ketotic hyperglycinemia, citrullinemia, argininosuccinic aciduria). Maple syrup urine disease (MSUD) typically presents 6–7 days after birth. A significant proportion of metabolic diseases with clinical onset after the 4th week of life are considered to be early or late infantile, childhood and juvenile, and are not therefore discussed here.

CLINICAL SIGNS AND SYMPTOMS

Neonates with metabolic disorders may present with dysmorphic features involving the mid-facial structures, for example in propionic and methylmalonic acidemias, multiple coenzyme A dehydrogenase deficiency or in peroxisomal disorders of neonatal onset but these may also develop later, for example the characteristic face in Cockayne and MSUD. In some of the diseases imaging studies may reveal malformations of the brain, for example cortical dysplasia in Zellweger syndrome, callosal hypoplasia in non-ketotic hyperglycinemia.

Malformations of the brain always suggest a profound metabolic derangement of prenatal onset. Abnormal odor of the skin, hair, earwax or urine is a frequent and often characteristic feature of metabolic diseases, for example 'sweaty feet' in glutaric aciduria type 2 and isovaleric acidemia, 'burnt sugar' in MSUD, 'cat urine' in multiple carboxylase deficiency. Ophthalmological abnormalities may provide useful additional clues to the diagnosis, for example cataract in rhizomelic chondrodystrophia punctata, retinal degeneration in Zellweger syndrome. Fatty acid oxidation disorders typically present with hepatosplenomegaly, myopathy and cardiomyopathy. On neurological examination, neonates with urea cycle defects, non-ketotic hyperglycinemia and peroxisomal disorders typically present with severe hypotonia. In a few other diseases, such as MSUD, episodes of hypertonia (opisthotonus) may alternate with hypotonia. In organic acidemias both hypotonia (e.g. in propionic acidemia) and hypertonia (e.g. methylmalonic acidemia, isovaleric acidemia) may be observed. Hypertonia (contractures) is characteristic in rhizomelic chondrodystrophia punctata.

Epileptic seizures, usually myoclonic in neonates (in urea cycle defects, non-ketotic hyperglycemia) with occasional grand mal seizures later during infancy (organic acidemias, Zellweger syndrome, Menkes disease) are frequent and represent severe neurological complications in metabolic diseases. In fatty acid oxidation disorders epileptic seizures are related to hypoglycemia.

Acute metabolic crises often mimic infection (meningoencephalitis) of the central nervous system but at the same time patients with organic acidemia, urea cycle defect and MSUD are prone to intercurrent infectious complications. This may result in confusing clinical presentations potentially leading to a delay in diagnosis and treatment.

LABORATORY FINDINGS

Laboratory analysis of body fluids (blood, urine, cerebrospinal fluid) is an essential part of the diagnostic work-up in metabolic diseases. Routine biochemical findings are often non-specific but may be suggestive or characteristic of certain disease groups or even disease entities. Analysis of blood pH, glucose, ammonia, lactic acid, urine ketone bodies and hepatic profile provides useful baseline information and guide any further diagnostic work-up.

One of the most important laboratory tests in neonates with a suspected metabolic disorder is the blood ammonia level. It is usually normal or borderline elevated in MSUD, and markedly elevated in both urea cycle defects and organic acidemias. If blood ammonia level is higher than 1000 mM, irreversible neurological damage is likely to occur. These two groups can be differentiated from each other by determining the blood pH, which will reveal a respiratory alkalosis in the former and a metabolic acidosis in the latter.

The metabolic acidosis can further be characterized by the presence or absence of lactic acidosis and ketosis. A blood sugar level assessment is also important.

Lactic acidosis with hypoglycemia is typically seen in HMG CoA lyase deficiency[14], in some subtypes of 3-methylglutaconic acidemia, glutaric aciduria type 2 and in medium- and long-chain fatty acid oxidation disorders.

Lactic acidosis with normoglycemia may be present in oxidative phosphorylation diseases (primary lactic acidosis). Determination of the pyruvate–lactate ratio may be helpful in identifying the different forms, such as pyruvate dehydrogenase deficiency (pyruvate/lactate <1/25) and pyruvate carboxylase deficiency or cytochrome c oxidase deficiency (pyruvate/lactate >1/35).

Ketosis with hypoglycemia is seen in patients with isovaleric, propionic and methylmalonic acidemia and in ketothialase deficiency. Adrenal insufficiency, sepsis, and dehydration may, however, also present with similar laboratory findings.

Ketosis with hyperglycemia is present in diabetic ketoacidosis.

Severe acidosis without lactic acidosis or ketosis may be seen periodically in 5-oxoprolinuria.

Hepatic function may be altered in inborn errors of metabolism of neonatal onset. Clinical and laboratory evidence of liver disease are typically present in fatty acid oxidation and oxidative phosphorylation disorders. High plasma levels of phytanic, pipecolic and very long chain fatty acids (VLCFA), as well as bile acid intermediates are typical findings in peroxisomal diseases.

More sophisticated biochemical techniques that may be needed to reach a specific diagnosis include; gas chromatography/mass spectrometry (GC/MS) of the urine, high pressure liquid chromatography (HPLC) and tandem mass spectrometry (tandem MS) of the blood. In addition there are specific enzyme studies, for example glutathione reductase assay of red blood cells in 5-oxoprolinuria, propionyl-CoA carboxylase or HMG-CoA lyase assay in white blood cells in propionic acidemia and HMG-CoA lyase deficiency and pyruvate carboxylase or cytochrome c oxidase assay in liver or muscle biopsy specimen in oxidative phosphorylation disorders.

Conventional MR imaging in metabolic diseases in the neonate

TECHNICAL CONSIDERATIONS

Sequence selection

Differences in the histochemical properties (water and myelin content) between the immature (newborns and infants) and the mature (children and adults) brain requires appropriate adjustment of some of the parameters of conventional spin echo or fast spin echo sequences. To compensate for the longer T2 relaxation time (due to the high water and lower myelin/lipid content) of the brain parenchyma in the newborn and infant, longer repetition (TR) and echo (TE) times are used in T2 weighted imaging.

To enhance signal differences between the myelinated and the non-myelinated structures 'myelin sensitive' inversion recovery techniques ('real' and 'modular') provide optimal results.

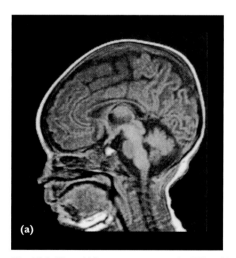 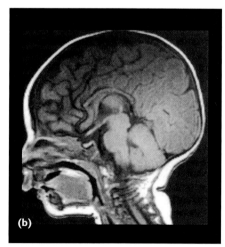 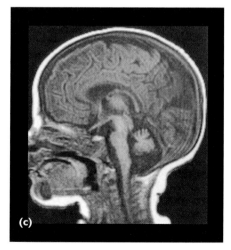

Fig. 17.2 The mid-line structures on sagittal T1 weighted spin echo images in metabolic diseases in neonates. **(a)** Normal corpus callosum and cerebellar vermis in a 7-day-old male neonate with primary lactic acidosis. Accurate analysis of the corpus callosum may be challenging in neonates because of its small size and lack of myelin. **(b)** Dysmorphic/hypotrophic corpus callosum in a 2-month-old female infant with non-ketotic hyperglycinemia. **(c)** Hypo- or dysplastic cerebellar vermis in a 40-day-old male infant with methylmalonic acidemia.

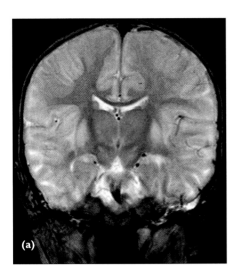 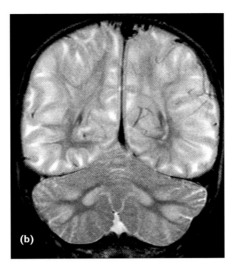

Fig. 17.3 Coronal T2 weighted fast spin echo images in an 18-month-old boy with propionic acidemia presenting with acute metabolic crisis. Predominantly the gray matter structures are involved. The cerebral cortex, the putamina, the tails of the caudate nuclei and the subthalamic nuclei **(a)** as well as the dentate nuclei and the cerebellar cortex **(b)** exhibit an abnormal hyperintense appearance. Most of these structures are best assessed in the coronal plane.

Spatial resolution

Accurate analysis and identification of the involved anatomical structures (especially in the cerebellum and the brain stem), which are indispensable for lesion-pattern recognition by MRI, may require the use of a high-resolution (512×512) matrix.

Slab orientation

The use of multiplanar imaging is necessary to detect and delineate lesions involving specific areas of the brain. Midline structures such as the corpus callosum and the cerebellar vermis are best assessed on sagittal images (Fig. 17.2). The cerebellar white matter, the dentate (Fig. 17.3) and subthalamic nuclei (Fig. 17.3) and the tails of the caudate nuclei are best imaged in the coronal plane. The brain stem structures, the basal ganglia, the internal capsules, the cerebral hemispheric white matter and the cortex are best visualized on axial images.

The baseline MRI work-up of a newborn, suspected to have metabolic disease should include sagittal T1 weighted spin echo, axial proton density and T2 weighted fast spin echo and axial fast inversion recovery sequences. Optional techniques include axial or coronal T2 weighted fast spin echo or modular inversion recovery sequences. Whenever possible, the use of a high-resolution matrix is preferred. Depending on the findings, additional axial or coronal diffusion-weighted echo-planar sequences and an MR spectroscopic study may be indicated to enhance the sensitivity and diagnostic specificity.

Intravenous contrast injection is usually not necessary in metabolic diseases of neonatal onset (except neonatal adrenoleukodystrophy, see later) but may be indicated where there is a suspicion of infection.

MRI findings in neonates with metabolic disorders are usually non-specific, even in those diseases, which eventually lead to fairly characteristic lesion patterns. Very few diseases present with suggestive or pathognomonic abnormalities in the immediate postnatal period. The combination of conventional and diffusion-weighted MRI as well as MR spectroscopy may however lead to a more specific diagnosis.

Diffusion-weighted MRI in neurometabolic disorders

Although the technique itself is not new, only recent improvements in MR gradient technology in the form of fast and powerful gradient subsystems have allowed the implementation of echo-planar diffusion-weighted imaging (EP-DWI) in routine practice. The short acquisition times (20–50 s) are particularly advantageous in pediatric patients. Diffusion-weighted MRI of the brain has already many well-established indications, including stroke and the assessment of normal and abnormal myelination[5]. Analysis of the type and pattern of diffusion abnormalities may enhance the sensitivity and specificity of the MRI work-up in neonates.

In non-myelinated white matter, some but not significant water diffusion anisotropy is present and the apparent diffusion coefficient is higher than in the mature brain. As the myelination process progresses, prominent diffusion anisotrophy develops, characterized by relatively free water diffusion along the fiber tracts and restricted diffusion across the myelin sheaths[29,42]. Besides the presence of extra- or intracellular barriers (myelin layers, cell or organelle membranes, fiber tracts) other possible causes of water diffusion restriction in the brain parenchyma include increased extra- or intracellular microviscosity, which is induced by the presence of macromolecules.

In cytotoxic (intracellular) edema water accumulates within the cells (due to intracellular retention of sodium), where its diffusion is restricted in all directions. Isotropically restricted water diffusion presents with hypersignal on diffusion-weighted images. In vasogenic edema excess water moves into the extracellular space. As a result, the apparent tissue water diffusion increases, isotropically in the gray matter, and with a preferential direction along the fiber tracts in the white matter.

In vivo demonstration of pathological water diffusion is clinically important because with conventional MRI techniques dys- or demyelination and all types of brain edema present with similar signal changes (hyposignal on T1 and hypersignal on the T2 weighted images). Differentiation between them based on T1 or T2 relaxation properties is almost impossible. By demonstrating abnormal water shifts between the extra- and intracellular spaces and the resultant apparent water diffusion changes, DWI has the unique potential to differentiate between vasogenic and cytotoxic edema[10]. Furthermore, different types and stages of myelin breakdown (dys- and demyelination) may also be identified based on water diffusion properties within the central nervous system[31].

A specific form of brain edema ('myelin edema') related to vacuolating (or spongioform) myelinopathy has a peculiar appearance on diffusion-weighted images. Histopathologically, vacuolating myelinopathy is found in some of the neurometabolic diseases, such as Canavan's disease, van der Knaap's disease[43], L-2-hydroxyglutaric aciduria and neonatal MSUD. In vacuolating myelinopathy water is probably trapped within vacuoles between the myelin sheet layers, leading to isotropically restricted water diffusion. This explains the markedly increased signal intensities in areas of active vacuolating myelinopathy on diffusion-weighted images in MSUD (Fig. 17.15). It is similar to the appearance in cytotoxic edema although the underlying pathological mechanisms are distinctly different (Fig. 17.4). Additionally, this also allows clear differentiation between

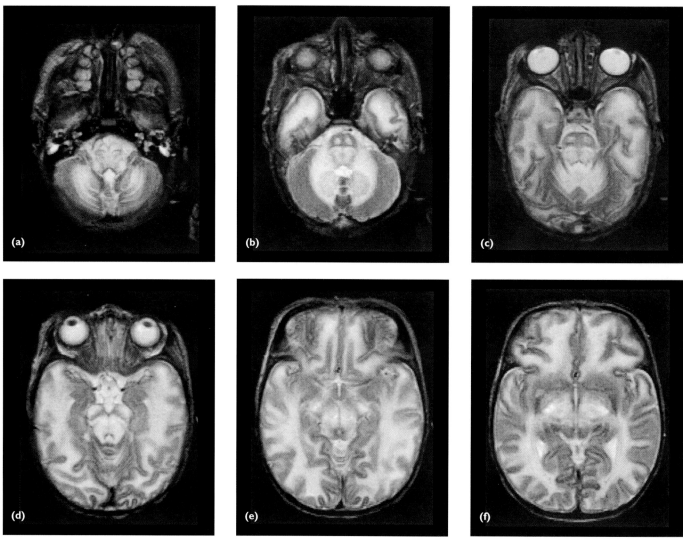

Fig. 17.4 (see overleaf)

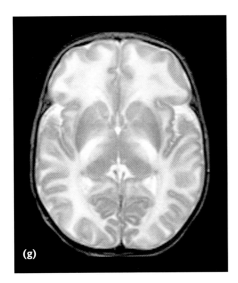

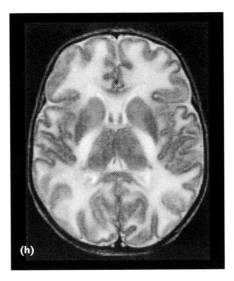

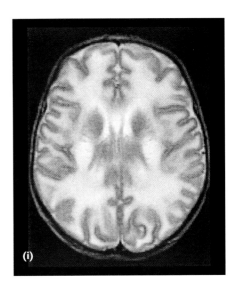

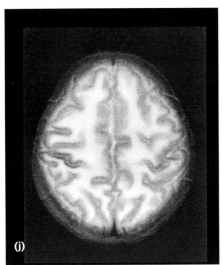

Fig. 17.4 Axial T2 weighted fast spin echo images in a 20-day-old male infant with MSUD. Marked T2 prolongation is seen in all of the structures, which are normally myelinated in the newborn (vacuolating myelinopathy). The non-myelinated white matter structures are relatively spared but diffuse brain swelling is clearly demonstrated (vasogenic edema) (see also Fig. 17.15).

myelinated and non-myelinated structures in the neonatal brain, since in MSUD vacuolating myelinopathy presents with isotropically restricted water diffusion (hypersignal) and the non-myelinated white matter with diffusion abnormalities (hyposignal) suggestive of vasogenic edema. Hence, as a by-product, a very accurate *in vivo* myelination map is obtained (Fig. 17.15).

It is noteworthy that histopathological studies describe vacuolating myelin changes both in the classical (neonatal) and atypical (late-onset) forms of non-ketotic hyperglycinemia. It is therefore possible that diffusion-weighted imaging would reveal changes (hypersignal related to isotropically restricted water diffusion) similar to those observed in MSUD, potentially causing a problem differentiating the two disorders.

Cellular swelling in non-ischemic conditions may also lead to significant anisotropical restriction of water diffusion and present with hypersignal on diffusion-weighted images (hyposignal on anisotropic diffusion coefficient (ADC) maps). This phenomenon is not infrequently encountered at the level of the basal ganglia in active metabolic diseases, in particular organic acidemias, indicating an on-going cellular dysfunction, potentially leading to cell death and extensive tissue necrosis. This, however, has not been observed in neonates presenting with acute neurometabolic disease.

Single voxel proton MR spectroscopy in neonates with inborn errors of metabolism

In a routine clinical setting the single voxel proton MR spectroscopy is the preferred technique. A more detailed account of the techniques used to obtain MR spectra has been given in the previous chapter. The spectroscopy findings in inborn errors of metabolism may be non-specific, although sometimes suggestive or characteristic, or specific.

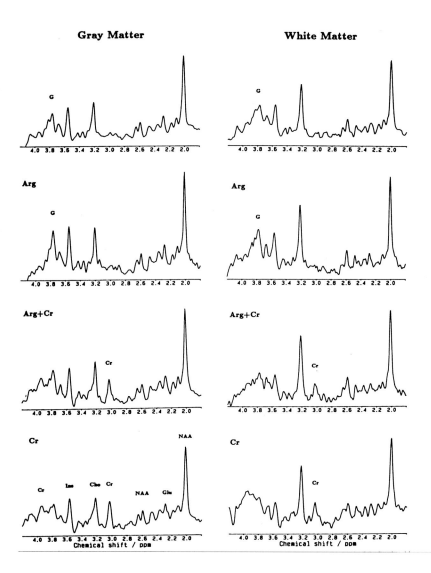

Gray Matter   **White Matter**

Fig. 17.5 Localized proton MR spectrum of parietal gray matter (*left:* 18 ml volume) and white matter (*right* 7.7 ml volume) in a patient with complete creatine deficiency (*top traces*), in the patient at 22 months of age after a 4-week substitution of L-arginine (*second row of traces*), and after a 6-week substitution of creatine (*bottom traces*). Resonances assignments are due to N-acetylaspartate (NAA), glutamate (Glu), creatine and creatine-phosphate (Cr), choline-containing compounds (Cho), *myo*-inositol (Im), and guanidinoacetate (G). (Reproduced with permission of International Pediatric Research Foundation, Inc. from Stöckler *et al.* Creatine deficiency in the brain: a new, treatable inborn error of metabolism. *Pediatr Res* (1994) **36(3)**, 409–413.)

NON-SPECIFIC FINDINGS

In most of the neurometabolic diseases with neonatal onset proton MR spectroscopic findings are non-specific. Nevertheless, they can provide useful additional information on the basic pathological processes occurring within the brain parenchyma. Alterations in the normal constituents of the spectra such as N-acetyl aspartate (NAA), choline (Cho), and creatine (Cr) may be identified, reflecting various degrees of loss of neuronal integrity, myelin breakdown and impairment of basic energetic processes.

Lactate in the brain parenchyma is a non-specific indicator of neurometabolic disease. However, in the neonate, particularly the preterm neonate, a small amount of lactate may be a normal finding (see Chapter 16).

SPECIFIC FINDINGS

Disease-specific metabolites are rarely present but may be occasionally identified in some of the metabolic disorders with neonatal onset. Branched chain amino acids (L-leucine,

L-isoleucine, valine) in MSUD, and glycine (Gly) in non-ketotic hyperglycinemia are the best-known examples. Other disease specific abnormalities include increased N-acetyl-aspartate in Canavan's disease[2,17,24] and absence of creatine in guanidinoacetate methyltransferase deficiency[38,40] (Fig. 17.5) but these disease are typically seen in the infantile age group.

Specific inherited metabolic disorders

ORGANIC ACID DISORDERS

Methylmalonic acidemia

Five discrete metabolic deficits may result in methylmalonic acid in the blood.

Enzyme deficiency

Methylmalonyl coenzyme A mutase partial or complete deficiency. Hydroxycobalamine reductase deficiency and cobal-

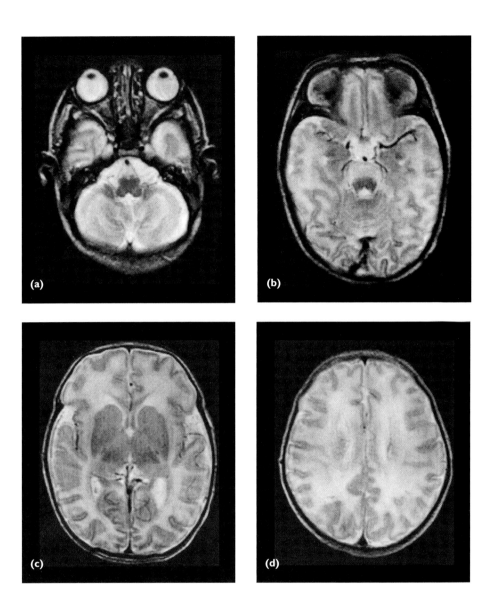

Fig. 17.6 Axial T2 weighted fast spin echo images in a 2-day-old female neonate with methylmalonic acidemia. Diffuse brain swelling and T2 prolongation of the non-myelinated white matter (e.g. ventral mesencephalic structures on **(b)** and hemispheric white matter on **(d)** are demonstrated.

amine adenosyltransferase deficiency, which are both related to an abnormality in vitamin B12 metabolism.

Inheritance

Autosomal recessive.

Genetics

The encoding gene for the mutase enzyme is located on chromosome 6.

Metabolic features

The excess metabolite, methylmalonyl coenzyme A, inhibits multiple other systems that are involved in gluconeogenesis (pyruvate carboxylase), the urea cycle (N-acetylglutamate synthetase) and the glycine cleavage system in the liver but not in the brain, unlike in non-ketotic hyperglycinemia. Neonates present with hyperglycinemia, hyperammonemia and ketoacidosis during the first few days of life (60%) or in early infancy (40%). Sixty per cent of the neonates present with hypoglycemia secondary to impairment in gluconeogenesis[30].

Clinical features

Vomiting, stupor, tachypnea and occasionally seizures. The clinical onset varies with the enzymatic defect. All infants with complete mutase deficiency present within 7 days of delivery.

Clinical course

Excess methylmalonic acid has effects on myelin and also on the external granular layer of cerebellum (Fig. 7.2c). In neonates presenting with complete mutase deficiency, 60% die and 40% survive with neurological impairment.

Treatment

The outcome may be improved in some infants if they are diagnosed and treated early with a low protein diet and with supplements of cobalamin and L-carnitine. Some patients may respond to high-dose vitamin B12.

Imaging

In neonates the disease presents with unremarkable or non-specific MRI findings. Mild swelling of the brain may be seen, in conjunction with T2 prolongation within the non-myelinated white matter structures, most probably related to vasogenic edema. The myelinated white matter structures; in the brain stem, the posterior limbs of the internal capsules, etc. appear to be spared. In one case hypoplasia of the cerebellar vermis was also observed. After the acute phase, atrophy of the brain may develop. In the chronic phase of the

disease, bilateral globus pallidus lesions are found. This, when present, is a fairly characteristic imaging finding, but unfortunately it is not conspicuous in the neonate (Figs 17.2c and 17.6).

Propionic acidemia

Enzyme deficiency

Propionyl coenzyme A carboxylase.

Inheritance

Autosomal recessive.

Genetics

This is a 'mitochondrial' disease since the deficient enzyme – propionyl coenzyme A carboxylase – is located within the

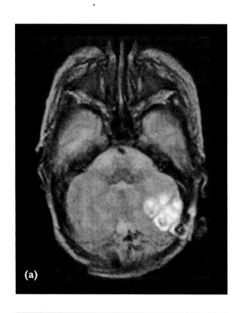

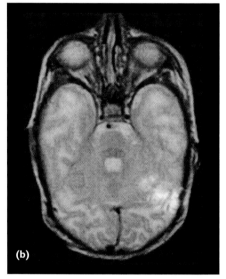

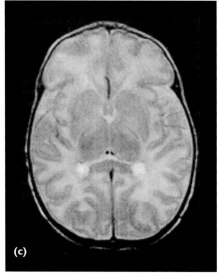

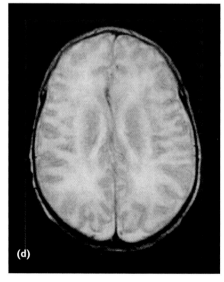

Fig. 17.7 Axial T2 weighted fast spin echo images in a 16-day-old female neonate with propionic acidemia. The findings are rather unremarkable and non-specific, only diffuse brain swelling is seen. Foldover artifacts project over the cerebellar hemisphere and the occipital lobe on the left side **(a)**, **(b)**.

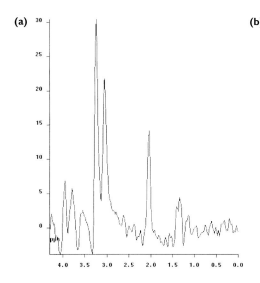

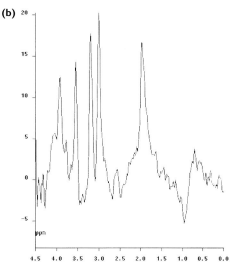

Fig. 17.8 Proton MR spectroscopy obtained with the PRESS technique at 270 ms echo time **(a)** and the STEAM technique at 20 ms echo time **(b)** in a 28-day-old infant with propionic acidemia. The sampling voxels (2 × 2 × 2 cm) were placed on the hemispheric white matter. Both spectra show significant decrease of the NAA (2.02 ppm) and elevation of the *myo*-inositol (3.55 ppm) peaks. Abnormal lactate (1.3 ppm) is demonstrated on the first spectrum **(a)**.

mitochondria. Encoding genes have been found on both chromosome 3 (beta subunits) and 13 (alpha subunits).

Metabolic features

The neonatal form presents with increased ammonia levels, erroneously suggesting a urea cycle defect. Ketosis, acidosis (metabolic and lactic) and hypoglycemia are found in conjunction with increased glycine levels (see above in methylmalonic acidemia). For the aforementioned reasons the disease is also called 'ketotic hyperglycinemia'. The co-factor of the enzyme is biotin; hence other enzyme deficiencies (multiple carboxylase deficiency, see later in 3-methylcrotonyl coenzyme A carboxylase deficiency) related to impairment of the biotin cycle (holocarboxylase synthetase, biotinidase) may cause diagnostic problems.

Clinical features

The disease has a severe neonatal (80–90%) and a milder infantile (10–20%) onset variant. Skin rashes, hypotonia, lethargy, dehydration, seizures and irregular breathing are seen in the neonate before severe acidosis leads to coma and death.

Clinical course

Prognosis in the late-onset form is much better. If the ketoacidotic metabolic crises which are often triggered by infection, fasting, constipation or high protein intake are successfully prevented, affected patients may reach adult age.

Treatment

Low protein diet with L-carnitine supplementation.

Imaging

In the infantile-onset form, propionic acidemia is a predominantly gray matter disease. Involvement, with swelling and signal intensity changes, of the dentate nuclei, the basal ganglia and the cerebral cortex is well appreciated on the MR images during the acute metabolic crisis. In the chronic phase, necrosis of the basal ganglia, diffuse brain atrophy and occasionally patchy white matter lesions are present. In the neonate these changes are not evident. Instead, diffuse brain edema and subsequently delayed myelination and atrophy are the most typical findings[6] (Figs 17.3 and 17.7).

Spectroscopy

A decrease in NAA and *myo*-inositol and an increase in glutamate/glutamine have been found with short echo time (STEAM) proton MR spectroscopy[6] (Fig. 17.8). MR spectroscopy may demonstrate lactic acidosis during a metabolic crisis.

PRIMARY LACTIC ACIDOSIS (OXIDATIVE PHOSPHORYLATION DISORDERS)

Lactic acid is the product of anaerobic metabolism of glucose. Lactic acidosis is frequently related to inborn errors of metabolism as either a primary or secondary lactic acidosis but it may also be acquired. Primary lactic acidosis may be caused by impairment of lactate and pyruvate oxidation, disorders of the Krebs cycle and of the respiratory chain. Secondary lactic acidosis is present in several metabolic diseases, notably in organic acidemias, urea cycle and fatty acid oxidation defects. Acquired causes of lactic acidosis include cardiopulmonary disease, severe anemia, malignancy, diabetes mellitus, hepatic failure and postconvulsion status or can be drug-related. Mitochondrial enzyme defects that cause primary lactic acidosis include pyruvate transcarboxylase, pyruvate dehydrogenase and cytochrome c oxidase deficiencies. These all have neonatal as well as later-onset forms. The remarkable phenotypic variability of the mitochondrial diseases is due to the segregation of the mutant mitochondria and the resultant heteroplasmy.

Pyruvate dehydrogenase deficiency

This is the most frequent cause of primary lactic acidosis. The enzyme has three subunits (E1, E2 and E3), which are all prone to mutations.

Inheritance

Depending on the chromosomal location of the gene encoding the defective subunit, the inheritance may be autosomal (E1-beta, E2, E3) or X-linked (E1-alpha subunit). Leigh syndrome, which usually presents in infancy but may also present in the late neonatal period, has an autosomal recessive inheritance.

Metabolic features

Lactic and pyruvic acidosis and hyperalaninemia.

Clinical features

There are three forms of presentation within the neonatal period:

(1) A severe neonatal form presenting within the first week and often within the first 24 h with fulminating lactic acidosis, stupor, tachypnea, hypotonia and seizures.
(2) An infantile form presenting with hypotonia, dysmorphic craniofacial features, mild acidosis and cerebral dysgenesis including agenesis of the corpus callosum and subependymal heterotopias. These infants are usually female and are heterozygous for the X-linked form of the disorder.
(3) An infantile form presenting with early-onset Leigh disease with hypotonia, respiratory difficulties, oculomotor abnormalities, facial weakness and seizures.

Clinical course

Almost all infants with the severe neonatal form die within 8 months. In the milder neonatal form with dysmorphic features there is usually severe neurological impairment and the development of microcephaly. In Leigh disease there is usually developmental arrest, later onset of movement disorders and developmental regression.

Treatment

Early recognition and treatment of the acidosis are vital. Long-term therapy includes a ketogenic diet to provide sufficient calories as fat. Fat, unlike carbohydrate, by-passes the enzymatic defect and provides a source of acetyl-CoA. Initially treatment with additional L-carnitine may be useful. A trial of high dose thiamine is also appropriate, as there have been reports of thiamine dependence.

Pyruvate carboxylase deficiency

Inheritance

Autosomal recessive.

Metabolic features

Infants present with lactic and pyruvic acidosis and ketosis. Hyperalaninemia, hyperammonemia, citrullinemia, hyperlysinemia occur secondary to disturbance of the urea cycle. Hypoglycemia is not a prominent feature despite the role of pyruvate carboxylase in hepatic gluconeogenesis. There is increased conversion of pyruvate to acetyl-CoA, which is converted to fatty acids and ketone bodies because of the disturbance in the Krebs cycle.

Clinical features

There are two clinical forms: a fulminant neonatal and a later infantile form. The fulminant neonatal form presents with stupor, coma, tachypnea and seizures.

Clinical course

In the neonatal form the resultant lactic acidosis is severe and rapidly fatal, in the infantile form the metabolic derangement may be milder and life expectancy is somewhat longer.

Treatment

Dietary therapy is difficult. A relatively high carbohydrate diet is recommended but with no substantial effects reported. A high fat diet is not indicated partly because ketosis is a prominent feature.

Cytochrome c oxidase deficiency

Cytochrome c oxidase is one of the five multi-subunit enzyme complexes forming the so-called respiratory chain located within the inner membrane of the mitochondrion and is responsible for the electron transport during the end-stage of oxidative phosphorylation.

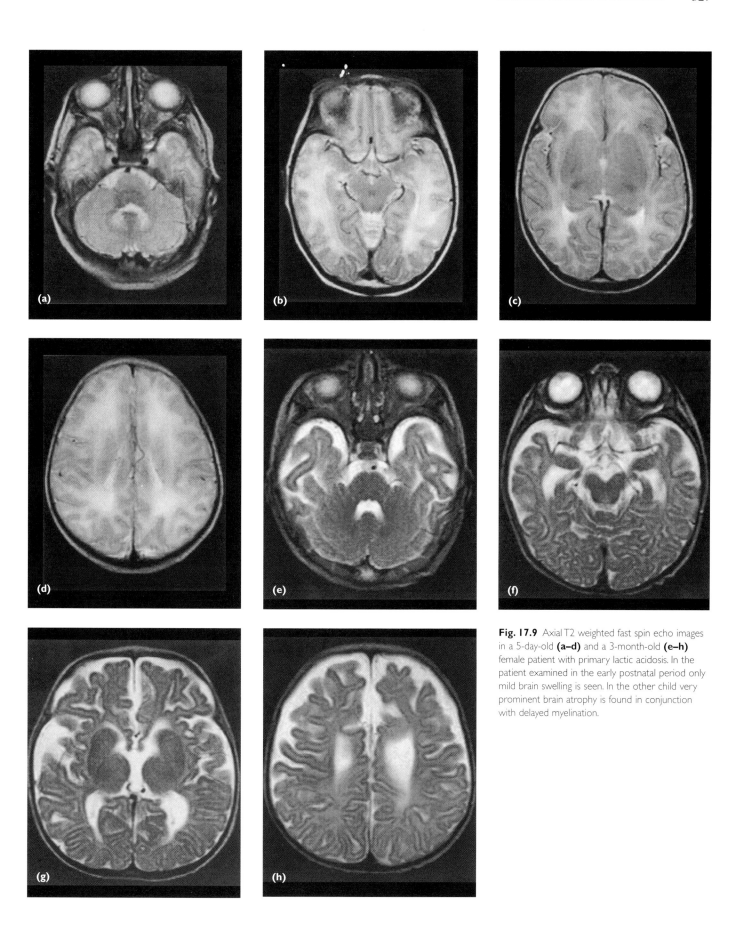

Fig. 17.9 Axial T2 weighted fast spin echo images in a 5-day-old **(a–d)** and a 3-month-old **(e–h)** female patient with primary lactic acidosis. In the patient examined in the early postnatal period only mild brain swelling is seen. In the other child very prominent brain atrophy is found in conjunction with delayed myelination.

Inheritance

Respiratory chain defects are mostly related to maternally inherited mitochondrial DNA mutations but since nuclear DNA also plays a role in the encoding of some of the complexes, autosomal and even X-linked forms are also known.

Metabolic features

Infants present with lactic acidosis and mild pyruvic acidosis. The creatine phosphokinase is only mildly elevated.

Clinical features

Neonatal forms present with severe hypotonia, weakness and hyporeflexia. Respiratory failure develops.

Clinical course

Infants usually die in early infancy. A benign form exists which presents identically but infants show gradual improvement and may be normal at 2–4 years of age. These forms may only be distinguished by identifying the subunits that are absent on muscle histochemistry.

Treatment

Intensive supportive therapy is warranted until the exact form of the disorder can be identified.

Imaging (in oxidative phosphorylation disorders)

Infants with the less severe neonatal form of pyruvate dehydrogenase deficiency may show congenital malformations such as callosal agenesis or disturbances of neuronal migration. The conventional MRI findings are otherwise non-specific in neonates with this group of disorders. Diffuse brain swelling is seen with prolongation of the T2 relaxation time within the white matter throughout the entire brain, perhaps with some predilection to the non-myelinated structures. At the early stage no definite structural or signal abnormality is seen within the basal ganglia although they may appear swollen. In survivors the disease leads to prominent cerebral atrophy and/or delayed myelination (Fig. 17.9). Basal ganglia disease with atrophy and signal intensity changes suggestive of necrosis also develops in the severe therapy-resistant cases.

Spectroscopy (in oxidative phosphorylation disorders)

The ability to detect lactate makes ^{1}H magnetic resonance spectroscopy (MRS) a useful tool to diagnose and follow these patients. Studies using combined ^{1}H MRS and ^{18}F deoxyglucose (FDG) positron emission tomography to assess two aspects of glycolysis (glucose uptake and lactate deposition) demonstrate that defects in oxidative phosphorylation cause a massive increase in glycolysis to cover energy requirements with corresponding accumulation of lactate in brain

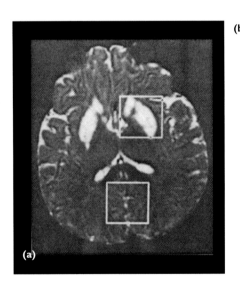

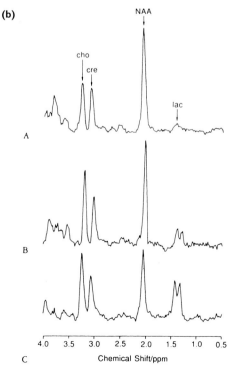

Fig. 17.10 **(a)** A T2 weighted axial MRI scan through the basal ganglia showing focal hyperintensity characteristic of Leigh syndrome (TR = 3000 ms; TE = 120 ms). The locations in this plane of 25-mm³ regions of interest chosen for spectroscopy from the basal ganglia and from a normal appearing region in the occipital lobe are shown. **(b)** Water-suppressed ^{1}H MR spectra obtained from normal cortex (**A**), occipital lobe in a patient with Leigh syndrome (**B**), and right basal ganglia in a patient with Leigh syndrome (**C**). Spectra are plotted on equal signal intensity scales. Singlet resonances from choline (cho, 3.2 ppm), creatine (cre, 3.0 ppm), N-acetylaspartate (NAA, 2.0 ppm), and the lactate doublet (lac, 1.3 ppm) are clearly resolved. Levels of lactate are elevated in both **B** and **C**, whereas N-acetyl aspartate is most markedly decreased in **C**. (Reproduced with permission of the American Neurological Association from Detre et al. Regional variation in brain lactate in Leigh syndrome by localised 1H magnetic resonance spectroscopy. Ann Neurol (1991) **29(2)**, 218–221.)

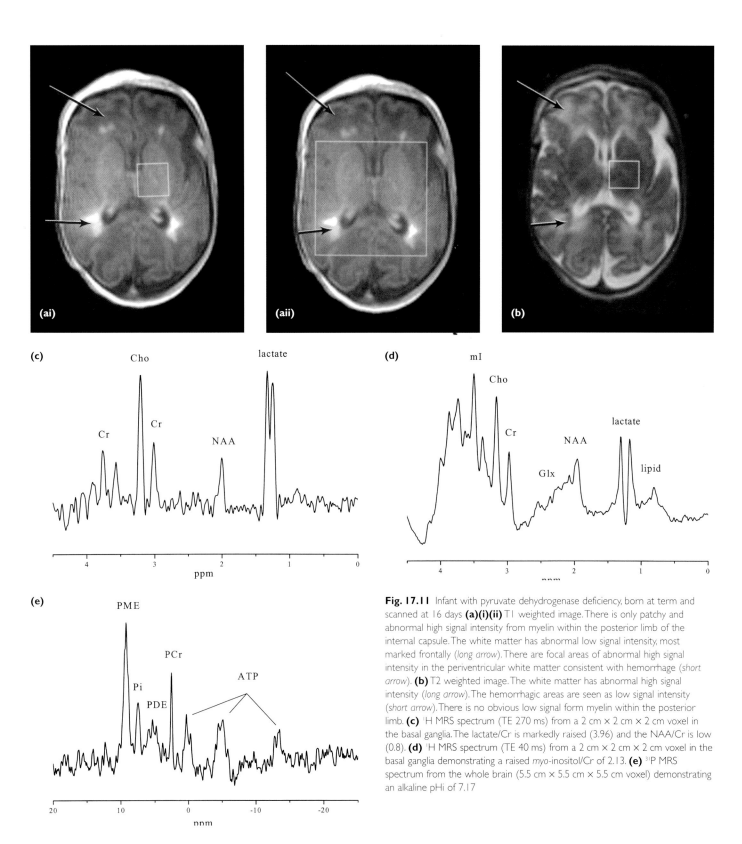

Fig. 17.11 Infant with pyruvate dehydrogenase deficiency, born at term and scanned at 16 days **(a)(i)(ii)** T1 weighted image. There is only patchy and abnormal high signal intensity from myelin within the posterior limb of the internal capsule. The white matter has abnormal low signal intensity, most marked frontally (*long arrow*). There are focal areas of abnormal high signal intensity in the periventricular white matter consistent with hemorrhage (*short arrow*). **(b)** T2 weighted image. The white matter has abnormal high signal intensity (*long arrow*). The hemorrhagic areas are seen as low signal intensity (*short arrow*). There is no obvious low signal form myelin within the posterior limb. **(c)** ¹H MRS spectrum (TE 270 ms) from a 2 cm × 2 cm × 2 cm voxel in the basal ganglia. The lactate/Cr is markedly raised (3.96) and the NAA/Cr is low (0.8). **(d)** ¹H MRS spectrum (TE 40 ms) from a 2 cm × 2 cm × 2 cm voxel in the basal ganglia demonstrating a raised *myo*-inositol/Cr of 2.13. **(e)** ³¹P MRS spectrum from the whole brain (5.5 cm × 5.5 cm × 5.5 cm voxel) demonstrating an alkaline pHi of 7.17

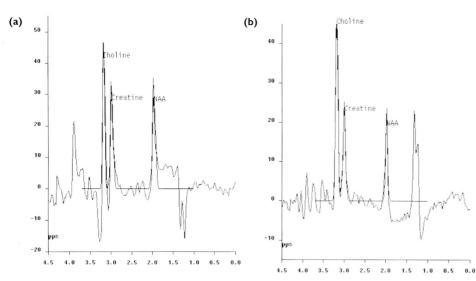

(a)

(b)

Fig. 17.12 Proton MR spectroscopy in a 7-day-old male infant with primary lactic acidosis (same patient as Fig. 17.2a). The spectra were obtained using the point-resolved spectroscopy (PRESS) technique, the sampling voxel (2 × 2 × 2 cm) was placed on the basal ganglia on the right side. With 135 ms echo time **(a)** a prominent negative doublet is seen at the 1.3 ppm level, which becomes positive at 270 ms **(b)** (J-coupling phenomenon).

tissue[19]. In Leigh disease high signal intensities are seen in the putamen and caudate heads on T2 weighted MR images[3] (Fig. 17.10) with high brain lactate concentrations on localized ¹H MRS. Regional variation in the concentration of cerebral lactate in mitochondrial disorders has also been demonstrated[9] (Figs 17.10 and 17.11) and lactate has been detected in areas of brain thought to be 'normal' on MRI[41]. ¹H MRS has been used effectively to monitor therapy in Leigh disease and appears to be a better measure of response than CSF or plasma lactate. In the latter case[39] brain lactate could be detected even when the CSF lactate level had normalized; continuing neuronal loss and breakdown of membrane phospholipids were reflected by a decrease in NAA/Cr and an increase in Cho/Cr (Fig. 17.12).

ABNORMALITIES OF THE L-LEUCINE BREAKDOWN PATHWAY

Several inborn errors of metabolism are related to enzyme deficiencies along the complex L-leucine breakdown pathway. These disorders include MSUD, isovaleric acidemia, 3-methylcrotonyl-CoA carboxylase deficiency, beta-keto-thiolase deficiency and (HMG)-CoA lyase deficiency. MSUD is the most common followed by isovaleric acidemia which accounts for approximately 15% of all organic acidurias.
(1) The first step of the catabolic process is the conversion of L-leucine into 2-ketoisocaproic acid by the branched-chain amino acid transaminase. No specific disease is known at this level.
(2) The second step is the conversion of 2-ketoisocaproic acid into isovaleryl coenzyme A by the branched-chain alpha-ketoacid dehydrogenase. Deficiency of this enzyme, which is also involved in the catabolism of L-isoleucine and valine, leads to MSUD (see later in amino-acidurias).

(3) Isovaleryl coenzyme A is converted into 2-methylcrotonyl coenzyme A. Deficiency at this level results in isovaleric acidemia.

Isovaleric acidemia

Enzyme deficiency

Isovaleryl coenzyme A dehydrogenase.

Inheritance

Autosomal recessive.

Metabolic features

The excess metabolite is isovaleryl coenzyme A. The disease is characterized by severe ketosis, lactic acidosis and hypoglycemia, due to the lack of gluconeogenesis, rapidly leading to coma. The associated thrombocytopenia may present clinically with disseminated intravascular coagulopathy.

Clinical features

An acute severe form accounts for about half the cases. Onset is usually between days 3 and 6 with vomiting, tachynea and stupor. The accumulation of isovaleric acid in body fluids results in a smell of sweaty feet.

Clinical course

Without treatment over half the neonates die and the remainder are left with neurological impairment.

Treatment

Aggressive acute treatment and long-term therapy with low protein diet and supplementation with carnitine and glycine

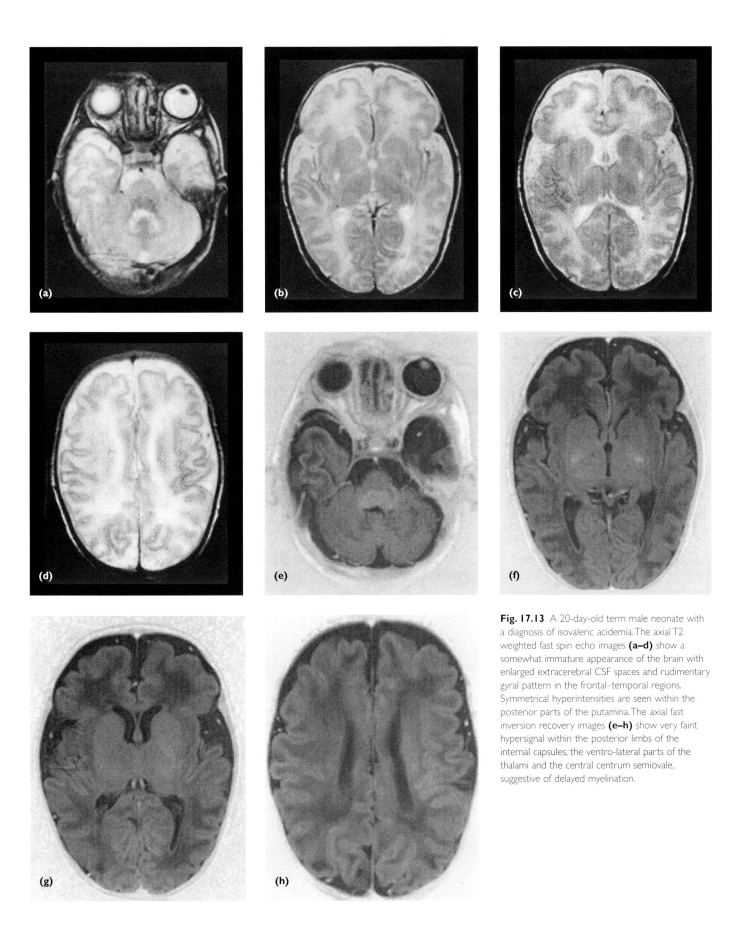

Fig. 17.13 A 20-day-old term male neonate with a diagnosis of isovaleric acidemia. The axial T2 weighted fast spin echo images **(a–d)** show a somewhat immature appearance of the brain with enlarged extracerebral CSF spaces and rudimentary gyral pattern in the frontal–temporal regions. Symmetrical hyperintensities are seen within the posterior parts of the putamina. The axial fast inversion recovery images **(e–h)** show very faint hypersignal within the posterior limbs of the internal capsules, the ventro-lateral parts of the thalami and the central centrum semiovale, suggestive of delayed myelination.

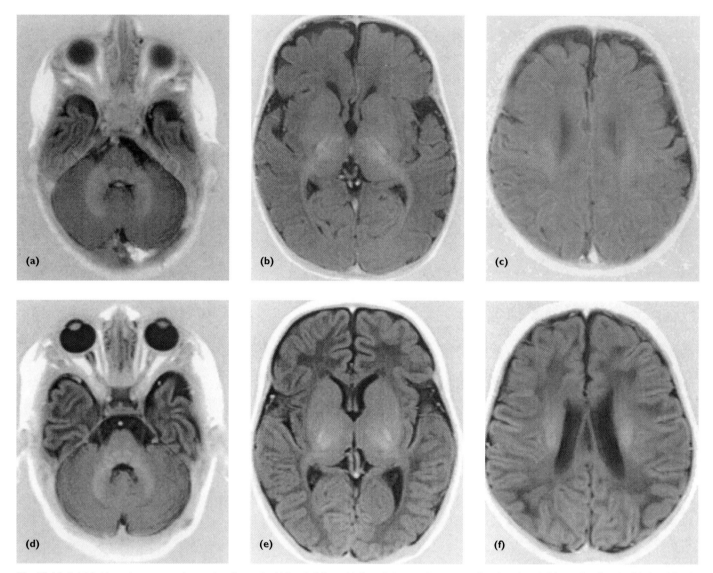

Fig. 17.14 Axial fast inversion recovery images in a 3-month-old female infant with 3-methylcrotonyl coenzyme A carboxylase deficiency **(a–c)** and a 50-day-old male infant with biotinidase deficiency **(d–f)**. In both cases the myelination of the supratentorial structures is delayed for the respective ages of the infants.

has increased survival rates and improved the neurological outcome of survivors. Glycine combines with isovaleryl coenzyme A and is readily excreted by the kidneys.

Imaging

In a case of a 20-day-old neonate, there was already atrophy of the brain with fronto-temporal predominance. Delayed myelination was also suggested. On the T2 weighted images bilateral symmetrical signal abnormalities were seen within the posterior parts of the putamen (Fig. 17.13).

Spectroscopy

In a 5-month-old patient with isovaleric acidemia and normal MRI findings, no abnormality was demonstrated by proton MR spectroscopy using 135 and 270 ms echo times[16].

(4) Isolated dysfunction of the 3-methylcrotonyl coenzyme A carboxylase, responsible for the conversion of 2-methylcrotonyl coenzyme A into 3-methylglutaconyl coenzyme A is a rare condition. The 3-methylcrotonyl coenzyme A deficiency more often develops in a specific metabolic disease group, referred to as multiple carboxylase deficiency. The enzymes involved in multiple carboxylase deficiency are pyruvate carboxylase, propionyl coenzyme A carboxylase, acetyl coenzyme A carboxylase and 3-methylcrotonyl coenzyme A, for all of which biotin is an essential co-factor (see primary lactic acidosis, propionic acidemia). Deficiencies of these enzymes, including the 3-

methylcrotonyl coenzyme A deficiency, therefore usually develop in conditions characterized by unavailability of biotin, notably in biotinidase or holocarboxylase synthetase deficiency.

Biotinidase deficiency

Biotinidase is responsible for the recycling of biotin released from the turnover of the different carboxylase enzymes. Biotinidase deficiency manifests with an insidiously developing progressive encephalopathy. In both the biotinidase and the rare isolated 3-methylcrotonyl coenzyme A carboxylase enzyme deficiencies delayed myelination was observed (Fig. 17.14).

Holocarboxylase deficiency

Holocarboxylase synthetase (HCS) is a biotin carrier, responsible for the attachment of biotin into the active center of 3-methylcrotonyl coenzyme A carboxylase or the other carboxylase enzymes. Holocarboxylase synthetase deficiency usually presents in neonates.

Inheritance

Autosomal recessive.

Genetics

The encoding gene is located on chromosome 21.

Metabolic features

Metabolic features include ketoacidosis, moderate hyperammonemia and hypoglycemia. The organic acidemia includes propionate, lactate, *B* methylcrotonate.

Clinical features

Neonates may present with vomiting, tachypnea, hypotonia and sometimes seizures.

Clinical course

Rare benign forms of the disease may be biotin responsive, otherwise the disease is lethal.

Treatment

Treatment is with high dose biotin, which may be given antenatally.

(5) Deficiency of the 3-methylglutaconyl coenzyme A (3-MGC) hydratase results in impairment of the conversion of 3-methylglutaconyl coenzyme A into 3-hydroxy-3-methylglutaryl coenzyme A (HMG-CoA). The resultant disease is one of the several forms of 3-methylglutaconic acidemia.

3-methylglutaconic acidemia

3-methylglutaconic aciduria (3-MGC) is a heterogeneous group of several biochemically and clinically distinct entities[1].

Enzyme deficiency

In some of them (type 1) the underlying enzyme deficiency is known (3-MGC hydratase deficiency), in others (type 2, 3 and 4) it is unidentified.

Clinical features

Some patients present with pyramidal, others with extrapyramidal tract signs (e.g. Behr or Costeff syndrome: optic atrophy, ataxia, nystagmus, extrapyramidal signs, urinary incontinence, mental retardation) or both. Cardiomyopathy is present in an X-linked variety of the disease (Barth syndrome: X-linked cardiac and skeletal myopathy, short stature and neutropenia)[4]. Since neonatal lactic acidosis with hypoglycemia represents one of the typical laboratory manifestations of the disease, it may actually correspond to a complex mitochondrial disease.

Clinical course

The disease is therapy resistant, leading to death during the first few years of life in most cases.

Imaging

No imaging data are available in the neonatal age group. Later the disease typically presents with cerebellar atrophy and bilateral necrosis of the caudate nuclei and the putamina. In a patient, whose clinical presentation was highly suggestive of Behr syndrome (Behr or Costeff syndrome: optic atrophy, ataxia, nystagmus, extrapyramidal signs, urinary incontinence, mental retardation) MRI examination at the age of 2 years showed ventricular dilatation, bilateral putaminal signal changes in conjunction with extensive cystic lesions within the subcortical white matter[26]. The cystic lesions were already demonstrated by cranial ultrasound at the age of 6 months.

(6) The final step of the pathway is the breakdown of HMG-CoA into acetoacetate and acetyl coenzyme A. Deficiency at this level leads to a specific disease entity, referred to as HMG-CoA lyase deficiency.

HMG-CoA lyase deficiency

Enzyme deficiency

HMG-CoA lyase.

Metabolic features

HMG-CoA is indispensable in many biochemical processes, including cholesterol synthesis and the formation of ketone bodies; the latter are important nutrients of the brain. Additionally, excess HMG-CoA also inhibits the normal gluconeogenesis.

Clinical features

The Saudi phenotype[32] of the disease typically (60%) presents in neonates, elsewhere the disease is characterized by infantile onset. The unavailability of endogenously synthesized ketone bodies and glucose has the potential to create a life-threatening hyperacute encephalopathy if glucose supply is restricted or the glucose demand is high, for example fasting, vomiting, intercurrent illness.

Imaging

In a 14-day-old neonate in our series no definite MRI abnormality was detected. In patients undergoing MRI examination during infancy or childhood, mild frontal atrophy and ventricular enlargement, bilateral basal ganglia and dentate nucleus and multiple patchy white matter lesions were described[51]. In the Saudi phenotype the white matter lesions appear to be predominantly periventricular[32], whereas in cases reported from North America the lesions were found in both periventricular and subcortical[12] or in exclusively subcortical location[15].

FATTY ACID OXIDATION DISORDERS

This group includes carnitine cycle defects (carnitine–palmitoyle transferase deficiency, carnitine translocase deficiency), beta-oxidation disorders (very long-, medium-, and short-chain acyl coenzyme A dehydrogenase, as well as long- and short-chain 3-hydroxy-acyl coenzyme A dehydrogenase deficiencies) and electron transfer flavoprotein dehydrogenase deficiency (multiple acyl coenzyme A dehydrogenase deficiency, usually referred to as glutaric aciduria type 2).

Very long-chain acyl coenzyme A dehydrogenase, long-chain 3-hydroxy-acyl coenzyme A dehydrogenase and glutaric aciduria type 2 may be encountered in neonates, the others have only later onset, infantile or childhood forms.

Fatty acid oxidation disorders – because of the resultant impairment of the aerobic energy metabolism at the mitochondrial level – are characterized by multi-organ (heart, liver, muscles) involvement. Dysfunction of the mitochondria within the myocardium, where energy is partially derived from fat, results initially in conduction problems and subsequently in global cardiac failure. On the other hand, fatty acid overload leads to steathosis at the level of the liver.

Very long-chain acyl coenzyme A dehydrogenase and long-chain 3-hydroxy-acyl coenzyme A dehydrogenase deficiencies

Metabolic features

Neonates present with hyperammonemia, hypoglycemia, lactic acidosis and cardiac arrhythmia.

Clinical course

The condition is usually untreatable and leads to death, except the Scandinavian phenotypes, which are compatible with life.

Treatment

Aggressive treatment of hypoglycemia and avoidance of fasting. A high carbohydrate and low fat diet is used.

Imaging

No imaging data are available in very long-chain acyl coenzyme A dehydrogenase and long-chain 3-hydroxy-acyl coenzyme A dehydrogenase deficiencies.

Multiple acyl coenzyme A dehydrogenase deficiency (glutaric aciduria type 2)

Glutaric aciduria type 2 has two neonatal and one later-onset phenotypes. This needs to be distinguished from glutaric acidemia type 1, which is secondary to an isolated deficiency of glutaryl-CoA deficiency and presents in infancy.

Enzyme deficiency

This disease is caused by deficiency of the electron transfer flavoprotein failing to transport electrons to intramitochondrial dehydrogenase enzymes. It therefore also represents a profound mitochondrial metabolic–energetic disorder.

Metabolic features

Onset is characterized by metabolic acidosis, organic (glutaric, 2-hydroxyglutaric, isovaleric, isobutyric, ethylmalonic) aciduria and hypoglycemia without ketosis.

Clinical features

There is a high incidence of premature birth. The neonatal form may present with or without congenital malformations. These include hepatomegaly, enlarged kidneys, abnormal external genitalia, rocker bottom feet, defects of the anterior abdominal wall and neuronal migration defects in the brain. Onset of metabolic symptoms is usually between 24 and 48 h of age with stupor, tachypnea, hypotonia and sometimes seizures. Hypotonia can be very marked and suggestive of a neuromuscular disorder.

Clinical course

Those infants presenting with associated congenital anomalies usually die within the first few weeks of life. Patients with the other neonatal phenotype develop progressive cardiomyopathy and die by the age of 1 year.

Treatment

Restricted fat and protein diet with riboflavin and carnitine supplementation has been generally unsuccessful. Treatment may need to be started antenatally.

Imaging

In a case report of the neonatal form, underdeveloped frontal and temporal lobes with enlarged Sylvian fissures (somewhat similar to glutaric aciduria type 1), delayed myelination and hypoplasia of the corpus callosum have been described at the age of 14 weeks[39].

Spectroscopy

Normal NAA, increased lactate were described in glutaric aciduria type 2, in conjunction with increased Cho/Cr ratio, interpreted as a sign of dysmyelination[39].

OTHER ORGANIC ACID DISORDERS

Pyroglutamic aciduria (5-oxoprolinuria)

Enzyme deficiency

In the classical form the underlying enzyme abnormality is glutathione synthetase deficiency.

Inheritance

Autosomal recessive.

Genetics

The encoding gene is located on chromosome 20.

Metabolic features

Acidosis without ketosis or lactic acidosis. The unavailability of glutathione causes membrane fragility of the erythro-

cytes presenting with hemolytic anemia and jaundice. The resultant hemolytic–acidotic crisis may be seen both in neonates and infants. It is, however, noteworthy that transient or constant 5-oxoprolinuria is a non-specific laboratory finding and can occur without defect in the gamma-glutamyl cycle (e.g. in GM2 gangliosidosis, urea cycle defects, tyrosinemia type 1, methylmalonic and propionic acidemias)[27].

Clinical features

Approximately half of neonates exhibit neurological signs usually stupor or coma. The disease may also manifest with a slowly progressive encephalopathy later in childhood.

Treatment

Therapy with glucose and sodium bicarbonate is vital acutely. Infants may remain well between intermittent episodes of acidosis.

Sulfite oxidase deficiency

This may occur as an isolated enzyme defect or in combination with xanthine dehydrogenase deficiency as part of molybdenum co-factor deficiency. Molybdenum co-factor is essential for the action of both enzymes.

Metabolic features

Sulfite, S-sulfocysteine, taurine and xanthine accumulate and are excreted in the urine. A sulfite strip test on fresh urine offers a useful screening test. Xanthine is found in molybdenum co-factor deficiency but not in isolated sulfite oxidase deficiency. Lactic acidosis may be present. Blood uric acid is depressed in the molybdenum co-factor deficiency form of the disease, the detection of hypouricemia is a valuable screening test.

Clinical features

Feeding difficulties, vomiting and seizures within the first few days.

Clinical course

Survivors develop spasticity, microcephaly and severe intellectual impairment. Seborrheic rash and dislocated lenses develop later in infancy.

Treatment

Dietary methionine restriction and cysteine supplementation has been tried, with one reported success.

Imaging

Studies show progressive destruction of cortex, basal ganglia, thalami, cerebellum and white matter. Cystic changes within the myelin may be found.

DISORDERS OF AMINO ACID METABOLISM

Maple syrup urine disease (MSUD, branched chain aminoacidemia)

Enzyme deficiency

Deficiency of the branched-chain alpha-ketoacid dehydrogenase enzyme (see earlier in abnormalities of the L-leucine breakdown pathway).

Inheritance

Autosomal recessive.

Genetics

The encoding genes of the three enzyme subunits are located on chromosomes 19 and 6 (E1 alpha and beta subunits), 1 (E2 subunit) and 7 (E3 subunit). It is noteworthy that the E3 subunits of the pyruvate dehydrogenase (see above in primary lactic acidosis), the alpha-ketoacid dehydrogenase (defective in alpha ketoglutaric aciduria, a metabolic disease with late infantile or childhood onset) and of the branched-chain alpha-ketoacid dehydrogenase are identical and encoded by the same gene (chromosome 7q31–q32) in prokaryotic cells.

Metabolic features

Owing to the underlying enzyme defect the metabolism of alpha ketoisocaproic, alpha keto-beta-methylvaleric and alpha-ketoisovaleric acids (intermediate metabolites in the breakdown of L-leucine, L-isoleucine and L-valine) is interrupted in MSUD. Biochemical effects of the marked elevation of branched-chain ketoacids and branched-chain amino acids in body fluids involve the metabolism of neurotransmitters and compounds important in energy metabolism (pyruvate and glucose) and the synthesis of proteins and myelin.

Clinical features

Four clinical phenotypes of MSUD have been identified. The classical form is the most severe, occurring in neonates. The intermediate and intermittent forms are usually of infantile or even later onset. The thiamine responsive form is encountered in all age groups. The classic variety presents at about 5–7 days after birth with poor feeding, vomiting, hypoglycemia, seizures, fluctuating ophthalmoplegia, coma and a characteristic odor of maple syrup.

Clinical course

Early diagnosis and an appropriate dietary regimen improve long-term outcome in patients with MSUD but intercurrent decompensation is a possible life-threatening complication.

Treatment

Diet that contains no or restricted branched-chain amino acids, according to blood levels.

Imaging

This disease presents with a highly characteristic, and practically pathognomonic MRI pattern if diffusion-weighted imaging is used in addition to the standard conventional sequences (see earlier section on diffusion-weighted MR imaging in neurometabolic disorders). Diffuse brain swelling is observed in the non-myelinated white matter secondary to vasogenic edema. Prolongation of the T2 relaxation time is seen within the cerebral white matter, more pronounced within the myelinated (due to vacuolating myelinopathy) than the non-myelinated (due to vasogenic edema) white matter (Figs 17.4 and 17.15).

Spectroscopy

The protons of the methyl groups of the branched-chain amino acids resonate at 0.9–1.0 ppm. In healthy subjects, with long echo time, there is no observable signal at 0.9–1.0 ppm. However, in patients with MSUD with acute metabolic decompensation where plasma, CSF and cerebral levels of branched-chain amino acids and ketoacids are elevated, a peak at 0.9–1.0 ppm may be detected using either short or long TE proton MR spectroscopy[11] (Fig. 17.16). A possible associated elevated lactate peak at 1.3 ppm reflects the impairment in energy metabolism and utilization of pyruvate in the citric acid cycle. These two peaks were seen to disappear on recovery[11]. The NAA peak may also be low during the acute decompensation and return to a higher level on recovery[48].

Non-ketotic hyperglycinemia

Enzyme deficiency

A defect of the glycine cleavage system. The glycine cleavage system is expressed in liver, kidney and the brain and its defect leads to an accumulation of glycine in body fluids. The defect of the glycine cleavage system in the brain and the resulting accumulation of glycine are thought to be critical in the neurotoxicity. There appear to be two neurotransmitter roles for glycine in the CNS – one inhibitory and one

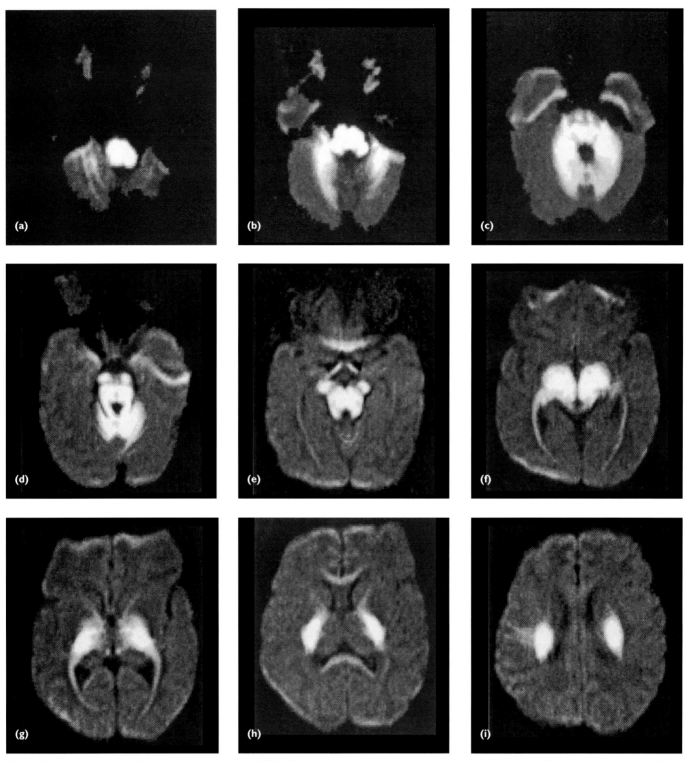

Fig. 17.15 Axial echo planar diffusion-weighted images (**b** = 1000, diffusion gradient in the slice selection direction) of the brain in MSUD (same patient as Fig. 17.4). Very prominent signal intensity is seen within the myelinated structures (compare with Fig. 17.4) consistent with isotropically restricted water diffusion. In contrast to the T2 weighted images, the non-myelinated white matter structures are hypointense with this technique, therefore vasogenic edema (characterized by increased water diffusion) is easily differentiated from vacuolating myelinopathy. At the same time an accurate myelination map of the newborn is also provided. *See also overleaf* (**j**).

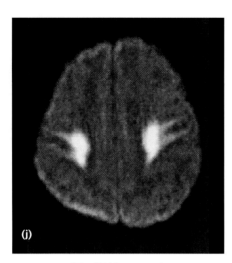

(Fig. 17.15 *continued***)**

excitatory and these roles are influenced by maturation. The classic glycine receptor is inhibitory and located in the spinal cord and brain stem. The second glycine receptor site is associated with the N-methyl-D-aspartate (NMDA)-receptor channel complex. Glycine acting at this site is excitatory and potentiates the action of glutamate, leading to glutamate-induced excitotoxic neuronal death.

Inheritance

Autosomal recessive.

Metabolic features

Marked accumulation of glycine in blood, urine and CSF occurs; the latter being particularly characteristic. Diagnosis is made with the ratio of the concentration of glycine in the CSF to that in the plasma and ranges from 0.1 to 0.3 (control values approximately 0.02).

Clinical features

Non-ketotic hyperglycinemia has four known clinical phenotypes: neonatal, infantile, late-onset and transient. The neonatal form (often referred to as classical, the others as atypical) is far the most common. The neonatal form of non-ketotic hyperglycinemia presents within the first 2 days of life with encephalopathy, lethargy, breathing difficulties leading to respiratory failure, multifocal myoclonic seizures (showing burst suppression pattern on the EEG) and quite characteristically with hiccups[23]. The pronounced hypotonia may be related to the inhibitory effect of glycine on anterior horn cells within the spinal cord.

Clinical course

Most children die in the first year of life while others display severe neurodevelopmental delay but may survive for many years.

Treatment

The disease is usually resistant to treatment.

Imaging

Diffuse cerebral atrophy, callosal hypotrophy and disturbed/delayed myelination constitute the imaging hallmarks of non-ketotic hyperglycinemia[33]. Assessment of the corpus callosum is difficult in the neonate, due to its small size and lack of myelin, but the underdevelopment of the corpus callosum becomes evident later. Occasionally, a true malformation (agenesis, dysgenesis) may also be encountered[50] (Figs 17.2 and 17.17).

Atrophy of the brain may already be present in the neonate but continues to progress. In surviving patients,

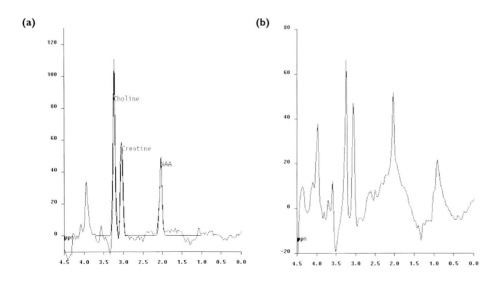

Fig. 17.16 Proton MR spectra obtained with the PRESS technique using 135 ms echo time **(a)** and the STEAM technique using 20 ms echo time **(b)** in a 1-month-old infant with MSUD. The sampling voxel (2 × 2 × 2 cm) was placed on the basal ganglia. The first spectrum shows a decreased NAA peak and a small amount of lactate at the 1.3 ppm level. On the second spectrum a rather prominent peak is seen at the 0.9–1.0 ppm level, corresponding to branched-chain amino acids.

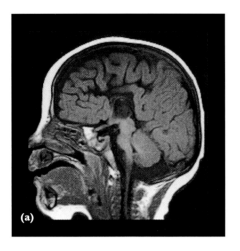
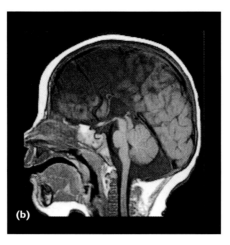

Fig. 17.17 Sagittal T1 weighted spin echo images in an 8-month-old infant with non-ketotic hyperglycinemia. The anterior components (genu and the anterior part of the body) are markedly hypotrophic but recognizable consistent with partial dysgenesis.

delay in the myelination process becomes increasingly conspicuous with age. Supratentorial structures appear to be predominantly involved; the brain stem and cerebellar structures may be relatively but not totally spared. Atrophy and delayed myelination are also quite common findings in other metabolic disorders, in particular in organic acidurias. Proton MR spectroscopy, however, by directly demonstrating abnormal amount of glycine within the brain parenchyma, provides specific diagnostic information (see below).

Spectroscopy

Proton MR spectroscopy of the brain at long echo times (e.g. TE = 135 ms) allows the non-invasive, direct demonstration of glycine in infants with non-ketotic hyperglycinemia. This signal at 3.56 ppm generated by the protons of glycine overlaps with the *in vivo myo*-inositol signal at short (e.g. 20 ms) echo times (glycine accounts for less than 20% of the 3.56 ppm signal in normal subjects). However, as the signal from *myo*-inositol significantly decays at longer echo times, a prominent 'residual' signal on a second sampling at a long echo time allows their reliable differentiation (Fig. 17.18).

Cerebral concentrations of glycine seem to correspond more reliably to clinical findings than CSF and plasma levels[20]. Serial proton MR spectroscopy studies have been found to be useful in following the therapeutic response to drugs aimed at reducing glycine in the CNS (e.g. sodium benzoate and dextromethorphan which have been shown to have beneficial effects in some infants with non-ketotic hyperglycinemia)[18,20].

UREA CYCLE DEFECTS

The urea cycle is involved in the synthesis of arginine and the elimination of excess nitrogen through the formation of urea.

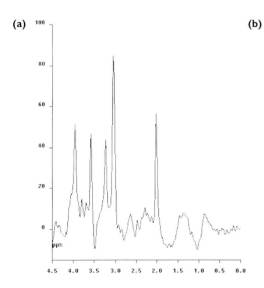
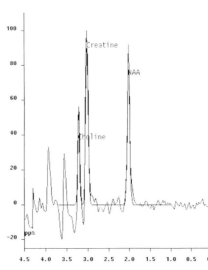

Fig. 17.18 Proton MR spectra obtained with the STEAM technique using 20 ms echo time **(a)** and the PRESS technique using 135 ms echo time **(b)** in a 9-month-old infant with non-ketotic hyperglycinemia. The sampling voxel (2 × 2 × 3 cm) was placed on the basal ganglia. The NAA and choline peaks are decreased. *myo*-Inositol and glycine are known to overlap at the 3.55 ppm level when short echo times are used **(a)**. Using long echo times the *myo*-inositol peak disappears, whereas glycine, which has a longer T2 relaxation time, remains apparent, if present in abnormal amount. In this case the persistent peak indicates that it mostly corresponds to glycine **(b)**.

Enzyme deficiencies

The involved enzymes are the carbamylphosphatase synthetase, ornithine transcarbamylase, argininase (hyperargininemia), argininosuccinic acid lyase (argininosuccinic aciduria) and argininosuccinic acid synthetase (citrullinemia). The carbamylphosphatase synthetase and the ornithine transcarbamylase are mitochondrial enzymes, the others are found within the cytosol.

Inheritance

Ornithine transcarbamylase deficiency has an X-linked recessive inheritance; the other diseases are autosomal recessive.

Metabolic features

Impairment of the urea cycle has significant consequences:

(1) Arginine becomes an essential amino acid (except in hyperargininemia).
(2) Severe hyperammonemia develops. Besides its direct toxic effect, it also leads to disequilibrium between the excitatory (glutamate) and inhibitory (gamma amino butyric acid (GABA)) neurotransmitters through stimulation of glutamate synthesis from glutamine and ammonia at the presynaptic level. Although the exact mechanism of the resultant damage to neurons ('glutamate suicide') is still poorly understood, this is felt to be one of the major factors behind the devastating effects on the brain parenchyma in urea cycle defects and in some of the organic acidurias, for example glutaric aciduria type 1.

Besides hyperammonemia, in urea cycle defects aminoacidemia and respiratory alkalosis are also typically seen.

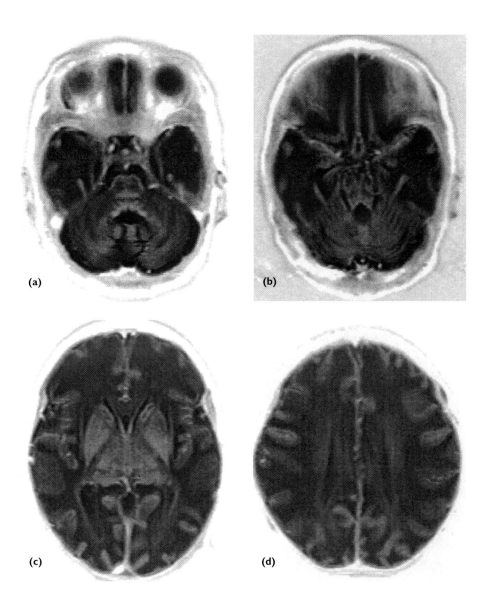

Fig. 17.19 Axial fast inversion recovery images in a 12-day-old neonate with carbamylphosphatase synthetase deficiency. Prominent diffuse brain edema is seen in conjunction with marked T1 prolongation predominantly in the non-myelinated white matter structures.

(a)

(b)

(c)

(d)

Clinical features

Ornithine transcarbamylase deficiency, carbamylphosphatase deficiency and citrullinemia are the most frequent forms to occur in neonates. Argininosuccinic aciduria usually has a few days later onset, whereas in hyperargininemia the typical presentation is slowly progressive encephalopathy. In the neonatal forms of urea cycle defects hyperammonemia leads to diffuse brain edema responsible for the signs of raised intracranial pressure at physical and neurological examination (hypotonia, vomiting, hypothermia, seizures, bulging fontanel, rapidly increasing head circumference). Hyperventilation results in the distinctly characteristic respiratory alkalosis.

Clinical course

Over half the infants die in the neonatal period. The majority of survivors show neurodevelopmental impairment.

Treatment

Immediate postnatal diagnosis and treatment of urea cycle defects is of utmost importance, since delay in appropriate management leads to death or severe and irreversible neurological deficit. Emergency procedures to reduce ammonia levels are followed by a low protein diet. Abundant non-protein calories and essential amino acids are required to reduce protein catabolism. The most encouraging results of appropriate short- and long-term treatment occur in infants with carbamylphosphatase synthetase deficiency.

Imaging

The most prominent MRI imaging finding in all neonatal forms of the urea cycle defects (carbamylphosphatase synthetase, ornithine transcarbamylase, citrullinemia, argini-nosuccinic aciduria) is the diffuse and marked brain edema. Analysis of the T2 weighted images reveals prominent signal changes within the non-myelinated white matter with relative preservation of the myelinated areas (Fig. 17.19). This is in clear contrast with MSUD, where signal changes predominate in the myelinated white matter. The underlying pathophysiological mechanism in urea cycle defects (vasogenic edema) is different from that in MSUD (vacuolating myelinopathy), as demonstrated by the distinctly different presentations on diffusion-weighted images. Gray matter structures, the basal ganglia and cortex may also be involved in the most severe cases.

The conventional MRI findings may be very similar to some of the organic acidurias; however, by proton MR spectroscopy they can be easily differentiated (see below).

Spectroscopy

Increase in glutamate and glutamine and a decrease in *myo*-inositol (mI) is typical, although non-specific findings in urea cycle defects using proton MR spectroscopy[8,47] (Fig. 17.20). Glutamine is usually easier to demonstrate with short echo time (20 ms), but high concentrations may be detectable at longer echo times (135 ms), too. Additional abnormal proton MR spectroscopic findings include decrease of NAA, choline and creatinine. Since similar changes occur in hepatic encephalopathy, these abnormalities are non-specific, but in the given clinical setting and when interpreted together with conventional imaging findings, they can be highly suggestive.

PEROXISOMAL DISORDERS IN THE NEONATE

Peroxisomes are cellular organelles. Peroxisomal enzymes are involved in multiple metabolic pathways, including lipid metabolism. They are therefore indispensable in the normal

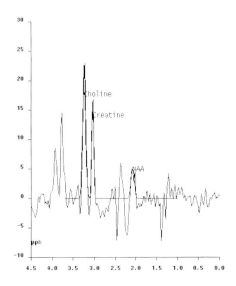

Fig. 17.20 Proton MR spectrum obtained with the PRESS sequence using 135 ms echo time in a 12-day-old newborn with urea cycle defect (same patient as Fig. 17.19). The sampling voxel (2 × 2 × 1 cm) is placed on the basal ganglia. Prominent decrease of the NAA peak is seen in conjunction with increased glutamine–glutamate peaks both at the 2.3 ppm and the 3.8 ppm levels. Abnormal amount of lactate is also suggested at the 1.3 ppm level.

myelination process. For this reason, peroxisomes are particularly abundant in oligodendrocytes in neonates and infants. Peroxisomal diseases typically present with involvement of the central nervous system with predilection of the white matter (hypo-, dys- and demyelination).

Peroxisomal diseases represent a continuum. Those caused by total absence of peroxisomal activity (peroxisomal biogenesis disorders) are characterized by neonatal or early infantile onset and represent the most severe forms. The resultant disease entities, such as Zellweger's syndrome and neonatal adrenoleukodystrophy, present with immediate postnatal onset of clinical signs and symptoms. These are generalized systemic diseases, in which involvement of the central nervous system is always severe but not exclusive. The infants present in the neonatal period with hypotonia, difficulty in sucking and swallowing requiring gavage feeding, myoclonic seizures, abnormal vision and abnormal facies. They typically lead to death within the first few months or years of life. Other forms with multiple peroxisomal dysfunctions are characterized by infantile or childhood-onset (pseudo-infantile Refsum disease, Zellweger-like syndrome) and the disease course is more prolonged.

If the metabolic abnormality is limited to the loss of a single peroxisomal function only (e.g. metabolism of phytanic acid in Refsum disease or degradation of very long-chain fatty acids in X-linked adrenoleukodystrophy (X-ALD)) the resultant disease may be of childhood, juvenile or adult onset. Some of them may be compatible with life (adrenomyeloneuropathy, Refsum disease); others (X-ALD) are not.

Zellweger (cerebrohepatorenal) syndrome

Enzyme deficiency

There is a lack of biogenesis of the peroxisomes, therefore practically all peroxisomal functions are absent. This is the most severe of all the peroxisomal diseases.

Inheritance

Autosomal recessive.

Metabolic features

Elevated very long-chain fatty acids in the plasma and fibroblasts, impairment of plasmalogen biosynthesis and abnormal patterns of bile acids.

Clinical features

Besides the rather typical facial dysmorphic features, the most severe abnormalities are seen at the level of the brain (cortical dysplasia and hypomyelination), liver and kidneys.

Clinical course

Infants with Zellweger disease fail to thrive and usually die before the age of 1 year.

Imaging

Conventional MRI findings alone are pathognomonic in this disease. Diffuse, markedly delayed myelination is easily appreciated in both the inversion recovery and the T2 weighted images. Careful analysis of the cortical ribbon in the temporo-parietal regions reveals extensive areas of polymicrogyria-like changes. These abnormalities are often easier to identify on the T2 than the T1 weighted images. The use of high-resolution matrix significantly enhances their conspicuity (Fig. 17.21). Subependymal, so-called germinolytic cysts are occasionally present along the frontal horns of the lateral ventricles[36]. Incomplete opercularization, verticalization of the Sylvian fissures, colpocephaly[28], cerebellar cortical dysplasia, hypo- or dysplasia of the inferior olives have been also described in this disease. The presence of both white and gray matter abnormalities as well as dysmorphic–dysplastic changes of the brain are in keeping with a profound metabolic abnormality with early intrauterine onset. Additional imaging work-up shows calcification within the patella and acetabulum (plain X-ray) and cysts within the kidneys (ultrasound, CT)[49].

Spectroscopy

A study comparing four infants with variants of Zellweger syndrome with normal controls, demonstrated a marked decrease in NAA in white and gray matter, thalamus and cerebellum. In two cases an increase in cerebral glutamine and a decrease in *myo*-inositol in the gray matter reflecting the concomitant effect on hepatic function were seen. Two severe cases also demonstrated an increase in mobile lipids in the white matter. A slight increase in lactate levels was seen. These findings are not specific to peroxisomal disorders but give insight into the metabolic effects on the developing brain (Fig. 17.22).

Neonatal adrenoleukodystrophy

Metabolic features

Typical laboratory findings include increased plasma pipecolic, phytanic acid and very long-chain fatty acid levels and lead to the correct diagnosis despite the non-specific clinical presentation.

Clinical features

These children do not have dysmorphic features or skeletal abnormalities but involvement of the central nervous system

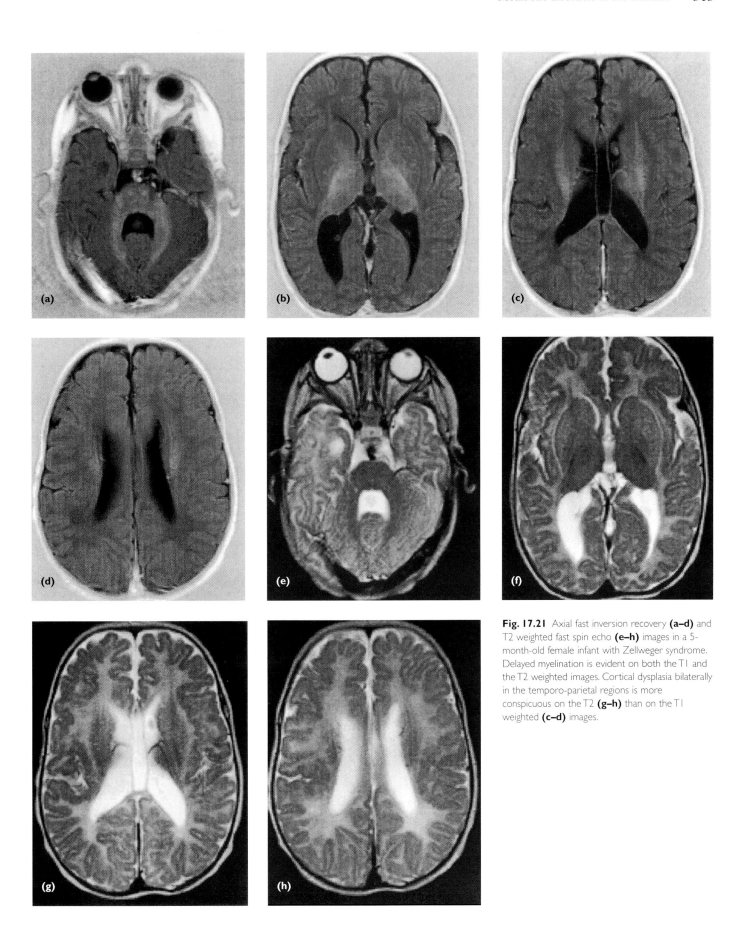

Fig. 17.21 Axial fast inversion recovery **(a–d)** and T2 weighted fast spin echo **(e–h)** images in a 5-month-old female infant with Zellweger syndrome. Delayed myelination is evident on both the T1 and the T2 weighted images. Cortical dysplasia bilaterally in the temporo-parietal regions is more conspicuous on the T2 **(g–h)** than on the T1 weighted **(c–d)** images.

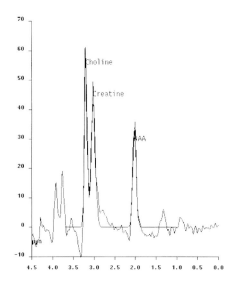

Fig. 17.22 Proton MR spectrum obtained with the PRESS sequence using 270 ms echo time in a 5-month-old female infant with Zellweger syndrome. The sampling voxel (2 × 2 × 2 cm) is placed on the basal ganglia. The NAA peak is markedly decreased, the glutamine–glutamate peak at the 3.8 ppm level is increased and a small amount of lactate is also detected at the 1.3 ppm level.

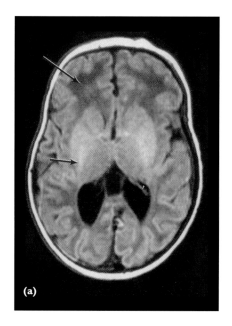
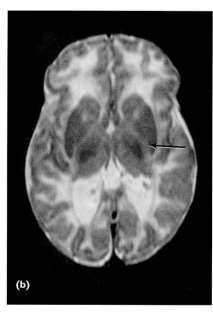

Fig. 17.23 Term-born infant with neonatal adrenoleukodystrophy. Imaged at 3 days of age. **(a)** T1 weighted images. There is low signal intensity within the white matter, most marked frontally (*long arrow*). The signal intensity from myelin in the posterior limb is indistinct (*short arrow*) **(b)** T2 weighted images. The white matter has a very high signal intensity, most marked frontally. The posterior limb is seen as a very broad high signal intensity (*arrow*). It is not possible to see any low signal intensity consistent with myelin.

is already apparent at birth by the presence of severe hypotonia, hearing loss, retinal degeneration and seizures.

Imaging

Imaging findings are compatible with dys- and/or demyelination within the cerebellar and cerebral white matter (Fig. 17.23) (see Chapter 14). Signs of a neuronal migration disorder may also be conspicuous. The presence of contrast uptake in the involved areas described on CT images suggests an active, perhaps inflammatory process, similar to that seen within the active inflammation zone in X-linked adrenoleukodystrophy[45].

Rhizomelic chondrodysplasia punctata

Enzyme deficiency

Multiple but not all peroxisomal functions are absent.

Inheritance

Autosomal recessive.

Clinical features

Dysmorphic features are evident at birth. Shortening of the proximal parts of the extremities is the most characteristic physical examination finding. Severe psychomotor delay, failure to thrive, ichthyosis and cataract complete the clinical syndrome.

Imaging

Besides the straightforward abnormalities of the extremities, plain X-ray examination reveals more profound skeletal abnormalities, including calcifications within the epiphyseal cartilage, metaphyseal cupping and coronal clefts in the vertebral bodies. MRI findings suggest a combination of delayed and dysmyelination[44].

Menkes disease (kinky/steely hair disease, trichopoliodystrophy)

Menkes disease is a metal metabolism disorder due to a defect in intracellular–intercompartmental copper transport (in contrast to Wilson's disease which represents an extracellular copper transport abnormality).

Enzyme deficiency

Several enzymes which require copper as a co-factor are deficient, the most important of which are those involved in catecholamine synthesis (dopamine-beta-hydroxylase), oxidative phosphorylation (cytochrome c oxidase) and elastin–collagen formation (lysyl oxidase).

Inheritance

X-linked.

Clinical features

The disease has neonatal and infantile-onset forms. Impairment of catecholamine (neurotransmitter) synthesis and oxidative phosphorylation may explain the neurological manifestations (hypotonia, seizures) of the disease, whereas the elastin–collagen formation disorder possibly causes intimal fragility and the characteristic tortuous elongated appearance of cerebral arteries. The typical hair abnormalities may not be apparent in the newborn.

Imaging

MRI studies during the early postnatal period usually do not reveal significant abnormalities. Subtle signal abnormalities within the cerebral cortex may be seen, the pathological significance of which is unclear[3, 21]. Later scans show progressive white matter disease with frontal and temporal predominance[7] and prominent cerebral and cerebellar atrophy. MR angiography was found to be useful in the demonstration of the characteristic tortuosity of the cerebral vessels[21]. In a patient treated with copper histidinate no cerebral atrophy or white matter abnormalities were seen, tortuosity of the cerebral arteries was however still conspicuous[1]. Patients with Menkes disease are prone to 'spontaneous', most probably 'ex vacuo' developing subdural hematomas which should not be misdiagnosed as a sign of child abuse.

Clinical management of inborn errors of metabolism in neonates

PRENATAL MANAGEMENT

Prenatal diagnosis is possible in many of the neurometabolic disorders, including propionic acidemia, Menkes disease, peroxisomal diseases, urea cycle defects and disorders of oxidative phosphorylation by demonstration of deficient enzyme activity in cultured amniocytes and chorionic villous samples and/or of abnormal metabolites in amniotic fluid.

Emerging new techniques, allowing for pre-implantation diagnosis by direct identification of gene and chromosome abnormalities or sex determination (in families with high risk for X-linked genetic disorders), represent new promising options in the prenatal management of inborn errors of metabolism.

In one case, prenatal ultrasound has been reported to be diagnostic in rhizomelic chondrodystrophia punctata by demonstrating the characteristic skeletal abnormalities[37]. Imaging techniques, however, have not been used systematically in the prenatal diagnosis of inborn errors of metabolism. With the increasing use of fast (HASTE – half-Fourier single shot turbo spin echo) intrauterine MRI imaging this may change and diseases presenting with malformations or morphological abnormalities of the brain (Zellweger syndrome, glutaric aciduria type 1) may be depicted.

POSTNATAL MANAGEMENT

Imaging work-up is an integral part of the postnatal management process. In this respect ultrasound and CT have a definite role as well, especially in ruling out other pathologies, such as hydrocephalus in neonates with progressive increase of head size and intracerebral bleeding in neonates with lethargy or coma. Ultrasound has been found to be useful in the demonstration of morphological changes suggestive of neurometabolic disease (e.g. bilateral Sylvian fissure abnormalities in glutaric aciduria type 1 or germinolytic cysts in Zellweger syndrome)[13,36].

Many of the neonatal metabolic disorders present with non-specific MRI findings during the early postnatal period. The characteristic imaging findings (basal ganglia disease, dys- or delayed myelination, white matter disease) may develop at a later stage. Therefore, in the case of non-conclusive initial work-up, follow-up MR examinations may be helpful.

Non-invasive monitoring of the effects of therapeutic measures by conventional MR imaging (e.g. progress of myelination) or MR spectroscopy (e.g. decrease of the brain concentration of abnormal substances) is another important indication of follow-up studies[8,20,25].

Conclusion

Management of neonates with metabolic disorders requires a multidisciplinary approach and close collaboration of obstetricians, pediatricians, geneticists, biochemists and radiologists. The age of onset, the presence or absence of dysmorphic features, skin manifestations, laboratory changes, neurological signs and symptoms, visceral and musculoskeletal abnormalities, MRI and spectroscopic alterations are all potentially important clues in the diagnostic work-up. Metabolic diseases may present with confusingly similar or distinctly different clinical, biochemical and imaging abnormalities, each of them representing a 'fingerprint' or 'pattern' of the disease, some of which may be therefore non-specific, others characteristic, suggestive or even pathognomonic[22,46]. The set of these 'stigmata' describes the clinical–radiological pattern, which is a function of the varying susceptibility and vulnerability of the various organ systems to the different metabolic abnormalities. Recognition of the clinical and imaging substrates of selective vulnerability leads to clinical–radiological pattern recognition, the single most important concept that needs to be systematically applied in the diagnostic management of inborn errors of metabolism.

MRI is the most valuable modality in the imaging assessment of the central nervous system manifestations of inborn errors of metabolism, due to its inherently exquisite sensitivity to demonstrate lesions in the cerebral parenchyma. Awareness and recognition of the most characteristic imaging and spectroscopic patterns (e.g. urea cycle defects, peroxisomal disorders, propionic acidemia, non-ketotic hyperglycinemia, MSUD) is important, especially in centers which have sparse clinical experience with metabolic disorders, and where the diagnostic burden is heavier on the radiologist.

Summary

- The age of onset is an important diagnostic and prognostic factor in the inborn errors of metabolism. It can be prenatal, neonatal, infantile, childhood, adolescent or later. As a general rule, the earlier the onset, the more profound the metabolic disorder.

- Most inborn errors of metabolism of neonatal onset fall into the category of devastating metabolic diseases with potentially severe systemic or neurological sequelae.

- MRI is the technique of choice in the imaging evaluation of metabolic disorders. Plain X-ray, CT and ultrasound may occasionally provide complimentary information.

- Conventional MRI of the brain in neonatal metabolic disorders usually shows non-specific abnormalities (brain swelling, atrophy, delayed or hypomyelination).

- More rarely, specific morphological changes (e.g. callosal, cortical abnormalities) or parenchymal lesion patterns (i.e. the imaging manifestations of selective vulnerability) may be identified.

- The complex MR evaluation of inborn errors of metabolism includes diffusion-weighted imaging and proton MR spectroscopy. These techniques may enhance the diagnostic sensitivity and specificity of the MRI work-up.

- Many metabolic disorders present with characteristic or specific clinical abnormalities, which together with the MRI and spectroscopic findings may delineate a suggestive or pathognomonic clinical–radiological pattern.

- The definite diagnosis of inborn errors of metabolism usually relies on laboratory tests.

- The diagnosis and therapeutic management of metabolic disease requires a multidisciplinary approach.

Acknowledgements

The authors acknowledge and thank the support, guidance and stimulating collaboration of Mohammed Al-Essa MD, Zuheir Al-Rahbeeni MD, Jehad Al-Watban MD, Enrique Chaves-Carballo MD, Sarwat Hussain MD, Pinar Ozand MD PhD, Jaap Valk MD PhD and Mary Rutherford before and during the preparation of this chapter. Special credit is given to Ghadheer Al-Thali, Jennifer Bryant, Christine Corcoran, Helen McQuillan, Abdullah Balfagieh, Craig Briggs and Edgardo Martinez for performing the MR studies and their help in putting together the photographic material and to Vivienne Kynoch for scientific secretarial assistance.

References

1. al Aqeel A, Rashed M, Ozand PT et al. (1994) 3-methylglutaconic aciduria: ten new cases with a possible new phenotype. Brain Dev 16 (Suppl), 23–32.
2. Barker PB, Bryan RN, Kumar AJ et al. (1992) Proton NMR spectroscopy of Canavan's disease. Neuropediatrics 23, 263–267.
3. Barkovich AJ, Good WV, Koch TK et al. (1993) Mitochondrial disorders: analysis of their clinical and imaging characteristics. Am J Neuroradiol 14, 1119–1137.
4. Barth PG, Scholte HR, Berden JA et al. (1983) An X-linked mitochondrial disease affecting cardiac muscle, skeletal muscle and neutrophil leukocytes. J Neurol Sci 62, 327–355.
5. Beaulieu C, D'Arceuil H, Hedehus M et al. (1999) Diffusion-weighted magnetic resonance imaging: theory and potential applications to child neurology. Seminars in Pediatric Neurology 6, 87–100.
6. Bergman AJIW, van der Knaap MS, Smeitnink JAM et al. (1996) Magnetic resonance imaging and spectroscopy of the brain in propionic acidemia: clinical and biochemical considerations. Pediatr Res 40, 404–409.
7. Blaser SI, Berns DH, Ross JS et al. (1989) Serial MR studies in Menkes disease. J Comput Assist Tomogr 13, 113–115.
8. Connelly A, Cross JH, Gadian G et al. (1993) Magnetic resonance spectroscopy shows increased brain glutamine in ornithine carbamoyl transferase deficiency. Pediatr Res 33, 77–81.
9. Detre JA, Wang Z, Bogdan AR et al. (1991) Regional variation in brain lactate in Leigh syndrome by localized 1H magnetic resonance spectroscopy. Ann Neurol 29, 218–221.

10. Ebisu T, Naruse S, Horikawa Y *et al.* (1993) Discrimination between different types of white matter edema with diffusion-weighted MR imaging. *JMRI* **3**, 863–868.

11. Felber SR, Sperl W, Chemelli A *et al.* (1993) Maple syrup urine disease: metabolic decompensation monitored by proton magnetic resonance imaging and spectroscopy. *Ann Neurol* **33**, 396–401.

12. Ferris NJ and Tien RD (1993) Cerebral MRI in 3-hydroxy-3-methylglutaryl-coenzyme A lyase deficiency: case report. *Neuroradiology* **35**, 559–560.

13. Forstner R, Hoffmann GF, Gassner I *et al.* (1999) Glutaric aciduria type 1: ultrasonographic demonstration of early signs. *Pediatr Radiol* **29**, 138–143.

14. Gibson KM, Breuer J, Kaiser K *et al.* (1988) 3-hydroxy-3-methylglutaryl-coenzyme A lyase deficiency: report of five new patients. *J Inher Metab Dis* **11**, 76–87.

15. Gordon K, Riding M, Camfield P *et al.* (1994) CT and MR of 3-hydroxy-3-methylglutaryl-coenzyme A lyase deficiency. *Am J Neuroradiol* **15**, 1474–1476.

16. Grodd W, Krageloh-Mann I, Klose U *et al.* (1991) Metabolic and destructive brain disorders in children: findings with localized proton MR spectroscopy. *Radiology* **181**, 173–181.

17. Grodd W, Krageloh-Mann I, Petersen D *et al.* (1990) *In vivo* assessment of N-acetylaspartate in brain in spongy degeneration (Canavan's disease) by proton spectroscopy. *Lancet* **336**, 437–438.

18. Hamosh A, Maher JF, Bellus GA *et al.* (1998) Long-term use of high-dose benzoate and dextromethorphan for the treatment of nonketotic hyperglycinemia. *J Pediatr* **132**, 709–713.

19. Heindel W, Kugel H, Herholz K (1999) H-1 MRS and 18-FDG-PET in children with congenital lactic acidosis. *Proc Intl Soc Magn Reson Med* (Abstract).

20. Heindel W, Kugel H and Roth B (1993) Noninvasive detection of increased glycine content by proton MR spectroscopy in the brains of two infants with nonketotic hyperglyclinemia. *Am J Neuroradiol* **14**, 629–635.

21. Jacobs DS, Smith AS, Finelli DA *et al.* (1993) Menkes kinky hair disease: characteristic MR angiographic findings. *Am J Neuroradiol* **14**, 1160–1163.

22. Kohlschlütter A (1994) Neuroradiological and neurophysiological indices for neurometabolic disorders. *Eur J Pediatr* **153**(Suppl 1), S90–S93.

23. Lu FL, Wang PJ, Hwu WL *et al.* (1999) Neonatal type of non-ketotic hyperglycinemia. *Pediatr Neurol* **20**, 295–300.

24. Marks HG, Caro PA, Wang ZY *et al.* (1991) Use of computed tomography, magnetic resonance imaging, and localized 1H magnetic resonance spectroscopy in Canavan's disease: a case report. *Ann Neurol* **30**, 106–110.

25. Martinez M and Vazquez E (1998) MRI evidence that docosahaenoic acid ethyl ester improves myelination in generalized peroxisomal disorders. *Neurology* **51**, 26–32.

26. Marzan KAB and Barron TF (1994) MRI abnormalities in Behr syndrome. *Pediatr Neurol* **10**, 247–248.

27. Mayatepek E (1999) 5-oxoprolinuria in patients with and without defects in the g-glutamyl cycle. *Eur J Pediatr* **158**, 221–225.

28. Nakada Y, Hyakuna N, Suzuki Y *et al.* (1993) A case of pseudo-Zellweger syndrome with a possible bifunctional enzyme deficiency but detectable enzyme protein. Comparison of two cases of Zellweger syndrome. *Brain Dev* **15**, 453–456.

29. Nomura Y, Sakuma H, Takeda K *et al.* (1994) Diffusional anisotropy of the human brain assessed with diffusion-weighted MR: relation with normal brain development and aging. *Am J Neuroradiol* **15**, 231–238.

30. Oberholzer VG, Levin B, Burgess EA *et al.* (1967) Methylmalonic aciduria. An inborn error of metabolism leading to chronic metabolic acidosis. *Arch Dis Child* **42**, 492–504.

31. Ono J, Harada K, Sakurai K *et al.* (1997) Differentiation of dys- and demyelination using diffusional anisotropy. *Pediat Neurol* **16**, 63–66.

32. Ozand PT, Aqeel A, Gascon G *et al.* (1991) 3-Hydroxy-3-methylglutaryl-coenzyme A (HMG-CoA) lyase deficiency in Saudi Arabia. *J Inher Metab Dis* **14**, 174–188.

33. Press GA, Barshop BA, Haas RH *et al.* (1989) Abnormalities of the brain in nonketotic hyperglycinemia: MR manifestations. *Am J Neuroradiol* **10**, 315–321.

34. Rashed MS, Bucknall MP, Little D *et al.* (1997) Screening blood spots for inborn errors of metabolism by electrospray tandem mass spectrometry with a microplate batch process and a computer algorithm for automated flagging of abnormal profiles. *Clin Chem* **43**, 1129–1141.

35. Rashed MS, Ozand PT, Bucknall MP *et al.* (1995) Diagnosis of inborn errors of metabolism from blood spots by acylcarnitines and amino acids profiling using automated electrospray tandem mass spectrometry. *Pediatr Res* **38**, 324–331.

36. Russel IM, van Sonderen L, van Straaten HLM *et al.* (1995) Subependymal germinolytic cysts in Zellweger syndrome. *Pediatr Radiol* **25**, 254–255.

37. Sastrowijoto SH, Vandenberghe K, Moerman P *et al.* (1994) Prenatal ultrasound diagnosis of rhizomelic chondrodysplasia punctata in a primigravida. *Prenatal Diag* **14**, 770–776.

38. Schulze A, Hess T, Wevers R *et al.* (1997) Creatine deficiency syndrome caused by guanidinoacetate methyltransferase deficiency: diagnostic tools for a new inborn error of metabolism. *J Pediatr* **131**, 626–631.

39. Shevell MI, Didomenicantonio G, Sylvian M *et al.* (1994) Glutaric acidemia type II: neuroimaging and spectroscopy evidence for developmental encephalopathy. *Pediatr Neurol* **12**, 350–353.

40. Stöckler S, Holzbach U, Hanefeld F *et al.* (1994) Creatine deficiency in the brain: a new, treatable inborn error of metabolism. *Pediatr Res* **36**, 409–413.

41. Takahashi S, Oki J, Miyamoto A *et al.* (1999) Proton magnetic resonance spectroscopy to study the metabolic changes in the brain of a patient with Leigh syndrome. *Brain Dev* **21**, 200–204.

42. Takeda K, Nomura Y, Sakuma H *et al.* (1997) MR assessment of normal brain development in neonates and infants: comparative study of T1- and diffusion-weighted images. *J Comput Assist Tomogr* **21**, 1–7.

43. van der Knaap MS, Barth PG, Vrensen GFJM *et al.* (1996) Histopathology of an infantile-onset spongiform leukoencephalopathy with a discrepantly mild clinical course. *Acta Neuropathol* **92**, 206–212.

44. van der Knaap MS and Valk J (1991) The MR spectrum of peroxisomal disorders. *Neuroradiology* **33**, 30–37.

45. van der Knaap MS and Valk J (1995) Zellweger cerebrohepatorenal syndrome, neonatal adrenoleukodystrophy. In: van der Knaap MS and Valk J (Eds) *Magnetic Resonance of Myelin, Myelination and Myelination Disorders.* Berlin, Springer, pp. 119–120.

46. van der Knaap MS, Valk J, de Neeling N *et al.* (1991) Pattern recognition in magnetic resonance imaging of white matter disorders in children and young adults. *Neuroradiology* **33**, 478–493.

47. Vion-Dury J, Salvan AM, Confort-Gouny S *et al.* (1998) Atlas of brain proton magnetic resonance spectra. Part II: Inherited metabolic encephalopathies. *J Neuroradiol* **25**, 281–289.

48. Wang Z, Zimmerman RA and Sauter R (1996) Proton MR spectroscopy of the brain: clinically useful information obtained in assessing CNS disease in children. *AJR* **167**, 191–199.

49. Weese-Mayer DE, Smith KM, Reddy JK *et al.* (1987) Computerized tomography and ultrasound in the diagnosis of cerebro-hepato-renal syndrome of Zellweger. *Pediatr Radiol* **17**, 170–172.

50. Weinstein SL and Novotny EJ (1987) Neonatal metabolic disorders masquerading as structural central nervous system abnormalities. *Ann Neurol* **22**, 406(Abstract).

51. Yalcinkaya C, Dincer A, Gündüz E *et al.* (1999) MRI and MRS in HMG-CoA lyase deficiency. *Pediatr Neurol* **20**, 375–380.

Imaging of brain function during early human development

18

Ernst Martin

Contents

Structure–function relationship

Cerebral structures mature in a predetermined and well-organized way[55]. Myelination of the central nervous system proceeds slowly during late intrauterine life and rapidly in the neonatal period. Initially there is a dramatic increase in the number of neurons and synapses, which is followed by a subsequent reduction in nerve cell density[7,15,24].

Structural brain maturation has been shown to correlate with behavioral and functional milestones which the neonate and infant attain at various stages of development[29]. However, our understanding of the brain–behavior relationship has been predominantly based on the correlation between alterations in behavior and changes in brain structure. The majority of our knowledge of localization has resulted from lesion studies in adults, where an intact and mature neural system has been destroyed. Because of the low incidence of focal lesions, this approach has shed little light on the structural variation and connectivity of normal brain development or on the physiology and pathophysiology of brain development. The location, extent and age of occurrence of such anomalies within the developmental trajectory, and the effects of plasticity, may all have implications for the resulting behavioral deficit. In the past, maturational changes have been monitored electrophysiologically and behaviorally, and have been related to age (for a review see Holmes[23]). Modern imaging techniques provide assessment of the developing brain *in vivo* at a macroscopic level[4,33,50]. Moreover, structural imaging methods have improved our understanding of developmental disorders such as the autistic spectrum and the developmental language disorders[13,25].

Imaging of brain function

In the mature brain specific functions are carried out at anatomically distinct cortical regions[42]. These areas are highly interconnected by a network of excitatory local circuitry. Corresponding anatomical and functional structures exist to varying degrees in the immature brain of neonates and infants. Detailed anatomical and functional mapping of the various sensory, motor and cognitive tasks the brain performs is necessary in order to understand how the brain works at the various stages of development. Co-registration of structural and functional images provides a platform for identifying the structures delineated by activation patterns in combination with morphometry to quantitatively map active brain structures.

Functional neuroimaging allows us to precisely describe *where* specific operations are carried out, *how* large and widely distributed these functional sites are, and *how* they are interconnected to form a *functional unit*.

Positron emission tomography (PET), single photon emission CT (SPECT), multidetector electro-encephalography and more recently magneto-encephalography are established techniques and have led to a better understanding of functional connectivity within the brain. Temporal and spatial relationships have been identified between the metabolic rate of glucose[11,12] the metabolic rate of oxygen[1,51] and cerebral blood flow[40,52] in distinct neuroanatomic regions during brain maturation. These processes are regulated in such a way as to meet the instantaneous energy requirements with changing cerebral activity of distinct regions that are functionally important during specific developmental periods[11,30,49].

The fact that neuronal activity and cellular metabolism are coupled to cerebral blood flow was postulated over 100 years ago[46]. However, the link between neuronal activity and local cerebral blood flow (CBF), whether in response to vasoactive neurotransmitters from the abundant perivascular nerve supply[32,44], or to other chemical compounds[27,45] still remains to be determined[32,39]. Thus, the underlying mechanisms leading to the MR signal and contrast changes especially during the initial phase after neuronal activation are not yet fully understood[20]. PET studies have shown that functionally induced increase in neuronal activity leads to a proportional increase in the local cerebral metabolic rate of glucose ($lCMR_{Gluc}$) and oxygen ($lCMR_{O_2}$), but to a disproportionate increase of the local cerebral blood flow ($lCBF$[17]). The consequences are an increase in the ratio of oxyhemoglobin to deoxyhemoglobin in the capillaries and small veins draining the active brain region. This causes a transient functionally induced hyperoxemia[53]. This non-linear relationship between oxygen consumption and oxygen delivery[9] has also been explained by an 'uncoupling' of the neuronal oxidative metabolism[18].

The signal arising from water protons can be used in functional MRI (fMRI) as well as functional spectroscopy (fMRS) to monitor cerebrovascular changes associated with brain function[5,28,40]. Whereas fMRI primarily makes use of the paramagnetic effect of deoxygenated hemoglobin as an internal contrast agent (see below), fMRS depends on local changes in proton spin density, magnetic susceptibility[21] and metabolite concentrations, for example lactate[43]. fMRI has distinct advantages over other functional techniques. It is non-invasive and makes no use of radioactivity, it permits simultaneous registration of functional and anatomical data within the same imaging modality, and is fast and has a superior spatial resolution compared to the other methods such as PET.

Blood oxygen-level dependent contrast (BOLD) reflects local changes in blood oxygenation that accompany brain activation. Changes in the relative concentration of oxy- and deoxyhemoglobin cause magnetic susceptibility variations which can be expressed as changes of $T2^*$ relaxation rates. BOLD contrast forms the basic mechanism underlying fMRI[28,41]. It has dramatically improved our understanding of brain function. However, several pitfalls limit the value of the

technique[19]. Both fast gradient echo and fast spin echo techniques have been used extensively in the past with success. The former offers a good signal to noise ratio, but greater sensitivity to larger vessels, the latter offers sensitivity to microvasculature but of a lower signal to noise ratio. Echo-planar imaging (EPI) is a very fast data acquisition technique which reduces intrabrain motion artifacts and allows whole brain imaging in multislice and even true 3D mode, with a high signal to noise ratio. However, it requires special and expensive hardware and software for data acquisition and postprocessing. 3D and multislice (more than 20 contiguous slices) techniques are essential to detect unexpected activation sites and complex interneuronal connectivity during higher order cognitive processing. Event related ultrafast echo-planar pulse sequences, with single plane imaging times of 40–80 ms, promises to resolve the stimulus-dependent vascular response function. This technique is able to deconvolve neuronal events with time scales of the order of the vascular response. An alternative strategy for investigating neonates and infants with fMRI is the use of completely silent pulse sequences allowing functional imaging without any gradient noise. These new methodological developments have improved BOLD contrast fMRI; so that it is now set to become the principle functional imaging tool (Fig. 18.1).

Developmental neuroimaging

Developmental neuroimaging extends the analysis gained from adults to include the temporal evolution of a structure and associated function. It provides monitoring of the physiological, structural and functional plasticity during early postnatal life by identifying the size and distribution of processing components of discrete elementary operations. The ultimate expectation is that it will reveal typical activation patterns that define sensory inputs, contribute to cognitive tasks and eventually lead to distinct behavioural operations in the child. Such measures of structure–function relationship may well need to be explored in the normal developing brain, as well as in cases of brain dysfunction and delayed maturation.

fMRI is completely non-invasive and allows repeated measurements to be taken from the same subjects to assess intra-subject reproducibility and perform longitudinal studies. It is well suited to the study of infants and children. There are, however, constraints in fMRI of neonates and infants. The images should provide high spatial resolution and good contrast, while the total imaging time should be low. Artifacts produced by head movements are a serious obstacle to successfully collecting functional data. The high level of acoustic noise from fast switching gradients in echo planar imaging sequences not only frightens children but is also a major

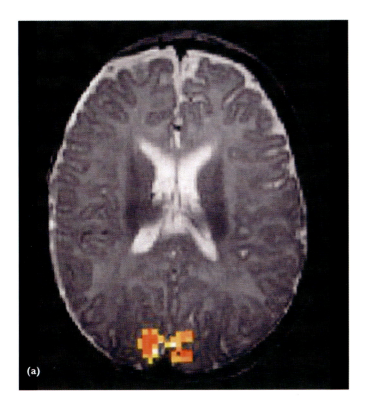

(a)

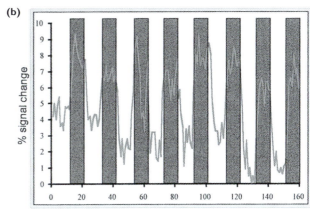

(b)

Fig. 18.1 **(a)** (*left*): Functional MRI of a 5-month-old child depicting visual activity in the striate cortex. The image is composed of a statistical image based on the result from the cross-correlation analysis, overlaid on an anatomical image. **(b)** (*right*) The change in the BOLD signal in the activated region during periods of stimulation (*boxed area*) and periods without stimulation.

source of anxiety for the attending parents. Moreover, typical fMRI experiments require that specific tasks be performed by the subject under investigation over an extended period of time. All these aforementioned points render

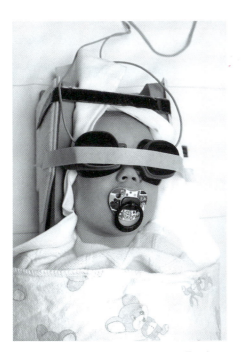

Fig. 18.2 An infant prepared for an fMRI measurement. The flicker-goggles are placed over the eyes and the tape serves merely to hold them in place. Care is taken not to apply excessive pressure on the goggles. The padded headhold provides the infant with the necessary head stability and prevents head movements.

neonates and infants poor candidates for MRI studies. A solution to this problem is to examine young children during natural sleep or under sedation. This requires the development of paradigms and fMRI methods that impose no demands on patient co-operation, for example visual stimulation through the closed eyes (Fig. 18.2). Pentobarbital and chloral hydrate are often used in children during clinical MR examinations to avoid movement artifacts and claustrophobia. In the past, barbituates have been shown to suppress the CBF and CMR_{O_2} in a dose-dependent manner[26,38]. More recently, thiopental has been shown to lower the amplitude of visually evoked potentials[10] and to reduce the increase in regional CBF (rCBF) in response to somatosensory stimulation in rats[31]. However, careful analysis of the cortical activity in response to visual stimulation in pentobarbital-sedated adult volunteers has revealed changes in neuronal activity and metabolism to be much smaller than to the reduction in rCBF[36].

To perform consistent and reproducible functional experiments with reliable results in neonates and infants, these issues need to be addressed.

Mapping visual processing in neonates and infants with fMRI

During the early postnatal months one of the most interesting areas of functional maturation is the development of vision[2]. For a long time, the accepted theory on visual processing was that the entire visual system was functional from birth, inefficient at first but maturing rapidly[6,22]. Research on animals then led to the conclusion that two visual systems co-exist[47]. Diamond and Hall[14] and later Bronson[8] proposed that a secondary, phylogenetically older, extrageniculate visual system, which consists of a number of subcortical structures such as the superior colliculi and thalamic nuclei, may play an important role in neonatal and infantile visual behavior, such as smooth tracking of a slowly moving object. However, this system is not capable of providing conscious visual perception in humans. This hypothesis is in line with early metabolic maturation of thalamic afferent pathways and thalamic CBF[11,52], indicating thalamic activity in neonates.

The secondary visual system mainly processes stimuli falling outside the central area of the retina and has direct connections to various extrastriate visual cortical areas. The involvement of this older subcortical system in visual perception of neonates has been described earlier[16,48]. Testing the visual performance of premature infants with hypoxic–ischemic and hemorrhagic brain lesions clinically it was found that lesions near the thalami, such as periventricular hemorrhage extending into the basal ganglia were more likely to affect visual behavior than substantial infarction of the occipital cortex. These findings have been confirmed recently[37]. Infants who later became cortically blind seemed to retain their ability to track and show pattern preference until about 2 months postnatally, depending on their gestational age. It is concluded that these functions do not require cortical integrity, but are most probably mediated through subcortical pathways. Moreover, the time when the affected neonates apparently lost their ability to track objects seems to coincide with the time at which binocular vision is first demonstrable. This is a function which is thought to be cortically mediated. Thus, cortically mediated visual processes, which involve cognitive processes in order to identify the target object in the foveated area, only start to function during the first 3 months of life. They are mediated via the *primary visual pathway* passing via the lateral geniculate bodies and entering the cortical visual processing area in V1. Nevertheless, different cortical mechanisms appear to be operational at different postnatal times.

Visual acuity, binocular vision and other visual attributes seem to mature in a predetermined manner[54]. Vision probably plays a relatively minor role during postnatal adaptation. However, it is rapidly developing during the first months of life and may become the most important sense with which the infant explores his or her environment and achieves social contact. Vision then forms the basis for perceptual and future cognitive, intellectual and social function[3]. It is not surprising that the primary visual area is one of the earliest neocortical structures to mature and to obtain specific func-

tions. Whereas cortical rCBF and $rCMR_{O_2}$ are lower in neonates compared to older children and adults, the respective ratio is greater than one in the primary visual area of neonates compared to adults[51]. In investigating visual processing during brain development, our interest focused primarily on where different visual tasks are processed in relation to the developmental stage of the brain and their relation to the complexity of the visual stimulus; that is, the developmental plasticity of vision. As the child grows older and starts to analyze and understand the visual input, the interrelation of visual and cognitive processes becomes of major interest. More recently, studies have concentrated on the reparative plasticity of the brain; that is, how the brain compensates for functional impairments created by various brain lesions affecting the visual system at different time points during development.

Our group has investigated developmental aspects of the human visual system that take place during early postnatal life by studying its cortical activity in response to visual stimulation using fMRI. This enabled us to elucidate the role of the primary visual cortex and prestriate areas in the processing of visual information at different stages of brain develop-

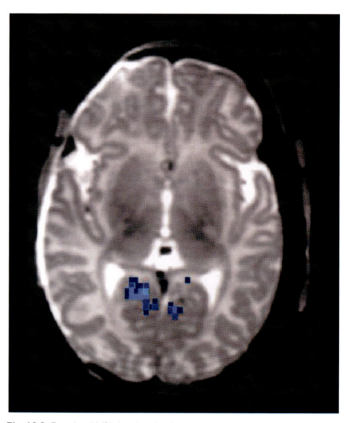

Fig. 18.3 Functional MRI showing visual activity in a neonate. Compared to the fMRI signal of older infant (see Fig. 18.1 **(a)**) the signal differs in both location and polarity. While the visual activity is more anteriorly located in the calcarine sulcus, the BOLD signal is lower during the periods of stimulation than during the rest periods, (i.e. negatively correlated as indicated in blue).

Primary and Secondary Visual Pathway

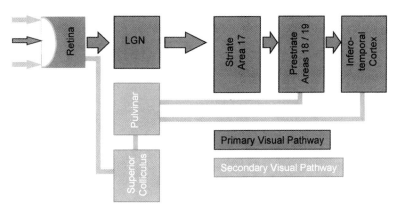

Fig. 18.4 Schematic representation of the primary and secondary visual pathway. In the primary visual pathway the signal from the retinal fovea is passed via the dorsal lateral geniculate nuclei to the striate cortex (V1) and subsequently to the extrastriate cortical visual areas. In the secondary visual pathway signals from more peripheral parts of the retina are passed via subcortical structures such as the superior colliculi and the pulvinar thalami directly to the extrastriate, cortical, visual areas.

ment. Seventy-five infants and children of different ages have been investigated during visual stimulation either with 8 Hz LED flashing goggles, or with computer controlled checkerboard paradigms presented to the subjects in the magnet via a video-goggle system[34]. The results of the cross-correlation analysis obtained from the children were compared to those of normal healthy adult volunteers, with specific emphasis on: (i) exact location of the response signals within the primary visual cortex and the prestriate areas; (ii) their spatial distribution; and (iii) the effect of anesthesia. The results can be summarized as follows: using the same stimulation paradigms, small children generally exhibit lower activity than older children and adults in V1. In neonates ($n = 12$) nine did not show significant stimulus related activation in the visual cortex, whereas two exhibited negatively correlated signal changes in the prestriate area (Fig 18.3). The characteristic positive BOLD contrast related signal change observed in adults during visual stimulation could only be found in two newborn infants in the pulvinar thalami. Among 12 infants, aged 1–12 months, four showed positive, and five negative activity. In three, no activity could be found. These findings contrast to a 100% positive stimulus related signal change observed in 12 children above the age of 6 years. In the instances where a negative BOLD contrast

signal was observed, the site of the activity was usually located more anteriorly in the calcarine sulcus compared to the positive signal changes in V1. From anatomical slices the exact locus of the negatively correlated signal change was judged to correspond to the extrastriate cortical visual area V2. In fact, the majority of toddlers showed stimulus-related activity in V2, rather than V1. The presence of a negative BOLD contrast signal in area V2 confirms earlier electrophysiological findings that activation of extrastriate cortex to visual stimulation can be detected from birth using fMRI. Moreover, careful investigations with fMRI and fMRS reveal activity-related signal changes not only in the prestriate cortex, but also in subcortical areas in some cases, indicating activity of the secondary visual pathway in the very young (Fig. 18.4). It is concluded that the process of postnatal visual development can be viewed as a progressive encoding of increasingly more complex aspects of information contained in the visual signal within different components of the visual network.

With recent developments of ultra-fast and silent imaging techniques fMRI has reached a point where functional maps of the cortical visual areas involved in processing the attributes of a stimulus, such as orientation, motion and color can now be determined in the very young.

Summary

■ Functional MRI can be produced by blood oxygen level dependent (BOLD) changes in the brain with neuronal activity.

■ Sequences may be too noisy to perform during natural sleep and therefore sedation is usually necessary.

■ The development of silent sequences will improve the rate of successful examinations.

■ The effects on brain activity as a result of sedation must be considered.

■ Functional imaging of the unco-operative newborn is restricted to those paradigms that can be performed with a sleeping infant.

■ Excitation of the visual system through closed eyes is the main paradigm to be used in the neonate to date.

■ The patterns of visual activation are distinct from those found in the adult.

References

1. Altman DI, Perlman JM, Volpe JJ et al. (1993) Cerebral oxygen metabolism in newborns. Pediatrics 92, 99–104.
2. Atkinson J (1984) Human visual development over the first 6 months of life. A review and a hypothesis. Hum Neurobiol 3, 61–74.
3. Atkinson J (1992) Early visual development: differential functioning of parvocellular and magnocellular pathways. Eye 6, 129–135.
4. Barkovich A, Kjos JB, Jackson OD et al. (1988) Normal maturation of the neonatal and infant brain: MR imaging at 1.5 T. Radiology 166, 173–180.
5. Belliveau J, Kwong K, Kennedy D et al. (1992) Magnetic resonance imaging mapping of brain function. Human visual cortex. Invest Radiol 27(Suppl 2), S59–65.
6. Bond E (1972) Perception of form by the human infant. Psychol Bull 77, 225–245.
7. Brody B, Kinney H, Kloman A et al. (1987) Sequence of central nervous system myelination in human infancy. 1. An autopsy study of myelination. J Neuropathol Exp Neurol 46, 283–301.
8. Bronson G (1974) The postnatal growth of visual capacity. Child Dev 45, 873–890.
9. Buxton RB and Frank LR (1997) A model for the coupling between cerebral blood flow and oxygen metabolism during neural stimulation. J Cereb Blood Flow Metab 17, 64–72.
10. Chi OZ, Ryterband S and Field C (1989) Visual evoked potentials during thiopentone–fentanyl–nitrous oxide anaesthesia in humans. Can J Anaesth 36, 637–640.
11. Chugani H and Phelps M (1986) Maturational changes in cerebral function in infants determined by 18-FDG positron emission tomography. Science 231, 840–843.
12. Chugani H, Phelps M and Mazziotta J (1987) Positron emission tomography study of human brain functional development. Ann Neurol 22, 487–497.
13. Courchesne E, Yeung-Courchesne R, Press GA et al. (1988) Hypoplasia of the vermial lobules VI and VII in infantile autism. N Engl J Med 318, 1349–1354.
14. Diamond I and Hall W (1969) Evolution of neocortex. Science 164, 251–262.
15. Dobbing J and Sands J (1973) Quantitative growth and development of human brain. Arch Dis Child 48, 757–767.
16. Dubowitz L, Mushin J, De Vries L et al. (1986) Visual function in the newborn infant: is it cortically mediated? Lancet 1, 1139–1141.
17. Fox PT, Raichle ME, Mintun MA et al. (1988) Nonoxidative glucose consumption during focal physiologic neural activity. Science 241, 462–464.
18. Frahm J, Kruger G, Merboldt KD et al. (1996) Dynamic uncoupling and recoupling of perfusion and oxidative metabolism during focal brain activation in man. Magn Reson Med 35, 143–148.

19. Frahm J, Merboldt KD, Hanicke W et al. (1994) Brain or vein – oxygenation or flow? On signal physiology in functional MRI of human brain activation. NMR in Biomedicine 7, 45–53.
20. Frostig RD, Lieke EE, Ts'o DY et al. (1990) Cortical functional architecture and local coupling between neuronal activity and the microcirculation revealed by in vivo high-resolution optical imaging of intrinsic signals. P Natl Acad Sci USA 87, 6082–6086.
21. Hennig T, Ernst T, Speck O et al. (1994) Detection of brain activation using oxygenation sensitive functional spectroscopy. Magn Reson Med 31, 85–90.
22. Hershenson M (1967) Development of the perception of form. Psychol Bull 67, 326–336.
23. Holmes GL (1986) Morphological and physiological maturation of the brain in the neonate and young child. J Clin Neurophysiol 3, 209–237.
24. Huttenlocher P, De Courten C, Garey L et al. (1982) Synaptogenesis in human visual cortex – evidence for synapse elimination during normal development. Neurosci Lett 33, 247–252.
25. Jernigan TL, Hesselink JR, Sowell E et al. (1991) Cerebral structure on magnetic resonance imaging in language-impaired and learning-impaired children. Arch Neurol 48, 539–545.
26. Kety S, Woodford R, Harmel M et al. (1947–48) Cerebral blood flow and metabolism in schizophrenia. The effect of barbiturate semi-narcosis, insulin coma and electroshock. Am J Psychiat 104, 765–770.
27. Kuschinsky W (1990) Coupling of blood flow and metabolism in the brain. J Physiol Pharmacol 1, 191–201.
28. Kwong K, Belliveau J, Chesler D (1992) Dynamic magnetic resonance imaging of human brain activity during primary sensory stimulation. P Natl Acad Sci USA 89, 5675–5679.
29. Langworthy O (1933) Development of behavior patterns and myelinization of the nervous system in the human fetus and infant. Contrib Embryol Carnegie Inst 24, 3–57.
30. Lassen NA, Ingvar DH and Skinhoj E (1978) Brain function and blood flow. Scientific American 239, 62–71 [Review].
31. Lindauer U, Villringer A and Dirnagl U (1993) Characterization of CBF response to somatosensory stimulation: model and influence of anesthetics. Am J Physiol 264, 1223–1228.
32. Lou HC, Edvinsson L and MacKenzie ET (1987) The concept of coupling blood flow to brain function: revision required? Ann Neurol 22, 289–297.
33. Martin E, Boesch C, Zuerrer M et al. (1990) MR imaging of brain maturation in normal and developmentally handicapped children. J Comput Assist Tomogr 14, 685–692.
34. Martin E, Joeri P, Loenneker T et al. (1999) Visual processing in infants and children studied using functional MRI. Pediatr Res 8, 1–6.

35. Martin E, Kikinis R, Zuerrer M *et al.* (1988) Developmental stages of human brain: an MR study. *J Comput Assist Tomogr* **12**, 917–922.

36. Martin E, Thiel T, Joeri P *et al.* (2000) Effect of pentobarbital on visual processing in man. *Hum Brain Mapp* **10**, 132–139.

37. Mercuri E, Atkinson J, Braddick O *et al.* (1997) Basal ganglia damage and impaired visual function in the newborn infant. *Arch Dis Child Fetal Neonatal Ed* **77**, F111–114.

38. Nilsson L and Siesjö BK (1975) The effect of pentobarbitone anaesthesia on blood flow and oxygen consumption in the rat brain. *Acta Anaesth Scand (Suppl)* **57**, 18–24.

39. Ogawa M, Magata Y, Ouchi Y *et al.* (1994) Scopolamine abolishes cerebral blood flow response to somatosensory stimulation in anesthetized cats: PET study. *Brain Res* **650**, 249–252.

40. Ogawa S, Lee T, Kay A *et al.* (1990) Brain magnetic resonance imaging with contrast dependent on blood oxygenation. *P Natl Acad Sci USA* **87**, 9868–9872.

41. Ogawa S, Tank D, Menon R *et al.* (1992) Intrinsic signal changes accompanying sensory stimulation: functional brain mapping with magnetic resonance imaging. *Proc Natl Acad Sci USA* **89**, 5951–5955.

42. Posner M, Petersen S, Fox P *et al.* (1988) Localization of cognitive operations in the human brain. *Science* **240**, 1627–1631.

43. Prichard J, Rothman D, Novotny E *et al.* (1991) Lactate rise detected by H-1 NMR in human visual cortex during physiologic stimulation. *Proc Natl Acad Sci USA* **88**, 5829–5831.

44. Purves MJ (1978) Control of cerebral blood vessels: present state of the art. *Ann Neurol* **3**, 377–383.

45. Raichle ME, Grubb RL Jr, Gado MH *et al.* (1976) Correlation between regional cerebral blood flow and oxidative metabolism. *In vivo* studies in man. *Arch Neurol* **33**, 523–526.

46. Roy C and Sherrington C (1890) On the regulation of blood supply of the brain. *J Physiol* **11**, 85–108.

47. Schneider G (1969) Two visual systems. *Science* **163**, 895–902.

48. Snyder R, Hata S, Brann B *et al.* (1990) Subcortical visual function in the newborn. *Pediatr Neurol* **6**, 333–336.

49. Sokolow L (1981) Localization of functional activity in the central nervous system by measurement of glucose utilization with radioactive deoxyglucose. *J Cereb Blood Flow Metab* **1**, 7–36.

50. Stricker T, Martin E and Boesch C (1990) Development of the human cerebellum observed with high-field-strength MR imaging. *Radiology* **177**, 431–435.

51. Takahashi T, Shirane R, Sato S *et al.* (1999) Developmental changes of cerebral blood flow and oxygen metabolism in children. *Am J Neuroradiol* **20**, 917–922.

52. Tokumaru AM, Barkovich AJ, O'Uchi T *et al.* (1999) The evolution of cerebral blood flow in the developing brain: evaluation with iodine-123 iodoamphetamine SPECT and correlation with MR imaging. *Am J Neuroradiol* **20**, 845–852.

53. Turner R (1994) Magnetic resonance imaging of brain function. *Ann Neurol* **35**, 637–638.

54. Weinacht S, Kind C, Monting JS *et al.* (1999) Visual development in preterm and full-term infants: a prospective masked study. *Invest Ophthalmol Vis Sci* **40**, 346–353.

55. Yakovlev P and Lecours IAR (1967) The myelogenic cycles of regional maturation of the brain. In: Minowski A (Ed.) *Regional Development of the Brain in Early Life*. Philadelphia, FA Davis.

Glossary of physics terms

A

- **Absorption**
  Transfer of energy from an electromagnetic field to tissue.
- **Acquisition**
  Electronic recording of an RF signal or data set of multiple signals.
- **Acquisition matrix**
  Set of signal data in a multidimensional array of pixels (e.g. two-dimensional set of data forming a single 256 × 256 voxel image). In 2D Fourier transform imaging, matrix size is in the number of data points acquired in the phase encoding direction × the number acquired in the frequency-encoding direction.
- **Artifact**
  A false signal on an image. A signal that does not correspond to an anatomical structure or one which has an inappropriate value.

  chemical-shift artifact These are bright or dark bands at fat water interfaces in MR images. Chemical-shift artifacts are caused by spatial misregistration (in the frequency-encoding direction) or spins with different chemical shifts, such as protons in water and protons in lipid.
  data-clipping artifact Artifact caused by the signal being too large to be digitized properly for a given attenuation setting.
  ghost artifact False images of a tissue or organ that propagate along the phase encoding direction. They are often due to motion.
  gibb's artifact (also truncation artifact) Artifact caused by the inability of a digital Fourier transform to reproduce faithfully an abrupt discontinuity at a boundary.
  metallic artifact Geometric signal distortions caused by local magnetic field inhomogeneity from a metallic object. This artifact is usually worse on gradient echo (compared to spin echo) images and is worse for ferromagnetic (compared to non-ferromagnetic) metals.
  motion artifact Spatial misregistration of signal usually along phase-encode direction caused by motion and typically resulting in ghosts.
  susceptibility artifact Signal loss and geometric distortion due to different magnetic properties of tissues or materials. May appear at the boundary of two tissues with differing diamagnetic susceptibility (e.g. brain and air-containing paranasal sinuses).
  truncation artifact Multiple bands of alternating high and low signal intensity that appear parallel to a boundary between two tissues with different signal intensities.
  wrap-around (aliasing) artifact Image located outside the field of view on the opposite side of the image. This is caused by an inadequate number of phase-encoding or frequency-encoding samples.
- **ATP**
  Adenosine triphosphate.
- **Averaging**
  Combining more than one data acquisition.

B

- **Bandwidth**
  Range of frequencies received (measured in **Hz** per pixel or ± kHz) by the receiver. The MR receiver bandwidth must be sufficient to process the range of frequencies in the data sampled or wrap-around artifact occurs.
- **Bird-cage coil**
  Whole-volume RF coil that has a cage-like design which is used at higher fields.
- **Blood oxygen level dependent (BOLD)**
  MRI techniques sensitive to the presence of deoxyhemoglobin in a tissue. Oxyhemoglobin is diamagnetic and has a lower magnetic susceptibility than deoxyhemoglobin, which is paramagnetic.
- **Bulk water**
  Water molecules whose molecular motion is determined solely by the interactions between water molecules (i.e. no macromolecular interactions are occurring).

C

- **Carr–Purcell sequence**
  T2 characteristics of tissue can be measured by applying a 90° RF pulse followed by a train of 180° pulses. This results in multiple spin echoes. It is technically difficult to produce perfect successive 180° pulses and this results in 'pulse error accumulation'. This accumulation can be reduced by altering the direction of 90° or 180° pulses with reference to one another in 3D space, i.e. altering the phase of these pulses in relation to the rotating frame of reference. Such modified sequences are known as Carr–Purcell–Meiboom–Gill (CPMG) sequences.
- **Chemical shift**
  Protons in different molecules may have slightly different Larmor frequencies due to the 'shielding' effect of adjacent electron orbits. This results in signals from the same voxel being mapped to different pixels causing false signal voids and hyperintensities around the edges of structures or lesions. These effects are exaggerated by higher field strengths and are seen in the frequency encoded direction. The amount of shift is expressed as parts per million (ppm) of the resonance frequency and is given the greek symbol Delta.
- **Chemical-shift cancellation effect**
  Pulse sequence that exploits the phase difference between two components (usually protons in lipid and protons in water) in the same voxel.
- **CHESS (chemical-shift selective)**
  Imaging sequence in which an RF pulse is applied at a frequency that saturates certain chemical components. If the conventional pulse sequence is then applied at a different frequency, only those chemical components that have not already been saturated will produce a signal. This imaging method can be used to differentiate fat from water.
- **Cine-MRI**
  Fast image acquisition with sequential looping of the resultant images which can be used to display dynamic processes. Cine-MRI has been particularly useful in studying CSF flow.
- **Coherence**
  Consider the old executive's toy, Newton's Cradle. If all five balls are pulled to one side and then let go, they will all swing together and the motion will continue for some time. This is because they are all swinging in phase and their motion is coherent. But if three balls are pulled to one side and two to the other, the balls will collide and soon cancel their motion out. They have been given opposite phase and

their motion lacks coherence. In a similar manner, MR signals from protons in tissue with similar frequency and identical phase are said to be coherent. But proton spin/spin interactions lead to loss of phase coherence and thus the MR signal will decrease with time. This is the basis of T2 relaxation.

- **Coil**
An electric current flowing through a wire will produce a magnetic field around it. Likewise, a changing magnetic field will induce a current in a wire. Specially shaped coils or wire are used in MRI to both produce the RF interrogating pulse and to detect the resultant MR signal from the protons. The voltage strength of these induced currents is proportional to the MR signal strength.

- **Computer**
If the magnet is the engine then the computer is the driver in MRI. Unlike CT where significant computer processing only occurs after data acquisition, MR requires powerful computation to provide appropriate RF pulses and gradients for signal generation. Overall command is provided by a central processing unit (CPU) which links into pulse and gradient generators, spectrometers, memory and data storage facilities and image generation/manipulation outputs.

- **Contrast**
Difference in signal intensity between two discrete regions of an image (e.g. two tissues), scaled to a reference such as signal intensity of one of the two regions (or tissues), their mean, another region (or tissue), the background noise level, or an external standard.

- **Contrast agent**
Any drug or material that alters the contrast of a region (e.g. a tissue) on an image. MR contrast agents usually shorten T1 and/or T2 relaxation times. In MRI the contrast agents work by altering the relaxation characteristics of the target tissue, e.g. enhancement is achieved by gadolinium decreasing the T1 relaxation time of abnormal tissue. MR contrast agents may be ferromagnetic, paramagnetic or superparamagnetic.

- **Contrast-to-noise ratio (CNR)**
Ratio of signal intensity differences between two regions, scaled to image noise. The ratio indicates the ability to detect low-contrast lesions.

- **Coupling**
Magnetic dipole interactions with local electric and magnetic fields created by neighboring nuclei. Atoms induce a relaxation because the motions of one particle are coupled to the motion of another. In general, only magnetic dipole–dipole coupling is important in proton MRI.

- **Cross-talk**
Efforts to reduce imaging times in MR resulted in multiple slice acquisition programs. Unfortunately, perfect accuracy is impossible and each slice may receive some of the RF pulse intended for adjacent slices which results in degradation of the signal from that slice or spurious echoes. Hence truly contiguous slices cannot be obtained without resorting to volume acquisition techniques.

- **Cryogen**
Superconducting magnets need to be kept at extremely low temperatures which are maintained by liquified gases or cryogens. The most commonly used are helium (boiling point = –269°C) and nitrogen (boiling point = –196°C). These gases need to boil off over time and can represent a major part of the running costs of a superconducting magnet unless a recycling system or cryosaver is employed.

- **CSE**
Conventional spin echo.

D

- **1D**
One-dimensional.

- **2D**
Two-dimensional.

- **3D**
Whole volume pulse sequence that uses phase encoding for two axes. 3D techniques are based on gradient echo sequences that employ short repetition times (TRs).

- **dB/dt**
Rate of change of the gradient magnetic field with time. Time-varying magnetic fields can induce electric currents in materials that have free charges or dipoles. Such currents are a potential safety hazard.

- **Dead time**
After sampling an echo, the central processing unit of an MR computer needs a finite time to process the next set of instructions before it can switch into signal generation mode. This is known as dead time.

- **Decay time**
After excitation, the protons gradually lose their transverse magnetism (T2) as they process back to their resting state. The time taken can be referred to as the decay time.

- **Deconvolution**
The frequency distribution of signals forming an image may not match the frequency distribution of signals from the object under study if, for example, spurious signals are incorporated. The frequency distribution can be 'cleaned up' by using a mathematical process called deconvolution. An example of its use would be in reducing wraparound by rejecting signals from part of the body not in the field of view of the image.

- **Decoupling**
This is a strategy used in MR spectroscopy to suppress the dominant signals from hydrogen protons to allow study of other nuclei such as carbon or phosphorus. This is achieved by applying a stream of pulses at the Larmor frequency of hydrogen whilst acquiring data of the resonant frequency of the nuclei under study. A drawback to this technique is the high amount of RF energy deposited which may cause a rise in temperature of the patient or sample.

- **Dephasing**
Loss of phase coherence within a voxel.

- **Depth resolved spectroscopy**
Given the acronym DRESS, this is a technique using field gradients to obtain MR spectra from predetermined depth in a sample volume.

- **Detector**
Also known as a demodulator, this device receives the MR signal and converts it into a lower frequency prior to image processing.

- **Dewar**
This is the name given to an insulated container for the storage of cryogens. These are bulky, and consideration must be given to their storage and access for exchange when designing an MR facility.

- **Diamagnetic**
If a substance placed in a magnetic field becomes magnetized in the opposite direction to that field, it will cause a localized decrease in the field and is said to have diamagnetic properties or negative susceptibility.

- **Diffusion**
Translational molecular motion caused by random thermal or Brownian motion. The parameter that characterizes diffusion, the *apparent diffusion coefficient*, describes the amount of translational molecular motion in a period of time for a particular material.

- **Dipole**
This is a term applied to any particle with a single pair of separated points of positive and negative charges of equal magnitude. When given spin this results in the particle behaving as a small magnet with a discrete field. Many dipoles together can have an effect on one another and this is an important contributing factor to the relaxation characteristics of tissues. These interactions can be modified by paramagnetic agents which is the basis of enhancement techniques in MR.

■ **Dipole electric**
Particle (nucleus, molecule, or larger) with a single pair of separated centers of positive and negative charges of equal magnitude.

■ **Dipole–dipole interaction**
Magnetic interaction between two spins with magnetic moments resulting from the magnetic field produced by one spin acting on the other. The proton–proton dipole–dipole interaction is the principal source of relaxation for nuclei.

■ **Dispersion**
The rate of relaxation of tissue will alter at different strengths of the external magnetic field (B_o). This variation is known as dispersion and it is an important quantity in the study of relaxation mechanics. Knowledge of dispersion profiles is important in the development of MR contrast agents.

■ **Display matrix**
This refers to the number of picture elements (pixels) which form each line of the image. A typical high quality image will have 512 pixels per line and 512 pixels per column – a '512 × 512' image. However, in order to see a high-quality image, the acquisition matrix must equal or exceed that of the display matrix. If the display matrix is greater than the acquisition matrix then data are calculated in adjacent pixels by a process known as interpolation. The final image would therefore lack detail.

■ **Dixon technique**
This is a chemical shift imaging technique which requires the acquisition of two images in order to resolve the chemical shifts of fat and water. The pay-off is excellent spatial resolution.

■ **Duty cycle**
A finished image for study is the product of interrogation, data collection, data processing and image formation. The period of interrogation by the RF pulses is an example of duty cycle within the overall function of image production. There is also a more rigid application of the term which refers to the time taken for excitation and data sampling for a single slice.

E

■ **Echo**
During spin echo imaging the free induction decay of the 90° pulses used to create the information signal is 'contaminated' by the effects of inhomogeneities in the main magnetic field and diffusion within the sample volume. This overall time constant is known as T2*. In order to separate out the T2 component of this signal a 180° rephasing or refocusing pulse is used and the residual signal from this pulse is collected. The residual signal is known as the echo and represents the pure T2 component. This echo can be sampled more than once in the multiple echo imaging techniques to give varied T2 weighting to the image and so increase the diagnostic yield.

■ **Echo planar imaging**
This is a fast scan technique which can create images of single slices in fractions of a second by rapidly switching the phase encoded gradient during the free induction decay of a single excitation pulse. This produces a train of gradient echoes which can be Fourier transformed into a single image. The process is virtually real-time and offers the prospect of interactive MR at the cost of increased RF energy deposition in the patient. The rapid rate of change of the magnetic gradients can also cause peripheral nerve stimulation, although the switching rates now used in image formation do not cause observable effects.

■ **Echo time**
See TE.

■ **Eddy currents**
Any conductor placed in a changing magnetic field will experience the induction of eddy currents. These can cause problems with image degradation and are a potential hazard to patients in high field systems with rapidly varying gradients. Their effects can be minimized by using specially shielded gradients.

■ **Effective transverse relaxation time (T_2^*)**
When the observed transverse relaxation time is faster than the normal T2 transverse relaxation time because of spatial inhomogeneity of the magnetic field, it is termed T2*. Spins at different locations experience slightly different magnetic fields, causing a loss of phase coherence, consequently the transverse relaxation decreases more rapidly than it would on the basis of T2 alone.

■ **Electromagnetic radiation**
This is the transmission of energy by variations in electric and magnetic fields in the form of waves. The frequency of the waveform gives the radiation its physical properties. Radio, light and X-rays are merely electromagnetic radiation at different frequencies.

■ **Electron**
Negatively charged particle with a mass $1/1864$ that of a proton and located in orbitals of discrete (quantized) energies surrounding the nucleus of atoms.

■ **Energy level**
In a magnetic field, nuclear spins can populate different energy states. The energy levels available to particular nuclei depend on the angular momentum of the spinning nuclear charge, which is normally designated by the spin quantum number, I.

■ **Enhancement**
In the context of nuclear relaxation, enhancement is an increase in the relaxation rate or a decrease in the relaxation time.

■ **Excitation**
Delivery of energy (in the form of a RF pulse or magnetic field change) into a spin system (e.g. a 90° transverse pulse).

F

■ **F**
See frequency.

■ **Faraday's law**
A changing magnetic field will induce a changing current in a conducting loop (circuit). A changing current in one circuit can create a changing circuit in another circuit field to which it is not physically connected except through the magnetic flux between the circuits.

■ **Fast Fourier transform (FFT)**
Fast computational algorithm for performing a Fourier transform that allows a periodic function to be expressed as an integral sum over a continuous range of frequencies.

■ **Fast spin echo (FSE)**
Long TR, multispin echo technique where each echo is separately phase encoded. Interecho times are short, and typically 4, 8 or 16 echoes are obtained per excitation, proportionally reducing scan time.

■ **Ferrite**
Iron oxide with the formula $Fe^{+2}_x M^{+3}_y O_z$ (e.g. magnetite Fe_3O_4). Ferrite magnetic properties are determined by crystal size and structure.

■ **Ferromagnetic**
Any substance that has a large, positive magnetic susceptibility and shows a magnetic memory or residual magnetization.

■ **Field distortion**
Local field inhomogeneity caused by presence of diamagnetic, paramagnetic or ferromagnetic substances and leading to artifacts in the image.

■ **Field strength**
Intensity of static magnetic field. In the context of MRI, low field strengths range from 0.02 to 0.3 T, medium field strengths range from 0.3 to 1.0 T, and high field strengths are greater than 1.0 T. These definitions are evolving.

- **Field of view (FOV)**
Size of anatomical region imaged, which may be square or rectangular (i.e. asymmetric). FOV is also the product of the acquisition matrix (e.g. 128×256) and pixel dimensions (e.g. 3.1×1.6 mm) (FOV in this example would be 40×40 cm).

- **Filling factor**
Ratio of the volume of sample within an RF coil to the volume of the coil. Filling factor affects the efficiency of irradiating the object and detecting MR signals, thereby affecting the signal-to-noise ratio. Achieving a high factor requires fitting the coil closely to the object.

- **FLAIR**
Fluid-attenuated inversion recovery.

- **FLASH (fast low angle shot)**
Gradient echo imaging technique that uses gradient reversal and a $180°$ rephasing pulse. Tip angles (excitation pulses) of less than $90°$ are generally used, leaving a substantial fraction of the longitudinal magnetization unperturbed.

- **Flip angle**
Angle of rotation of the macroscopic magnetization vector produced by an RF pulse. Flip angles are measured relative to the longitudinal (z) axis of the main magnetic field (B_0). For example, a $90°$ flip angle rotates the magnetization vector into the transverse (xy) plane. The flip angle is proportional to amplitude and duration of the RF pulse.

- **Flow artifacts**
Both artifactual signal voids (time of flight signal loss) and hyperintense areas (flow-related enhancement) can be caused by flow phenomena in body fluids. Flowing matter can take signal away from an area of data acquisition to cause a void and it can equally bring signal into an area from adjacent excitations in multislice acquisitions.

- **Flow-related enhancement**
Increase in signal intensity of flowing blood or cerebrospinal fluid relative to stationary tissue caused by entry of unsaturated spins.

- **Flow void**
Signal loss observed with rapid flow caused by a combination of high-velocity signal loss, turbulence and intravoxel dephasing. Rapidly flowing arterial blood usually appears dark, whereas slowly flowing venous blood appears bright.

- **Fourier transform**
This is a mathematical tool which is used to convert the raw MR signal into its frequency and phase components. In multiple-slice imaging frequency and phase are the x and y coordinates for the final image. Hence 2 Fourier transformations will be sufficient (2-DFT). However, if data have been acquired from a volume rather than a slice then a third coordinate will be needed which requires a third Fourier transformation (3-DFT).

- **Free induction decay (FID)**
When a gyroscope is tipped away from its vertical spinning axis it will return to its upright position in a spiralling motion and the amount of this precession around its axis will decay with a characteristic time constant. In the same way a spinning proton tipped from the main magnetic field of an MR magnet by the interrogating RF pulse will return to alignment with the main magnetic field (in time constant T2*).

- **Frequency (f)**
Number of repetitions of a periodic process (cycles) per unit time. Electromagnetic radiation frequency (radiowaves, microwaves, X-rays, etc.) is measured in Hertz (Hz) with units of inverse seconds.

- **Frequency encoding**
In a flat plane any point on that plane can be described by its x and y coordinates. In a 2-D MRI image slice the equivalent of the x and y coordinates are the frequency and phase characteristics of each point. If the x scale is to be the 'frequency' characteristics then a range of frequency values across the slice must be provided by 'encoding' the MR signals from protons along the slice.

G

- **Gadolinium**
The first clinically available contrast medium for MRI was the chelate of this metal from the lanthanide series with diethylenetriamine penta-acetic acid (DTPA). The ion of gadolinium has the greatest paramagnetic effect of any ion but is highly toxic in the unbound state. Its chelation provides safe bioavailability without removing its paramagnetic properties.

- **Gating**
In order to remover the effects of physiologic motion from tissues or fluids MR data can be acquired at the same point in each motion cycle. Successful gating requires regular or cyclical motion. Thus gating cannot overcome artifact due to bowel movement.

- **Gauss**
A Gauss (G) is a unit of magnetic flux density. This has been replaced in the SI system by the Tesla (T), where 1 T = 10 000 G. The Gauss is still used as a convenient method of describing very small fields such as the stray field around an MR system.

- **Gradient**
Spatial variation of some quantity, such as magnetic field strength.

- **Gradients**
In order to localize MR signals emanating from protons in three dimensions a series of three magnetic field gradients are superimposed on the external magnetic field (B_0). This results in each point in a volume of tissue experiencing a unique magnetic field strength. Thus the Larmor frequency of precession will be unique for each point which allows for selective excitation or detection. The three gradients are: slice selection gradient; phase encoding gradient; and readout gradient.

- **Gradient coils**
Coils producing a magnetic field gradient. Proper design of the size and configuration of the coils is necessary to produce a controlled and uniform gradient.

- **Gradient echo**
Echo produced by reversing the direction of the frequency-encoding (readout) magnetic field gradient so as to cancel out the position-dependent phase shifts that have accumulated because of the gradient.

- **Gradient echo imaging**
Spin echo imaging achieves T2 weighting by nullifying the effects of the magnetic field in homogeneities with a $180°$ 'rephasing' pulse. Unfortunately, this tactic increases scan times and quadruples the amount of RF power deposited in tissues. However, T2 weighting can also be achieved by rapid reversals of the readout gradients and acquiring the resultant echoes. The contrast in these images are dependent on the T2* signal (the sum of T2 and the effects of magnetic field inhomogeneities) and so they are sensitive to unstable or impure static fields. Image acquisition time is reduced by both the deletion of the $180°$ rephasing pulse and by the ability to reduce flip angles owing to the rapidity with which gradient reversals can be applied.

- **Gradient-recalled echo (GRE)**
Pulse sequence used in fast-scanning techniques in which the free induction decay is dephased and subsequently rephased into an echo via a gradient.

- **Gradient reversal**
Pulse sequence that has both a negative dephasing gradient and a positive rephasing gradient. In gradient echo sequences the gradient reversal is applied along the slice-selection and frequency-encoding directions.

- **GRASS (gradient-refocused or recalled acquisition in the steady state)**
Gradient echo imaging technique with rewinder gradient in which the transverse magnetization is not spoiled, allowing persistence of the steady state.

- **G_x, G_y, G_z**
Symbols for magnetic field gradients. Used with subscripts to denote spatial direction of the gradient in cartesian coordinates.

- **Gyromagnetic ratio (γ)**
Ratio for the magnetic moment to the associated angular moment of a nucleus. A constant for all nuclei of a given isotope. For example, γ is 42.58 MHz/T for ^{1}H, and 17.24 MHz/T for ^{31}P.

H

- **Helmhotz coil**
Paired RF coils having a uniform sensitivity along their central axis. The distance between two single wire loops is set equal to their radius.
- **Hertz (Hz)**
SI unit of frequency (equal to the cgs unit of cycles per second).
- **High-velocity signal loss**
Signal loss of moving spins that were not in the selected slice to receive both 90° and 180° RF pulses required to generate a spin echo.
- **Homogeneity**
Homogeneity of the static magnetic field is an important criterion of magnetic field quality. *Inhomogeneity* is measured in parts per million (ppm) over a specified diameter spherical volume (DSV).
- **Hybrid magnet**
Type of magnet in which the magnetic field is composed of two or more different types of magnets (i.e. resistive, permanent, superconducting) to form a more homogeneous or stronger field.

I

- **Image acquisition time**
Time required to obtain MR data necessary for image reconstruction. For a 2D Fourier transform acquisition, the total image acquisition time equals the product of TR, the number of signals averaged (NSA or NEX) and the number of phase-encoding steps.
- **Image noise**
Non-anatomical fluctuations in voxel signal intensity. Random or statistical noise (white noise) has a broad bandwidth and no phase coherence and appears at all points in the images as 'graininess'.
- **Image reconstruction**
Mathematical process of converting the composite signals obtained during the data acquisition phase into an image.
- **Induction**
The term induction is used in two senses in MR, not entirely unrelated, but worthy of distinct explanation.
  (1) Magnetic field strength is denoted by the symbol H and has the units of amperes/meter. Any object inserted into this field will have a magnetic flux induced within it. Magnetic induction, denoted by the symbol B, has the units of Tesla. The extent of the magnetic induction is dependent upon the magnetic permeability (μ) of the material which is usually compared to the value for free space ($μ_0$). Strictly we should be concerned with the magnetic induction B since this will depend on the nature of the material or body within the field H.
  (2) A constant current passed through a wire loop generates a magnetic field along the axis of that loop. This is the basis upon which the static field B_0 is generated. The converse, that a magnetic field applied to a coil generates a current, is *not* true. In order to generate any current in the coil the magnetic field must be varying in time and this is an expression of Faraday's law of magnetic induction. Strictly it is required that the magnetic flux cutting through the conductive loop varies in time in order to generate a time varying current. Transverse magnetization and its

associated magnetic flux lines precess at the Larmor frequency with respect to the magnet and receiver coil. A time-dependent current is induced, with the small variations in precessional frequency being reflected by commensurate changes in current in the receiver coil. This signal is subsequently amplified prior to digitization and further processing within a computer.

- **Inhomogeneity**
The term inhomogeneity can be applied to the applied static field B_0 and the radiofrequency (RF) or B_1 field employed in MR. In each case the quality of the respective magnetic field over the extent of the imaged region is of relevance.
The local magnetic field can be varying due to spatial variations caused by imperfections or inhomogeneities in B_0. A magnet system would usually have some corrective mechanism, called shimming, that allows field imperfections to be reduced. This procedure would be done at the time of installation of the magnet and would not require further attention as long as the environment of the magnet was not changed significantly.
- **In-phase image**
Spin echo image acquired with 180° pulse at TE/2, so that temporal rephasing from the gradient reversal occurs simultaneously.
- **Inversion pulse**
A 180° RF pulse that causes precessing nuclei to shift to the opposite spin state. This pulse causes the net equilibrium longitudinal magnetization vector, if in the low-energy state parallel to the applied magnetic field (B_0), to invert to the higher-energy state (antiparallel).
- **Inversion recovery sequence (IR)**
The IR sequence is specifically employed to measure the longitudinal magnetization following the initial 180° pulse. If a series of inversion recovery sequences is employed this can allow the relaxation behavior of the longitudinal magnetization to be measured and its associated time constant T1 calculated. In MRI it is simply employed as a means of emphasizing T1 by selecting a single TI.
As its name implies the sequence commences with a 180° or inversion RF pulse. It is usually assumed that the nuclear spins are all aligned along B_0 prior to this pulse. As a result there is no signal directly after the perfect inversion pulse since no transverse components of magnetization are generated. The magnetization is rotated from +z to −z. Following the inversion the nuclei are free to re-establish themselves as they please which will be to restore their orientations with respect to the magnet. The longitudinal component of magnetization becomes less negative, passes through zero and heads towards +z. Since longitudinal magnetization can not be seen directly we must apply an observing 90° pulse to take a look at the extent of the relaxation along B_0. The 90° pulse occurs at time TI after the 180° or inversion pulse. This 'look' can involve the image gradients to allow the construction of an image if required. The resultant image will contain a heavy weighting toward the T1 process.
- **Inversion time (TI)**
The interval TI denotes the interval between 180° inversion pulse and subsequent 90° observation pulse in an inversion recovery pulse sequence.
- **ISIS (image-selected *in vivo* spectroscopy)**
Surface-coil B1 gradient method that uses frequency-selected inversion pulses in the presence of magnetic field gradients to provide 3D localization of an image volume.

K

- **K space**
Mathematical (transform) space whose coordinates are frequency and phase as opposed to physical space.

L

- **Laminar flow**
  Non-turbulent, linear flow with a parabolic velocity profile. The fluid at the center of the vessel moves twice as fast as the average; the fluid in contact with the wall has zero velocity.

- **Larmor equation**
  Larmor frequency (F) of precision of a nuclear magnetic moment is proportional to the magnetic field (B) and the gyromagnetic ratio (γ):
  $$F = \gamma B.$$

- **Lattice**
  As used in NMR, lattice refers to the chemical environment.

- **Line shape**
  Distribution of the relative amplitude of resonances as a function of frequency, which establishes a particular spectral line. Common line shapes are Lorentzian and Gaussian.

- **Line width**
  Spread in frequency of a resonance line in an MR spectrum. A common measure of line width is Hz at full width half maximum (FWHM) for a specific field strength.

- **Localization technique**
  Techniques for selecting a restricted region from which a spectrum is desired. These can include the use of surface coils, magnetic field gradients, or a combination of both.

- **Longitudinal magnetization (M_z)**
  Component of the macroscopic magnetization vector along the static B_0 magnetic field. Following excitation by an RF pulse, M_z will approach its equilibrium value, M_0, with a characteristic time constant, TI, according to the equation $M_z/M_0 = 1 - \exp(-t/TI)$.

- **Longitudinal relaxation**
  Return of the longitudinal magnetization to the equilibrium value after excitation. Energy is exchanged between the nuclear spins and the lattice.

M

- **M**
  Conventional symbol for macroscopic magnetization vector.

- **M_0**
  Equilibrium value of the magnetization, directed along the static magnetic field. At a given temperature the value of M_z is proportional to spin density (N), the gyromagnetic ratio (γ), and the static magnetic field (B_0).

- **Magnet**
  The magnet is the central piece of equipment of the MR scanner. It should provide a field (B_0) whose strength is stable over a period of time and spatially homogeneous over a region that must compare in size with the object to be imaged. The homogeneity is expressed as parts per million (ppm) figure for a defined volume of space, say a 30 or 50 cm diameter sphere.
  Magnets may be permanent, resistive or superconducting in construction. For higher fields, above 2.0 T, the superconducting magnets present the only choice. Permanent magnets are built from blocks of ferromagnetic alloys of metals such as nickel, iron and cobalt. The source of ferromagnetism is the unpaired electrons within the component elements of these alloys. Resistive magnets consist of many windings of copper wire and the field is maintained by the permanent supply of electrical current from a suitably stabilized power supply. Superconducting magnets are similar in the respect of having many windings. However, rather than copper, alloys of metal such as niobium and tin are employed whose characteristic is that they lose all electrical resistance when reduced in temperature. Once energized a superconducting magnet will maintain a field without additional

power consumption. The catch is that incredibly low temperatures have to be maintained usually in the region of 20K (20° above the zero [approximately –273°C]). The electricity bill is replaced by the expense of the cryogenic (cooling) gases nitrogen and helium, although many magnets now require helium only.

- **Magnetic dipole**
  Effective separation of magnetic north and south poles in a sample. An electric current loop, including the effective current of a spinning nucleon or nucleus, can create an equivalent magnetic dipole.

- **Magnetic dipole–dipole coupling**
  Small increment or decrement in the static magnetic field strength caused by a neighboring nucleus.

- **Magnetic dipole moment**
  Measure of magnitude and direction of the magnetic properties of a nucleus that has an $I \neq 0$. From a classical viewpoint, a rotating nucleus (or charge) behaves analogously to an electric current flowing in a loop and thus possesses a magnetic dipole.

- **Magnetic field**
  The field is in the region surrounding a magnet in which magnetic properties can be detected. One property is that a small magnet in such a region experiences a torque that tends to align it with the magnetic field. The direction of the magnetic field is defined by a vector that points from south pole to north pole.

- **Magnetic field gradient**
  For example G_x, G_y and G_z consist of a magnetic field B, the strength of which varies linearly along one or more coordinate (spatial) directions. Magnetic gradients are used in MRI for selection of a region being imaged (slice selection) and to encode the in-plane location of MR signals received from the object being imaged.

- **Magnetic moment**
  Magnetic moment is a descriptive term employed interchangeably with, for example, nuclear spin, nuclear magnet or nucleus.
  A conventional bar magnet will align itself within a magnetic field, a concept we are familiar with in the compass. The magnetic moment is strictly defined as the force required to keep the bar magnet or compass needle at right angles to this preferred alignment along the field. The greater the strength of the bar magnet or field, the greater the magnetic moment.
  The *nuclear* magnetic moment when placed in a magnetic field can take only a small number of orientations and can never perfectly align itself along this field. The energy differences between these orientations are the basis of the magnetic resonance phenomenon. The size of the nuclear magnetic moment is directly proportional to the magnetogyric ratio of the element (or more specifically isotope) under investigation.

- **Magnetic interactions**
  These interactions or couplings are the basis for the MR phenomenon. Time independent or motionally averaged interactions determine the positions of nuclear resonances in the frequency spectrum. Fluctuating or time dependent magnetic couplings, particularly when they are varying at a rate close to the Larmor frequency, have a significant role in the relaxation of the nuclei under investigation.
  The primary magnetic interaction is between the applied magnetic field (B_0) and the nuclear magnetic moment, the nuclear Zeeman effect. The size of this interaction is dependent upon the B_0 field strength and would be most commonly expressed as the Larmor frequency that lies in the range 5–64 MHz for whole body MRI systems.

- **Magnetization**
  Magnetization is the bulk equivalent of magnetic moment and is defined as the density of magnetic moment per unit volume (of tissue in clinical MRS). There are various contributions to the overall magnetization induced when a body is placed in a magnetic field. These include the diamagnetism of the electrons and the paramagnetism of the nuclei.

Nuclear magnetism is generated by the alignment of atomic nuclei within the applied field. It represents one of the smaller components of the total magnetization.

The induced magnetization (M) generated is proportional to field (B) and this is expressed by the equation

$$M = \chi B.$$

where χ is the (nuclear) susceptibility and will vary between tissues.

■ **Magnetic ratio, γ**
The magnetogyric ratio (γ) relates the magnetic field strength (B) to the nuclear precessional or Larmor frequency (ω). This is summarized by the Larmor equation

$$\omega = \gamma B.$$

Note that ω is the angular frequency which is simply the usual Larmor frequency expressed in Hertz multiplied by 2π.

■ **Magnetic resonance (MR)**
Resonance phenomenon resulting in the absorption and/or emission of electromagnetic energy by nuclei or electrons in a static magnetic field after excitation by a resonance frequency pulse. The resonance frequency is proportional to the magnetic field and is given by the Larmor equation. Only unpaired electrons and nuclei with a non-zero spin exhibit MR.

■ **Magnetic resonance imaging (MRI)**
Use of magnetic resonance to create images of hydrogen (protons), sodium, fluorine, phosphorus, etc. The image signal intensity depends on the density of the nucleus.

■ **Magnetic resonance spectroscopy (MRS)**
Use of magnetic resonance to obtain spectral information in the form of spectral peaks. Peaks are analyzed according to their frequency or chemical shift (depending on substance being imaged), peak amplitude, and area under the peak (depending on number of nuclei).

■ **Magnetic shielding**
Reduction of magnetic field outside imaging area by passive 'architectural' measures, such as the Faraday cage for B_1 shielding and steel plates in the walls of the imaging suite for B_0 shielding.

■ **Magnetic susceptibility**
Ratio of the intensity of magnetization induced in a substance to the intensity of the magnetic field to which the substance is exposed; often expressed as a dimensionless quantity times 10^{-6}.

■ **Magnetite**
Fe_3O_4; a cubic, close-packed crystal. It can be superparamagnetic or ferromagnetic.

■ **Magnetization**
Magnetic polarization of a material produced by a magnetic field. Magnetic moment per unit volume.

■ **Magnetization transfer**
Magnetic labeling of spectroscopic peaks and subsequent observation of chemical transfer of the magnetically labeled nuclei to other peaks.

■ **Magnitude image**
Form of image presentation, which is reconstructed from magnitude data. Magnitude data = $([\text{Real data}]^2 + [\text{Imaginary data}]^2)^{1/2}$. The magnitude image is generally used because of its insensitivity to phase errors.

■ **Magnitude reconstruction**
Image reconstruction technique that yields a modulus image.

■ **MIP**
Maximum-intensity projection.

■ **Misregistration**
Incorrect spatial mapping of an acquired MR signal. This artifact may be secondary to motion (flow, pulsation, respiration) chemical shift or aliasing.

■ **M_0**
Vector representation of the equilibrium value of the magnetization that is parallel to the static magnetic field. The value of M_0 is proportional to spin density. See also **spin density**.

■ **MT**
Magnetization transfer.

■ **Multiple echo imaging**
Imaging using a series of echoes acquired as a train following a single excitation pulse. In spin echo imaging, each echo is formed by a 180° pulse at $TE_n-1 + (TE_n - TE_n-1) \div 2$. Typically, a separate image is produced from each echo of the train.

■ **Multislice imaging**
MRI pulse sequences must be separated in order to build spatial encoding into the signals. The spatial encoding process is short, say 10.50 milliseconds (ms), in comparison to the relaxation delays (TR) that are conventionally employed to manipulate image contrast (2000–1500 ms). It is apparent that there is plenty of time when there is nothing to do except wait for relaxation to take place. If all radiofrequency (RF) pulses are made slice-selective then this 'dead time' can be usefully employed to acquire data from different slices in an interleaved fashion.

■ **M_{xy}**
See **transverse magnetization**.

■ **M_z**
See **longitudinal magnetization**.

N

■ **NAA**
N-acetyl aspartate.

■ **Negative enhancement**
Signal intensity loss induced by a contrast agent (e.g. ferrite).

■ **NMR**
Nuclear magnetic resonance. See **magnetic resonance**.

■ **Noise**
This is comprised of electronic and acoustic forms. The random motions of electrons within conducting media constitute small, random electric currents. These currents give rise to spurious signals that can be detected by the sensitive MR receiver system. Electrolytes within the body, the copper within the receiver coils and its associated cabling and connectors and electronic components all contribute to the overall noise level. The aim would always be to be limited by noise generated in the patient rather than the equipment.

■ **Non-selective pulses**
RF pulses whose bandwidth contains all Larmor frequencies produced within the imaged object (i.e. the entire object is excited by the pulse).

■ **NSA**
Number of signals averaged together to determine each distinct position-encoded signal to be used in image reconstruction.

■ **Nuclear magnetic resonance (NMR) signal**
Electromagnetic signal in the RF range produced by the precession of the transverse magnetization of nuclear spins. The precession of transverse magnetization induces a voltage in a coil, which is amplified and demodulated by the receiver. The NMR signal may refer only to this induced voltage.

■ **Nuclear spin quantum number (I)**
Property of all nuclei related to the largest measurable component of the nuclear angular momentum are quantized (fixed) as integral or half-integral multiples of $h/2\pi$, where h is Planck's constant. The number of possible energy levels for a given nucleus in a fixed magnetic field is equal to $2I + 1$.

■ **Nucleon**
Particles found in the nucleus of an atom (i.e. neutrons and protons).

■ **Nucleus**
The nucleus is the positively charged center of an atom composed of a number of protons and neutrons (generically known as nucleons). Hydrogen, the simplest atom, contains only a single proton. The arrangement of these nucleons, both of which individually possess magnetic moments, determine the total nuclear magnetic moment of the nucleus.

- **Null point**
  In the context of inversion recovery imaging, term used to describe the point in time at which the net magnetization passes through zero after the initial 180° pulse.

P

- **^{31}P**
  Phosphorus-31.
- **Paramagnetic**
  Substance with a positive magnetic susceptibility. Individual paramagnetic moments, non-aligned in the absence of an external magnetic field, become aligned in the presence of a magnetic field. Addition of small amounts of paramagnetic substance may greatly reduce relaxation times of water.
- **Paramagnetism**
  The component atoms of a paramagnetic material possess permanent magnetic moments. The total moment of an individual atom has contributions from the unpaired orbiting electrons and from the central nucleus. Nuclear paramagnetism is several hundred times weaker than the electronic component. However, the dominance of either will depend upon the particular atomic configuration. The atoms or ions of transition metals are typical examples of an electronic paramagnetic substance.
- **Partial saturation**
  When the time between radio frequency (RF) pulses is less than or comparable to the longitudinal relaxation time (T1) then a material is said to be partially saturated. Since there is insufficient time for full T1 relaxation between RF pulses, the signal is currently less than the equilibrium magnetization (M_0) of the tissue. The various extents of saturation amongst a variety of tissues with different T1's are the basis for generating contrast in MR imaging.
- **Parts per million (ppm)**
  Measure of the relative difference between an observed quantity and a reference value in units of one-millionth the reference value. For example, a measured frequency of 64.001 MHz differs from a reference frequency of 64 MHz by $[(64.001-64)/64] \times 1\,000\,000 = 15.625$ ppm.
- **PCr**
  Phosphocreatine.
- **Peak area**
  Area encompassed by a spectroscopic peak and the frequency axis. If relaxation effects are taken into account, the peak area is proportional to the concentration of the chemical species producing the peak.
- **Permanent magnet**
  Magnet whose magnetic field originates from permanently magnetized (ferromagnetic) material.
- **Phantom**
  A test object to assess performance of the scanner. The phantom may contain water doped with paramagnetic Cu^{2+} or Mn^{2+} ions in order to control the relaxation times. As an alternative, gels may be included since they may closer approximate to tissue where longitudinal relaxation times (T1) are significantly longer than their transverse counterparts (T_2).
- **Phase**
  The components of magnetization constituting the MR signal can be imagined as the hand of a clock. It has a magnitude, the length of the hand, and a phase, how far it has rotated from the 12 o'clock position. In MRI we usually calculate an array of magnitudes only, display them on a two-dimensional grid and call them an image. Alternatively, the phase of the signal may be computed, formatted to a gray scale and be presented as an image. Such practices have been useful in velocity phase encoding, where phase is linearly related to the velocity of blood for example, and field mapping where the phase is directly related to the magnetic field.

- **Phase angle**
  Phase difference of two periodically recurring phenomena, expressed in angular measure.
- **Phase encoding**
  The two-dimensional Fourier transform (2-DFT) imaging method has emerged as the dominant technique by which MR images are generated. Following slice selection magnetic field gradients are employed to localize the signal into a two-dimensional array of pixels. In the 2-DFT scheme of imaging, one direction, which we can arbitrarily call the horizontal axis, is called the frequency encode axis. The vertical direction is called the phase encode axis. The frequency encoding can be envisaged as a number of phase encode steps collected in rapid succession during one pulse cycle.
  Each phase cycle under the 2-DFT scheme employs a different phase encode gradient. Usually 128×256 different values would be employed to generate the image. A complete scan would then take 128×256 times the TR of the sequence.
  For a static object the differences between phase and frequency directions are minimal. However, for breathing or moving objects the fact that the phase encoding points are acquired every TR, rather than the faster rate of the frequency encoding, means this direction is the more sensitive with respect to movement.
- **Phased array coil**
  Two or more RF coils, connected to separate pre-amplifiers are used simultaneously to image a larger area, with higher SNR, than is possible with a single coil.
- **pHi**
  Intracellular pH.
- **Photon**
  Elementary quantity, or quantum, of radiant energy.
- **Pi**
  Inorganic phosphate.
- **Pixel**
  Shorthand form for picture element. Each pixel within an MR image has a thickness, say 5 mm, and this can lead to partial volume effects. Under these circumstances the term voxel (volume element) is perhaps more suitable.
- **Planck's constant**
  Constant of proportionality (6.626×10^{-27} erg-second) that relates the amount of energy emitted or absorbed by a photon to its oscillation frequency.
- **Planar imaging**
  MR signals are generated from the volume enclosed within, or in close proximity to, the receiver coil. By employing slice selective RF pulses, signals may be limited to planes within this volume. Additional field gradients are then employed to further spatially localize these signals in order to generate images. Planar imaging requires a decision as to the best imaging plane prior to the acquisition of the data. However, if sufficient numbers of narrow slices are produced, they can be employed to produce further oblique images.
  As an alternative the signal from the volume may be manipulated without slice selective pulses. This is the volume scan which, once the data has been acquired, can be reformed to generate any arbitrarily oriented image plane.
- **PME**
  Phosphomonoester.
- **Population**
  Total number of nuclei or electrons in different energy levels. At thermal equilibrium the populations of the energy levels will be given by the Boltzmann distribution.
- **Power**
  Rate of energy flow, expressed in watts (W).
- **ppm**
  Parts per million.
- **Pre-amplifier**
  The MR signal is very weak and can be easily swamped by noise. The

pre-amplifier is an exceptionally low noise subsystem whose role is to magnify the basic MR signal (and noise) from the receiver coil without degrading it with additional noise. This initial amplification is the most critical and subsequent stages of the signal processing are more tolerant of lower quality components.

Precession

The precession of nuclear magnets lies at the center of the classical description of the nuclear magnetic resonance phenomenon. The static magnetic field (B_0) has a twisting effect upon the individual nuclear paramagnets. These magnets trace out a conical path around the direction of the field B_0 and this is known as precession. The nuclear precessional frequency is given by γB_0, and this is known as the Larmor frequency.

Precession angle (β)

Angle between the axis of gyration of a spinning body and the static magnetic field.

Pre-emphasis

The close proximity of the gradient coil system to the structures of the magnet ensure that there is always a limited rise-time to the required changes in the gradient waveform. The changing currents in the windings of the gradient coils induce currents within the bore of the magnet via magnetic interaction. This induced, or eddy current in the magnet structure generates additional magnetic field gradients which are in opposition to those actually required. This non-ideal response can be reduced by pre-emphasizing the initial sections of the input gradient drives.

Proton

Positively charged nucleon.

Proton density (ρ)

Number of protons per unit volume.

Proton density-weighted image

Spin echo technique with a long TR and a short TE. Also, a gradient echo technique using very small flip angles ($\leq 10°$) and long TR values (>100 ms).

Proton relaxation enhancement (PRE)

Enhancement of the signal intensity of hydrogen spectra or images using contrast agents.

Pulse sequence

An MR pulse sequence consists of a series of radiofrequency (RF) and the gradient pulses spaced by well-defined time intervals. The RF pulses generate the MR signal. When applied simultaneously with a magnetic field gradient the RF pulses are slice selective, that is, MR signal is produced from only a slice of tissue. The signal can be further encoded with spatial information by the application of magnetic field gradients alone.

Pulse sequences repeat themselves with the periodicity of TR (seconds). Additional commonly occurring intervals are also defined; TE, the echo time and TI, the inversion time.

The MR pulse sequence may also include locking or synchronization to physiological features such as the heart beat or respiratory motion.

Pulse, 90° ($\pi/2$ pulse)

RF pulse designed to rotate the macroscopic magnetisation vector 90° about its axis, as referred to the rotating frame of reference. If the spins are initially aligned with the magnetic field, this pulse will produce transverse magnetization.

Pulse, 180° (π pulse)

RF pulse designed to rotate the macroscopic magnetization vector 180° about its axis, as referred to the rotating frame of reference. If the spins are initially aligned with the magnetic field, this pulse produces an inversion.

Pulse repetition time

See **TR**.

Pulse shape

Profile of amplitude versus time for magnetic gradient pulses or the profile of amplitude versus frequency for RF pulses. RF pulse shape corresponds to the slice profile.

Q

Q

Q is the symbol for the quality factor of a tuned resonant circuit. A receiver coil, which is tuned to the nuclear Larmor frequency, with a high Q will resonate over a smaller range of frequencies than that of a low Q system. The signal-to-noise (SNR) of the detected MR signal is related to the Q of the coil; a high Q coil being most desirable in this respect. The proximity of a patient, or any conducting medium, to a tuned coil system will degrade its quality factor (and also SNR). The realistic measurement of Q will require 'loading' of the coil with a suitable conducting material (or piece of anatomy).

Quadrature coil

A quadrature coil can be considered as two separate coils in close proximity to one another. Ideally, they do not couple together so that the noise detected in each coil is uncorrelated. When these two noise signals are combined or averaged then the noise level in increased by $\sqrt{2}$.

The two coils are arranged to be perpendicular (90°) to one another. If the two signals are combined, taking into account this 90° in the receiver electronics, then overall signal is improved by 2. The net advantage of the quadrature coil is an improvement which if it were sought by signal averaging alone, would increase the scan time by a factor of 2.

Quadrature coils

Phase-sensitive detector or demodulator that detects the components of the signal in phase and at 90°.

Quadrature excitation

Transmission of RF energy that produces a single rotating magnetic field vector (i.e. circular polarization) resulting in a more uniform distribution of RF and less RF power deposition.

Quadrature detection

Phase-sensitive detector or demodulator that detects the components of the signal in phase and 90° out of phase with a reference oscillator.

Quench

If the superconducting windings of a magnet were to become partially resistive then they immediately start to generate heat in the manner of an electric fire. The liquid helium bath, which maintains low temperature for a superconducting state in the windings, starts to evaporate rapidly and this further accelerates the charge of the magnet into a resistive state. This process is known as the quench of the magnet. There is a collapse of the magnetic field and large quantities of helium gas are released from the magnet cryostat. This would usually be vented to the atmosphere in order to reduce hazards.

Quenching

Loss of superconductivity in the current-carrying coil causing loss of magnetic field in a superconducting magnet. Change from superconductivity releases heat, boiling off cryogenic liquid.

R

R1

Longitudinal relaxivity or efficiency, per unit concentration of solute, of an agent that alters T1 relaxation rates. R1 is 1/TI and is expressed in units of $(mM\text{-}s)^{-1}$. See also **relaxivity**.

R2

Transverse relaxivity or efficiency, per unit concentration of solute, of an agent that alters T2 relaxation rates. R2 is 1/T2 and is expressed in units of $(mM\text{-}s)^{-1}$.

Radiofrequency (RF)

The relationship between frequency ω and the magnetic field B is given by the Larmor equation ($\omega = \gamma B/2\pi$). For protons (^1H) at 1

Tesla the frequency is 42.6 MHz and, for the range of currently available magnets (say up to 12 Tesla for smaller bore systems), This puts the NMR frequency in the radiofrequency (RF) band of the electromagnetic spectrum. The RF band is usually defined to lie in the frequency range of 10–100 MHz. NMR is often referred to as an RF spectroscopy technique. The related technique of electron paramagnetic resonance (EPR) operates in the microwave portion of the electromagnetic spectrum.

The energy involved with each quantum of photon of RF radiation is low compared to typical molecular bond energies and this underlies the intrinsic safety aspects of MR when compared to X- and γ-rays towards the higher end of the electromagnetic spectrum.

The widespread use of RF in radio and television systems can lead to problems unless measures are taken to shield the MRI scanner from all interfering sources.

Radiofrequency (RF) coil
Used for transmitting RF pulses and/or receiving NMR signals. For MRI, saddle-shaped coils or coils with solenoid configurations are most frequently used.

Radiofrequency (RF) pulse
Timed burst of RF energy of amplitude B_1 is delivered to an object by the RF transmitter. For RF frequencies near the Larmor frequency, the RF pulse will result in rotation of the macroscopic magnetization vector in the rotating frame of reference or a more complicated nutational motion in the stationary frame of reference. The angle of rotation will depend on the strength B1 and duration of the RF pulse.

Rapid imaging
Methods employed to reduce the total scan time are termed rapid imaging techniques. In general, these methods reduce one or more of the following: (i) number of excitations; (ii) pulse repetition time; and (iii) number of phase-encoding steps.

RARE (rapid acquisition with relaxation enhancement)
Multiple RF or gradient echo sequence with echo-encoding, multiple phase steps.

Readout gradient
Magnetic field gradient applied for frequency encoding of the object being imaged.

Receiver
Detector for an RF signal. Receivers consist of electronic demodulators, preamplifiers and amplifiers.

Receiver coil
The detector of the MR signal is the receiver coil which would usually be defined to be fairly closely fitting to the anatomy in order to improve sensitivity. The receiver coil is tuned to the Larmor frequency which is defined by the field strength. The coil connects to a low noise pre-amplifier in order to boost the intrinsically low signals prior to meeting the outside world.

The receiver coil may physically be the same coil as the transmitter. In such cases additional electronics will be included in the transceiver system to switch between the high power transmit and low power receive phases of its operation.

Refocusing
Restoration of phase coherence by application of magnetic gradient(s) or RF pulses.

Relaxation rates
Reciprocal of the relaxation times, measured in inverse seconds.

Relaxation
The initial equilibrium polarization of nuclear magnets or spins takes a finite time to evolve following positioning within the magnet. This time period is known as relaxation. Any non-equilibrium state of the nuclear magnetization can only exist for a transitory period since relaxation processes are always working to maintain or restore the magnetization along the B_0 field. These non-equilibrium states could be achieved by rapidly changing the magnitude or direction of B_0; in this case rapid means fast compared with the timescale of the relaxation processes. A more elegant approach is to apply RF pulses to realign magnetization away from its preferred orientation

along B_0. The relaxation behavior of nuclear spins, and in particular that of water (^{1}H), underpins the diversity of image contrast available in MRI.

Relaxivity
Efficiency of relaxation enhancement expressed in units of $(mM\cdot s)^{-1}$.

Repetition time (TR)
The time between consecutive repetitions of a pulse sequence is labeled as TR. It is usual to say that if TR exceeds the five times the longitudinal relaxation time T1 then full relaxation has occurred and the spin system has no 'memory' of its previous history. Variations in the TR of a particular sequence can be employed to vary the T1 contrast in the resultant image.

Rephasing
By applying a 180° pulse, out of phase spins are returned back into phase.

Resistive magnet
Magnet whose magnetic field originates from current flowing through an ordinary, non-superconducting conductor.

Resolution
The smallest distance between distinct objects or features in an image. For a fixed field of view image higher resolution requires a longer data acquisition period. The resolution of the acquired data is a function of the amplitude of the gradient pulses and their duration. The appearance of the processed image may be improved by interpolating the data to a finer matrix; however, no additional detail results. Routine resolution in the plane of the image may be in the range 1–2 mm and it might have a depth or slice thickness, of perhaps 5 mm.

Resonance
A mechanical system such as a child's swing has a natural frequency at which it will oscillate if left to its own devices. If such an oscillatory system is driven by some periodic force then it will undergo forced oscillations. When the driver is at the natural frequency then resonance is said to have occurred; the amplitude of the oscillation builds up rapidly as energy is absorbed from the driver, in this case the exhausted parent. At other frequencies, slower and faster than the natural frequency, there is a flow of energy back and forth between oscillator and driver with no net gain by either system.

Resonance frequency
Frequency at which resonance phenomenon occurs, given by the Larmor equation for MRI.

RF spoiled FAST
Gradient echo technique that provides superior T1 contrasts. The technique removes effects of steady-state contributions without gradients by RF spoiling.

RF spoiling
Component of several fast scanning techniques having 'digital' RF systems. RF (as opposed to gradient) spoiling randomizes the phase of sequential RF pulses such that any residual transverse magnetization does not contribute to the subsequent signal.

Rotating frame of reference
Frame of reference that is rotating around the axis of the static magnetic field B_0 (with respect to a stationary ['laboratory'] frame of reference) at a frequency equal to the nuclear precessional frequency. Although B1 is a rotating vector, it appears stationary in the rotating frame during resonance, leading to simpler mathematical formulations.

S

Saddle coil
RF coil design (resembling a saddle) frequently used when the static magnetic field is coaxial with the axis of a magnet (i.e. typically used solenoidal type of superconducting magnets).

Sampling
The MR signal is a continuous voltage waveform that must be sampled

or digitized into discrete steps for input into a computer prior to processing into an image. The sampling occurs at intervals in time during the evolution of the signal. During an MRI data acquisition the signal may typically be sampled every 10 μs. The voltage, which may now have been amplified to somewhere between –10 and +10 V is digitized, for example, into one of 16 384 discrete levels.

■ **Saturation**
Non-equilibrium state in which equal numbers of spins are aligned against the magnetic field so that there is no net magnetization. Saturation can be produced by repeated RF pulses at the Larmor frequency with a TR much less than T1.

■ **Saturation pulse**
Technique for decreasing flow artifacts by selectively saturating spins located outside the image volume. For example, blood or CSF spins flowing into the image volume are so heavily saturated that they do not cause flow artifacts arising from flow-related enhancement.

■ **Saturation recovery (SR)**
Pulse sequence characterized by two sequential 90° pulses, a saturation pulse and a detection pulse, with signal collected after the detection pulse. In this manner, magnetization builds up exponentially from zero to a value determined by the interpulse interval (time between saturation pulse and detection pulse). Short TR spin echo pulse sequences in clinical use are occasionally referred to as SR sequences.

■ **SE**
See spin echo imaging.

■ **Selective excitation**
A RF pulse, by virtue of its limited duration, contains only a restricted range of frequencies, and as such can only excite a portion of the MR spectrum. Narrow excitation bandwidths are achieved with longer RF pulses. A pulse of duration t_p seconds will have an approximate bandwidth in the region of $1/t_p$ Hertz, a 1 ms (10^{-3}s) pulse has a bandwidth in the region of 1 kHz (10^3Hz). By carefully tailoring the exact pulse shape and its carrier or center frequency it is possible to selectively excite a given portion of the MR spectrum.

■ **Sensitive volume**
Region from which an MR signal is acquired because of strong magnetic field inhomogeneity elsewhere.

■ **Shielding**
The interference caused by external RF sources such as hospital paging and computer systems can introduce artifacts and seriously degrade the signal-to-noise ratio of resultant MR images. The MR scanner is protected from its RF environment by Faraday shielding. ECG leads and other patient monitoring equipment that may breach the Faraday shield will have to be RF filtered to prevent interfering signals propagating through the wires.

■ **Shim coils**
Electric coils used to correct for inhomogeneities in the static magnetic field of an MR system.

■ **Shimming**
The process of improving the quality or homogeneity of the static polarizing field B_0 is known as shimming. The intrinsic inhomogeneity of a magnet in a particular hospital site can be improved at the time of installation with additional current carrying coils within the construction of the magnet itself. These shim coils may take currents of several amperes in order to generate additional corrective magnetic fields. As an alternative small pieces of ferromagnetic material can be accurately positioned within the bore of a magnet to produce a similar compensating and shimming effect.

■ **SI**
International standard of physical units and measures which supersedes the meter–kilogram–second (MKS) and centimeter–gram–second (CGS) systems.

■ **Signal averaging**
Repetition of signal acquisition in an imaging plane. As more signals are averaged, signal-to-noise ratio increases (as the square root of the number of averages) and artifacts are reduced. However, scan time increases to obtain the additional signals.

■ **Signal-to-noise ratio (SNR, S/N)**
Describes the relative contributions to a detected signal of the true signal and random superimposed signals ('noise'). SNR can be improved by increasing the number of signals averaged by increasing field strength, or by increasing the size of the imaging voxels.

■ **Sinc pulse**
RF pulse modulated by a sinc function, i.e. $\sin(x)/x$.

■ **Slice**
Physical extent of the planar region being imaged.

■ **Slice profile**
Spatial distribution of sensitivity of the imaging process in the direction perpendicular to the plane of the slice.

■ **Slice selection**
When an RF pulse is applied at the same time as a magnetic field gradient the frequency excitation can be expected to be heavily spatially dependent. If all pulses within an MR sequence are slice selective then during the necessary relaxation delays additional slices can be excited.

■ **Slice-selective excitation**
Exclusive excitation of protons in one slice. Slice-selective excitation is performed by applying a gradient magnetic field G_z and a narrow bandwidth or slice-selective RF pulse. The range of frequencies in a slice-selective pulse, via the Larmor equation relationship, corresponds to a specific range of magnetic field strengths along the slice-selection gradient G_z.

■ **Slice thickness**
Thickness of an imaging slice. Since the slice profile may not be sharply edged, a criterion such as the distance between the points at half the maximum value (FWHM) or the equivalent rectangular width (the width of a rectangular slice profile with the same maximum height and same area) is generally used.

■ **Software**
Set of instructions and programs (supervising 'executive' programs, data acquisition programs, data-processing programs such as image reconstruction, display programs) that controls the activities of the computer.

■ **Solenoid coil**
Coil wound in the form of a cylinder. When a current is passed through the coil, the magnetic field within the coil is nearly uniform.

■ **Spatial frequency**
Signal frequency related to the spatial coordinate.

■ **Specific absorption rate (SAR)**
Electromagnetic radiation can deposit energy by inducing small currents in the electrolytes of the body. The absorbed energy manifests itself principally in the form of heat. The specific absorption rate is defined as the energy deposited per second into a kilogram of tissue. It has the units of watts per kilogram (W/kg).

■ **Spectral line**
Frequency or narrow band of frequencies, depending on resolution, that corresponds to a particular chemical shift.

■ **Spectral width**
Width of frequency (in Hz) that is selected for a particular NMR spectrum to be observed.

■ **Spectrometer**
MR apparatus that actually produces the NMR phenomenon and acquires the signals. Components of a spectrometer include the magnet, the probe, the RF circuitry, and the gradient coils.

■ **Spectroscopy**
In the general sense spectroscopy is the separation of a signal into its component frequencies. The decomposition of white light into seven distinct colors is the common example. Spectroscopic techniques now exist throughout the electromagnet spectrum from the lower radiofrequencies (NMR), electron paramagnetic resonance (EPR), infrared, optical and ultraviolet and beyond. The methods are employed as probes to molecular and atomic structure.

■ **Spectrum**
Array of the frequency components of the MR signal. Nuclei with

different resonant frequencies will show up as peaks at their corresponding frequencies.

- **Spin**
Intrinsic angular momentum of an elementary particle (nuclei, electrons, etc.) that is also responsible for the magnetic moment of the particle. Spins of nuclei have characteristic fixed values. Pairs of neutrons and protons align, thus canceling out their spins, so that only nuclei with odd numbers of neutrons and/or protons will have a net non-zero rotational component characterized by an integer or half-integer quantum nuclear spin number (I).

- **Spin density**
Density of resonating spins in a given volume. Spin density is one of the principal determinants of the strength of the MR signal (i.e. the higher the spin density the higher the signal received).

- **Spin echo imaging**
Imaging of a spin echo formed by sequence of RF pulses and gradient reversals. The standard spin echo sequence uses an RF pulse sequence consisting of a 90° excitation pulse followed by a 180° echo-rephasing pulse.

- **Spin lattice relaxation times**
See T1.

- **Spin–spin coupling**
Interaction between nuclei in the same molecule, resulting in a splitting of a single resonance line into two or more lines. For example, a carbon nucleus with one directly bonded proton will be a doublet.

- **Spin–spin relaxation time**
See T2.

- **Spin tagging**
Nuclei retain their magnetic orientation for a short time (on the order of the corresponding T1 value) even in the presence of motion or chemical exchange. If nuclei have their spin orientation changed, the altered spins serve as a 'tag' to trace the motion of any fluid.

- **Spin warp imaging**
Most common form of Fourier transform imaging in which phase-encoding gradient pulses with constant duration but varying amplitude are applied to one of three spatial dimensions; the second dimension is frequency encoded and the third dimension is defined by slice selection.

- **SPIO**
Superparamagnetic iron oxide.

- **Static magnetic field**
Constant magnetic field in an MR system (B_0).

- **Statistical noise**
Point-to-point variation in signal intensity caused by random fluctuations (e.g. Brownian motion) at each voxel. This is contradistinction to non-random fluctuations from macroscopic motion and flow.

- **STIR (short T1 inversion-time recovery)**
Inversion recovery technique that produces images in which T1- and T2-dependent contrasts are additive. STIR imaging is used to suppress the signal of short T1 tissues such as fat.

- **Superconducting magnet**
Device that creates a magnetic field by use of electric current flowing through a superconductor.

- **Superconductor**
Substance whose electric resistance disappears, usually at temperatures near absolute zero. A frequently used superconductor in MR system magnets in niobium–titanium, embedded in a copper matrix.

- **Superparamagnetic**
The magnetic susceptibilities of superparamagnetic materials are similar to ferromagnetic materials and are much larger than paramagnetic materials. Unlike ferromagnetic materials, superparamagnetic materials do not exhibit residual magnetism when the external magnetic field is removed.

- **Suppression**
It is not uncommon in MR for there to be very strong signals in close proximity to more interesting but weaker areas. In MRI the intense lipid signals, exacerbated by the use of a surface coil, can dominate the image. In MRS the strong water resonance, representing 100 M ^{1}H, totally overwhelms the weaker spectroscopically interesting metabolite resonances. In both cases signal suppression techniques can be employed to reduce the amplitude of the offending signals.

- **Surface coil**
RF that is placed close to the surface of the object being imaged. Surface coils increase signal-to-noise ratio for regions close to the coil, permitting increased resolution, and sometimes help decrease motion artifacts.

- **Susceptibility imaging**
Gradient echo sequence that relates fluctuations of the actual tissue susceptibility to the measured field deviations.

T

- **T1 or T1** ('T-one')
Spin lattice, thermal, or longitudinal relaxation time measured in milliseconds. T1 reflects the characteristic time constant for spins to align themselves with the external magnetic field. Starting from zero magnetization in the z direction, the z magnetization will grow to 63% of its final maximum value M_0 in a time T1 (i.e. $M_z/M_0 = 1 - \exp[-t/T1]$).

- **T1 shortening**
Decrease of the spin lattice relaxation time or increase in relaxation rate caused by MR contrast agents or macromolecular binding.

- **T1 weighted**
MR sequence such as short TR/short TE spin echo or inversion recovery designed to distinguish tissues with differing T1 relaxation times.

- **T2 or T_2** ('T-two')
Spin–spin or transverse relaxation time. T2 reflects the characteristic time constant for loss of transverse magnetization M_{xy} and MR signal. Starting from a non-zero value of the magnetization of the xy plane M_0, the x magnetization, decays to 37% of its initial value in a time T2 (i.e. $M_{xy}/M_0 = \exp[-t/T2]$).

- **T2*** ('T-two star')
(1) Effective spin–spin relaxation time (faster than T2, it includes effects of static field inhomogeneities, intrinsic to tissue or B_0 imperfections).
(2) Observed time constant of the free induction decay.

- **T2 shortening**
Decrease of the spin–spin relaxation time caused by molecular diffusion, paramagnetic molecules, ferromagnetic particles, or local magnetic susceptibility effects.

- **T2 weighted**
MR sequence such as spin echo with a long TR/long TE designed to distinguish tissues with differing T2 relaxation times.

- **T1, T_2, T_2***
The time constants associated with longitudinal (T1) and transverse (T_2) relaxation. These relaxation processes are usually assumed to be exponential in character and are given by the analytical solution to the Bloch equations. In cases where this is not true then a sum of exponential relaxation processes may physically be a realistic model to allow characterization of the relaxation behavior.
Following a 90° RF pulse there is no component of magnetization aligned along the applied field B_0; after a period of T1 there will be 63% growth of the magnetization along B_0 towards the equilibrium M_0. During T_2 transverse components of magnetization decay by 63% from their value towards zero. Usually five times the relaxation time, either T1 or T_2 is taken to be the time necessary for the respective components of nuclear magnetization to fully relax.
T_2* is employed to denote the actual observed decay in transverse relaxation. The distinction is required since T_2* depends upon the experimental conditions under which the signal is observed to be decaying. In the simplest case, in the absence of imaging field gradients

following a single RF pulse for example, this merits that the field inhomogeneity (δB_0) can also contribute to the decay of the MR signal.

- **TE**
Echo time. Time between the center of the 90° pulse and the center of the spin echo. For multiple echoes, TEs are designed numerically as TE1, TE2 and so on.

- **Tesla**
Named after Nikolai Tesla (1870–1943), the Tesla is the SI unit of magnetic flux density and is given the symbol T. Commercial MR scanners usually operate in the range of 0.2–2.0T. One Tesla equates to 10 000 Gauss, the equivalent CGS unit.

- **Three-dimensional Fourier transform (3-DFT)**
Mathematical technique that constructs a 3D image from acquired MR data. Two dimensions are constructed using the standard 2-DFT technique. Positional information for the third dimension is obtained in the same manner as the second dimension of the 2-DFT (i.e. by using phase encoding gradients in the z direction).

- **TI**
Inversion time (used in inversion recovery). Time between the inverting (180°) RF pulse and the subsequent exciting (90°) pulse.

- **Time of flight signal loss**
Phenomenon of the decreased signal resulting from protons travelling through a selected slice too quickly to acquire the 90° excitation pulse and subsequent 180° rephasing pulse. These protons are therefore unable to emit signal.

- **Tip angle**
Angle between bulk magnetization vector before and after an RF excitation pulse.

- **Tissue characteristics**
Tissues parameters that determine MR signal intensity, such as spin density, relaxation times, chemical shift and motion.

- **TR**
Repetition time. Time between the beginning of one pulse sequence and the beginning of the succeeding pulse sequence at a specified tissue location. See also **imaging cycle**.

- **Transmitter**
Portion of the MR systems that produces the RF current and delivers it to the transmitting coil.

- **Transmitter coil**
A coil system capable of handling high RF current. The current, as it flows around the coil, generates a time dependent of RF magnetic field; this is generally referred to as B_1 to compare with the static polarizing field B_0. The current in the transmitter coil is switched on and off, or pulsed, under computer control in order to generate the required RF pulse sequences.

- **Transverse magnetization (M_{xy})**
Component of the macroscopic magnetization vector in the right angles to the static magnetic field (B_0). Precession of the transverse magnetization at the Larmor frequency produces the detectable MR signal, which decays to zero (with a characteristic time constant of T2 or T2*) when the externally applied RF magnetic field is switched off.

- **Transverse relaxation**
The equilibrium magnetization is aligned along the z-axis, defined by the static magnetic field B_0 and there are no components in the transverse or xy-plane. Following an RF pulse any transverse magnetization must decay to zero and this occurs at the molecular level by transverse relaxation mechanisms.

- **Tuning**
The adjustment of the frequency to a specific volume where resonance can occur is known as tuning. The concept is familiar when selecting a specific radio station. In MR terms the RF system must be matched to the Larmor frequency. Individual coils within the MR system, be they high powered transmitter coils or receiver coils, must also be tuned to the Larmor frequency for optimum performance.

- **TurboFLASH**
An ultrafast imaging technique that employs a separate magnetization preparation (MP) period before a standard FLASH sequence with a short TR (5–10 ms).

- **Two-dimensional Fourier transform (2-DFT)**
MR technique in which data are reconstructed mathematically into a 2D image. Brightness of pixels is proportional to the intensity of MR signal from the corresponding region of the imaged object.

V

- **Vector**
Mathematical quantity having both magnitude and direction. Vectors are represented by an arrow whose length is proportional to the magnitude and an arrowhead indicating the direction.

- **View (projection)**
Data obtained from sampling of the free induction decay or spin echo. For the generation of an image, multiple views must be acquired (e.g. 128 or 256).

- **Volume averaging**
MR technique in which signals are received from the whole object being imaged rather than from a slice. Advantages of volume imaging include improvement in signal-to-noise ratio.

- **Volume imaging**
In the absence of any magnetic field gradients all parts of the body within the transmitter coil are excited by an RF pulse. If the receiver coil surrounds a large volume of this excited region then the signal can be manipulated for volumetric imaging.
Volume imaging can be achieved with frequency encoding and two phase encode axes – a three dimensional Fourier transform (3-DFT) technique. A volume scan will take n times longer than its planar equivalent, where n is the number of points required in the third dimension. Unless n is large then a multislice dataset may be competitive in terms of coverage of the required anatomy.

- **Voxel**
Shorthand form for the volume element of an image. Voxel emphasises that the smallest image element not only has an in-plane dimension but also has a thickness or depth.

W

- **Water-suppression techniques**
Elimination of a water signal by saturation of the water resonance or by selective excitation of the non-water region.

- **Wavelength**
Distance between points of corresponding phase of a periodic wave.

- **Weighting**
A variety of tissue characteristics interact with any selected pulse sequence to influence the signal intensity of reach tissue and thereby determine image contrast. When one tissue characteristic is the major determinant of the image contrast, the image is said to be weighted by that tissue characteristic.

X, Y, Z

- ***x,y,z***
These refer to the three principal axes in a Cartesian coordinate system, that is the usual rectangular system that can be applied to rooms, buildings and the like. x, y and z are said to be in the laboratory frame of reference if they are attached to the system hardware associated with the MR scanner. Convention has it that the applied magnetic field defines the z-axis of the coordinate system, Since the majority of systems today are based upon the superconducting solenoid magnet this means that z usually runs from

head to foot in the patient. The x and y axes are not only perpendicular to z but also at right angles with respect to each other.

■ x^*, y^*, z^*

These also refer to a Cartesian system of coordinates but the inclusion of the superscript prime indicates that these axes refer to a rotating frame of reference. The choice of the 'rotation' is entirely arbitrary but is selected to simplify the description of the movements of nuclear magnetization. This is true for the visualization in the mind and also the underlying mathematics. In MR the rotating frame is usually taken to be attached to the precession of a particular group of nuclei in the magnetic field. As such the z and z^* axes are one and the same and the x, y and x^*, y^* axes are simply rotating with respect to one another. The literature is apt to be rather loose about the coordinate system or frame of reference in which nuclei or magnetization are being discussed.

■ **Zero filling**

Dummy data points (usually zero) added to the actual sample values to increase digital resolution before the Fourier transform is processed.

■ **Zeugmatography**

A term coined from Greek roots to mean MRI. Positively the last word in Magnetic Resonance Imaging.

References

1. Bryant DJ and Blease S (1997) *A Glossary of MR Terms.* Bristol, Clinic Press.

2. Floyd LJ, Williams RF and Stark DD (1999) Glossary. In: Stark DD and Bradley WG (Eds) *Magnetic Resonance Imaging*, 3rd edn. St Louis, Mosby.

Index